THE ENGINES
OF HIPPOCRATES

Wiley Series on Technologies for the Pharmaceutical Industry

Sean Ekins, Series Editor

THE ENGINES OF HIPPOCRATES

From the Dawn of Medicine to Medical and Pharmaceutical Informatics

BARRY ROBSON
Director of Research and Professor of Biostatistics, Epidemiology, and Evidence Based Medicine, St. Matthew's University School of Medicine and Chief Scientific Officer, The Dirac Foundation

O.K. BAEK
Senior Enterprise Solution Architect, Medical Informatics, Clinical Genomics, eScience and Emerging Industry Solutions

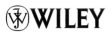

A JOHN WILEY & SONS, INC., PUBLICATION

Copyright © 2009 by John Wiley & Sons, Inc. All right reserved

Published by John Wiley & Sons, Inc., Hoboken, New Jersey
Published simultaneously in Canada

For general information on our other products and services or for technical support, please contact our Customer Care Department within the United States at (800) 762-2974, outside the United States at (317) 572-3993 or fax (317) 572-4002.

Wiley also publishes its books in a variety of electronic formats. Some content that appears in print may not be available in electronic formats. For more information about Wiley products, visit out web site at www.wiley.com.

Library of Congress Cataloging-in-Publication Data

Robson, Barry.
  The engines of Hippocrates : from the dawn of medicine to medical and pharmaceutical informatics / Barry Robson, O.K. Baek.
     p. ; cm.—(Wiley series on technologies for the pharmaceutical industry)
  Includes bibliographical references and index.
  ISBN 978-0-470-28953-2 (cloth)
  1. Medical informatics. I. Baek, O. K. II. Title. III. Series.
  [DNLM: 1. Medical Informatics Computing. 2. Health Services–trends. 3. Man-Machine Systems. 4. Medical Informatics Applications. W 26.5 R667e 2009]
  R858.R615 2009
  610.28—dc22

                                                                                    2008045094

Printed in the United States of America

10 9 8 7 6 5 4 3 2 1

To our parents and children,
who share our DNA.
To our wives,
who shared theirs with us.
To our nearly seven billion relatives,
and the engines that are coming to protect us.

CONTENTS

PREFACE

Information technology is poised on the brink of transforming healthcare. IT is entwined with the continuing evolution of the molecular and physical sciences, and rather than dehumanizing us, IT has the potential to continually transform healthcare by the power of its information sharing and processing capabilities. IT particularly has the power to restore good aspects of healthcare based on a personalized and holistic approach, which has been progressively lost, and increasingly so since the Industrial Revolution and the escalating patient-to-physician ratios of the last century.

This book is built on those premises to examine the task ahead, with emphasis on six key considerations required for a transformation that must realistically plan for construction on the historical foundations, opportunities, challenges, and controversies associated with medical advances. First, there is the new awareness of human individuality as the diversity of the human genome that evolved over many thousands of years, responsible for the uniqueness of us all through our differing risks of developing diseases and differing responses to pharmaceutical drugs. Second, there are our no less diverse cultural heritages, belief systems, concerns, and prejudices. They are epitomized by the still significant split between Western medicine rooted in Hippocrates and Galen, and the enduringly popular systems of alternative, Eastern medicine, despite the long standing opportunities of the Arabic medicine to mediate between the two extremes. Here, the broad definition of health by the World Health Organization encourages us to ponder the nature of, and strategy messages for, mental and spiritual well-being, including the strangely contrasting

The views expressed in the book are those of the authors and not necessarily those of the IBM Corporation or any other previous employer of the authors.

and essentially impartial disciplines of Eastern Zen and Western existential-ism. Between these two opposites modern neurology and information technol-ogy are finding a common thread. Third, there is a delicate balance between privacy and autonomy, or self-interest balanced against solidarity, and sharing and participating for the common good, which became a prominent and some-times disturbing issue in the twentieth century. Fourth, there is a pragmatic issue of timeliness of waves of new industry and economy, which is attributed largely to the rise of the Internet and may now be working to improve health-care. Fifth, coupled increasingly to that there is an issue of the healthcare and health insurance systems of today, the often entrenched and bureaucratic Towers of Babel beset by mountains of paper, high rate of medical error, and the challenge of the aging Baby Boomer population and internationally polar-ized between managed healthcare and socialistic philosophy. Sixth, bringing us in closure with the first issue, there is not least the role and mode of practice of the pharmaceutical companies, currently caught in the early twenty-first century in transition between the revenue model of one blockbuster drug for everyone and the multiple personalized approaches that our differential genomics demands.

To tell that story with its many diverse aspects of broad human importance, the authors have sought to mix a journalistic and scientific style along with factual data and projected scenarios and use cases, along with short illustrative anecdotal snapshots. It was considered to be a lost cause from the outset to render in *exactly* the same style a description of the coding principles of the US health provider billing system and the future impact of nanotechnology on human destiny in any event. To maintain continuity so that the reader is not constantly flipping pages, we have sometimes allowed a degree of duplica-tion with each portion to be complete in itself with the appropriate focus, and given references explicitly in situ, in the text. Additionally, at the end of the book, we give sources, bibliography, and a guided further reading, the latter with reference to both broader topic source books and example original sci-entific papers. Research papers are personal favorites due to the breadth of matters covered, but there should be enough information in the text for the reader to use the increasingly powerful Internet and find relevant material in seconds.

Barry Robson
O.K. Baek

ABOUT THE AUTHORS

Barry Robson PhD DSc, has a background originally briefly in surgical and psychiatric nursing, subsequently in both medical science and computational chemical physics, and then in helping start up biopharmaceutical R&D companies. He is probably best known academically for early contributions to bioinformatics and in industry for helping design and use integrated R&D systems to realize biopharmaceutical agents and diagnostics (including the mad cow disease diagnostic marketed by Abbott). He has also been active in healthcare informatics, receiving the Asklepios Award for outstanding vision at the Future of Health Technology Congress in 2001. He has published some 220 scientific papers and patents, and a standard textbook "Introduction to Proteins and Protein Engineering" (B. Robson and J. Garnier, 1988). He is Director of Research and professor of biostatistics, epidemiology, and evidence-based medicine in the Department of Behavioral and Integrated Medicine at St. Matthew's University School of Medicine, Grand Cayman. He was associated with IBM for more than 10 years after originally being hired by IBM research headquarters as strategic advisor. For some 5 years he advised IBM business in the role of chief scientific officer, IBM Global Pharmaceutical and Life Sciences, and IBM Distinguished Engineer. He continues since 1995 as founder and chair of The Dirac Foundation, formed to honor Nobel Laureate Paul A. M. Dirac at the behest of his widow Margit Dirac, by helping promote understanding of the applications of theoretical physics and chemistry to human and veterinary medicine.

O. K. Baek is a senior enterprise IT architect specialized in end-to-end solution design for emerging industries and associated sciences and technologies at

IBM, such as health science, biomedical engineering and life sciences, with a background in electronics, computer engineering, computer science, and bioinformatics. He has been particularly active in regard to the integrated healthcare system and medical centers for "translational" biomedical research and continues to collaborate with Barry on a number of occasions. In addition to his commitment to Western medicine, he has also a deep interest in the history and principles of Eastern traditional medicine, and is a strong advocate of combining the better features of mainstream and alternative medicine in modern healthcare with emphasis on using new architectures to enable personalized, preventative and holistic approaches. His recent contributions have notably included the idea of data-centric computing by which massive amounts of medical data or sensitive data protected by the privacy laws can be shared securely and in compliance to the statutory requirements for protection of personal privacy by software roaming dynamically to the data to be analyzed. The processed results are then created along with automatically generated metadata so that the analytical results or discoveries can be shared among the collaborators to enable multidisciplinary, cross-institutional, and translational research. He is currently developing a molecular diagnostics solution for presymptomatic analysis to help realize the concept of predictive and preventative wellness-oriented healthcare through an early detection of minute symptoms of a disease. He has filed more than a dozen international patents related to the technology innovation.

1

A SHORT PREVIEW OF MANKIND, MEDICINE, MOLECULES, AND MACHINES

Between wisdom and medicine there is no gulf fixed.
—Hippocrates, *The Decorum*

THE ACCELERATING PACE OF LIFE

No one interested in the life sciences can fail to notice how the pace of life always quickens. This seems so whether we look back a few years of our own lives, or millions of years of the evolution of life. The story starts slowly. But whatever evolutionary phase of pre-human life or human lifestyle that we look back on, the last small fraction always represents a new explosion to a previously unparalleled sophistication. Some 3 billion years ago, there were the first complex cells, some 550 million years ago, the first complex multicellular life, some five million years ago, the hominids (the Homo species). A million years ago, the early protohumans, *Homo erectus*, were chipping away at stone to make their first crude devices, developing the technology of fire. Just short of 200,000 years ago, anatomically modern humans were living, dying, and leaving their bones in Ethopia, the earliest known *Homo sapiens* bones at the time of writing. There were accelerating waves of migrations out of Africa to colonize the world about 50,000 to 80,000 years ago, a new, literally "cutting edge," technology arises: humans begin to develop *new blade tools*, fashioned from bone and antlers as well as stone. Armed with their New Stone Age blade

The Engines of Hippocrates: From the Dawn of Medicine to Medical and Pharmaceutical Informatics, by Barry Robson and O.K. Baek
Copyright © 2009 by John Wiley & Sons, Inc.

technology, a few thousands of humans began a new diaspora out of Africa, their descendants displacing the Neanderthals and all previous modern ex-African humans, to the extent of wiping all modern traces of their genetic heritage and leaving only their own. Over the past 8,000 to 20,000 years the fixed-locale, agricultural lifestyle began the city era, the formation of the first towns, and cities, including such sites as those at Jericho and Catal Huyuk. In this progression from tribes to villages, and villages to cities, tribes-folk became citizens, and began to specialize into sophisticated craftsmen, warriors, administrators, thinkers, spiritual leaders, ... and physicians.

This quickening pace continues into the historical period (which can also be considered as due to biological and evolutionary forces). In the past 3,000 years, we have seen the rise of logical thought processes, including some 2,400 years ago the birth of modern public and private medicine and healthcare due to the philosophy of Hippocrates. Some 700 years ago, there was the European Renaissance, and the beginning of the spread of European civilization across the world. Then some 300 years ago, there was the Age of Enlightenment, leading rapidly to the Industrial Revolution 200 years ago, with its flux of populations into the great cities. There were the much less enlightened slave trades, representing the last great diaspora out of Africa, except that this time *millions* of Africans spread their genes across the world. Some 150 to 100 years ago, there was the consolidation of modern science in the form of most disciplines now established in academe, and of engineering using electricity. In the past 80 years came electronics, and 50 years ago, computers, software, increasingly pervasive smart devices, and then the Internet developed, all of which we call IT or information technology. This technology and not least the democratic structure of the Internet was crucial to support the international genome projects, the sequencing, or "readout" of the DNA in the genome of living organisms.

The Internet is a global network connecting millions of computers in more than 100 countries, and exchanging data, news, and opinions originally among scientists, and later the public. It is worth reminding, however, that unlike centrally controlled online services, each participating computer, sometimes called a *host*, is independent and of equal rank. It is amazing, and perhaps to many unexpected, that out of that democratic chaos has emerged order and vast utility.

"Future shock" arose as an issue in the twentieth century when the accelerating pace of the transitions described became very significantly shorter than the period of a typical human life. Indeed, at the start of the current millennium, new discoveries capable of transforming healthcare were emerging on an almost daily basis. A particularly watershed day was June 26, 2000. The world formally completed its first draft of the human genome, and life on Earth began to look back and within, understand its origins and nature, and to contemplate itself in detail.

Of course, when progressing at an ever-quickening pace and looking backward contemplatively, it is all too easy to trip over one's own feet! Most of the themes in this book relate to the dizzying pace of progress, especially in information technology, and how we should watch out for its consequences for healthcare. For the most part we believe that progress is good, even great, news. However, the pace has caused some problems in recent history. These problems need to be put right, and there is some justice in the fact that accelerating developments in other areas, especially IT (again, *information technology*), can help us do just that. For example, the major theme for this book is that in the industrialized Western world, at least, many of us transiently lost something of importance in the twentieth century. The accelerating pace of medical technologies yet poor communications between those technologies, increasing dominance of economic considerations, and a much higher ratio of patients to physicians than in early village culture, lost the ancient personalized, holistic (i.e., whole-life-embracing) touch of medicine. US doctors, in particular, often lost their bedside manner, and patients began to be processed as if on a conveyer belt that passed through a physician's office. Yet this has been a production line whose high-throughput aspirations have been in marked contrast to the miserable inefficiency with which data are passed back and forth almost every time the patient is the primary source of all data about past medical history. But the big message here is that information technology has precisely the ability to restore the dissemination of useful information from few physicians to many and back again, to help us all spare more time for each other. It can help us restore these proven ancient personal and holistic approaches, and spread them, laced with new science, to the whole, still largely underprivileged, world.

To consider how to approach this ideal, we must address in this book six main issues that set the stage. None of these issues can be considered in any meaningful sense as positive or negative. That is, with the exception of number 5, whose gloomy situation yet represents a glowing opportunity for the IT industry, they represent things just as we find them at this moment in the human story. But that should detract nothing from the excitement of the challenges.

1. **Genetic diversity.** The recent awareness of the extent of human individuality is seen in the diversity of the genomics of the human race that has evolved over many thousands of years, and that is responsible for the uniqueness of all of us through our differing risks of developing diseases and differing responses to pharmaceutical drugs.

2. **Cultural and intellectual diversity.** Our no less diverse cultural heritages, belief systems, concerns, and prejudices epitomized by the still significant split between Western medicine rooted in Hippocrates and Galen, and the enduringly popular systems of alternative and Eastern medicine.

3. **Patient rights.** The delicate balance between privacy and autonomy, or self-interest and solidarity, and sharing medical data and participating in studies for the common good.
4. **The economy.** The issue of timeliness of waves of new industry and economy that may now be working in healthcare's favor, thanks largely to the rise of the Internet.
5. **Legacy healthcare systems.** The healthcare and health insurance systems of today, which are often entrenched and bureaucratic Towers of Babel and yet typically beset by mountains of paper, high rate of medical error, and the challenge of the aging baby boomer population, and internationally polarized between managed healthcare and socialistic philosophy.
6. **Pharmaceutical industry transition.** The genetic diversity and the role and mode of practice that are currently caught in the transition between the revenue model of one blockbuster drug for everyone and the multiple personalized approaches that our differential genomics demands.

Despite the huge global economic downturn of 2008, the president-elect of the United States, at time of writing, is giving high priority to modernizing the healthcare system with leverage of the 21st-century technology. Building the new healthcare system is not a one-off computer deal but a basis for an information technology that will continue to become more and more part of our lives.

Prehistory and history, ancient and modern, is important for the *provenance* or historical origin and justification of the moral issues to be addressed. If we are not to trip up, and to avoid wrong turns and rough ground, we must often look forward, and practice some futurology. So another theme of this book relates to the fact that life on Earth has not only begun to look back and within and contemplate its nature in detail but has begun to look forward into the distant future to see *no visible limits to the growth of technology*. As pointed out by science fiction writer and visionary Arthur C. Clark, any sufficiently advanced civilization is indistinguishable from magic. If we do not consider our scientific potential and the kind of scenarios it can ultimately create, we may find ourselves in a dark future, with a very alien definition of well-being. To build well at the boundary of tension between the past and the future and try and understand what human society most generally considers *right* and *wrong*, it helps to draw insight both from mythology and ancient teachings and from science fiction, as we will do from time to time.

Recent revelations have been the incredible vision of what technology can do for progress of medicine. But both in our current *and in our projected* modes of thinking, ethical considerations are vital to guide us. The nature of medicine, after all, is that it can potentially change what we are, hopefully for the better, and our ethics may, and perhaps must, similarly evolve. In the future of health care, we are our own moving target.

Vision is not the sole prerogative of the modern world. This is manifestly obvious in regard to great engineering feats. Stonehenge had to be planned. Yet the cautionary biblical story of the ill-fated Tower of Babel reminds us that grandiose engineering aspirations were seen occasionally even in very ancient times, while also cautioning us that if we are to look forward, we should try to do so with the best possible clarity and avoid miscommunication. Indeed the ancient Greeks were no slouch in architecture and engineering: if *communication* had been better and they had got their act together between the human-powered chariot and the spinning steam-powered sphere, they would have had steam engines. Such is the importance of *translational research*, namely mobilization of latest research and discovery, and for the purpose of healthcare benefit, this represents concept that will be discussed in some detail from the IT perspective.

SCIENTIFIC ADVANCEMENT ACCELERATES MEDICINE

Modern IT depends critically on mathematics and physics. The calculations in support of healthcare and pharmaceutical research involve mathematics, physics, chemistry, biology, epidemiology, sociology, and even, by helping in compliance, ethics. Computers are becoming more quantum mechanical *and* biological: prototypes of quantum mechanical computing and DNA computing already exist. Controversially, humans could progressively become more hardware than machine: right now implanted computer chips could aid in treating epilepsy and Parkinson's disease, and have already helped correct hearing loss. The barriers between the sciences are breaking down, and in a few hundred years divisions between the sciences will be meaningless. In the far future perhaps, as discussed in the last chapter, the distinction between humans and computers may have less meaning than it has today.

Not surprisingly, almost all great contributors to science have left a legacy that is having or will have an impact on future health care. If we are to name the greatest scientists in the human history, we need to start with the Greek philosopher Aristotle or Aristoteles (384–322 BC) whose works are the foundation of Western physics, poetry, botany, zoology, physics, astronomy, chemistry, and meteorology, geometry, zoology, logic, rhetoric, politics, government, ethics, and biology. We need to include as well Johannes Kepler (AD 1571–1630) who discovered (in 1609) that the planets revolve around the Sun in elliptical orbits. Galileo Galilei (1564–1642), a physicist, astronomer, and philosopher, developed the first two laws of motion and also in astronomy, the telescope, and he is considered the father of astronomy. Next is the physicist, mathematician, astronomer, alchemist, and natural philosopher Isaac Newton (1643–1727) who is best known for his explanation of universal gravitation and three laws of motion that he used to prove that both the motion of objects on Earth and of celestial bodies are controlled by the same natural laws. Our understanding of laws of motion, governing bodies from atoms to planets and stars, are essential today for the computer simulation and design of drugs acting at their targets in the body. Charles Robert Darwin (1809–1882) is best known for the *Origin of Species by Means of Natural Selection* (1859). His thinking is the cornerstone of modern biology—without it, the new sciences lack assessment based on genetics—and of pharmacogenomics. Without Darwin's theory, our understanding of human differences that underpin personalized medicine and are rooted in recent human evolution would have no sensible foundation. But not all matters of health are inherited: Louis Pasteur's introduction of germ theory has became the base of today's microbiology, and his invention of the process called "pasteurization" has helped destroy harmful microbes while preserving taste and nutritional value.

Albert Einstein (1879–1955) is considered as the great scientist of the twentieth century. He is most notable for his theory of relativity, and he received the Noble Prize in Physics in 1921 for his explanation of the photoelectric effect and for his research in theoretical physics. He was followed closely by Paul A. M. Dirac (1902–1984), who perfected quantum mechanics, a new way of perceiving the world in terms of fundamental uncertainty that Einstein helped create but finally could not accept. Yet quantum mechanics fundamentally underlies electricity, electronics and IT. Neither can we omit the founders of electrical engineering. Thomas Edison (1847–1931) is the great inventor whose over 1,000 patents and inventions include the phonograph, the electric bulb, the telegraph system, the carbon telephone transmitter, and the carbon microphone that was used in telephones until 1980. Nor can we forget Alessandro Giuseppe Antonio Anastasio Volta (1745–1827) an Italian physicist who had much earlier developed the electric battery. He is regarded as the founder of the electric age and consequently the electric unit Volt is named after him. Today the British physicist Stephen Hawking is considered by most as the greatest scientist since Dirac for his big bang and black hole theories; he is famous for his book *A Brief History of Time* in which he sets out a truly cosmological vision in quantum mechanical terms.

With accelerating speed toward the midtwentieth century, there were among the band of actual and mental engineers. Imhotep (c. 2600 BC), Leonardo da Vinci (1452–1519), Jules Verne (1828–1905), H. G. Wells (1866–1996), Isambard Kingdom Brunel (1806–1859), Isaac Asimov (1920–1992), Arther C. Clark (1917–2008), Alan Turing (1912–1954), and Marvin Minsky (b. 1927) who envisioned progressively more incredible devices that could shift great rocks, move unaided, fly and drill, think for us, conquer space, and even time.

Naturally the same dizzying pace in engineering applies to the repair and engineering of human life, and hence to health care. Medicine has been practiced, based on long-standing opinion, as an art; medicine, however, is a science and effectively an engineering science! Physicians are, in a sense, bioengineers; it is just that the state of knowledge until recently has been limiting their activities to maintenance and repair. It is only recently that it has become possible to think of medicine as a kind of engineering because it is only recently that we have been able to "see" the molecular cogs and wheels. New technology allows us images at the molecular level, so we can think of ourselves as repairable and improvable machines, which is to think in an engineering sort of way. Our cogs and wheels are, of course, very small. Access to our molecular scale selves provides us with matter that we cannot see and manipulate directly, and vast amounts of information too complex for traditional methods to handle. Knowledge of, and influence over, the molecular world is indirect, and IT is required to mediate. Many other engineering disciplines have come to benefit from IT, but they also managed without it. As medicine becomes increasingly molecular, IT is becoming indispensable.

WHAT ROLE IS IT STARTING TO PLAY IN MEDICINE?

For centuries we have been using observation and theory for medical research as these were the two pillars on which science was built. The third pillar of science, "computation," and hence "simulation," was adopted a few decades ago for science and engineering disciplines. The HIV protease inhibitors, the AIDS drugs, have been among the first important pharmaceutical molecules to be based partly on rational molecular design on computers, and work continues using the same laws of motion of Newton, often refined by quantum mechanical calculation.

The healthcare industry is lagging behind other industries such as the financial industry in terms of leveraging IT. Computers used by medical staff are largely confined to recording appointments and basic local patient information, word processing, and email. Most patient records are still in paper form. It seems to be the norm for *the patient* to fill out a form with personal details and medical history every time he or she visits a new physician or a medical center, even if it belongs to the same medical organization as does the primary physician. We are in a time of transition where the digital patient record and vigilance of patient health still has a long way to go, but things are accelerating rapidly. The overall goal set forth in Section 905 of the US 2007 Food and Drug Administration Amendment Act is to create a current and available active surveillance system on the health and response to drugs of a hundred million people by the year 2012 (25 million patients by 2010). It was motivated by apparent under-reporting of adverse reactions to drugs. Such adverse reactions, or sometimes simply lack of beneficial effect, are probably due in large part to the genetic differences between us that demand a more personalized medicine: clinical trials required for approval of new drugs represent, after all, a small and hence unrepresentative sample of the diverse population for which the drugs will ultimately be prescribed. The FDA must submit a report to Congress by 2011, on how it is *using* this vigilance system.

Today, IT is mostly used in the local management of patient records and medical images. IT has brought massive amounts of geographically dispersed medical information *together* for the common good, from patient records, medical images, and basic research. Systems are being requested to integrate feedback from physicians and patients, the US Food and Drug Administration, and the pharmaceutical industry. The importance of this accelerating acceptance of IT is its ultimate smooth integration with the simulation, prediction, and design of molecules. Indeed as was noted by Tony Hey, former director of the UK national e-science program, a new (fourth) pillar of science may be emerging—data-centric science—to enable research that is data intensive, computer-intensive collaborative and multidisciplinary. One of the authors made an assertion that advancement in medical science calls for leverage of the fourth pillar and has filed ten patent applications related to the new pillar of science.

MEDICAL FUTURE SHOCK

Healthcare administration has often been viewed as one of the most conservative of institutions. This is not simply a matter of the inertia of any complex bureaucratic system. A serious body with an impressive history and profound responsibilities cannot risk unexpected disruptions to public service by changing with every fashionable new convenience, just for the sake of modernity. A strong motivation is needed to change a system on which lives depend and which, for all its faults, is still for the most part an improvement on anything that went before. However, this is also to be balanced against the obligation of healthcare, as an application of science and evolving human wisdom, to make appropriate use of the new findings and technologies available. This is doubly indicated when significant inefficiencies and accidents look as if they can be greatly relieved by upgrading the system. Sooner or later something has to give, and the pressure of many such accumulating factors can sometimes force a relatively entrenched system to change in a sudden way, just as geological pressures can precipitate an earthquake. An Executive Forum on Personalized Medicine organized by the American College of Surgeons in New York City in October 2002, similarly warned of the increasingly overwhelming accumulation of arguments demanding reform of the current healthcare system. Later in 2008, healthcare administrators and IT providers listened, with baited breath, to news about the "healthcare impact of the Obama presidency" with expectations of imminent great revisions. In a sense, the large magnitude of the changes, now beginning, needed to be voluntary: if there is to be pain in making changes to an established system, then it makes sense to operate quickly, to incorporate all that needs to be incorporated and not spin out too much the phases of the transitions, and lay a basis for ultimately assimilating less painfully all that scientific vision can now foresee. But scientific vision is of course not known for its *lack* of imagination and courage, and is typically very far from conservative, still making an element of future shock inevitable in the healthcare industry.

As the accelerating pace in medicine continues into the future, what precisely do we expect to see? As argued in this book, there is reason to believe that the union of IT, telecommunication, genomic and postgenomic sciences within the past half-decade will have profound life science and healthcare applications. Wonderful machines, submicroscopic processors and devices, robot guardian angels, and complex IT infrastructures will be dedicated to our care, down to the very molecular level. It may be that Earth will run hot again in a new accelerating cycle of evolution, as life turns back not only to contemplate itself but also to repair, improve, and evolve itself, at dizzying speed.

Stop the clock! This is future shock indeed. This expectation of things to come begs some introductory explanation because in a sense many things never change, except in form and sophistication.

ON PLANTS AND STONES: THE EVOLVING MARRIAGE OF TECHNOLOGY AND MEDICINE

Modern medicine consists of plants and stones. The utility of molecules and tools (including computers) is a basic underlying concept that has gone unchanged since ancient humans chewed on their first herbs and appreciated the beneficial result, and chipped their first rocks into axes. What leads to discovery is science that is, rooted in empirical observation, but what *transforms* it into a social force is *innovation*.

While it is one thing to speak of discovery and invention as the scientific roots of modern medicine, actual adoption requires innovation and acceptance on a large scale, via marketing and sales. The impact of medicine on society transcends the spark of scientific insight, which many times in history has failed to fuel the fire (where we lack evidence of this, it is probably because it is lost to history!). Innovation does not have to be a radically different scientific world view or even sophisticated high tech, and for most of prehistory it was not: a stone or plant used a new way, or with the birth of ceramics a pot used the first time as a chimney pot, is innovation. Even today, in terms the process of innovation and impact, our technological marvels amount to the same impact as stones and plants. The point is that innovation has to spread and be broadly utilized. Even today there are many things that are done in the mind or laboratory but not on an industrial scale because communicative, distributive, cultural, ethical, and often legal processes are required.

The life sciences and emerging technologies have always had an intimate relationship. New tools enabled agriculture and hence the motivation to master biology, as well as astronomy and meteorology, and predict the course of agriculture. Obsidian blades facilitated ancient surgery, and over the next 3,000 years new technology enabling more sedentary lifestyle turned human thoughts from by the minute survival to more scholarly contemplations of mortality and conquest of disease.

Necessity, it is said, is the mother of invention, and environmental pressures shape cultural views and acceptance of, or desire for, the good life. Herb science is a kind of technology of huge prehistorical, historical, and continuing importance to medicine. The technology of proactively learning to recognize, collect, and cultivate plants with beneficial effects, rather than simply gather or grow extensive fields of plants as sources of metabolic energy, came as a result of a more settled agricultural life. Less varied food groups caused nutritional problems, largely through crops rich in starch but poor in protein, mineral, and vitamin, compared with the earlier hunter-gatherer period, and the distinction between beneficial effects of animal and plant material for nutrition could not have been well distinguishable from other pharmacological effects. From the Chinese whose food-based medicine can be equated to the emerging science of "nutrigenomics," we learn that for as long as history an entanglement of herbs in some pharmaceutical awareness *dominated* medicine for millennia. Monastic gardens kept the science alive through the European Dark Ages. Shakespeare's plays give several now-obscure references to herbs that indicate medieval and Elizabethan medicinal practices. We now know that certain medicinal plants were efficacious because of the molecules they contain. In that sense through the ages people were practicing a crude technology of active ingredients, essences or "principles" that would await Thomas Sydenham (1624–1689) to clarify in words, early organic chemists to purify and put into bottles, and the pharmaceutical industry of today to redesign, synthesize, and put into pills.

Today, molecular and computer technology are two convergent technologies for medicine. Computers are a kind of sharper stone tool, and the drugs they help design are a modern purified and refined form of the herb. Today, as in the evolution from stone blade to electronics, few of the latest tools have failed to be pressed somehow into the service of agriculture and medicine. In the recent past we have seen new tools necessitate other tools. X-ray machines, magnetic resonance imaging (MRI) machines, positron emission tomography (PET), and other electronic medical devices of twentieth-century medicine are all partly computer operated. Computers additionally process the complex data, help diagnose the medical problem, and even recommend treatment.

As IT has increasingly transcended its purely supportive role, IT's *transtechnological* role has put technology as we understand it to human power less as "slave devices" and more as peers of humankind. Devices become smarter, and if we are careful, kindlier. Caring and kindliness required for medicine demands a degree of human-equivalent stature and independence. Who would want a dumb or slavishly obedient physician or nurse? Already in the field of artificial intelligence, mainly due to Marvin Minsky's initiative at MIT, robots and IT systems, computers and their software, sensors, and so forth, are being designed to be "caring agents" who understand the principle of how to look after us. An important influence in this regard was science fiction writer Isaac Asimov who coined "robotics" in his book *I, Robot* and defined three laws of robotics that give human-care an ultimate priority over all other responses to instructions. Actually robots do not always walk or look like a human, and they may not walk at all. From present-day trends, we can expect computer processors to become smaller and smaller, down to the molecular scale, but this will be more than compensated by their insidious incorporation into all things in our environment. Effectively the net mass of computational power working to protect us will increase dramatically.

THE SHARPNESS OF STONES: THE STATE OF ART OF COMPUTERS

A mere 50 years ago computers were cumbersome. By the 1990s, they were powerful enough to be used in routine medical image analysis, and by 2000, IBM was announcing the construction of a powerful new class of supercomputer, Blue Gene, intended to overcome key problems in molecular medicine by running at petaflop speed of 1,000,000,000,000,000 or 10^{15} mathematical calculations per second. Another IBM machine, also with molecular and medical applications, recently broke that barrier first (see Chapter 10).

Petaflop speed amounts to 10^{15} complex mathematical (floating point) operations per second. For readers not of a numerical or engineering disposition, 10^{15} is 1,000,000,000,000,000; that is, the number one followed by 15 zeros. Most often here we will say things like "1000 … 000, where there are 15 zeros." Scientists think that too unwieldy and choose. 10^{15} instead. The engineer's briefer style of writing is to put it all on one line as 10E15, where "E" means "exponent" or "power," here just the exponent of 10 (writing 11015 on one line where E is replaced by 10 would have obvious problems). There is about 3×10^7 or 3E7 seconds in a year, actually 31,536,000 (allowing for leap year seconds, which must be accounted in "time-stamped" medical events on the digital record). Expressions like 3×10^7 or 3E7 inevitably imply a degree of approximation, that it is closer to 3×10^7 than 3×10^6 or 3×10^8. Typically numbers with exponents are even rougher than that: an exponent like 7 means the number is more like somewhere between 6 and 8. To express the number of seconds to a higher level of precision, scientists write 3.6552×10^{17} and engineers write 3.6552E17. Both are 36552000 … 000, where there are 13 zeros, as four of the 17 were used up with the ".6552".

By 2010, computer-based medical and health-care information management may well rise to 60%. In late 2003 we estimated that the Earth will have some 30 to 800 petabytes (1 petabyte is 10^{15}, i.e., 1,000,000,000,000,000 bytes) of medical information on computers. Today, this may be an underestimate as more than 400 petabytes of medical images (X rays, magnetic resonance images, etc.) could be generated annually (see chapter notes and bibliography at the end of this book).

A "byte" is a package of bits, usually eight of them. Each "bit" (short for "binary unit") is coded by an on/off state of some electrical switch or up/down of some magnetic element, and is usually represented by 1/0. Bytes can mean one of a lot more things than can a bit, which means just one of just two things. A byte of eight bits can stand for 256 different things, in fact allowing one to code the whole alphabet in lower case a, b, c, ... , z and upper case A, B, C, ... , Z, numeric digits like 0,1,2, ... , symbols like "+" and "@", and various control characters for computer equipment. "00100001" is a byte that represents an exclamation mark "!" in ASCII code, the American Standard Code for Information Exchange. In most computer languages (the programming language Perl is an exception) numbers like 6.4 intended for rapid calculation are represented differently than by the byte for 6 followed by the byte for "." followed by the byte for 4. A byte can instead be a binary number 00100001 that stands for its decimal equivalent, 32. Several bytes can stand for very big or very small decimal numbers to a specified level of precision.

For comparison and to get a reference point, let's take a pause to review the situation right now, at the time of writing. It's actually quite a bit more advanced than when we first thought of writing this book, and will be more advanced again by the time you read this book. Things are accelerating incredibly rapidly. IT is being used right now for medical imaging, intensive care, and less invasive surgery (e.g., robotic surgery, laparoscopy). One might argue that these are still the only aspects of medical practice that are making really sophisticated use of IT. Even in the relatively industrialized and high-tech US and circa 2005, only 31% hospital emergency departments made extensive use of computers other than, for example, intensive care equipment, and only 27% outpatient departments and 17% physicians made use of computers (the source for most data in this paragraph is David Laskey of the New York-based Markle Foundation, which has a special interest in "digitalizing the US health system"). The situation is only improving in other sectors and EU countries with more social medicine, where there are no fees for service, and in veteran hospitals, departments of defense, small medical groups that interact vigorously internally, and high prices of liability for harming patients.

NOW IS THE CRITICAL TIME FOR IT-BASED HEALTHCARE

The truth is medicine and healthcare and their IT are in a time of transition, and so too is the pharmaceutical industry undergoing transformation, with an increasing eye on using IT to help develop drugs for personalized medicine, that is, for each major different genomic group or "strata" of the patient population. Why do we assume that things are "improving" with more widespread use of computers? Putting aside the thorny issue that some recent systems could have been improperly designed or improperly used, and thus making things worse, computers even in the least sophisticated applications help greatly in holding or recovering information rapidly, and communicating among many centers. To see the scale of the problem, let us take the example of the United States. It is not a typical example, but it is nonetheless the big spender. The annual healthcare spending in the United States exceeded $2 trillion and is expected to grow to $4 trillion or 20% of GDP in 2015 according to the nonprofit organization for National Coalition on Healthcare (www. nchc.org). Right now the US scenario, which computers must address, is that medically important paperwork is escalating, in other words, getting hard to locate when you need it, and rarely locatable in time in a medical emergency. For example, five days in intensive care produces a 100-page document, not to mention the medical images like X rays and magnetic resonance imaging (MRI). In the United States there are 300 million people, and each person could have at least such a record over several years. There are about 5,500 hospitals with 2 million nurses, and about 700,000 physicians, 70% of who are in small groups of 3 to 4 physicians at a time. There are about 1,800 health insurance organizations to which 6 million employers make contributions, and 50 different state medical aid programs (every one is different). There are 43 million uninsured people, 24% of who are under 65 years of age. Despite this massive number of players, all who ideally want the perfect healthcare system, most are drowning in paper, hard copy medical images, and telephone calls, causing confusion and mistakes. There are approximately 100,000 preventable deaths in US hospitals, and optimal care is delivered only 55% of time. Overall, the present medical system represents an archaic and inefficient service model. As some counterbalance for this bad news, one might point out that the United States does compensate because of the money invested in research to provide patients, at a price, with the cutting edge technology. US residents have a better chance of having good treatment than most if they can afford it. But "translational research," meaning the basic scientific research that moves out of the research laboratories to ultimately benefit the patient, takes 15 years to do so. Soon, unless something is done, the curves will cross, and the US citizen will be back in the dark ages as far as his or her healthcare is concerned.

Of course, one hopes that this will not be allowed to happen. We can look at the distant future and compare the present status, and we can hope that positive progress will be made in the *imminent* future to prevent deterioration of the health system. What will be the key technical issues in the imminent future? Certainly as introduced above, medical images will be important. There will in general be a need for storing, recovering, moving, and displaying large amounts of data in regard to medical history ("digital patient record"), lab results, diagnoses, prognoses, prescriptions, and procedures. An additional important concept, however, is that right now we are said to be in the "post-genomic era," as we are just at the period when, after the completion of the first draft DNA readout of the human genome, information about patient genes and proteins (proteomics, expression arrays, etc.—to be discussed below) is coming in. The illustrative fact that there are some 32,000 human genes, which are translated into many more kinds of proteins, makes the ability to handle enormous amounts of data a clear priority. The data that the health informatics or life sciences informatics solutions have to deal with on a daily basis are mind-boggling in terms of the volume in addition to the heterogeneity and multidimensionality. The human genome of about 50 terabytes grows somewhat in information as it is represented in fragments, annotated, and variants are included. One single genome can generate 300 terabytes (i.e., 300 trillion bytes) of trace files. Today a typical pharmaceutical company already generates over 20 terabytes a day of new data. Yet even these numbers pale before the amount of storage, transmission, management, and analysis required for medical and research images. Institutions now consider a cluster of virtual servers and storage systems to manage petabytes of data and beyond.

HEALTH CARE DEMANDS AN EVER SHARPER STONE

So medical data is accumulating in massive amounts, not only in terms of sheer bulk but also in terms of the numbers of parameters and descriptors of things and how they relate. Computers may be millions of times faster than humans at processing medical data, but they cannot always process things on demand and in real time, for example, as in the case of medical emergency. So an issue is computer power, which for the most part means the number of processors or chips running at particular speeds. If you have more chips of greater speed, you have more computer power. But different problems, namely different types of study, analysis, or processing, need different power even when the same data are used as input. So one important aspect of the difficulty of computation is the *order* of any computational problem, and roughly speaking, this is how rapidly computation gets harder as the data increases. The order of computation determines effectively "the sharpness of the stone" that is needed. In many of the common operations involving medical images and DNA, the bytes of information do not interact much. They involve one-to-one copying: they are said to be "processes of order 1." The degree of difficulty will merely double if you double the amount of data. The expected "3D and 4D" analyses by sophisticated new medical imaging machines may account for much of the predicted activity, certainly more than a half. These "D" terms, by the way, have nothing *directly* to do with the order, just the nature of what the data represents. Here 3D means three-dimensional; 4D means three-dimensional motions of the body and its organs, plus motions in time. It does have an effect, but image analysis tends to be of a nature that this is not so much. The computer programmers know how to keep the problem under control. However, operations on the raw data will include not only basic image analysis, but soon also the simulation of body motions including the elasticity, plasticity, and coefficients of friction of nerves, vessels, muscles, and organs to help interpret images. These dimensional components of the data will bring us up to computer calculations approximately of order 2. Today, new waves of stand-up imaging machine are arriving somewhat ahead of schedule, and at the time of writing, the managed healthcare in the United States appears to be having trouble keeping up. While the problem of the time scale of the relaxation of nuclear spin used in magnetic resonance imaging has to be overcome to get "movies" in real time, sonograms, which might be combined, are already there. Other kinds of computation may, however, be of still higher order, as discussed below.

The very large amounts of medical data generated by the variety of technologies, advanced medical imaging, DNA and protein analyses, and so on, have to be stored for long periods. At any point in time a large amount will be constantly moving around the Internet or other wide-area network. Figure 1.1 on page 17 shows an estimate of the data volumes devoted to medicine and related matters up to 2010. The lower curve is a base estimate. It assumes clinical and biomedical use will be at least 30% of total world storage in 2010, conservatively set at several hundreds of petabytes. It downplays advanced imaging capabilities. The upper curve, in contrast, represents the case where advanced medical imaging takes off. This is an optimistic projection with an assumption that 50 million (5×10^7) adult population require 82×10^9 bytes of medical image data for each adult by 2010. It is primarily based on an assumption of advanced 3D (three-dimensional images) and 4D (plus the dimension of time, as in the movies). Such imaging capabilities could hold approximately 80% of all medical storage and a sizable fraction, maybe 40% to 60%, of all storage. But this may be an underestimate. At the time of writing over 400 petabytes of new medical images are created each year these are currently held locally and not all accessible to all concerned via the Internet; overall, there are believed to be over 150 petabytes (1.5×10^{17}) of medical data and laboratory animal data that researches are interested in accessing, especially if combined with other data such as genomic data (see the chapter notes and bibliography for this chapter at the end of the book).

Orders of computation of about 2 may seem moderate compared with other types of calculation considered below, but the real difficulty of a calculation requires how long the calculation takes for a fixed amount of input data, not just how rapidly things get harder as the data increase. Medical imaging is crucial to healthcare and may dominate it in 2010. But as a scientific challenge today's computation doesn't even scratch the biological and medical molecule problems that IBM's Blue Gene supercomputer is supposed to tackle. Blue Gene is intended (but has found many other applications) to help delve into another much deeper and more fine-grained world. It was conceived to simulate the motion of individual atoms in the proteins of our bodies, and ultimately the interactions of those proteins with drugs. Add to the figures above the fact that it takes more than 10^{21} (i.e., 1000 ... 000 where there are 21 zeros) of complex mathematical calculations in a second to fold a single protein *ab initio*, as is calculated by the basic principles of physics, and we have on our hands a further massive amount of data being generated continuously that didn't even go into the calculation in the first place. *Ab initio* means that it simply got deduced from a small number of basic laws. Computers can themselves create a lot of data for computers to analyze. That data is important to the pharmaceutical drug industry. Pharmaceutical drugs must have their ultimate efficacy or otherwise because the protein molecules that they target typically interact with other protein molecules, and these in turn pass on the information about the interaction to other proteins, and other molecules, of the body. How would we therefore simulate the whole body at the level of every atom? The good news is that, forgetting quantum mechanics for the moment and remembering the mathematical physics due to Sir Isaac Newton, these kinds of calculations may take nothing more, or less, than analysis of the forces within each and every *pair* of atoms, atom with atom, in a system of one or more molecules at a time. That is, we recall, a calculation of order 2. This may sound like a lot of computation, and it is. It takes a long time to simulate in a computer what can take a fraction of a second in the real world. For example, one of the early reasons for IBM's petaflop computer project was that there was some reasonable chance of achieving in a year the development of a computer capable of processing the complex mathematical calculations required to simulate the folding up of a protein molecule to achieve its biologically stable functional structure, a process often taking a second or less in the real (biological) world.

Yet such medical computations may not be the only demanding computations. A real challenge to computer power comes from using the vast archives of patient medical records to discover new associations between laboratory results on disease and the most effective therapies. This looks much less like science fiction, and at least to some tastes to represent digital-clerical boredom of the worst kind. Yet the counter to this boredom is that lives are saved by aiding diagnosis, prognosis, physician decisions, epidemiology, biothreat defense, and medical research.

Mathematicians are appreciating that computational needs can dwarf current protein and drug interaction modeling into insignificance. Unlike the calculated rules about the energy and behavior of molecules, rules on medical relationships cannot be always be deduced from pairwise interactions or repeated multiple bivariate analyses alone. The computer can look at far more than pairs of things at a time. For example, early programs deem to inform us that anemic males are not uncommon, and anemic pregnant patients are very common, and these are pairwise, "order 2," relationships. But unless it has the benefit of a full artificial intelligence (AI), and it specifically looks and counts, a computer cannot deduce from such pairwise things that three-way things such as anemic pregnant males are a different story. It has to look at these "order 3" things specifically. And it isn't the case that the most complex rules need be just of order 3. In fact complex diseases, like cardiovascular disease or cancer, may involve analysis problems that require the complex rules in the order of 100 or more. Let's imagine that we put each patient record on a

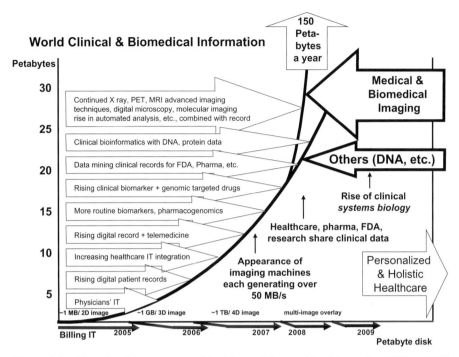

Figure 1.1   Growth of data generated by biomedicine and healthcare for 2000 to 2010

spreadsheet, one patient per row, with $N = 100$ columns to hold all the interesting data to analyze. This kind of data structure is among the least troublesome to analyze. Generally the number of possible rules to consider is about x^N (i.e., x times x times x times x … done N times), where x is often a lot bigger than 2. But for a spreadsheet x equals only 2, and that is bad enough. Let's say N equals just a 100 (i.e., 2^{100}). That means that there are potentially 10^{30}, or 1000 … 000 with 30 zeros, potential rules to consider. On a medical record 2,000 basic features may be more common, and may even be a lot less than many would like.

How can we estimate the computer power needed for the vast data of future? See Figure 1.1. It is believed that each and every petabyte will require roughly a day's work by a machine, with the kind of processing speed available to Blue Gene to process it. This implies thousands of computers, even hundreds of thousands and maybe more in the years 2010 to 2020, and the heat generated by those massive numbers of computers will require huge amounts of energy for cooling. Certainly, in building this new era, we are acutely aware of the natural tendency of work to degrade to heat, as were the engineers of the first Industrial Revolution. Yet we have only very recently solved the problems of heat production and dissipation for petaflop machines, and certainly not beyond (e.g., exaflop machines, which will be a thousand times faster than the petaflop machines). "Hot" is, however, rather overstated. The human race will certainly not allow itself to be baked on a world resembling the hot rock that it was before the evolution of life. At least, it will not do so as a consequence of computing! Still we can reasonably expect hundreds of thousands of such superprocessors of some kind to be needed for medicine and healthcare in 2010 to 2020.

Beyond 2020, unless there are profound changes in computing based on subtle analysis of the thermodynamic principles deduced in the industrial revolutions, heat will become an even bigger challenge as in the distant future the mass of the world becomes converted more and more to computer processors. In addition to the heat, we also need to deal with the electric power required by the massive number of processors. A supercomputer of million processors will require 100 megawatts of electricity as an Intel Pentium processor takes 100 watts at the time of writing this book. Also we need to be concerned about the size and space required by those systems as a system with such large number of processors for massively parallel processing (MPP). To minimize the potential leaks of electrical currents out of the connectors and the electrical cross-talk on the adjacent connectors between the transistor gates within the integrated circuits of a silicon chip, the connecting wires must be kept within a certain distance and therefore miniaturization of silicon chips has a limit. However, there is a slight hope that the embryonic concept of photonic computing, using movement of photons instead of electrons, or molecular computing, often referred to as DNA computing may help with those problems.

Quantum technology may provide the ultimate and "sharpest possible stones" of the medical toolkit. Quantum computing holds great promise, not least in the ability to do many calculations at the same time. And quantum technology in general may be so important for medicine that medical physicists at research hospitals are contributing to it. Marke Brezenski and Bin Liu of the Center for Optical Coherence Tomography and Optical Physics, Department of Orthopedic Surgery, Brigham and Women's Hospital, recently published the paper "Non-local quantum macroscopic superposition in a high-thermal low-purity state" (*Phys. Rev. A* 78 (2008): 063824). There are many potential medical applications of the curious fact of the quantum world that many things can go on, and exist at multiple places, at the same time, if only the quantum mechanical phenomena, well known in the tiny worlds of both particle physics and molecules, can be stabilized and tamed in the large-scale world of everyday human experience. The medical Internet news service Healthorbit (http://healthorbit.ca/, December 2008) was excited by the possibilities: "Imagine a computer chip so fast, it is capable of doing calculations it would take current computers a billion years to replicate. Imagine the ability to kill a cancer tumor by taking some of its cells and destroying them outside the body and, in turn, cells from that tumor still inside the body would die. Is either example possible? In the case of the computer chip, researchers suggest that by 2025, the chip's ability to perform more functions at a faster rate will come to an end. … [The above workers] … using principles related to quantum teleportation, [have] made an important step which not only opens the way for computer chips to increase the processing rate indefinitely, but information processing and telecommunication in general." We shall see. While quantum computing is widely accepted as theoretically possible, the idea for selectively killing cancer cells seems most unlikely for several reasons. They include the relatively large scale and complexity of the cancer system, its interaction with the environment, and the very different way that cells have entangled histories compared with much simpler and tinier particles that could show comparable possibilities. But at least now we have an authoritative good guess at a date: 2025. It is not so far off in "healthcare time" even for such Star Trek–style possibilities: if the healthcare continues to modernize, the majority of the older people among us of the "Baby Boomer" generation will live to see if these predictions come true.

KEEPING OUR HUMANITY

All this new medical technology, advanced biology practiced by advanced IT, has the potential to profoundly alter the way we live, the very nature of what we are, and how healthy we are. It gives us myriad ways to improve the way we live in our relationship with the world. The very boundaries of life can become blurred, and so in consequence may the nature of what we mean by "health." Until recently we have been able to work with the ancient dialectic of *secundum naturam* (natural, normal) and *praeter naturam* (unnatural, abnormal). But what will "normal" be? Until recently health could not be associated with the unnatural, the different, and the artificial, except in rather limited ways. This all will change as concepts of genetic engineering, gene therapy, prosthetics, robotics, bionics, and bio-nanotechnology begin to arise, when it is at least *glimpsed* how one could modify life and extend life capabilities. New classes of life might even need to be created that challenge the very definition of life. In the last chapter we will take this vision into the distant future to imagine minute devices within us, monitoring and even modifying the functions of the organs inside our body, and ultimately vast swarms of minute nanoscale robots, or nanobots. In short, our every need will be nurtured at the molecular level, as powerful, incredibly smart, internal (i.e., implanted) and external computing devices all communicate and direct the show.

Is this blazing technology really what the human race needs? Each of us must assess that for ourselves. But since it seems that wealthy nations will almost certainly take us in the direction of ever-improving medicine, we must be prepared as to how we are going to face it.

If this seems at all a disconnect from our inherent sense of our humanity, the reader may be pleased to learn that we are also going to explore a little the role of *alternative medicine*, that is, alternatives to current mainstream medicine that are often considered more caring and respectful of the patient, and focusing on wellness and disease prevention rather than reacting upon a clinical event, that is, when a symptom of disease presents. In particular, we will touch on two further fundamentally interrelated humanistic approaches in this book, the whole life approach called *holistic medicine* and the more personal touch of *personalized medicine*. There is absolutely nothing wrong with these intertwined principles of great antiquity and in very recent time they have become accepted terms of mainstream healthcare. It is the twentieth-century medicine that got it wrong by trying to tackle healthcare based on fragmented (i.e., nonholistic), episodic (i.e., lack of continuum of services), and external symptom-based (as opposed to dealing with the root cause of illness) diagnostics and treatments, mostly depending on the one-fits-all approach and yet on the trial-and-error method for treatments. Alternative medicine was adopted as a complementary measure, but in the twentieth century it was not adequately armed with science and technology. But that was no great loss, since the science and technology were not yet up to the standard to be fundamentally personal and fundamentally holistic. Today, with deepening molecular insights and advanced IT, medical treatment can become more personalized. We will show that IT can be respectful of these alternative disciplines and even enhance their capabilities.

Some issues discussed above (and others below) relate to *medical ethics*. The most routine use of that term in the twentieth century was in developing the first steps of a strong *regulated* concept of good and bad medical practice, to be discussed in regard to the ethical issues and IT in a later chapter. After the Nazi experiments during the Second World War there were strong movements in regard to patient's rights, medical research, privacy, and so forth. Public reaction to subsequent and persistent moral failures concerning human experimentation in the United States (discussed later) spurred even stronger legislation. Examples of common ethical topics today include how to respect an individual's wishes in medicine and range from what kind of lifestyle an individual wants to have through to matters of a living will and consent for use of medical data for research.

Advances in biological technology, of course, raise new issues. Matters of ethics relate to the sanctity of life and issues on when life begins in regard to stem cell research. With scientific progress the boundaries of life that seemed so crisp when viewed on the macro scale can become blurred under the scientific microscope. So does individuality when it comes to cloning. Just how far we can or we should go with engineering of life? We mentioned above how we have until recently been able to work fairly well with the ancient ideas of *secundum naturam* (natural, normal) and *praeter naturam* (unnatural, abnormal). The new medical technologies and the new power of biology are beginning to strip away these arbitrary divides. It has become clearer why it never was easy to define health objectively without getting trapped in a cyclic argument. The science of medicine, as we understand it, has its province of the treatment of disease or pathologies. The word medicine is from the Latin *medicina*, that is, *ars*, art of healing, and *mederi*, to heal. Disease and pathology are states of being on which medicine acts. A current and growing goal of medicine is the issue of *health*, to prevent disease before it strikes and to build well-being and fitness. Health appears to be a "correct state," "sound state," or "vigorous state" of life. These terms invoke an impression relative to the counterpart of health, a state that is unsound and nonvigorous. Pathology and disease have no deeper penetrable meaning.

It seems enough of a paradox that medicine will progressively disappear from dominance in healthcare, which will be about, literally, care of health, and prevention of disease, not management of it. But it also opens the new question of what health is, in the current world, when no one is perfect and almost all of us believe we are capable of improvement. There is a market for it. Witness the advertisements and amount of email spam about improving body build, losing fat, enhancing sexual performance, sharpening memory, and improving interpersonal skills. The economics of medicine is in many ways fundamentally different from the economics of other industries. Few people would put limits on the resource that is needed to achieve the *goals* of medicine, health, happiness, and longevity. In 1968 British Minister of Health Enoch Powell stated in a speech "there is virtually no limit to the amount of health care an individual is capable of absorbing." If asked, most of us who would choose ambitious goals would primarily go as far as possible on the continuum of a potential that leads from (1) relief from pain, despair, hopelessness, and cure from disease and insufficiency, at one end, through to (2) eternal health, well-being, excellence, and bliss at the other. Why stop arbitrarily at a present point of time when moving on to the future would make today look like a relatively cruel and inhumane Dark Age? We may not all like the world as it is right now, but it is an odd individual who does not want to be happy and productive for as long as he or she can.

Indeed, what do we have as the definition of health by the World Health Organization? Is it that the level of pathogens below a certain load? Is it that laboratory blood and biochemical results are in normal ranges? Is it that your weight and heart behave themselves? Unfortunately, nothing so clinical! The World Health Organization defines health as *a state of complete physical, mental, and social well-being. Health does not consist only of the absence of disease or infirmity.* Good health is in fact an ambitious goal that most of the world, even the industrial world, does not meet. We will constantly touch on this WHO vision.

Ethical issues in social and political science effectively relate to the potential for society to mess things up. How might our goals get messed up? For keeping our humanity, recent debates over matters such as stem cell research and human cloning are barely a glimpse of the controversies to come. That society is at least excited by the challenges is proven because the possible impact of biomedical knowledge has been a mainstay of fiction and speculative essays since the nineteenth century. It has created a market that competes vigorously with the enduring human interests in love and family relationships. It is hardly surprising, bearing in mind that many or all of these fundamental literary themes can be wrapped into a good biomedical thriller. As the essential point of the story, many books and films describe how new biological and medical technology might go wrong, or lead to questionable accomplishments for humankind. They are basically healthcare-philosophy in biomedical futurology, in fictional form. Glitches of biomedical technology are a constant theme in the works of Michael Crichton: *The Terminal Man, The Andromeda Strain, Jurassic Park, Prey*, and so on. *The Terminal Man*, for example, was written in response to real experiments in electrical stimulation of the brain such as those of Jose Delagado. One showpiece was described in the New York Times of 17 May 1965: " *'Matador' with a Radio Stops Wired Bull. Modified Behavior in Animals the Subject of Brain Study.*" Crichton's stories typically describe one-off events that even within the stories told give the human race time to speculate and prevent problems arising again. Some people write about how civilization could soon be transformed, for better or worse, by biomedical progress: *GATTACA* is a movie about a genetically engineered elite, and Bernard Wolfe's *Limbo* is a long-standing classic about prosthetic replacement by superior robotic limbs as a preferred practice for almost all.

And what is the perfect life and well-being anyway, if the nature of reality itself is in question? Others address the possibility that well-being can be engineered on demand, and in some cases well-being could mean discarding reality for an *illusion* of a whole world of peace or bliss, chemically, neurologically, or computationally. The drug *soma* of Huxley's classic *Brave New World*, the humorous science fiction stories of Lanislov Lem, the movies *The Matrix* and *Vanilla Sky*, pithy passages from the works of Robin Cook and Larry Niven address such issues. Related issues even arise for the pharmaceutical industry today, say as to whether a drug which improves the sense of well-being and management of an Alzheimer's patient is as important as a drug which might restore the patient to a less euphoric normality. But apart from the voices of those who advise strict adherence to the guidance in ancient authoritative works, there is no single popular and certainly no agreed ethical system about those things that will increasingly affect the lives of our children.

The authors do not think that the answer to perfect human existence necessarily lies in a future idyllic village or garden life like that portrayed for the (ill-fated) Eloi in H. G Wells' *The Time Machine*. Phases of biological and social evolution already passed are not necessarily the best models for biological and social evolution to come, even if we could have total control of the process. But we do think that that the ancient principles of village life, when personal differences and all aspects of life were under the watchful eye of the shaman, do provide some principles for the future of medicine. As we will see, it is in the hands of some great thinkers such as the ancient Greek Hippocrates that the road of medicine split into two paths, at least in the Western world. Still, it could be argued that these two paths, though distinguishable, have been intertwined up to the nineteenth and twentieth centuries, when mainstream medicine became more organized, but relied on a few highly trained individuals to administer to growing populations. The first doctrines, ideas, and approaches of medicine arose in ancient times when Shamans, folk physicians, and other medical wise men had a lot more time to spend on individuals in their small populations. The ancient wise men, in misty prehistory were born with brains essentially the same as ours. They were probably as smart as physicians today; there was just less data of the kind that we have today on atoms, molecules, and cells. With fewer details like that to think about, they applied (at least in many cases) a lot more effort to considering the whole life, diet, and sense of well-being, including spiritual life. So the ancients derived much wisdom for us by having their minds focused on the personal and holistic view, developing proven approaches for which the analytical science and overburdened and thinly spread health-care system of the twentieth century had little time. IT can help with that logistic problem.

Today, a *re-emergence* of ancient holistic and personalized approaches to medicine is raising their own challenge about how information should be shared between the patients and the providers of patient care. For example, a tension is developing between autonomy—the concern of the patient for maintaining privacy—and *solidarity* or *cooperation*—what the patient is willing to share to be pooled for the common good. Personalized medicine, with its focus on the individual, emphasizes autonomy, but it critically depends on solidarity too, as we will see later.

As we move toward the kind of future envisaged here, being ultra-healthy does not mean languishing in some kind of perpetual vacation or even perpetual orgasm. We humans are a restless species. We are always looking to improve our lot in the world. The ability to change is freedom, and that sense of freedom is part of what is needed for contentment. *We may feel cramped by the present,* but we humankind always want to move on, to migrate, and to improve technologies, and not least the care of our health.

OUR ETHICALLY THERMODYNAMIC FUTURE

So we believe that consideration of the long term is important in formulating the ethics of more imminent future medicine. There are challenging ethical issues in what we mean by life and well-being. However, these ethical and philosophic matters seem to lie far outside the realm of anything that information science and technology can contribute other than, it seems, creating in the first place the opportunities and risks that need to be addressed. But this is not entirely true. There are insights from information science and related disciplines of mathematics physics which give us a rock of cool logic on which we stand and examine the liquid larva that is streaming past us and that will solidify into the future. This is important when the future being considered is still too controversially alien for our current "gut feelings" and everyday frames of reference to apply. The wisdom of the ancients also cannot help us, unless part of that wisdom can be re-expressed in modern mathematical terms. Strictly speaking, the following is not formally required to appreciate the benefit of information science, but it somehow really seems to help: many modern physicists and mathematicians, such as Gregory Chaitin and Charles Seife, would even hold that *everything* is information, an intellectual and no less quantifiable extension of Einstein's proof that all matter is energy ($E = mc^2$). That includes life, as illustrated by the following, but which, it must be confessed, raises its own new ethical issues. Our great grandchildren may decide to opt out in hope of rebirth for a better era and leave all relevant details for their reconstitution, such as their DNA sequences and brain pattern connections, in digital form. A person who might delete such a record could be tried for murder, or another could steal it and copy or modify the information to some dark, or even intended good, purpose, such as removing the genetic defects and enhancing others' performance. These are complex ethical issues outside our present frame of ethics.

Our answers may come from our consideration of the sibling sciences of thermodynamics and information technology, and include even cosmology. Our medical future may be on a grand cosmic scale. Earth alone, or any future new Earth, will not last forever. As we move forward and evolve, or sicken and die, we all play that life-and-death game within the current laws of what we currently call physics. *Entropy* and disease are intuitively intertwined. A prominent nineteenth century scientific-philosophical theme since the industrial revolution has been the inevitable increase of entropy, or disorder and decay, in the universe. It is, at least statistically and overall, a force so fundamental that it is believed by many physicists to define the direction of time. Entropy may seem like a wooly concept when described as disorder and decay, but it can be measured by the methods of thermodynamics (the principles of heat engines, and indeed any system) just as much as quantities like energy, pressure, and temperature. Moreover we now know that an increase in entropy corresponds to a loss of information, so entropy is a kind of negative information. If dropping your computer somehow lost you one gigabyte of memory chip, its entropy went up by one gigabyte from that perspective. While that isn't the unit that the steam engineers used, we could use it equivalently, with a single conversion factor. It also is why running massive computers to keep us alive and well, and away from disorder and decay, necessarily involves a compensating price in terms of heat production. The damaged computer got slightly hotter because the motion of the parts of the memory chip suddenly stopped accelerating smoothly together in a concerted way to the floor, and on hitting the floor, the memory chip started going off somewhat randomly in a less concerted way. Such a disorganized form of energy (motion) appears to us as what we call heat. In addition it seems impossible, at least in practice, to do computations without converting at least some organized energy to heat. In fact doing anything is difficult without degrading something to heat, with the exception of certain idealized processes (including in computing) that are said to be fully reversible.

From such quantitative considerations we learn that life seems to reverse that process of disorder, at least a bit and at least locally. *This is an important concept because it reveals an essence of health and healthcare, since without that constant reversal, we have disruption, disease, and ultimately death.* We do know from modern thermodynamics that entropy is negative information, meaning that if the information in a system—such as us—goes up, the entropy goes down.

Yet animate things can look pretty messy and complicated. We need to distinguish the simple everyday dialectic of order and disorder from what is meant here. If information is associated with order, how can it be that the digital pulses encoded on a CD (compact disk) or DVD (digital video disk) can look pretty random. Crystals, on the other hand, have high order and low entropy. Who, however, would want to be something like a crystal of table salt (sodium chloride)? Such crystals are too regular and too frozen in space and time to contain any further information than that the crystal is sitting there with that regular structure! Such regimented lack of disorder seems closer to death than life. The great theoretical physicist Erwin Schrödinger put the relevance of crystals very well. He said that the basis of life and heredity had to be some kind of *aperiodic crystal*, that is, without a repeating pattern. By this he predicted what we now call DNA. The trick is to understand that the kind of order that interests us is paradoxically and typically a disordered looking mess, but it is *one particular* disordered looking mess that serves a particular reference point, goal, or purpose, in regard to which we say it has *meaning*.

The astute reader will note that mathematically and philosophically some fundamental questions remain as to what really is information, what is randomness, what is knowledge, what is consciousness, what purpose means for any string of binary digits, what is a computer program, can it be conscious, what are data, and what is output. These and other relevant questions still defy the best brains, and are far-reaching, intertwining with issues of the apparent direction of time and the nature of space. Ultimately they may turn out to be unanswerable or to have incomprehensible answers, because we are asking the wrong question.

In promoting and maintaining this reversal with health and well-being, what forces will fight that battle for us? Since entropy is negative information by the physicist's own definition, and if information is something to do with good and entropy something to do with bad, *a reasonable answer is that IT will fight that battle for us*. IT versus the forces of darkness, the great game of the universe, with human healthcare at stake, is not a bad background story against which to touch on the sometimes seemingly drier issues such as of health insurance and billing systems, federated data bases, data analytics, and computer-aided compliance. They are all essential challenges or tools on the road to a grander vision.

Thus big picture puts the *sanctity of life* in perspective. While our views on entropy have stayed solid since the nineteenth century, our other views of cosmology have changed throughout the ages. These days, and since the mid to late-twentieth century, cosmologists believe that the universe began with the Big Bang roughly 12 to 15 billion years ago. Then, some five billion (i.e., a five thousand million) years ago, the hot Earth cooled and life began. That is a reasonably measured pace of interesting events: it seems sobering to many to think that terrestrial life is something between as much as a quarter to a half of the age of the entire universe. Those of us who subscribe to a literal interpretation of the Old Testament Bible like to think that humans are about as old as the universe, and of central importance in it, and so find the new view disturbing. Others may take comfort in believing that the universe is vastly older, perhaps eternal, and life started only in the last tiny fraction, which the latest evidence shows not to be so. But this view also means that if *intelligent* life took so long to appear, it may be rare. In that view we may be unique, as life is precious. It behooves us to live on, and ultimately that may be among the stars.

STEPS TOWARD A GOOD END?

In the late twentieth century such thoughts about computers ensuring our survival were incorporated by some scientific philosophers into visions of the very distant future. This idea of healthcare ultimately placed in the context of computers that will sequester the universe and ourselves with it, will be resurrected in Chapter 10, along with mention of such thinkers as the Jesuit teacher Paul Teilhard de Chardin's thesis on the "Omega Point," and other thinkers specializing in *eschatology*, the destiny of the universe, and see a role for humankind in that.

Probably one of the best known contemporary works by a physicist addressing these issues is that of Frank J. Tipler, with the remarkable title of *The Physics of Immortality: Modern Cosmology, God, and the Resurrection of the Dead* (Doubleday, 2007). Tipler feels that cosmology and what is effectively transforming the universe by, and to, computers, will give us, and all the dead who ever lived, a second chance. It is, in effect, a rather extreme Christian physicist's view of healthcare IT on the cosmological scale. But suppose he is wrong; how much time do we, or rather our descendants, have before death holds dominion over everything? And if he is even half right, how much time do we have to secure our immortality? We opened this chapter with consideration of how the pace of life, in every interpretation of that word, quickens. But this is not so of the cosmological stage on which the game of life is acted: here the reverse is true. In the first 10^{-43} seconds, an atom-size entity explodes and space is created. In the first 10^{-32} seconds, which is incredibly slower than the above step, quarks, electrons, and fundamental particles are formed. Atoms form in 300,000 years, and in a billion years the stars form, and ten billion years later life appears. The stage on which we are players now changes the scenes ponderously slowly, and increasingly slowly, compared with the speed at which the actors change and the plot develops, and the speed of that change *increases*. It is as if life feeds on the pace of the universe, diminishing it to its own ends. But ultimately if Tipler and others are right, living entities will control everything, and not only move the scenery but redesign the scenery. As an evolving complex system, we are moving faster and faster than the universe of which we are made. Looking even a million years in the future the work ahead seems too huge and incomprehensible a task, but we still have billions of years to get it right. That is, as we used to say during the Cold War, assuming that we do not "blow ourselves up first" or, in contemporary terms, destroy our ecosystem.

BACK TO THE BEGINNING

Now to start our journey in this book, we have to go back and retrace our steps. We need to discuss in more detail what makes us the humans, and the patients, that we are, with our different tendencies to various diseases, and our different responses to herbs and drugs. We need to consider where common infectious diseases really came from. This story goes back only on a few tens of thousands of years, to the single human beings who left descendants today. Based on analysis of mitohcondrial DNA (mitochondria are cellular organelles passed down through the female line), Eve is the name given to the woman who is defined as the most recent common ancestral mother for all currently living humans. She is believed to have lived about 140,000 years ago in an area that is now Ethiopia in Africa. The time she lived is calculated based on understanding of the rate of changes of her descendant's DNA, as perceived by genetic differences in the current living branches of her family tree of descendants. Her "significant other" was not the genetic Adam of us all. By analyzing Y-chromsomal DNA from people in all regions of the world, geneticist and anthropologist Spencer Wells, who is leading the Genographic Project, has concluded (not uncontroversially) that all humans alive today are descended from just one male who lived in Africa around 60,000 years ago (see the bibliography at the end of the book.). And just about that long ago, a mere blink in evolutionary time, most of us came from just a tribe or two.

2

FROM PREHISTORY TO HIPPOCRATES

I swear by Apollo Physician and Asklepios and Hygeia and Panaceia and all the gods and goddesses. ... ,

—Hippocrates, "The Oath"

THE MEDICAL RECORD OF THE HUMAN RACE

Having made a fast transit of the medical adventure of the human race until the end of time in Chapter 1, we will step back a little to pick up the record for the entwined story of civilization and medicine so that we can consider how the human infectious diseases arose. This will allow us to look at another kind of medical record: the record of human history and its well-being and survival that we carry within our genes, as DNA, and its profound impact on modern medicine, especially molecular medicine. Our genetic history is also entwined with the migration of people and the rise of civilizations. We are the molecules of which we are made, and the story of migration and survival is the story of both.

Our mission, in part, is to trace (at least roughly) the descent of the great Hippocrates, legendary founder of Western medicine. We will start with essentially modern humans, which biologists classify as follows:

- kingdom Animalia
- subkingdom Metazoa

The Engines of Hippocrates: From the Dawn of Medicine to Medical and Pharmaceutical Informatics, by Barry Robson and O.K. Baek
Copyright © 2009 by John Wiley & Sons, Inc.

- phylum Chordata
- superclass Tetrapoda
- class Mammalia
- subclass Theria
- infraclass Eutheria
- order Primates
- family Homidae
- genus *Homo*
- species *Homo sapiens*

Except for those pathogens that infect us, or the vector animals like mosquitoes that carry them, or the animals that we have domesticated and that gave many diseases to us, we are interested in *Homo sapiens*. Primarily we are interested in human, not veterinary, medicine (though most principles discussed here hold for veterinary medicine too). For comparison of classifications we will mention one animal that once competed heavily with man but whose relatives became a great domesticated friend of man: the wolf which belongs to the different order Carnovora, family Canidae, genus *Canis*, and species *Canis lupus*. Important for our purposes it is also worth noting that other human species *Homo erectus* and *Homo heidelbergensis* coexisted with modern humans. More, important, *Homo neanderthalensis* (Neanderthal man), and humans who were modern but not our direct ancestors, coexisted with a major migration of our ancestors out of Africa that we will talk about here, essentially representing competitors who by some means or other our ancestors vanquished. *Homo florensis* is the elfin or "hobbit" human in Indonesia who lived until very recently and was discovered even more recently (in 2004), hinting that rumors of "Bigfoot" and the Himalayan "Yeti," or "the wood folk" or "the little people" of modern legend could also represent other human species still living in less accessible sites—though with humans now treading on almost every spot of land across the world, it is more likely that at best, like *homo florensis*, they died out recently.

The ancestral Adam and Eve of everyone, in and out of Africa, makes us all brothers and sisters even more than we have recently thought. But to trace the line of descent to Hippocrates, we need to consider just a few Africans. These were Africans who began their new diaspora out of Africa a mere 50,000 to 80,000 years ago, perhaps at most 100,000 or so. We can track the journey out of Africa by mutations that survive today, called *biomarkers*. For example the Y chromosome of many non-Africans, called marker M168, defines "Eurasian Adam," whose male ancestor lived 30,000 to 79,000 years ago but whose ancestors are still found in Eastern Africa and the Southern Middle East. Similarly a descendent of his acquired M45 in Central Eurasia north of India, but his descendants moved on west. So, though some of the descendants of these men still live in the vicinity of the places where the mutations occurred, they have spread to colonize northern Europe. The geographical distribution of peoples with these markers defines the journey of man. Similarly the DNA of the mitochondrion, an organelle within the cell and acquired from our female ancestors, defines the journey of woman.

Many if not all the people from this exodus were descended, probably from even well before the migration, from an African with a mutation that enhanced the power of the brain, making a new kind of *Homo Sapiens*, an innovative *Homo Sapiens*, who is our intellectual equal. They showed dramatic improvement in symbolic thought. Armed with a new stone blade technology, spear-hurling projectile devices, and a real flair for trade, they competed with Neanderthals and modern humans outside of Africa, and with any other peoples also emerging from Africa, to the extent that all non-Africans today are their descendants. Migrations took place in all directions in various times, spreading the advantageous new mutation across the world. These great African migrations continued up until fairly recent time including that of the Bantu going south and starting from south of the Sahara Desert, and taking over some 2,000 years in the process. The Bantu, a linguistically related group of tribes of about 60 million people, were responsible for one of the largest and last great migrations in human history. The impetus for this movement is uncertain, but it is a model for the impacting factors of other migrations in that it involved efficient food production and innovative new crops such as in the Bantu case yams, oil crops, and banana. The banana, native to south Asia, is a mystery that brief comments like "banana diffusion" (occasionally encountered in the literature) do not wholly resolve!

Migrations do not mean that everyone is always on the move. Some humans dropped out of the march and settled regions as they moved out of the hunter-gatherer mode. There were splinter groups, and these branches can be tracked by genomic sampling of populations that have not moved much since they settled there. Migrations some 50,000 years ago or more seem in some ways incredibly fast, but they were slow enough to leave many mutations and footprints in populations today of how populations have progressively spread. As mentioned above, all humans have genetic markers; there is a simple difference in their DNA (see Chapter 3 for details), say a G (guanine) where others have a C (cytosine) or A (adenine) where others have a T (thymine). This allows Europeans to trace their ancestry back to one of seven women who lived between 45,000 and 10,000 years ago and to learn roughly where they lived. The footprints of the journey are found in the geographical locations of their descendants alive today. The past very few years has seen the tendency of these genetic differences to be called *genomic biomarkers*, and as we will see, especially in Chapter 9, they have a continually increasing and profound effect on choice of prescription and on the pharmaceutical industry.

All said, it was not the biggest, fastest, nor last diaspora from Africa. Whereas the first would have involved a few hundred individuals, many millions of Africans exported in the slave trades over the past few hundred years made a massive contribution to the modern world, leaving genetic markers in many non-African people alive today. But, in comparison the latter great diaspora was an incredibly rapid leapfrog into other populations, with no or few stops on the way. That does not mean that the ultimate origins of Africans brought out of Africa by the slave trade cannot be traced. For example, a Bristol, UK, woman who came to Britain from America and was able to trace her ancestry back more than a few generations. Gene tests identified her as a descendant of the Kikuyu tribe in Kenya. Actually one in every hundred Britons is descended from an African or an Asian, according to a genomic sampling study by Bryan Sykes of Oxford University. Possible sources include African soldiers in the Roman legions, and Moors among the Spanish Armada wrecked by storms on the Irish coast.

Such genomic sampling, or genotyping, has become a popular pursuit, though sometimes yielding some unpopular findings. Many people have a view of their ethnicity that they do not easily give up. A staunchly Scottish school teacher who could trace back her British ancestry for 400 years was found to have Polynesian DNA. While writing this paragraph, there occurred one of those small personal watershed points in history: one of the authors (BR) and his wife sent off swabs from the inside of their cheeks to The Genographic Project, a collaboration between National Geographic magazine and IBM to track the different branches of modern humanity.

Author BR wrote, "we are proud of a strong Scottish and Viking ancestry … but who knows what the DNA will yield!" In fact the Y chromosome DNA result came out quickly, and identified the author as belonging to group R1b, the Cro-Magnon lineage defined by a marker point in the DNA known as M343. The ancestors of this group took the same route, at least in the earlier stages, as the peoples with the markers discussed above. They are also heavily responsible for much DNA in the United States, with the exception of the massive late African and Hispanic immigrations, a smaller but influential significant Asian immigration, and the lamentably low representation form Native North Americans due to massive suppression in the nineteenth century which the US government has only slowly moved to correct.

Being descendant of the "out-of-Africa" M168 marker and still carrying that marker too, author BR also carries M89 mutation associated with 90% to 95% of all non-Africans that arose in North Africa or the Middle East. The ancestors carrying this gene followed the grasslands through Iran to the steppes of Central Asia, enticed by herds of woolly mammoths, buffalo, and antelopes. In Iran 40,000 years ago a mutation gave rise to marker M9, and then some 35,000 years ago a further M45, whose people moved further to the Eurasian north. Remember that when the later markers appear by mutation, the earlier ones are retained. Although, in theory, the older markers on other points of the DNA could be changed again, the odds for that are small. Then an ancestor acquired M173 in Europe fairly early in a sharp turn west in the long march west to the Atlantic coast. His companions and descendants created the famous cave paintings at Lascaux and Chavet, and competed with and outlasted the last of the Neanderthals in the extreme challenges of the last great Ice Age. With the glaciers extending down to northern France, the author's ancestors weathered much of the Ice Age out in Spain and spread north as the ice retreated. The marker is very high in northern France and the British Isles. But the path of the migrating peoples carrying the M343 marker passed very close to Denmark, a distance away from the migration route which is 5% or less from the journey since M343 began. A Scottish and Viking ancestry is still possible and indeed likely for the forefathers. However, the mitochondrial DNA determining the "foremothers," the maternal line of descent and its history, is still not done because author BR misread and failed to fill in the "female" box on the form, thinking it referred to current gender, not female line of descent! In contrast author OB has not yet had his DNA analyzed, but could have several markers, M122, M174, or even M130 on route via Korea on the heroic mission across the frozen straits to colonize America.

Although such particular genotyping projects are deliberately not focused on medical aspects, they do provide genetic mappings called haplotypes (patterns of genetic differences) that have application to disease diagnosis and therapy. As we will see, such patterns correlate with tendencies to different types of disease and different responses to drugs, but not necessarily because the difference in the DNA directly causes the disease. Typically the gene tends to be inherited that causes the disease, somewhere on the DNA, even if we do not yet know what that gene is. Genes can gang together, though not necessarily at the same time in the same ancestor. It is precisely the tendency for gene variations to travel together that represents a haplotype, the set of traveling companions.

The concurrence of many diseases and many familiar genetic markers in an individual that keep showing up together purely on a statistical basis is useful to anthropological scholars. Another correlation is that between our ancestral tree, which is deduced from specific genetic differences that earmark populations, and the family tree of languages. Indo-Europeans have characteristic genetic markers, and they speak a characteristic type of Indo-European language. Indo-European languages have their markers two, since words with common meaning and common elements of pronunciation (e.g., the word for mother starts with "M") occur in both Europe and India. But there is no Indo-European gene that is a direct cause of speaking an Indo-European language. If there were, future genetic engineers could put Berlitz, the famous language teaching company, out of business. Human language, customs, beliefs, and many modes of thought just travel in packages, represented by our ancestors who carried them along together, whether it is part of their inherited biology or their passed-on habits, culture, and world view. There is a word which makes clear the distinction between what is genetically transmitted and what is culturally transmitted. A *meme*, as opposed to *gene*, is a component of cultural ideas, skills, symbols, or practices that transmit from one mind to another through examples, rituals, or anything that other humans can imitate. It is a unit of information storage and transmission rather less than a byte, more like an entire program as a set of instructions. Memes are not digitally encoded in our DNA nor were they originally coded in writing, but are analogous to genes in that they replicate and are subject to Darwinian selective pressures. Richard Dawkins coined the word in his book *The Selfish Gene* (Oxford University Press, 1976) to describe how one might extend evolutionary principles to explain the spread of ideas and cultural phenomena, including language, but the word is from the Greek *mimema* meaning mimic. Ideas and cultural phenomena also include tool-making, hunting, agricultural, trading, architectural, engineering, scientific, and medical skills, and writing, an early step in human-made information storage technology. The meme of writing would transform the nature of the selective pressure on human knowledge, and Caxton's printing press would much later transform it yet again, creating the world of publication with its selective pressure of scholarly analysis, debate, peer review, correction, and refinement of the ideas over many generations.

Before genomic science, the only plausible equivalent biomarker in health care was *ethnicity*. But because ethnicity is also a matter of cultural and religious differences (sometimes catching many different genetic origins under one label), because the highly diverse African nations tend to be pooled as "African," and because many nations are a genetic melting pot anyway, ethnicity is not a good indicator. One might say that it is our molecular ethnicity that matters. Appearance is not everything.

Still there are well-known correlations of geographic location not only with fine details of anatomy and physiology but particular diseases and disease risks in many cases. So medicine has focused on peoples in different geographic regions well before the detailed genomic data became available. Consider Finland. Mutations have arisen in Finland since the occupation of the region, and these mutations do not appear in the same form elsewhere in the world. These genetic mutations materialize as the congenital flat cornea, a Finnish type of congenital nephrosis (a severe renal disorder), and diastrophic skeletal dysphasia. Moreover these occur differently in various parts of Finland, the first to the northwest, the second to the south with a slight prevalence to the southwest, and the third to southeast. The different distributions make no sense in this case except that they arose by chance and reflect only the geographical location and relative moment in time, historic or prehistoric, of the persons in which they occurred. It is much the same story all over the human-occupied world, with some qualifications. One that is described below is that the environment *can* have an effect on which mutations are retained in the population, a kind of Darwinian natural selection.

The above reference to geographic genetic differences that are also genetic diseases raises interesting issues when we ask: where do these differences in DNA, these biomarkers, come from, and how do they survive? Well, again, the answer is as mutations that have been passed down. They are simply the same errors of DNA copying that are responsible for human evolution, the explanation of random variation that Darwin showed must take place along with natural selection of the organisms arising from them. However, the chances of an advantageous mutation are very small, which is why evolution is so slow.

One would think that the mutations will either be neutral in effect or have at least some slightly bad effect that is neither so bad nor so common as to prevent propagation through breeding. Detailed analysis of the patterns of mutations has shown, however, that this view is simplistic. Mutations are of different types, essentially according to the statistical features of DNA sequences.

Importantly, many common markers are *founder mutations* that are embedded in sections of DNA that are usually identical in all who have inherited the mutation. Because of chance swapping of sections of DNA (called *crossing over*) that occur in sexual reproduction of organisms, these sections do however become progressively eroded through the generations. Their length can be thus an indication of how many generations elapsed since the founding mutation appeared. In contrast to these founder mutations, there is a more random spread of mutations, some of which might be ancient founder mutations of which the surrounding stable section of DNA has long been dispersed. Some of them, however, certainly represent "hot spots" where is seems that the DNA is almost unstable. Achondroplasia, a form of dwarfism that keeps reappearing in populations, is such a hot spot mutation. In contrast, some founder mutations seem advantageous, such as LCT, which allows lactose tolerance and allows humans to drink cow's milk.

But most founder mutations are *also* considered fairly serious genetic diseases, and these do not just keep popping up from nowhere. So one wonders how they ever survived natural selection and got passed down. The answer is certainly not clear for some mutations, such as mutation GJB2 from a founding ancestor in the ancient Middle East, and responsible for deafness. But for most mutations, a good argument can be made that they have some beneficial effect in a particular environment, and typically when they occur on one chromosome (the *heterozygous* state) from a parent such that, with one gene copy still functioning, the bad effects are less severe. These possible beneficial effects are discussed later in this chapter, in a discussion of what "bad" and "good" means, if anything, for much genetic disease.

Colonization of areas by very few people, or an initially very small population even if different lines of descent are well represented, has its own predictable effect on the statistics of DNA. In relatively genetically isolated communities, where some 200 to 400 years ago there were relatively few founding fathers and mothers, with some ancient mutations that could occur in *homozygous* form with more serious effect. In the Caribbean Cayman Islands, diseases such as ataxia, lactose intolerance, and other disorders may show higher than average incidence, while other islands in the Caribbean have a different disease spectrum. In many places around the world it can be the luck of the draw in the DNA lottery, sometimes through new mutations but often genetic concurrence depends on the founding forefathers and foremothers in the colonization of a particular region. A few mutations may be beneficial.

In our human journey to fill the world, we have therefore inadvertently kept a travel journal, with the changes written or etched into the DNA that we can read today. The study of all this, outside and inside Africa, is precisely genomics. The study of the important medical impact is the differential risk for diseases, and in regard to the different actions of pharmaceuticals on different people, it is the relatively new science of pharmacogenetics or *pharmacogenomics.*

This etching has not been so drastic as to turn humans into new species or even into fundamentally different races. It provides no rationale for extreme right wing elitism. But it has been sufficient to create varieties of *patients,* in other words variations of different medical importance. So it is in the interest of healthcare, not just twenty-first century anthropology, that we may summarize the position as follows. As we hinted above, it appears to have adhered religiously to either pure chance or to the Darwinian principle of mutation and natural selection. A significant number of mutations can survive to be inherited. In just 200,000 years, and of course even in the last 50,000 to 80,000 years, we, African and non-African, differ in about 1 to 2 in every thousandth of our DNA because of this inheritance of mutations. These mutations and population movements can be deduced from DNA sampling studies on the surviving populations today. The differences in the DNA that researchers follow, by sampling current populations, are typically not changes of medical importance but get inherited as useful markers. Many of the changes that are of *direct* medical importance, and happen to travel along with these markers in our chromosomes, have yet to be identified.

PREHISTORIC MEDICINE

Cave paintings of some 17,000 years ago depict men in animal masks performing ritual dances that may be the first indications of early medical practice, albeit based on magic. Were they treating diseases of genetics? Not entirely!

First, there were the obvious effects of injury, including use of sticks as crutches and later splints. The new blade technology allowed rudimentary surgery. Obsidian blades used for trepanning skulls between 17,000 and 7,000 years ago (and still used in refined form in surgery today) could have been used for genetic-based disorders, including madness, and for treating abscesses, minor tumors, and disorders of ear, nose, teeth, and eyes and even cataracts at a much later stage.

Second, there was, of course, malnutrition. Agriculture provided quantity but not quality. Bones found from this period are stunted and show evidence of rickets. Pellagra, kwashiorkor, marasmus, scurvy, and the other deficiency diseases were probably rampant.

Third, part of the human story is its relationship with pathogens—viruses, bacteria, protozoans, worm parasites, and so on. In the great diasporas humankind was on the move, typically into unoccupied or sparsely populated territories. For such dispersed moving populations with no constant dangerous contact with animals save by hunting and carcass processing, *infectious diseases*

TABLE 2.1 Some Great Milestones of the Human Race up to Hippocrates

Years Ago	Development
1,000,000	Diaspora of *Homo erectus* out of Africa
750,000	Crude stone tools
500,000	Crude blade tools
400,000	Wooden spears
290,000	Grindstones, pigment processing
285,000	Massive use of ochre
280,000	Earliest possible date for beads
250,000	Pointed tools, start of Middle Stone Age. "Levalloisian technique" of striking flakes from a lump of rock.
233,000	Wooden human figurine found in Israel
200,000	First anatomically modern humans in Africa. First ostrich egg-shell beads.
170,000	"Mitochondrial Eve" the female ancestor of all modern humans in Africa.
140,000	Shell fishing. First evidence of long-distance exchange of goods.
130,000	Fishing. Obsidian tools in Tanzania.
120,000	Advanced use of pigments, especially ochre
100,000	Bone tools. Mining. Possibly etched records (of trade?). Evidence of trade of decorative objects. Scraped, heat-treated ochre.
100,000	Earliest accepted date for start of significant diaspora of modern humans out of Africa
80,000	Barbed harpoons
79,000	Earliest records of very sophisticated ochre art
75,000	Large numbers of tiny beads produced. Possibly engraved ochre.
50,000–70,000	Diaspora of modern humans out of Africa. No descendents today of earlier emigrants.
60,000	Drop in temperature. Monoliths. Advanced beads. In Africa, burning of grassland to cultivate tubers.
40,000–50,000	A mutation in one *Homo sapiens* individual giving rise to a new innovative variety of modern human (argues Kate Wong in *Scientific American*, June 2005)
50,000	Colonization of Australia
43,000	First appearance of intricate bone and stone carvings, jewelry, figurines
40,000	Images on cave walls. Great variety of narrow stone blades, clear signs of dominance of Neolithic culture.
35,000	European cave paintings
30,000–35,000	Sophisticated carved animal figurines
30,000	Last remnants of Neanderthals
20,000	Ice age at peak
15,000	Sophisticated spear-throwing devices
12,000	Ice age ends
12,000	Earliest evidence of villages and agriculture
11,000	Colonization of Americas

TABLE 2.1 *Continued*

Years Ago	Development
11,000	Stone buildings
10,000	Last mammoths
8,000	Earliest known use of plough
8,000	Large stone houses, "mansions"
7,500	Signs of bureaucracy (seals, etc.)
7,000	Earliest known writing
6,000	Rise of first cities
5,700	City of Uruk
5,400	Major colonization of Mesopotamia
5,200	Evidence of trade between cities
5,000	Earliest known wheeled carts
5,000	Bronze age begins
4,900	Earliest known money
4,570	Peak of Old Kingdoms of Egypt, pyramids at Giza
4,500	Stonehenge in England
4,000	Abraham in Canaan
3,200	Iron age begins
2,780	Flowering of Greek civilization, first Olympic games
2,450	Hippocrates

would have been relatively scarce but parasitic worms dominant. Progress has its price. Malnutrition and increasing population densities prepared the ground for susceptibility to infections diseases. So did the clearing of forests. An important sub-story of early origin is that malaria is not an infectious disease but the microscopic parasite spread by the mosquito is. Land cleared of forests to make villages, towns, and cities could not absorb rain water, and in the warm furrows and water holes that resulted, mosquitoes started to breed. Malaria has remained a major scourge to this day, killing millions, and at the time of writing malaria is still resistant to modern science. Nevertheless, malaria has not, in general, been as devastating as the pathogens that began to emerge from a new source.

THE ORIGINS OF INFECTIOUS DISEASE

What was the new prolific source of infectious disease? It is from no constant dangerous contact with animals, nor from the dangers of fang and claw. It is, as Edward Jenner (1749–1823) the father of vaccination had it more or less right: "The deviation of man from the state in which he was originally placed by nature seems to have proved to him a prolific source of diseases. From the love of splendor, from the indulgence of luxury, and from his fondness for amusement he has familiarized himself with a great number of animals, which may not have originally been intended as his associates. The wolf, disarmed of ferocity, is now pillowed in the lady's lap. The cat, the little tiger of our island, whose natural home is the forest, is equally domesticated and caressed. The cow, the hog, the sheep, and the horse, are all, for a variety of purposes, brought under his care and dominion" (Edward Jenner, *An Inquiry into the Causes and Effects of the Variolae Vaccinae, Known by the Name of the Cow-Pox,* 1798).

With the emergence of the early settled cultures, the great infectious diseases of the human race arose, starting as animal pathogens (hence *zoonotic disease*, meaning disease of animal origin). They transferred to humans via the new human proximity to domestic animals: cows with their very similar cowpox must have given rise to smallpox, horses may have given us the common cold, and dogs perhaps gave us measles, and so on. In the more ancient emergent diseases, the animal source may be lost lest a scientist hits on it by chance, and in some cases the source may be extinct. Scientists are better at tracking the origins of the more recent troublesome diseases: pigs and water birds gave us influenza, chickens and birds can directly give us avian flu (which is of concern because it does not require the pig as intermediate host), the civet and others give rise to SARS, sheep and cattle give us the prion diseases, primates gave rise to HIV, the deer (via the tick vector) gave us Lyme disease, and the rodents give us Ebola, The list runs on for some 50 or more examples. As humans began to live increasingly in wooden and thatch huts, the rodents increased the load and variety of a further long-standing itchy curse to the human race— fleas—along with the diseases they can carry.

The disease-jump process from animal to human is called *escape from restriction*, and it happens all the time (and between animals too). In the UK foot-and-mouth disease epidemic, a human was infected. In 1988, a person became ill with swine influenza virus (swine flu) and died after visiting the display area of the pig barn at a US county fair. Three healthcare personnel treating the patient also developed flu-like illness with laboratory evidence of swine influenza virus infection.

The zoonotic disease or zoonoses is thus the rule not the exception. Mumps and rubella too likely came from animals. A list of others of current concern is long, and includes anthrax, avian influenza (bird flu), Bolivian hemorrhagic fever, brucellosis, borrelia (Lyme disease and others), Borna virus infection, bovine tubercolosis, campylobacteriosis, Chagas disease, Creutzfeldt-Jakob disease (vCJD) a transmissible spongiform encephalopathy (TSE) from bovine spongiform encephalopathy (BSE) or "mad cow disease," Crimean-Congo hemorrhagic fever, cryptosporidiosis, cutaneous larva migrans, Dengue fever, Ebola, echinococcosis, Glanders, hantavirus, hendra virus, henipavirus, Korean hemorrhagic fever, Lábrea fever, Lassa fever, Leishmaniasis, leptospirosis, listeriosis, lymphocytic choriomeningitis virus, malaria, Marburg virus infection, monkey B virus, Nipah virus, ocular larva migrans, ornithosis (psittacosis), orf (animal disease), Oropouche fever, plague, Q-fever, psittacosis called "parrot fever," rabies, Rift Valley fever, ringworms (Tinea canis, mainly), salmonellosis, SARS, Sodoku, toxoplasmosis, trichinosis, tularemia called "rabbit fever," typhus and other rickettsial diseases, Venezuelan hemorrhagic fever, visceral larva migrans, and Yellow fever.

In addition, at an early stage, as pigs and other animals began to be kept and work began bare foot in tilled fields and paddy-fields, the parasite burden of humans began to rise, ascaris, helminthes, hookworm and filarial worm, the bilharzia fluke (schistosoma[1]), and so on. In modern industrial society there is a tendency to forget these kinds of "conquered" parasitic diseases in comparison to the continued threat of (mainly) bacteria and viruses. The parts of our immune system dealing with parasitic worms, and the like, would be dormant in industrial society today were it not for its (accidental and unfortunate) involvement in causing allergies (because the external sugar and protein surfaces of spores resemble the coats of parasitic worms). However, they must once have represented a major drain on health of most of humanity, as they do in parts of the third world today. For large visible parasites, fortunately, a kind of basic surgery was possible. For example, the rotation in the hands of the early medicine man (or woman) of sticks, so as to draw parasitic worms from surface blood vessels, is the basis of the "wand and worm" logo of Asclepios (or Asklepios) described below and of most Western physicians ever since.

Infectious diseases became an important part of the medical record of humans in a general sense. But is it fair to consider them as relevant to the DNA record within us? Our DNA is our natural digital storage medium transforming human prehistory into a written history of sorts, and an unambiguous record of inheritable disease. But is there an analogous record of infectious disease? Can viruses, for example, all of which are by definition nothing much more than a nucleic acid delivery package (except when replicating in a host), leave a direct DNA footprint that becomes a part of our genomics? The idea is not so silly. One argument in favor is that it is known to be common that microorganisms can exchange DNA via viruses. Another is that viruses must have come *from* the so-called "junk DNA" of complex organisms like us, so doing the reverse may not be so hard. Some of the "junk DNA" seems to be a seething ferment of nucleic acids being copied in and out. Recent research reveals that we are bathed (in air, sea, and on land) in a much higher dose and vaster range of viruses than previously thought, representing "DNA or RNA packages" that might provide a means of accelerating evolu-

---

[1] The schistosomes are unusual trematodes in that they are dioecious, meaning the sexes are separate. They reside in the blood vessels of the definitive host, and there are no second intermediate hosts in their life cycles. There are a number of species of schistosomes that can infect humans, but most human infections are caused by one of the three following species: *Schistosoma mansoni*, *S. haematobium*, and *S. japonicum*. Schistosomiasis is distributed throughout almost all of Africa, parts of Southeast Asia, parts of northwest South America, and some islands in the Caribbean Sea. It is estimated that approximately 200 million people are infected with schistosomes, resulting in 1 million deaths each year.

tion by carrying genes between organisms. This also could leave a footprint in our DNA. Recent research has also rocked the idea that most viruses have very little capacity for carrying extra DNA "payload" as a kind of transportation service. True, many viruses are very small packages, many with just the minimum of four genes required for viruses to exist (as exemplified by the MS2 and Qβ viruses). But there are viruses that do have enough capacity to carry extra DNA. For example, there are the enormous *mimiviruses*, bigger than some bacteria, carrying 911 protein-coding genes and with at least some 10% "junk DNA," which implies very significant extra DNA transporting capacity.

But whereas there *is* evidence of gene exchanges between complex organisms by such means on the long-term evolutionary scale, the last few 50,000 years or so interests us here. The tiny probabilities of the factors required to be just right for exchanging DNA by virus infection tend only to crop up over millions of years. The truth is that a virus outside a host cell is dead, and therefore cannot mutate to infect human beings for the first time without an interplay involving living host organisms. Even less likely than the interplay happening is that it could carry genes that have some chance to be incorporated as radically new genes into the host. There must be a path of species as stepping stones, as when the influenza viruses jumped from bird to pig, and to human. And note also that while viruses like influenza are incredibly dangerous because they are constantly changing their genetic material (actually RNA in the flu case), they are basically still *influenza genes* or parts of such as raised and mutated in an animal or human host, and not usually a radical exchange or extension with genes from non-influenza sources. In this game of probabilities there are always exceptions, but they are not common. This is even so for retroviruses, a type of virus that would seem to have the dice loaded in its favor as far as leaving a direct footprint DNA is concerned. Retroviruses like HIV (human immunodeficiency virus), which can lead to a condition in humans in which the immune system begins to fail and to life-threatening opportunistic infections, insert genes into our DNA thereby have some small chance, theoretically, to breach the laws of Darwinism. But passing on of HIV is not generally by inheritance via the sex cells, it is merely by transmission during pregnancy.

The mark left on our DNA record must usually be by indirect means. For that indeed to happen, the effect can be a strong one. Notably a group of some six genes called the HLA (human leukocyte antigen) genes, a kind of molecular medical insurance, is fundamentally concerned with response and resistance to infection. HLA genes reside on chromosome 6 and encode cell-surface antigen-presenting proteins, among others. These genes seem to change more rapidly and be more diverse than most other genes, giving a variety of different types of "protective cover." It is thought that HLA genes guarantee at least a small fraction of the population to survive an attack by a pathogen. Clearly, those humans who die out and do not pass on their HLA genes are those for whom the response was inappropriate or inadequate. Conversely, the near-absence of A and B blood groups in American Indians has been proposed to be due to an association with negative effect on the chances of survival to syphilis spread by the conquistadors. Hence HLA genes are very valuable for tracking the recent evolution and journey of humankind.

As civilization and knowledge advanced still more, so did disease. Some 5,000 years ago the great mega-city empires of Mesopotamia, Egypt, the Indus Valley, and the Yellow River began to arise, and in some intensely populated areas problems of sanitation posed the first issues of public health, but more important, these cities were supported by huge livestock, which in the case of cattle herds gave us diseases like smallpox.

VILLAGE AND THEN CITY LIFE GAVE RISE TO MODERN MEDICINE

Living together with animals is not all bad news. Agriculture and then city life drove the development of science and computation. The early human recognized the importance rhythm of the stars and seasons in relation to agriculture and disease (and also the epidemics and recycling of those infections of zoonotic origin!). Complex stone tokens in the forms of spheres, cones, pyramids, and disks were once thought, when first found, to be of magical significance. However, in the 1970s it was realized that they formed part of a sophisticated computation system, with the tokens probably used in the trading of livestock, food, and valuable herbs. Also, complex use of the hands and fingers would allow amazingly rapid calculation in trade and barter. Other calculations, like those of the much later Mayans in mezzo-America, were probably used judiciously to wage wars, and to predict epidemics. Medical science progressed too. Increasing sophistication in considered responses to pathogens would be complemented soon by observations not only of inherited characteristics like hair color but also of physical disorders that ran in families. That is, there was increasing awareness (but not understanding) of genetic disease.

In the earliest large and relatively settled groups there arose the tribal shaman, a combination of healer, sorcerer, teacher, and priest combined, allowing specialization of skills and passing-down of skills that enhanced the shaman's power and reputation. In the giant city-states of Mesopotamia, Egypt, and probably elsewhere too, the shamans began to subspecialize. They formed into typically three kinds of group, into healers, priests, and sorcerers or seers. In Mesopotamia these were the *asu*, *ashipu*, and *baru*, in Egypt the physicians were the *swunu*. These two healer types began to subspecialize: Iri was the Pharaoh's enema expert, Peseshet the head female physician. Without doubt the greatest *swunu* was Imhotep, chief vizier to the Pharaoh Zozer (circa 5,000 years ago) and a great all-rounder outside of medicine whose achievements included being architect of the pyramids. Imhotep's wisdom was among the first such written down in detail, and his postcontemporaries continued the growing tradition of deifying great thinkers.

In ancient Greece there arose two figures of comparable stature, who were almost certainly mere mortals who became immortalized as gods. The first was Apollo, later god of healing. The second was *Asclepios* (mentioned above, and actually spelled more variously as Esklapios, Esclapios, Askleopios, etc., or Aesculapius in Latin), although Homer shows him to be more of an early tribal shaman. More strictly it should be said that he was made a patron saint, and dubbed "a son of Apollo" and only because the appropriate god-spot was already taken. He is depicted with a staff and a snake twined round, undoubtedly a depiction of the means of removing parasitic worms from surface blood vessels mentioned above. This logo is the unchallenged origin of the modern caduceus sign: two snakes entwining a winged wand. He was also occasionally depicted with two daughters, *Hygeia* health, and *Panacea* (cure-all). His supposed sons the *Asclepiads* were at very least his intellectual off-spring: they became the first Greek physicians.

THE WESTERN WORLD AND THE ANCIENT GREEK HERITAGE IN PERSPECTIVE

We will continue our story of Greece after we loop out quickly to another example, that of oriental civilization. Civilization indeed is not synonymous with what the Greeks gave us, however important that contribution is. The term *civilization* basically refers to a level of development at which people live together peacefully in communities. No less noble civilizations have arisen in Mesopotamia and Egypt in the Middle East, in the Indus Valley region of modern Pakistan, in the Huang He (Yellow River) valley of China, and later in Central America, as well as the early Aegean basin civilization and notably that beginning on the island of Crete in the Aegean Sea. Probably all these civilizations, certainly China, developed complex systems of medicine that are inherently rational, even if the available facts were sparse and there was, from modern perspective, much erroneous extrapolation.

Rightly or wrongly, Western civilization as embodied in both Europe and America has had a powerful influence on the modern world by both imperialism and commerce. Ancient Greece is considered the birthplace of modern Western civilization and hence of much of a way of thinking that dominates the world today. "The search for truth is in one way hard and in another way easy, for it is evident that no one can master it fully or miss it completely. But each adds a little to our knowledge of nature, and from all the facts assembled there arises a certain grandeur" said Aristotle. Who originally penned this particular quotation popular with modern business people and attributed it reliably to Aristotle is not clear, but it appears in T. Goodman's *The Forbes Book of Business Quotations: 14,266 Thoughts on the Business of Life* (Black Dog & Leventhal Publishers, 2005) and *The Wiley Book of Business Quotations* (Wiley, 2000). It is also the civilization of Hippocrates (see next chapter). It is the culture that shaped his thoughts, and is therefore arguably the birthplace of modern medicine. Fundamental to ancient Greek and modern thought, as discussed in the next section, is a way of modeling the world.

There is some (apocryphal?) legendary reluctance of the Greek philosophers to actually lift up an urn to see what is under it, but instead to show a preference for heated intellectual debate over the matter. Yet, when change was forced on them, and they were faced with drought, famine, pestilence, and war, they had a remarkable ability to adapt and refine their models to a level in which they often had predictive and corrective power. As well as by the inventions of Archimedes (e.g., the "Archimedes screw" for raising water for irrigation) and others, their adaptive proclivity is well illustrated by their contributions to scientific medicine, and it is what distinguishes Greek from Chinese science. It may be that in ancient Greece the ability to adapt became pretty much of a sport anyway. Greek philosophers delighted in rhetoric and philosophical debate at the Olympic Games. While the Greek intellectuals did not always get it right the first time, in such a visible contest of intellectual abilities, it pays to constantly review that you are right.

In order to address the large picture, including the contributions from other genetics and other cultures, the medical contributions of China, India, and the Arab world will be discussed in various contexts later. But despite their differences that resulted in different medical thinking to be discussed below, their genes and memes have a degree of similarity, and ancient Greece, convenient for us as the land of Hippocrates, is not a bad ambassador as our first example for most of the world. The similarity occurs because of the relatively short time for the common descent from a tiny fraction of the African population. But if there is one place that is outstanding in showing our greatest diversity, it is Africa. Africa occupies a special position that cannot be neglected, even apart from the fact that it gave rise to all humankind in the first place. Over the past 200,000 years Africans have their own internal prehistoric civilizations and mass migrations, the Bantu, forest dweller and bushman cultures migrations being the major migration examples. In fact Africans and their more recent descendants from the slave trades have a larger variation because their heritage goes back to common ancestors some 200,000 years ago. This makes their genetics an important medical issue and, in view of the more extensive variation, an even more challenging one. Not least, the few thousand who were involved in the new Stone Age out-of-Africa event is a number that is negligible compared with the millions exported in the slave trades, and their more recent genetic impact in the world. A special effort is being made to ensure that all Africans, not just the minor tribe or two of a thousand or so that came out of Africa 50,000 to 60,000 years ago and gave rise to the rest of us, are given due attention as to the medical implications.

THE GREEK GATE

While the non-African descendants of the new Stone Age exodus are a remark-ably large slice of the population of the world, in the story of that slice, Greece and its neighbors play a special role in our thinking about the impact of the prehistoric world on modern molecular medicine. The geographical regions of Greece, Turkey, and India had an early beginning, with at least some genetic roots perhaps going back 35,000 years, and at latest its beginning could be reasonably considered as around the time of the transition of the Stone Age hunters to farmers. Incredibly we have quite a bit of insight even into the prehistoric period from molecular studies of DNA.

The answer is that sooner or later part of the diaspora of the new Stone Age peoples had to pass through the vicinity of modern Greece and Turkey, through the *Greek Gate* so called because of the impact much of the popula-tion had on the modern world. Only recently has the importance of migrations through India and to Europe via Northern Europe become clearer, but the Greeks stand large in modern Western perception as not just contributing their genomics but giving rise to three pillars of Western culture, *Western* philoso-phy, *Western* science and mathematics, and *Western* medicine, in a kind of unified package. The fourth pillar, due to the Romans, is *Western* bureaucracy. We italicize Western here throughout because India and the Orient had all these in great measure too, but with a different flavor that still endures today under the Western rubric of alternative medicine.

Since the Mediterranean origins of European genomics were the most prominent in our thinking before the more recent genomics studies, the extent to which that view still survives should be mentioned. There seems (at the time of writing) to be a slight discrepancy between studies of the DNA in our Y chromosomes (again, the male chromosome, inherited from our father line) and DNA in a special chromosome in the mitochondria of our cells (as noted earlier, inherited from our mother line), as to whether the original indigenous peoples of Greece and some of the genes they left today came up in the early phase of the out-of-Africa diaspora, or down via India and Northern Europe at a slightly later phase. These patterns of course are evident in the descen-dants of the male and female lines that survived, but they need not concur with each other.

The mitochondrial DNA, unlike the DNA in the nucleus of our cells on the main chromosomes, is a structure in the cell (i.e., a cellular *organelle*) outside the nucleus. The mitochondrion's multiple copies (convenient for extraction and analysis) were derived from a guest ancestral microbe entering our cells long before organisms became multicellular. It is responsible for our energy metabolism, and why we breathe oxygen. Unusual by representing genetics outside the main chromosomes of the cell nucleus, it said to carry extrachro-mosomal inheritance. What makes it a purely maternal thing in terms of passing down this information is the nature of fertilization. Since most of the mitochondria are in the tail of the sperm, which is discarded, and since any that do get into the egg appear to be selectively destroyed, we cannot inherit our father's mitochondrial DNA. It is a small genome and easily sequenced from a blood sample in a couple of hours, serving as a very useful standard tag to show the "genome family of a patient" as much as is relevant to understanding one's genome and providing the best health care. Y chromosomes (again, derived only from the father) may have similar benefits. But correlations with mitochondrial DNA early showed what language and even the dialect an ancestors spoke. As mentioned above, this is not because there are different genes for different languages but because the family tree of humanity can be deduced in broad terms from the different degrees of similarity between one population's mitochondrial DNA and another's. Such a tree can be compared with the tree drawn for the relationship between languages, and it is a darned good fit.

So how do we fulfill our promise of the plotting the story of human descent down to Hippocrates? Not so easily! Roughly speaking, in comparing human prehistory based on the Y chromosome and on the mitochondrial chromosome, the issue is one of whether the human race had to pass through the eastern Mediterranean, and the so-called Greek gate, or, by taking advantage of the lower sea levels at the time, took a Eurasian coastal route, spinning off other peoples on the march (and occasional boat trip) to Australia. Professor Cavelli-Sforza's student, Spence-Wells, who has performed the Y-chromosome-based studies, is less concerned by these differences. Males and females spread out in the same directions, it is just that in some cases the sampling tends to pick up one or the other.

In any event we do know that major fluxes of immigration came into Greece from the north between 1900 and 1600 BC, and that these peoples had important effects, genetic and cultural, on the Mediterranean region. These new immigrants entered the peninsula from the north, one small group after another. That is, at that relatively late time the Greeks or Hellenes, as these peoples called themselves, were not indigenous to the Aegean basin and what we now think of as the country of Greece. In fact scholars surmised this even before genomic studies: the Greek language demonstrated to prehistorians that these Hellenes (and incidentally the Hittites too) were a branch of the Indo-European-speaking peoples. They thus came down to Greece from the grasslands east of the Caspian Sea, nomadic tribes driving their flocks and herds before them. There is no conflict with the genomic record. *Au contraire*, we now know that language is intimately linked to the genomic history, to the extent of even being of value to analyzing the relationship between linguistics and genetics.

Moreover this more recent Hellenic immigration did *not* mean that the earlier peoples of the Aegean failed to leave their cultural and, importantly, their genetic heritage. The land that the Hellenic tribes invaded the Aegean Basin was the site of a remarkably well-developed civilization, with cities and palaces, gold and bronze, and pottery and paintings. The Greek invaders were still in the barbarian stage. They plundered and destroyed the Aegean cities, but gradually, as they settled and intermarried with the people they conquered, they absorbed some of the Aegean culture.

The Aegean-Hellenic transition period was followed by the great civilizations of the Minoan and Mycenaean kings, but sometime after 1450 BC the civilization of Crete was overcome by the Mycenaean[2] from mainland Greece. The time of Greek expansion from 1450 to 1100 BC was an era of great prosperity in Greece.

Also, as mentioned above, an important cult, that of Asclepios/Asklepios (well, we like the latter) flourished around 1200 BC. We recall that Asklepios appears to have been a real historical figure, described as a tribal wound healer by Homer. Asklepios may thus have been a kind of shaman, and the cult based on him was essentially magical, though there would have been much home wisdom and doubtless also some lore that diffused in from Mesopotamian and Egyptian medicine. This practice would have certainly included some use of herbs as well as spells: "Chiron was learned in the use of herbs and gentle incantations and cooling potions. But his pupil surpassed him. He was able to give aid in all manner of maladies. Whoever came to him suffering, whether from wounded limbs or bodies wasting away with disease, even those who were sick unto death, he delivered them from torment" (Edith Hamilton, "The Myth of Asklepios," in her *Mythology*, 11th ed. (Back Bay Books, 1998)).

It was from this society that the ancient Greeks emerged to conquer Troy in about 1186 BC, thereby also assuring their colonization of the coast of Asia Minor. Tablets found at Knossos, the oldest known Indo-European writings, reveal extensive undertakings in agriculture, trade, and war (as well as worship of the gods of Mount Olympus).

In short, we may be able to assign to the Greeks not only the wellsprings of Western civilization but, by their early military and marine supremacy, much of the world's genetic heritage. Moreover, particularly by conquest, ancient Greeks seem to have tended to export their genes rather than import them. This relatively pristine record of post–new Stone Age diaspora DNA is at least of direct consequence to modern Europeans.

The story of the Greek heritage is not without its glitches, however. There was, in particular, a major dark age comparable with that in Europe. Although the history discussed above spanned a period when still further technologies (and systems of thought) had been rapidly evolving, much competition between groups led to a dark age starting when Greece was invaded by the Dorian in approximately 1100 BC. This was a time period characterized by many such invasions and wars, and possibly loss of writing. A mere generation or so after the triumph of Greece in the war against Troy, it marks the end of the phase of Greek civilization called the Mycenaean civilization. It was not confined to

[2] When the Minoan civilization ended, the Mycenaean Greeks of the mainland dominated the Aegean as the Minoans had done before them. Like the Minoans, they engaged in overseas trade, especially in obtaining metals, such as copper and tin to make bronze. They probably also resorted to piracy and coastal raids. Distinctive Mycenaean pottery has been found over most of the eastern Mediterranean region and also to the west of Greece.

Greece: there was a general collapse of civilization in the eastern Mediterranean world during this period. The Hittite civilization collapsed; cities from Troy to Gaza were flattened. It is a classic example of how memes, those cultural ideas and technical skills conveyed by example, get lost, if nobody cares to use, demonstrate, and share them: artifacts become much cruder (for example, Greek Dark Age pottery has simpler geometric designs). The population seems to have been greatly reduced, with sparser and smaller settlements, suggestive of famine and depopulation. In view of clear evidence for devastating plagues of unknown nature in the later classical periods, it is not unreasonable to conjecture that it was all ultimately due to one of the first great plagues of civilization, pandemic to at least the Mediterranean world. (This unproven plague is not what is referred to in the title of the next section. The plague of our title is a well-authenticated horror yet to come in 430 BCE). The Dark Age of the Greek region otherwise tempts comparison with the mysterious collapse of the recent Mayan civilization of Mesoamerica, a sudden collapse from city state to jungle huts and isolationism between small groups. It was previously thought that contact was similarly lost between Greece and the outside world. However, artifacts from excavations on Euboea (an island to the east of mainland Greece) suggest that there were significant cultural and trade links with the east, at least with the area that we now call Turkey but probably further East too, possibly reflecting an increased embracing by the Greeks of ancient trade routes. It seems almost as if in this time there was a putting to one side, for a period, of Greek cultural arrogance, and a refocus on the East as the source for the essence and trappings of civilization. If so, this may have done significant good, allowing introduction of new memes (and perhaps even new herbs). It may have had profound effect on medical practice and thought.

FROM THE ANCIENT GREEK RENAISSANCE TO HIPPOCRATES, VIA A GENETIC DISORDER AND A PLAGUE

By around 700 to 800 BC Greece had survived its dark age and undergone its Renaissance. It was developing its modern writing system and seeking to record history. Thus much of Western history arguably began at this point.

In the period from 500 to 336 BC Greece was divided into small city-states, that is, a unit consisting of a city and its surrounding countryside. Relative peace, stable agriculture and the beat of the seasons, with alternating periods of arduous labor and relative rest, gave food for thought.

In the fifth to sixth centuries BC between these two periods, the seeds for that food for thought were generated. The *Axial Age* (700–200 BC) is defined by a burst of fresh thinking and intellectual pursuits that occurred worldwide in other civilized nations (in China, India, Iran, Near East). Anaximander (c. 610–546 BC) was a contemporary and possibly a co-student of Pythagoras whose birth and death dates are somewhat vague. Predating Socrates (469–399 BC), who gets much of the Medieval and modern press as a founder of Western intellectual thought, Anaximander is the better to be seen as *the* original true scientist of Western civilization. He was the first of the Greeks to think in terms of scientific origins and processes governed by laws and mechanisms (in fields ranging from astronomy to biology), to do experiments, *and* to put down his thoughts and findings in writing. Sadly, all but fragments are lost. He is credited with the first to think about biological evolution, that life was formed from sea and mud, and that humans are descendants of fish. His strangest concept, that originally humans grew to maturity in the mouth of a fish, came from a telling intellectual dilemma. How could mankind have evolved with its children so vulnerable and unprotected in the dangerous and chaotic world prior to Greek civilization? He did not extend his ideas to an answer in terms of social evolution; the world would have to wait many years for Occam's razor, the principle attributed to the fourteenth-century English logician and Franciscan friar, William of Ockham, that the simplest explanation is the most likely to be correct!

And so, in the fifth to sixth centuries BC, the Greeks pioneered a new kind of technology, namely theoretical techniques for explaining phenomena in the natural world by some understanding of mechanical processes. They could summon analogies that enabled them to view the world with an inner eye, and thereby to model it. For example, the ancient Greeks had notions of energy of atoms and of heat as motion of atoms, a model that helped them think about the world. In speaking about arrangements of atoms and what they did, they came awfully close to the concept of molecules. "Atom" comes from the Greek word for indivisible, hence that there are fundamental particles that are no longer reducible to any smaller conceptual model. The power of this general period in regard to Greek thought, and the words and durability of the language and the new Greek writing script, were such that a Greek philosopher transported from it by a time machine could probably pick up a modern Greek newspaper, and with only a little help make some sense of it. This is even in regard to news about modern scientific topics. For example, "splitting the atom" would at least convey that something very difficult and remarkable is going on.

As a biomedical example, the writings from the ancient Greeks or their subsequent documenters make it clear that they had some notion of genetics and the microscopic basis for our individuality, the model in this case being the passing on of some kind of seed, which made us tend to resemble our parents. The ancient Egyptians had earlier had recognized a relation between testes, phallus, semen, and pregnancy. The details in fact seem to have been hotly debated by different schools of Greek philosophers. Aristotle appears to have had a correct awareness that seeds of the mother and father were mixed at conception, whereas Aeschylus favored the then politically important view that the father produced the seed and the mother was a mere carrier. Hippocrates (discussed below) had yet a slightly different view.

By coincidence, and not so surprising, the earliest well-detailed case, that of a constitution *with a different individual responses to food and drugs*, concerned the arch-exponent of the new logical model of the world. Pythagoras modeled the world in terms of lines, circles, triangles, and so on. He also appears to have had favism, a genetic condition that rendered him allergic to fava beans (also known as koukia, broad bean, or Vicia Fab. The fava beans were a major source of beans in Europe before the discovery of the American continent. In roughly 20% of the people with this inherited disorder, eating fresh fava beans triggers a severe hemolytic anemia. They exhibit symptoms of jaundice and anemia and excrete blood in their urine. Even today, death follows in days for almost 10% of those who suffer this reaction. At the very least Pythagoras's problem is the first well-recorded case of *favism* or *fauvism*, a hemolytic anemia disorder that affects some 100 million persons worldwide. Consuming red wine, blueberries, all legumes, soya products, quinine, camphor, and certain barks, and these days oxidative drugs such as aspirin, vitamin C supplements, antimalarials (quinacrine), and some sulfonamides (e.g., sulfanilamide), can lead to severe anemia, headache, dizziness, diarrhea, nausea, vomiting, stomach pain, fever, and death. Since some of these products occurred in plants known to the ancients, there may already have been the possibility of the ancients knowing of a differential reaction of a patient to a standard medicine. As well as favism, the Greeks were probably aware of two other genetic disorders of sickle cell anemia and thalassemia. But before returning to these later (because they are well-understood examples even down to the molecular level), it is appropriate to consider whether there is other evidence of ancient awareness of the effects of foods and drugs, and ask whether there was some kind of recorded information playing at least an informative role like a kind of ancient food and drug administration. What written records of herbs and foodstuffs and their possible differential effect, other than fava beans, survive from the Mediterranean cultures at that time?

Sadly, the earliest known written Greek herbal by Diocles of Carystus dates back merely to the third century BC, and did not survive well. A few fragments from an illustrated herbal of one Krateuas have survived from the first century BC and suggest herbs common to Greeks and Egyptians. A familiar example is wormwood, actually a class of substance from a number of different plant sources, and similar quinine-like substances (quinine is among other things a reasonable anti-malarial, although the quinine often spoken about today was first brought to Europe by the Jesuits after being originally discovered by the Quechua Indians in Peru). This suggests that one can gain some appreciation of Greek understanding by examining surviving Egyptian texts; these are much more extensive and go back much further in time. Ancient Egypt was, after all, "just across the Mediterranean" from Greece and represented one of the worlds' most long-lived and important cultures, with agricultural foundations starting around 5000 BC and with a continuous 6000-year record. The Greeks must often have felt like "new boys on the block" and a very provincial, uptown block at that (in the New York City uptown/downtown sense). They may not have like Egyptian religion and philosophy, but they must be looking to the Egyptians, as the ultimate establishment, for much scientific and medical input. From 4000 to 3000 BC people in the Nile valley had already established highly advanced farming technology. Egyptian civilization as we know its familiar and unique style began with hieroglyphs around 3200 BC and the unification of Upper and Lower Egypt around 3100 BC. Apart from changes in mere details of that style in the three divisions of Egyptian history known as "Kingdoms," it endured almost unchanged up to and even through the invasions by the Assyrians in 671 BC, and started to transform in a more fundamental way, interestingly enough, only with the invasions of the Greeks around 320 BC.

One important Egyptian document measures one foot by sixty-six feet. It is probably the earliest *complete* book known of any kind, an update on Egyptian medicine written about 1550 BC but with material dating back to 3700 BC, copied from much earlier papyri, particularly from about 3400 BC. It was looted from a tomb of the XVIII dynasty in 1862, and then acquired by a German Professor, George Ebers, for the (then) fabulous sum of $8,000, and is hence called the "George Ebers papyrus." It contains disease indications and recipes for approximately 700 herbs. Many of these would have been known to the Greeks, but in any event it is probably indicative of the number of herbs know to an ancient civilization. The number in surviving ancient Chinese herbals combined runs into thousands, of which about 500 are still in use today worldwide. Compare this with modern Western medicine: at first glance it seems very different. There have been roughly 8,000 to 9,000 new drug launches a year averaged since 1980, and with no fewer than 150,000 preparations now in use, of which 90% did not exist 25 years ago, and 75% did not exist ten years ago. Much of this however is merely different molecular tweaking, different "packaging," and combinations of the same molecules. Similarly the George Ebus Papyrus and traditional Chinese medicine refers to different methods of extraction and preparation, and different mixes of herbs. There are in fact only about 300 FDA-approved distinct drug molecules in reasonably common use, and maybe 400 more much less so. At the rarest end of the spectrum, orphan diseases exist, that is, rare or pharmaceutically less profitable diseases affecting (by US definition of orphan disease) less than 200,000 of the US population, or of dubious merit for terminal diseases. According to Tan Nguyen speaking at the FDA at the eighth European Platform for Patients' Organisations, Science and Industry workshop in Copenhagen 2007 (http://www.orpha.net/actor/EuropaNews/2007/071030.html), for 200 applications for 2007, approximately 70% are granted; in the United States, an average of 14 ODs (i.e., orphan drugs, drugs treating orphan diseases) are authorized each year. Of these in the US 70% are chemical products, versus 30% biologics, and so effectively more directly of "herbal" origin; the fraction of those of herb origin is much higher in Europe. The bottom line is that things are not so fundamentally different today in terms of the number and perhaps variety of offerings.

With such commonness in the numbers that matter, then one might expect a similar spectrum of diseases treated and similar diversity of patient responses over several civilizations. Ancient records, therefore, could *in principle* not only provide evidence as to efficacy of drugs for different patients, but perhaps even give fresh information about responses to drug molecules in use today, or alternatively help discover new drugs. There are two caveats of particular importance.

First, this assumes at least a comparable or scalable level of efficacy of *some* of the herbs in ancient medical use, compared with drugs today, and that it is not all due to the famous placebo effect, that patients get better just because they believe they are being treated. This effect may be an in-built mechanism instructing the body to self-repair and reject disease when there is a sense of being cared for. There is even a genetic component that would confuse any attempt of pharmacogenomic analysis regarding action ancient herbs. Tomas Furmark and colleagues in the *Journal of Neuroscience* (2008: 2534–2538) have discovered that the ability to do this is likely determined genetically in 30% of the population. Note that according to the above source on orphan drugs, many rejections by the FDA are on grounds of lack of scientific rationale, but that a 2004 study in the *British Medical Journal* of physicians in Israel found that 60% deliberately used placebos in their medical practice, most commonly to "fend off" requests for unjustified medications or to calm a patient. But many natural products do work in the normal pharmaceutical sense. Also, it is likely that many classes (if not exactly equivalent) of biological molecules appear to have been in the Greek and Egyptian herb armory and survive in use today, albeit some times with chemical modifications. There is the ubiquitous aspirin from willow bark. Quinine (e.g., from the bark of the cinchona tree), has been a fairly effective anti-malarial. It is also used to treat nocturnal leg cramps and arthritis, and there have been attempts (with slight success) to treat prion diseases from beef infected with bovine spongiform encephalopathy (BSE). Artemisinin is a compound derived from the sweet wormwood plant and has been used for centuries in traditional Chinese medicine to treat fever. As artemether and combined in tablet with lumefantrine it becomes Novartis' highly effective antimalarial Coartem. "Absinthe wormwood" or grand wormwood has been claimed to remedy indigestion and gastric pain, and acts as an antiseptic and a febrifuge. Traditionally also, the herb is used to make a tea for helping pregnant women during pain of labor, and a dried encapsulated form of the plant has been extensively used as an anthelmintic. Extracts from the bark and leaves of witch-hazel are used for treating bruises and insect bites. It is the active ingredient in many hemorrhoid medications, and a traditional treatment for postpartum tearing of the perineum. There is also penicillin from moulds tweaked chemically to make it stable to stomach acid, glychorrhizic acid from licorice root used to treat inflammation and stomach ulcers, and chemically tweaked to become carbenoxolone, reducing risk of birth defects and other unfavorable reactions.

Second, it assumes that we can read these ancient documents properly. The problem with such sources as ancient Greek fragments and Egyptian papyri is that even when one can identify the plant, it is in many cases very difficult to translate what the disease was, and what the benefits and risks were, let alone how these varied from patient to patient. The George Ebers papyrus is not only arguably the best encyclopedic source from that part of the world at that time, but equally notoriously, it is terribly difficult to translate. This is partly a technology problem that astronomers and NASA have to be mindful of when planning how to communicate with alien civilizations. It is not much help to inform the reader that W causes X that usually benefits from Y and that results in Z if, say, W, X, and Z are taken for granted and not defined, even if Y is well defined, say in the present relevant case, as a clearly described species of herb. Such a difficulty is a common feature of historical medical documents, and even of translating fairly recent, say, English Victorian, medical documents concerning causes of death. That is, even when they are otherwise in very readable English. This is a pursuit of considerable importance because we can link causes and responses to the genealogical and hence genetic record. So, we can quote several examples of difficulties that must be greater still in translation of ancient Greek and Egyptian. *Senile decay* on a Victorian death certificate was a catch-all that not only covered many diseases of the elderly, but actually translates better as "no suspicious causes," as perhaps did *puerperal fever* in the case of maternal fatalities from childbirth. What did a death certificate mean describing the death of one Donald Tollett as *due to a stythe*? The word "stythe" was used for the appearance of asphyxiation that could be a medical condition such as severe allergic reaction, but that more often meant as due to substances called *choke damp* and *blackdamp* in coal mines. These words require further Internet research to identify the nature of this material as carbon dioxide or methane, but phrases "killed by a stythe" could mean that the methane exploded, or even that oxygen was sucked out of a mine by a fire or meteorological change, none of which are the same thing, not least from a public and industrial health perspective. And while some common disease terms like *apoplexy* survive till very reasonable time such that most people would translate it today as *stroke*, it earlier meant any sudden death including internal and in some cases even external bleeding. Similarly *inflammation* meant many things including sepsis, but most often, for certain periods and in certain areas, it meant gout. There is indeed a genetic propensity to gout as the tendency to form uric acid crystals in joints, from certain foodstuffs rich in certain nitrogenous substances, so it would be good to know when that meaning of gout is intended. But with the best will in the world by pre-twentieth-century physicians, it would not be easy to distinguish it from pseudo-gout, a condition which is due to the tendency to form phosphate crystals in joints with a risk factor dependent on different genetics and often confused with "true gout" even by physicians today. Unfortunately, diagnostic difficulties, broad catch-all terms, and shifting difference in meaning of early times obscure the written record of the diversity of human responses to diseases and therapies. Ancient texts stand in stark contrast to the rigorous medical taxonomic codes used today in, particularly, US patient billing systems.

But we can be reasonably sure that ancient recognition of different responses to herbs and foods by different patients was not confined to cases of patients having favism or not, because diversity of response is the expected norm, part of the human condition, and hence a valid scientific "null hypothesis" meaning that we are rather required to prove it is not the case, not that it is. Variance of patient response and need for personalized tailoring and re-tailoring of herbal treatments is a persistent theme of traditional Chinese medicine which survives to modern websites (e.g., http://www.ancientacu.com/whatsnew/20041022-1.htm). It is part of the human condition on chemical grounds *a priori*, because of our genetic diversity which governs the diversity of our protein molecules that interact with food and drug molecules and their metabolic products. As discussed in greater depth in the next chapter, the difference between all of us (one or two in a thousand base pairs in DNA) means that that a typical protein sequence will contain one or two amino acid residue differences. Even as recently back as our own parents three new mutations on average might have occurred in the eggs or sperm cells to a harmful effect on most probably three on average of the 30,000 or so genes in our bodies. But, favism itself is especially prevalent in the old Magna Graecia, the region ruled by the ancient Greeks. As much as 30% of the population in some areas is affected. That genetic effect would be hard to miss.

Although the prize goes to the Greeks for the first clear account of what we now see as a genetic disorder (but this is not entirely uncontested because of the accounts given by very ancient Chinese medicine; see below), in the interests of historical accuracy it must be said that Pythagoras does not seem to have been himself aware that this was a genetic condition. Aristotle said that Pythagoras denounced fava beans "either because they have the shape of testicles, or because they resemble the gates of hell, for they alone have no hinges, or again because they spoil, or because they resemble the nature of the universe, or because of oligarchy, for they are used for drawing lots" (for sources of this and quotes below see particularly *Pythagoras: His Life, Teaching, and Influence* by Christoph Riedweg and Steven Rendall (Cornell University Press, 2005)). More convincingly, Diogenes proposed that the Pythagorean school as a whole rejected favas "since they are full of wind and take part in the soul, and if one abstains from them, one's stomach will be less noisy and one's dreams will be less oppressive and calmer." In any event, Pythagoras thought that fava beans were generally a bad idea. It became a part of the spiritual movement that bears his name. Iamblichus tells of the time a group of Pythagoreans were being pursued by their enemies. They came across a field of favas in bloom. Rather than disobey the Pythagorean dictates and escape through the field, they stood ground and most were slaughtered. (When the captured were questioned about their beliefs, they refused to answer. One Spartan bit off her tongue rather than "spill the beans").

There seemed nonetheless to have been a growing awareness among the ancient Greeks that favism was one of those many things that did seem to correlate between parents and children. "Eating fava beans and gnawing on the heads of one's parents are one and the same," was one of the sayings of the Orphics. This may be presumed to be a rhetorical comment on inheritance: only in the case of Kuru (a "prion disease" among cannibals of Papua New Guinea and closely related to mad cow disease, and Kreutzfeldt-Jacob disease) might it literally be true. It was also noticed that favism is three times more common in males, but that children of affected women were likely to either die very young or be susceptible to adverse reaction to the bean in later life. Frequently cases of hemolytic disease of the newborn are associated with the disorder. Medical science has only recently understood why only women who carry the gene from both sides of the family are susceptible, but it was long known that attacks of severe anemia tended to occur among the infants of affected families who consumed the beans even when the infants were too young to eat the beans themselves (the reason given was that the poison can be passed in the mother's milk).

Only at the very end of the nineteenth century was it proved to be a genetic disorder. More recently it was found to be caused by a mutation of the gene for producing the glucose-6-phosphate dehydrogenase (G6PD) protein. The details are now known in precise chemical and three-dimensional molecular-structural terms. It is thus plausible that we know something about Pythagoras as an individual, down to at least a handful of his trillions of atoms. G6PD is, as readers with biochemistry background will know, an *enzyme*, meaning a protein with catalytic properties, and more specifically the first enzyme in the major metabolic pathway called the hexosemonophosphate shunt. This is a part of metabolism from which red blood cells derive most of their metabolic energy. Red blood cells are mainly bags of hemoglobin molecules, the red proteins responsible for carrying oxygen, and pretty well stripped down as far as metabolism is concerned, so this loss of function is serious. The function of this part of metabolism is to service other enzymes, glutathione reductase and glutathione peroxidase, that protect the red cells against damage due to oxidation. The mutant G6PD enzyme activity is present at about 15% of the normal level, so this protective mechanism is crippled, and certain drugs, in sufficient concentration, can seriously injure the erythrocyte. This is likely to have been what also troubled Pythagoras. As we noted, he was not alone. The deficiency is inherited as an X-chromosome-linked disorder with a high frequency among Black Africans. In Caucasians only the normal B type enzyme is found and the deficient type is also B (B-). In West and East Africa about 20% of males and about 4% of females (homozygous for the abnormal gene, i.e., carrying it on both paired chromosomes, being X chromosomes in this case) are affected. Heterozygous females have two populations of red cells, one deficient, and the other normal. The deficiency in Caucasian and Asian populations is more severe, with the enzyme activity being less than 1% of normal. Other rare types of G6PD biochemically different from the above may be associated with congenital nonspherocytic hemolytic diseases, and these occur sporadically in all races.

Carefully recorded observations on diseases like favism, at least within intellectual circles, were combined with more widespread unwanted opportunities to observe the effects of new epidemics. Epidemics were increasing in variety and severity with the explosive increase in population. Before the rise of agriculture, the world population was probably around a million. By the golden age of Athens in 500 BC, it had leapt to 100 million. That is quite a leap, and the population has increased 61 times since then. In 430 BC a particularly extensive and dreadful plague arose. The nature of this has not been identified today, but those afflicted presented with blistering skin, vomiting, convulsions, and often death. The plague traveled across North Africa and the Greek region, and brought to an end the ascendancy of Athens.

It wasn't the only plague of that period: one from the north was to follow a mere ten years later. It may not have been as severe as the plague discussed above that helped bring about the Greek Dark ages, if that was the cause, and it may not be as great as plagues yet to hit the human race, but one may note that the case/fatality rate was believed to be 25% (Phillip A. Makiowiack, *Post Mortem: Solving History's Great Medical Mysteries* (ACP Press, 2007)). That would have dramatic social effect. If between 15% and 35% of the US population could merely be *affected* by an influenza pandemic, the economic impact could range between, say, $71.3 and $166.5 billion. But imagine that in the crowded cities where exposure to infection is almost guaranteed, that one in every four people you know is not only sick, but dying! Such a plague could collapse a less hardy civilization. Even though it may have been more devastating in some areas than others, the legendary city of Athens was among them, giving rise to the name "the Athenian Holocaust." Its importance here is that could not have passed unknown or failed to inspire a few Greeks of that time who were planting the seeds of modern Western medicine.

INTRODUCING HIPPOCRATES

A Greek observer of this devastating plague was Hippocrates of Cos (460–377 BC). If not observation, at least awareness of the plague, combined with the new logical way of thinking, and matched by the careful keeping of written and verbal records, must have been factors that drew the great philosopher to make deductions that found modern medicine. Hippocrates matured general science and philosophy, and the earlier magical healing cult of *Asklepios*, to establish the tight ethical and scientific system that we know as modern medicine. Hippocrates was associated with the Asklepium of Cos, Cos being island off the coast of Asia Minor, near Rhodes. The Roman writer Celsus said: "Hippocrates Cous primus quidem ex omnibus memoria dignis ab studio sapientiae disciplinam hanc separavit." That means, Hippocrates first gave the physician an independent standing, separating him from the cosmological speculator, or nature philosopher (sources: see box).

A note on sources about Hippocrates and his historical reviewers: the Internet currently represents the convenient accessible compendium of such quotes (see, for example, http://publicquotes.com), but following the scholarly tradition of reporting back to published, print-on-paper sources requires research that reveals as interesting a history of publication about Hippocrates as it does about Hippocrates himself. The ultimate origin of "Hippocratic" quotes in our present text is presumed to be the Hippocratic Corpus (Latin: *Corpus Hippocraticum*), a collection of around seventy early medical works written in Ionic Greek, probably all (if not mainly) by Hippocrates' followers. In fact many reviewers and critics, such as the Roman Celus and later including the Monks of the European Dark Ages, have collected and transcribed these works and increasingly ascribed them to Hippocrates. A common more recent source for quotes of or about Hippocrates, including those by the Roman author Celus, was distributed by publishers R. Bonwick et al. in 1708. It was modestly said, by one C.J. Sprengell, to be edited by himself, but with Hippocrates and Celsus attributed as the authors. The publication is entitled (in the Baroque style of that time) "Aphorisms of Hippocrates, and the Sentences of Celsus; with Explanations and References to the Most Considerable Writers in Physick and Philosophy, Both Ancient and Modern. To Which are Added, Aphorisms Upon the small-pox, measles, and Other Distemper. ..." In considering this tradition of quoting Hippocrates as author, it might be recalled that it is not clear that Hippocrates himself actually wrote anything down. These have also been subsequently collected, by W.H.S. Jones (1868) in *Hippocrates Collected Works I* (Cambridge: Harvard University Press). There was much subsequent dispute as to what came even from the Hippocrates school of disciples (let alone Hippocrates) and what did not, so Francis Adams subsequently wrote *The Genuine Works of Hippocrates* (William Wood and Company, 1981). This follows the tradition of making Hippocrates author, plus now a new appearance by certain Dr. Emerson Crosby Kelly as author of the introduction, and then followed by Francis Adams of the original 1891 work and described as translator. The 2006 edition is unlikely to be a first edition of the new format, because Dr. Emerson Crosby Kelly was a notable medical historian who lived from 1899 to 1977 (see his obituary by Helen A. Frazer in *Bulletin of the Medical Library Assoc.* (1977) 65(4):499).

Hippocrates, as is held by tradition and later writers, based his medical practice on observations and on the study of the human body. He held the belief that illness had a physical and a rational explanation. Hippocrates held the belief that *the body must be treated as a whole and not just a series of parts,* which is the underlying concept of the recently emerging *systems biology*. He accurately described disease symptoms and was the first physician to accurately describe the symptoms of pneumonia as well as epilepsy in children. He believed in the natural healing process of rest, a good diet, fresh air, and cleanliness. He noted that there were individual differences in the severity of disease symptoms and that some individuals were better able to cope with their disease and illness than others. Hippocrates was also the first physician that held the belief that thoughts, ideas, and feelings come from the brain and not the heart as others of his time believed.

Hippocrates is generally credited with turning away from divine notions of medicine and using observation of the body as a basis for medical knowledge. Hippocrates did have a philosophical infrastructure to support all this knowledge, a metaphysical view of life. However, it was not inherently religious in tone and resembled somewhat twentieth century "systems theory," a useful scientific view of the world yet with a philosophical basis to it. He considered life to be a fundamental aspect of the dynamical nature of the universe, a great principle embodied in the balance between being and not-being, life and death. "There is one common flow, one common breathing, all things are in sympathy. The whole organism and each one of its parts are working in conjunction for the same purpose ... the great principle extends to the most extreme part, and from the most extreme part it returns to the great principle, to the one nature, being and not-being." These and other quotes below are indirectly from the Hippocratic Corpus (Latin: *Corpus Hippocraticum*)—see box. Prayers and sacrifices to the gods did not hold a central place in his theories: changes in diet, beneficial drugs, and keeping the body "in balance" were key. Chinese medicine is based on the same concept of keeping the body in balance (see the next section). To be sure, there was an associated theory of humors (blood, choler, phlegm, and black bile) not a million miles removed from those of other cultures. Although strange to our modern ears, such theories are not unscientific: there was simply inadequate data and an as-yet inadequate accumulation of scientific knowledge. It would not be until the Age of Enlightenment and the Industrial Revolution before the necessary cellular and molecular insight could be provided.

In particular, Hippocrates rejected the views of his contemporary society that considered illness to be caused by possession of evil spirits and disfavor of the gods. He remained respectful of the gods, but in a text known as the *Regimen* he is attributed to the saying "Prayer indeed is good, but while calling on the gods, a man should himself lend a hand." In another, known as the Law, there are implications of perhaps an even stronger position: "There are in fact two things, science and opinion; the former begets knowledge, the latter ignorance." (On the contrary, much of today's patient care is *opinion*-based, and not outcome-driven nor information-based, and as such disregards Hippocrates's position that *opinion* begets *ignorance*.) So for the practical purposes of medicine, Hippocrates largely discarded the gods, or at least the punitive or malicious role of the gods, in disease. Hippocrates's less emotive use of 'good' and 'bad' in medicine stands in particular contrast to a revival of the Asclepios cult in the early Christian era, and in medieval Christian medical philosophy (see below). In the medieval Christian philosophy, although the use of logic was far from reglected, the issue of the forces of 'good' and 'bad' were the core model.

MEANWHILE: THE CONTINUING CHINESE CONTRIBUTION TO MEDICINE

It cannot be denied that Eastern medicine must historically stand side by side with that of the Western world. Several cultures, including later the Arab culture (see the next chapter), also made huge impacts. One very good reason for pausing to look at the Chinese story is because it is extraordinarily well documented for over two millennia, and it shows how much they understood the relationship between the biology of animals and plants, as foods and herbs, and the biology of the human body (as well as the relation of the body to the stresses, physical and psychological, and the environment).

The first recorded use of the term "velvet" as medicine in ancient times dates back over two thousand years to a Han tomb in Hunan Province where a silk scroll was recovered a listing of over 50 different diseases for which antler velvet was prescribed. Velvet refers to the soft covering of deer antlers while they are growing and still in a cartilaginous state, before they harden into bone. Every year the stag's antlers grow with remarkable swiftness and every year, after the roar and mating season, the antlers are cast off to begin the cycle again in the spring. Velvet has been an enduring mainstay of Asian medicine. Li Shezan's much later great text the *Bencao Gangmu* (see below) devotes several pages to deer products including velvet, which was prepared as powders, pills, extracts, tinctures, and ointments.

Earlier we noted that herb and food practice across the ancient world constituted a hugely important form of technology that was, in modern hindsight, a biomolecular pharmacological technology. Such was most of medicine. Although there is evidence in skulls and bones of early forms of surgery, the main reasons for visiting any surgeon would be to fix bones and dislocation, to treat surface injuries, and to remove parasitic worms. Foods and herbs were the much safer and much preferred practice.

According to Chinese legend, Shen Nung, the Chinese father of agriculture and leader of an ancient clan, took it upon himself to test, one by one, hundreds of different plants to discover their nutritional and medicinal properties. Many plants turned out to be poisonous to humans. Over the millennia the Chinese used themselves this way to continue testing plants for their properties.

The start of the Chinese story goes back to the New Stone Age diaspora. Humankind must have at least passed through China 15,000 to 35,000 years ago on the long trek round the world, and it would be surprising if many did not stop in China. However, at least toward the end of that period, it was much wetter. All of northern China was covered by lakes and marshes, and central China was covered in an enormous lake. There is solid evidence of extensive settlement a bit later, about 14,000 years ago. That phase of population lasted until about 2000 BC and was characterized by a spread of settled agricultural communities, although hunting and gathering was still the norm. The largest concentration of agriculture was below the southern bend of the Yellow River, and millet was the main crop. The Xia dynasty was the arguably earliest dynasty. Its existence was long thought to be a myth until excavations in 1959 in the city of Yanshi uncovered a likely capital. The subsequent Shang dynasty of 2100 to 1800 BC is nevertheless considered to be the first true dynasty of China. The Shang dynasty too was originally considered to be a myth, but the dispelling has a definite pharmacological connection: the Shang dynasty was discovered because Chinese pharmacists sold, as therapeutic dragon bones, the oracle bones that the Shang had carved.

As with the ancient Greek revival described below, the second half of Zhou rule set the final stage for a period of intellectual and medical development when Qin unified the warring states (and hence China) and declared himself to be the first true emperor of China. This intellectual expansion occurred despite the fact that the Qin dynasty, although the strongest warring state militarily, was not the most culturally advanced. Be that as it may, a great deal of ancient medical knowledge was preserved in the period 221 to 207 BC, not so long after Hippocrates and to some extent for some 200 years afterward. The "Inner Cannon" (*Nei Ching*) is a comprehensive record of Chinese medical theories up to that time. A practical guide, even to the present day, on the treatment of illness, the "Treatise on Diseases Caused by Cold Factors" (*Shang Han Lun*) by Chang Chung-ching, was developed in the Han dynasty (206 BC–AD 220).

Chinese medical theory was used to describe the system of body functions, and recognized the concept of what we might see as a lasting effect of the environment. In some terms such as those of stress and immunological and chemotoxic effects to exposure to environment, diseases, and foodstuffs, its huge importance is just becoming realized in the West, by means of the analysis of complex medical data. The Chinese medical system was essentially a combinatorial description, a "spreadsheet" or "graph" view. Seven emotions combined with six external disease-causing factors, and then coupled with the theory of latent phenomena, are still used to perform diagnoses.

With this kind of infrastructure for the use of herbs and other medical practices, the Chinese developed over thousands of years a different conceptual medical system from their Western counterpart and seemingly maintained at least a common flavor throughout. Chinese medicine contrasts with the sharp discontinuity in Western medicine due to Hippocrates. It could be argued that because the Chinese got it roughly right the first time, it was harder to "upgrade" much later on (see below). Similar criticism was once made of the technical superiority of the European over the US telephone system, simply because the United States developed its telephone system most extensively first.

This possible criticism must be tempered by the very ingenious and effective character of the system. The system was, within the limited data then available, scientific. In the absence of a modern physics, chemistry, and molecular biology, a logical Chinese system was attempted based on the Ying (the female, passive, receding and intellectual aspect of nature) and Yang (masculine, active, advancing aspect), which are believed to contain all material life functions. These functions comprised:

1. heart, or mind (*hsin*): corresponding to Western consciousness and intelligence;
2. lungs, or respiratory system (*fei*): corresponding to the Western early twentieth-century concept of homeostasis concerning maintenance by feedback of the constancy of the internal milieu (in Chinese medical thinking, illness is only one manifestation of an imbalance that exists in the entire person);
3. liver (*kan*): the limbs and trunk, corresponding to the Western hypothalamic and autonomic system, are the response to the external environment, and the response of organs;
4. spleen (*pki*): corresponding to Western anabolism and using nutrition to build up the body; and
5. kidneys (*shen*): analogous to Western notions of metabolic catabolism, energy production, and removal of the waste products of this process.

These analogies are, of course, approximate, but what is remarkable is that, they are identifiable with modern Western medical philosophy. More important is the relation of the Chinese system to the emerging focus in Western medicine on the overall health of the person, as in the analogy regarding the lungs. The object of Chinese medicine effectively is not just the illness but the whole person.

The holistic aspect of medicine with its close affinity to the philosophy of modern Western systems biology can be illustrated by accounts of some great Chinese physicians. A number of stories are recorded in classical Chinese on the practice of medicine in the Qin dynasty in *The Record of the Warring State*, and these stories are included in the chapter note.

More recent Chinese medical works and contemporary Chinese medical practice, in general, are reminiscent of ancient experiences with plants as cures. The Chinese love affair with plants reached its peak of development during the Sung period (AD 960–1280), when there were great ornate herb gardens as described by Marco Polo. We can assume that such extensive screening continued to produce some amazing pharmaceutical cures. The great sixteenth-century herbal work by Li Shezan is discussed in the next chapter. Today, a Chinese pharmacist in the Republic of China filling a drug prescription ordered by a traditional Chinese doctor may not do it so differently from his counterpart in very ancient China. The pharmacist's shop would be like a micro version of the London or New York Museum of Natural History. In endless rows of drawers are plant and animal products. Cinnabar and amber relax the nerves. Safflower and peach pits ("stones") better the blood circulation. Various barks, leaves, and galls contain aspirin-like compounds and relieve pain and tranquilize. Cassia bark is considered warming in nature, and is useful in treating colds. Mahuang induces perspiration.

Ginseng stimulates alertness and cardiac function. The stem of Chinese ephedra is a sudorific, and its roots can halt perspiration. Mint is considered, as in the West, cooling and comforting in nature, and is used to relieve colds and fevers. Often, the pharmacist selects a few ingredients that the patient is expected to process as food and boil into a soup.

Chinese herbal medicine seems to have come to the West in part by Arab physicians, and later by the efforts of explorers like Marco Polo and the spice traders. For example, ginseng, used in China for over 5,000 years, was known to nineth-century Arab physicians, and later Marco Polo wrote of this prized, "wonder drug." Today US companies and researchers in China are going back to the texts of Chinese medicines, even in some cases copies of very ancient manuscripts, identifying the plants, analyzing the extraction and preparation procedure, evaluating pharmacological effectiveness and safety, and formulating concentrated dosages of Chinese pharmaceutical products for commercial sale.

As the traditions of Oriental medicine become more accessible to the Western world, many potent new herbal tonics and formulas are appearing on the market. While new to us in the West, many of the herbs have a history of continuous use that dates back thousands of years. They are still in use today for one reason—because they work.

We will return soon to ancient Greece. The difficulty in fitting the Chinese contribution into a larger chronological tale is that it began very early but performed a kind of pincer movement, affecting the West long after the contributions of the ancient Greeks. While we did not wish to break the flow by jumping too far forward in time, it must be said that the Chinese system of medicine has also enjoyed enduring impact. The personal, firm, and authoritative psychological approach, and efforts in specific areas like obstetrics, were pioneering; they might have had their roots in Chinese wisdom before the golden era of ancient Greek medicine and might have percolated to the West in the late Middle Ages. A testament to the wisdom of Chinese culture and medicine is the significant modern impact on Western *everyday* life of tea, ginseng, and other herbs, as well as Chinese systems of exercise and relaxation. Also, acupuncture has made a significant contribution to recent Western culture. The World Health Organization in 1980 released a list of 43 types of pathologies that can be effectively treated with acupuncture.

With these Chinese successes in mind, what about the difficulty, alluded to above, of "upgrading" what already seems to be a reasonably working system?

In 1810–1840, the West launched its great program of understanding molecules and cells and cultural themes, of course, flow both ways. Besides the kind of natural fusion of East and West noted above, the Chinese government has put great efforts into promoting the modernization of Chinese medicine. As a result there are now people trained in both traditional Chinese and modern Western medical arts, and they have made commendable contributions to the treatment of hepatitis, high blood pressure, cancer, and other diseases that even today remain difficult to treat. It is noteworthy that in this partnership the more proven ancient ways of Chinese medicine continue, essentially unchanged. We need an introduction of the molecular perspective to move it forward. Ultimately this should prove no barrier. The Chinese proved their metal in early insulin research, and continue to do in many areas of modern biology.

BACK IN GREECE: A CONTRASTING KIND OF MEDICINE?

Back in time and space in ancient Greece, while China was forging a holistic approach and its relation to the plants and relationships around us, the Greeks were applying their developments in philosophy, science, and mathematics drawn from nature but applied, in a somewhat more inward, drill-down, analytic way. This is not at all to say that the East was unscientific. Although the following statements are necessarily sweeping and simplifying, the Chinese and their neighbors tended to take a pragmatic and experimentalist approach, a kind of vast set of clinical trials over several thousands of years, bringing in theories that were essentially highlighting classification of their observations with the minimal requirement to make sense out of the world as required for practical use. The Greeks, who were purportedly preferring to philosophize and argue about what was in an urn rather than look in it, were emphasizing a theoretical but analytical approach, drilling down into reality as far as their thinking and limited drill-down experimental techniques could allow. Hippocrates and some of his followers were nevertheless atypical innovators in Greece in developing some early principles of modern biology based on scientific observation, seeing logical thought, not magic and religion, as part of medicine. *Between wisdom and medicine there is no gulf fixed*, wrote Hippocrates, in *The Decorum*.

ATOMS OF INHERITANCE?

Thinking about health, which depends on inherited factors as well as accidents and infectious disease, has to involve at least some basic appreciation of genetics and inheritance of features. Even the Old Testament has some appreciation of the principles: "and in Thy book all my members were written, which in continuance were fashioned, when as yet there were none of them" (Psalms 139;16). The Greeks with their view of philosophy and science, and an interest in controversies as to whether atoms composed the world, would be interested in what "elements" composed the "words" instructing inheritance.

The ancient Greeks knew nothing of ... GATACAGATTAC ..., but they recognized that some kind of seed is passed on that makes children resemble their parents. So the children tend to suffer some of the same kinds of disorder, or sometimes advantage. At one time Hippocrates or the Hippocratic School even attempted to address the inheritance of multiple features by suggesting that each body part gave rise to a seed, or part of the seed. And by this construct they had a notion of genetic disease. Witness "... for the semen comes from all parts of the body, sound from the sound parts, and unhealthy from the unhealthy parts" (*Airs, Waters, and Places* attributed to Hippocrates). This theory is incorrect in the sense that only the sex cells pass on genetic information. Still it captures the right spirit: the inherited DNA does give rise to our tissues, organs, and limbs, and "homeobox" genes control body part and organ development. Natural selection of certain random variations in our features (caused by mutations in the DNA of our sex cells) enables those variations "good for survival and reproduction" to be passed on to future generations, such that they tend to become the characteristics of descendants.

The Hippocratic School had a great deal of awareness about, and put a great deal of thought to, inheritable characteristics, and to inheritance of sound and unhealthy body parts. Had Hippocrates had more data, might he have considered Pythagoras while recognizing all his other redeeming features as having *bad* blood in respect to favism?

The emphasis here is on 'bad' in relation to unhealthy. That did not necessarily appeal to all the ancient Greeks, and certainly less so to the Hippocratic School. Discarding the notion of disease as some form of divine evil in favor of an objective assessment reflects to some extent the fundamental nature of the Greeks departure from the earlier religiously based medical healing cult of Asklepios. We restate the developing Hippocratic notion (not perfect, but developing) that in regard to the consequences of that seed, one should abandon the notion of *normal* being inevitably 'good' and *different* being inevitably 'bad' (this is discussed further in regard to Galen, and the Middle Ages, below).

The Hippocratic view turns out to be the more correct even from a modern molecular perspective, as follows. Consider the modern evidence about the different red blood cell disorders of favism, sickle cell anemia, thalassemia, all believed to be known (at least to some extent) to the ancient Greeks. The point is that it is impossible to use the notion of 'bad' here for the simple reason that these almost certainly conferred an advantage to survival at some stage in history, and prehistory.

We do not know for certain whether or not the Greeks knew of the advantage. Writings attributed to Hippocrates are rich in allusions to what we would interpret today as population genetics, and they contain many astute observations that imply general philosophical principles of biology. In principle, the

Greeks had all the tools required to collect and interpret the data, though not to interpret data in detail at the molecular level.

The notion that certain genetic disorders may have had prehistorical or historical benefits cropped up in discussion of founder genes earlier in this chapter. Recall that founder genes are mainly *defined* as having carried a surrounding chunk of DNA with them, a haplotype, from the founding father or mother who first had that mutation. But most founder genes may also have persisted because of the benefits. HFE is a founder gene mutation from an ancestor in northwestern Europe that causes the subject to sequester too much iron, but is advantageous when food is in short supply, so causing anemia. For reasons of famine, anemia is still the most common non-infectious disease in the world. According to latest World Health Organizations it must be joined by depression. These are then followed in order by respiratory tract infections (bronchitis, pneumonia, colds, and influenza), AIDS, malaria, diarrhea, tuberculosis, measles, whooping cough, tetanus, meningitis, syphilis, and hepatitis. It is easy to see how such a founder gene could survive and propagate if it can help the sufferer resist or fight off one of these major diseases. For AIDS, it is (as far as we know) not appropriate to discuss founder genes because this disease is of very recent origin (believed to be from primates—see earlier discussion on the zoonotic nature of most or all infectious diseases). Nonetheless, there is an analogous protection against the HIV virus by a mutation that most of the world did previously have, except largely in the genes propagated the Roman Empire. For protection against malaria, sickle cell anemia (mutation HbS) from the Middle East and Africa is an example of the "once beneficial" founder gene. However, the same mutation in hemoglobin occurred some five times because the haplotype DNA, the section carried with that mutation, is of five different types: four of African (Senegal, Benin, Cameroon, and Bantu origin) and one from the Arabian gulf and India area. For diarrhea, there is the cystic fibrosis mutation (CFTR) originating from a founder in South Eastern Europe or the Middle East that seems to confer some protection. For effects of injuries though not tetanus itself, mutation LVLeiden from West Europe and causing blood clots may have provided protection from bleeding or sepsis following infection, following findings that it seems to counter the lethal effects of blood infections. Mutation ALDH2 may confer resistance to hepatitis B.

ALDH2 is better known, however, as responsible for built-in intolerance to alcohol, especially in far eastern Asia, thus protecting against the effects of alcoholism. That needs some comment, as at first sight an excessive love of wine or beer seems unlikely as a significant evolutionary force some many tens of thousands of years ago. Some founder genes are old. A mutation for not being able to taste phenylthiocarbamide as bitter may have conferred an advantage by switching to being able to detect a major toxic substance in plants more than 100,000 years ago. But many founder mutations are quite recent: the HFE gene has kept quite a length of the original DNA around it, and may have occurred about AD 800. The ADH2 mutation is harder to date because it is actually a number of variants, but one variant may have derived from ancient Qiang population of China several thousand years ago. Still, the threat of alcoholism would have to come first to select for those with that mutation. For industrialized nations the WHO's addition of depression adds by implication its consequences, namely drug abuse, smoking, and alcohol addiction, which seem to be modern diseases. The prevalence of malaria in Africa is about 9% while that of smoking is 18% and growing rapidly, and it is said to be in many remoter places far easier and nearer to buy a packet of cigarettes (at average cost of equivalent of US $3.30 to $3.60 in Africa) than a bag of sugar. Nonetheless, outside the Americas, smoking is too recent to be an explanation for any founder gene. "Herb abuse" could perhaps be an explanation, prehistorically, as in opium addiction today. And risk of alcohol abuse certainly could be. Some of the earliest writings refer to the production and distribution of beer: the Code of Hammurabi included laws regulating Mesopotamian "pubs," and "The Hymn to Ninkasi," a prayer to the Mesopotamian goddess of beer, was basically a chanted beer recipe. Even before earliest agriculture, alcoholism poses a very real ancient risk since alcohol arises naturally in fermenting fruit in storage, or lying on the forest floor. A very strong reason for plants having evolved to bear fruit is that animals will like it and disperse the seeds. Fermenting fallen apples are apparently particularly delicious if one can catch them at the right early stage, or stomach the appearance. Forest deer drunk from fermenting apples are extremely common, and the occasional horse has been known to need rescuing after an "apple binge" (see http://www.dvorak.org/blog/2008/10/15/swimming-pool-rescue-for-a-drunken-pony/).

The advantageous aspect of what might otherwise be considered a genetic disease is well illustrated by sickle cell anemia (SCA). SCA is an autosomal recessive disease. That means, if it occurs only on one chromosome from mother or from father (i.e., if the person is *heterozygous* with respect to the gene), it has a less serious effect than if it occurs on both (i.e., if that person is *homozygous* with respect to that gene). The concept of "recessive" is not hard to understand: it simply means that if there is one working gene, the effect of a nonworking gene does not show up so much (the working gene is dominant, and the broken gene is recessive). About 8% of the African American population carry an SCA gene. It is transmitted genetically (i.e., carried), as a mutation in the hemoglobin beta gene (HbB) found on chromosome 11, a change of just one base pair (causing just one amino acid, glutamic acid, to be replaced by another, valine, six amino acids along from the start of the β-chain in hemoglobin). This molecular change produces a new form of hemoglobin called HbS, which causes red blood cells to crumple and assume sickle shapes at reduced oxygen pressure or high concentrations. SCA is the most commonly inherited blood disorder in the United States affecting about 72,000 Americans (1 in 500 African–Americans). On the face of it, this inherited mutation definitely does not have much going for it, especially in the homozygous form. Under certain conditions, like low oxygen levels or high hemoglobin concentrations, or with certain drugs, it can trigger unfortunate consequences. In individuals who are homozygous (i.e., carrying it on chromosomes from the mother and the father) for HbS, these deformed and rigid red blood cells become trapped within small blood vessels and block them, producing pain and eventually damaging organs. SCA is therefore characterized by episodes of pain, chronic hemolytic anemia, and severe infections, usually beginning in early childhood. Those who are heterozygous may show relatively mild symptoms. The production of some "normal" HbB makes up for the production of the "faulty" HbS.

However, we are preaching here that in population genetics, "disease" can sometimes mean "prevention of disease." Inspection of the worldwide distribution of malaria shows that is has a very similar distribution to that of the HbS gene, in the Mediterranean, West Africa, Sub-Sharan Africa, East Africa, the Nile Valley, and Asia. This geographical distribution suggests that the HbS mutation was originally useful in the contexts like the swamps of Africa, where it conferred some resistance to malaria and possibly other blood parasites. Apparently even being heterozygous will promote some resistance, so the unfortunates suffering from the full homozygous load are the price that humans have paid for the protection from malaria. This very ancient inherited mutation may thus go back well before the out-of-Africa diaspora.

It is interesting that SCA is the disease most often quoted in regard to the distribution of malaria. However, the genes for favism and another disease of hemoglobin, such as thalassemia, show a similar distribution. Thalassemia is not so often mentioned because it is more than one disease, genetically speaking. A variety of mutations affecting the quantity and quality of hemoglobin production are classed as "thalassemia." However, putting all these red blood cell diseases together, favism, sickle cell anemia, and the various thalassemias, one can obtain a map that more closely approximates the distribution of malaria. The inheritance of favism could have saved Pythagoras from a worse fate.

Similarly, in modern times, a change in the CCR5 gene, which makes a protein found on the surface of cells of the immune system, confers resistance not to malaria nor to other blood parasites, but to the HIV virus. It has been assumed that the CCR5 mutation is a relatively recent beneficial mutation or an older mutation of previously little consequence (of course, HIV could have entered the human population from African primates in several waves before historical documentation). Let us keep in mind that regardless of whether the genetic difference is considered a "fault," there are plenty of opportunities for mutations to occur, and under most circumstances inherited mutations seem to have no ill effects whatsoever except when certain pharmaceutical drugs are given. Humans evolved by exposure to mutation and natural selection long before medicine was around to exert a selective pressure. Sometimes what has good or bad consequences when a physician writes your prescription today was of zero genetic consequence just a few years ago.

Such one-time advantages may explain why so many genetic changes became genetic markers (i.e., survived to be passed on). Other variations in DNA may not be diseases by any stretch of the imagination. Indeed most are neutral because most of our DNA does not contain what we normally think of as genes. Even those genes that confer some minor disadvantage or inconvenience may not be all bad. Some inconvenient genetic differences are simply what physicians used to dismiss as "idiotypic" variations in response to drugs.

The term "polymorphism," as opposed to general use of "mutation," has recently become the politically correct term, although *genomic biomarker* still tends to be the generally preferred term. On the whole, inherited mutations are best thought of as polymorphisms, with single nucleotide polymorphism (SNP) used for straightforward differences in single base pairs (one of G, C, A, or T) or very few base pairs (see Chapter 3). So whether genetic differences are entirely neutral in their effect or have some 'good' or 'bad' impact, they should be considered with scientific due diligence as a matter of degree and variable with time, place, and circumstances. This is not unreasonable, and indeed there is evidence that the ancient Greeks and particularly Hippocrates had some sense of it, as mentioned above.

But Hippocrates and his followers wanted to go beyond taking medicine out of consideration of disease as offending, or as a punishment by, the gods, and beyond being bogged down in basic 'good' equals health, 'bad' equals disease, ethics, and beyond abstract philosophical and scientific thinking. They wished to apply it as *engineers of health*. Such a practical perspective brings in many *practical* ethical considerations of how to best practice and propagate that discipline. Which brings us to the Hippocratic Oath.

THE HIPPOCRATIC OATH

It is not clear that Hippocrates left any genetic descendants surviving today (despite some claims), but he left us his intellectual children ... and an oath. Based on accumulating empirical observations on inherited and infectious disease, interpreted by intellectually modeling the world, Hippocrates had achieved a convincing worldview and, apparently, convincing medical successes. Hippocrates thus had many protégés, and he formed them into a new order. From the fifth to the fourth centuries BC, the *Hippocratic Corpus* was composed. As discussed above, these collected writings, attributed to Hippocrates, comprise about 60 works on a variety of medical topics, including diagnosis, epidemics, obstetrics, pediatrics, nutrition, and surgery. It is not clear how much of the large amount of medical writings attributed to Hippocrates by Plato, Aristotle, and others really came from his hand. The probability that several authors were involved in the Hippocratic works, perhaps over several centuries, is raised by the variety of explanations for diseases. They could have in part been pulled together for the great library built by the Greeks at Alexandria. In the main, however, they are similar in looking for natural explanations and treatments of illness and rejecting sorcery and magic. They

prove that the Greeks had learned to describe the details of a disease scientifically. This was combined with an emerging humanitarian and ethical perspective that moved the patient to the central focus. At around the same time,
sophists begin teaching knowledge and rhetoric and spread over the known
world. This new diaspora of knowledge was carried out to the world by the
itinerant Hippocratic physicians.

The Hippocratic Oath that they took with them is one of the oldest binding
documents in history. As genuinely written down at some time in antiquity, its
general principles are more or less held sacred by doctors to this day: treat the
sick to the best of one's ability, preserve patient privacy, teach the secret arts
of medicine to the next generation, and so forth. The American Medical
Association's *Code of Medical Ethics* (1996 edition) holds that "The Oath of
Hippocrates has remained in Western civilization as an expression of ideal
conduct for the physician." The Hippocratic Oath has been updated by the
Declaration of Geneva, and the General Medical Council of the UK captures
the principles as a basis for best practice in the form of its *Duties of a Doctor*
and *Good Medical Practice* guidelines (that in the case of malpractice or complaint have some force of law). Yet in the 1970s, cultural and social forces
induced many US medical schools to drop the Hippocratic Oath from gradu-
ation ceremonies. Nonetheless, there is inevitably some equivalent form
intended to capture the spirit of the original oath. US schools usually substitute a version modified to be specific about aspects considered more politically
correct and up-to-date, including for example an explicit reference as to impar-
tiality to race, gender, and sexual orientation. There may be an alternate pledge
like the Prayer of the Jewish scholar Maimonides, possibly adjusted to be of
similar modern form. Of the remaining schools adhering to the more traditional form of the Oath of Hippocrates, few in any event use a form that much
resembles the original. The notions of not taking advantage of the patient in
any way, and in particular the notion of *primum non nocere*, that is, "do no
harm," are persistent strong features, although ironically the latter is said by
many authors not to be in the original oath and more likely due to Galen (see
the next chapter).

The following is the translation from the Greek by Ludwig Edelstein, *The
Hippocratic Oath: Text, Translation, and Interpretation* (Baltimore: Johns
Hopkins Press, 1943).

I swear by Apollo Physician and Asclepius and Hygieia and Panaceia and all the
gods and goddesses, making them my witnesses, that I will fulfill according to my
ability and judgment this oath and this covenant:

To hold him who has taught me this art as equal to my parents and to live my
life in partnership with him, and if he is in need of money to give him a share of
mine, and to regard his offspring as equal to my brothers in male lineage and to
teach them this art—if they desire to learn it—without fee and covenant; to give
a share of precepts and oral instruction and all the other learning to my sons and
to the sons of him who has instructed me and to pupils who have signed the
covenant and have taken an oath according to the medical law, but no one else.

I will apply dietetic measures for the benefit of the sick according to my ability and judgment; I will keep them from harm and injustice.

I will neither give a deadly drug to anybody who asked for it, nor will I make a suggestion to this effect. Similarly I will not give to a woman an abortive remedy. In purity and holiness I will guard my life and my art.

I will not use the knife, not even on sufferers from stone, but will withdraw in favor of such men as are engaged in this work.

Whatever houses I may visit, I will come for the benefit of the sick, remaining free of all intentional injustice, of all mischief and in particular of sexual relations with both female and male persons, be they free or slaves.

What I may see or hear in the course of the treatment or even outside of the treatment in regard to the life of men, which on no account one must spread abroad, I will keep to myself, holding such things shameful to be spoken about.

If I fulfill this oath and do not violate it, may it be granted to me to enjoy life and art, being honored with fame among all men for all time to come; if I transgress it and swear falsely, may the opposite of all this be my lot.

Despite the above mentioned revision or rejection in the 1970's, oath taking by medical students is practiced in some form in most schools of medicine, and has now risen to near uniformity. If it is ever seen as a step back for recognition of Hippocrates, it is a situation which must be compared with a mere 24% of US medical students taking the oath in 1928. The oath's limitations and relevance in the modern world are implictly (and sometimes explicitly) subjects of further following chapters, including consideration of medical and research ethics.

The oath and the teachings of Hippocrates are ultimately a *meme*, an innovation inherited by teaching and learning, and of a complexity that biological evolution and our DNA could never create and propagate, yet supplementing hugely the message in that DNA that makes us modern humans. The meme became quickly embedded in the information technology of writing, and in law as well as lore, and in the practices of our schools and healthcare institutions. The oath is more relevant, not less, in the information technology of the computer age. Its guiding principles serve well for the planners of the new technology, as IT becomes ever more a record, servant, scout, and watchdog. By automating the flow of medical work, and in providing guidance to physicians, the IT of which we would hope Hippocrates would approve will facilitate security, privacy, governance, compliance, responsibility, and best practice by all healthcare professionals.

BEYOND THE OATH

For the most part what is good and correct to do in near future medicine will be fairly clear, because Hippocrates and many generations of his reviewers, helped make it so. Until recently the ancient philosophies of the Greeks and others can be applied because the world has not, in the very basic essence of everyday life, changed too much. As mentioned earlier, the ancient Greeks and hence Hippocrates could probably pick up a Greek newspaper of today and make sense of much of it. This is thanks to the persistence of the Greek language in Greece, its use in science worldwide, and by the time of Hippocrates his probable familiarity with many modern scientific concepts, such as matter being particles in motion, or the idea of evolution. Such ideas were at least one theory from one of the Greek philosophers. Above we mentioned that splitting the atom would convey some sense (and it may be added that the sense conveyed would be at least the poetic one of some fundamental processes of great difficulty, because the word *atom* comes from a Greek word άτομο meaning indivisible). But also in some cases even advanced medical technology terms like μαγνητική τομογραφία, that is, *magnetic tomography* and modern Greek for magnetic resonance imaging (MRI), would probably translate reasonably well in context to look like something the engineering followers of Archimedes could conceivably come up with, rather than magic. But such is the acceleration of pace that soon the world will be less familiar to us and hence to Hippocrates. Ethical truths will be held by fewer and fewer people to be self-evident. As ancient Greeks argued over the early technology of induced abortion (with Hippocrates against it), and as recently the world argued over the consequences of stem cell technology and cloning, people will disagree on how to meet new technological challenges to ethics. Considerations will similarly arise about the promises and woes of bionic humans and nanotechnology. Increasingly there will seem more ways to do harm, and even to question what might be meant by good and by harm, than ever before. The legacy of Hippocrates will guide us less. But for a long time to come the spirit of the words of the Hippocrates school will work just fine: the core message is that all is for the good of the patient, in terms of health, the non-abuse of medical privilege, and privacy.

In the next step of the story, the oath must find its way to embracing the application of new medical technologies and the insight from a new and almost alien molecular science. But before that stage is reached in our story, Hippocratic medicine will first have to endure a revival of the Asklepios cult, and the subsequent Dark Ages that fell upon the largely Christian Western world.

3

THE ROAD TO THE NEW MEDICINE

The aim of the art of medicine is health, but its end is the possession of health. Doctors have to know by which means to bring about health, when it is absent, and by which means to preserve it, when it is present.

—Galen (c. AD 130–200)

There is virtually no limit to the amount of health care an individual is capable of absorbing.

—Enoch Powell, British Health Minister

THE ROAD FROM GALEN

All medical systems, like any other system, are new when they first arise, and seem exciting and innovative in their time. Here we consider primarily "mainstream" medicine as it evolved from Hippocrates via Galen. Galen, *Claudius Galenus*, was a Greek physician born in Pergamos (Pergamum) in Asia Minor in the year AD 129, 130, or 131. After receiving medical training in Smyrna and Alexandria, he gained fame as a surgeon to the gladiators of Pergamos. He was eventually summoned to Rome to be the physician of the Emperor Marcus Aurelius. Galen spent the rest of his life at the Roman court writing an enormous corpus of medical works until his death in AD 201.

Why mainstream? To put it briefly, there were medical systems in other lands, in popular culture, that took alternative views. They lie on another path.

The Engines of Hippocrates: From the Dawn of Medicine to Medical and Pharmaceutical Informatics, by Barry Robson and O.K. Baek
Copyright © 2009 by John Wiley & Sons, Inc.

Although they have an ancient common origin before Hippocrates, and many times historically they have been entwined with the mainstream road (sometimes indistinguishably), western medicine was "on site" to embrace the rise of western technology.

The most direct road to what we mean by the "new medicine" began in the same way that it continues today: in discovery of a new system for storing and processing medical information. The merits of the storage of information about medicine, mathematics, and science, in order to capture the wisdom of the ancients, were not lost on the entrepreneurial political powers of the established and emerging great centers of civilization. Libraries were the new technology. Several great libraries were created, the most famous being that at Alexandria. Pergamos, a part of the ancient Greek kingdom in Asia Minor, and later a Roman province, contained a library second in importance only to the great library in Alexandria.

If the work of Hippocrates can be taken as representing the foundation of Greek medicine, then the work of Galen, six centuries later, is the apex of that tradition. Using an entrepreneurial approach in many modern senses of the word, Galen crystallized and popularized all the best work of the Greek medical schools that had preceded him. Looking back, we can see that legacy of Greek medicine spread in three major phases, in a pre-Roman period, with the Roman empire, and via the Holy Roman empire and Christianity (incidentally, the spread of the Roman culture also carried with it a series of serious plagues, notably in the reign of Julian). It is primarily as Galenism that Greek medicine was transmitted to early scholars.

Galen was the Howard Hughes and Bill Gates of his time. He was born the son of a wealthy architect in Pergamos; he had access to the great technology of the period, the great library, as well as all the other intellectual trappings of Pergamos that went with it. Throughout his career Galen was not only a well-informed physician but a devout philosopher and empirical researcher. He inherited and created wealth, but wealth was not his motivation. He specifically decried the role of money in what he saw as creating a new future for humankind. The profit motive, Galen argued, is incompatible with a serious devotion to the art. Galen frequently accused his colleagues and peers of greed.

Galen's first professional appointment was as surgeon to the gladiators in Pergamos: in that tenure he must have gained much anatomical experience. After four years he moved to Rome, where he practiced medicine and became famous for his public demonstrations of anatomy. Three emperors were among his clientele.

Galen's learning (and wisdom and public relations skills) seems to have been second to none. Galen was a master of promoting himself, but on the whole his personal moral sensitivities and ethics are thought to be incontestable. Galen was also well known as a philosopher and training in philosophy is, in Galen's view, an essential part of being a doctor. He praised and built upon Hippocrates, although there was something slightly pre-Hippocratic about the philosophy of Galen and his followers in regard to the sense of good and evil as part of medical philosophy. The emotive use of concepts like "good" and "bad" had been a feature of the Asklepios cult since 350 BC, and Hippocratic medicine had somewhat rebelled against it as having religious or magical connotations. It was natural for Galen to return somewhat to that way of thinking. He had been raised as a *therapeutes* or "attendant" of the healing god Asklepios whose sanctuary was an important cultural center not only for Pergamos, but also for the entire Roman province of Asia. The increasingly prestigious cult association of *therapeutai* included senators, magistrates, highly ranking civil servants, and intellectuals from all over the Asian province. The *thereputai* took disease to be a departure from the line of health. The first requisite of medicine became an extensive and intimate acquaintance with the norm of the body. Accordingly it became a norm to speak of the life of the body either as proceeding with nature (*secundum naturam*) or as overstepping the bounds of nature (*praeter naturam*). The medieval world inherited this view.

The intellectual confusion over the issue of the natural and unnatural by Galen and his followers seems to be due of a growing awareness of the importance of *homeostasis* of the body, namely, the need to maintain the constancy of the internal physiological environment. Homeostasis is a powerful concept, and there was much accumulating data to support it. Not least, injury as in the gladiatorial arena must have well illustrated the undesirability physiological effects of "trauma" in departures from the anatomical norm.

But this information was not converted correctly to knowledge until many hundreds of years later Charles Darwin pointed out that there is no model of the norm to which species are formed nor even to which they tend to evolve. Rather, there is a random component in inheritance, a throw of the genetic dice, followed by a natural selective process of survival, that tends to favor the survival of the fittest to whatever circumstances and environment exist at the time. Physiological homeostasis and the stabilities of communities of organisms, when achieved, is in fact a consequence of that process. Unfortunately, the interpretation in terms of normal equals good, abnormal equals bad, became entrenched in the medieval Christian position. The Church in Rome, in its effort to promote the Christian model of the time against "pagan" (i.e., Hippocratic) interpretations, adopted a Roman-filtered version of the revived Asklepian view. Be that as it may, the concept does not seem to serve so well in certain areas of medicine such as the history of genetics. At that time patients dealt a particular genetic hand, or contracting incurable disease such as leprosy, had to live with their woes. Sometimes charity was abandoned; the sick were viewed with subjective cruelty, and neglected as an embodiment of evil.

DARKNESS FALLS: MEDIEVAL EUROPE

"Empires rise and fall" and "States cleave asunder and coalesce" are the first and last sentences of *Romance of the Three Kingdoms* written by Luo

Guanzhong 600 hundred years ago. Jared Diamond's *Guns, Germs and Steel: The Fates of Human Societies* (Norton Company, 1997) is perhaps its modern counterpart. But throughout such turbulence, agriculture, a degree of local law, protection, religion or world-view, and medicine must persist. Medicine did not immediately bond 100% with Christianization of the Roman Empire that marked the transition to the Dark Ages, partly because Hippocrates was considered pagan, partly because of the essentially revived Asklepios cult view of disease and the notion of *secundum naturam* and *praeter naturam*, and partly because of the new Christian focus on spiritual health, redemption, and resurrection in perfect form after death. As in the Dark Age of Ancient Greece and the Mediterranean described in Chapter 2, the focus at the start of social decline would be on survival, and a degree of contraction to a village life. Even very early in the Dark Ages, there were always forms of hospices, which were shelters or way stations operated by religious orders for pilgrims and for the dying, but one notes that this would typically mean for those of "proven worth," not for those "touched by the Devil."

It is not of course that the sick were left dropped and to rot in the streets; the question of who were the "Good Samaritans" who picked them up may lead to explanation of why early medieval medicine in Western Europe was a boundary of tension between pagan medicine and new spiritual influences. These the great anthropologist Claude Lévi-Strauss identified as the "shamanistic complex" and "social consensus". (*Anthropologie structurale* (1958; Penguin Press, 1968)). The choice for most that got sick was to pray or get the only help available, and when one fell sick, family, friends, and neighbors would stay supportive. It may be argued that this triggered a shift in attitude that might not only have caused the village shaman or wise woman to rise again, but also increasingly caused such persons be seen as witches, companions of the Devil. As with the original "Good Samaritan," who was from a hated group, the more medically skilled amongst friends and neighbors were not favored by the official consensus. There was also a sense of medical competition too. Christian miracles and laying on of hands abounded with the faith of the patient supplementing and supplemented by the placebo affect in perhaps 30% of cases (see Chapter 2). But ancient healing wisdom also thrived to good effect in frequently skilled but less approved hands. Village herbal remedies, similar or occasionally superior to that of the later monasteries, may have been seen as competitive to God's power. It may thus be that medicine for a period helped spawn the polarization between Christian practice and the "Black Arts," and even the long-standing historical tension between Christianity and science.

Quickly, however, in the early Christian era of Europe and even throughout the Dark Ages, true adherents to Christian concepts ensured the enduring (though occasionally faltering) Christian force of charity. Hospitals and infirmaries arose. In the earliest Christian period these included, prominently, Eastern establishments for the cure of the sick, the Infirmary of Monte Cassino and the Hotel-Dieu at Lyons in the sixth century, the Hotel-Dieu at Paris in the seventh, and many smaller refuges for the sick that sprang up in every part of Europe.

From the Dark Ages we have a curious inadvertent contribution to medicine due to the Vikings. Viking sagas contained strong information about heritage, and their colonization of Iceland led to a relatively isolated genetic community. The largest biotech company in Iceland, deCODE Genetics [www. decode.com], has focused on linking the genetic constitution of the population to their inherited medical disorders, and using this as a basis of computer-based healthcare for the nation. About 90% of Icelanders agreed to have their DNA sequenced and added to the national Biobank data bases.

In the twelfth century Arabic texts made a significant impact on medicine. These texts were brought back by the medical orders of the crusaders and later by a steady stream of intellectuals from the far more advanced Arabic world. There were great charitable organizations translating these texts into Greek like the Order of St. John of Jerusalem. Universities were founded for translating and interpreting Arabic and Greek texts. Arduous seven-year courses in medicine were imposed to distinguish real physicians from quacks. But the philosophy of charity and the spirit of professionalism did get lost at some stages along the way. Later medieval medicine was a business as well as a charity, and for the most part it was rather indifferent about, and very forgiving of the quality of, whoever practiced. Clergy and laymen, men and women, were all allowed to practice medicine.

Naturally, monks and nuns were prominent throughout as guardians of knowledge, protectors of the sick, and the physicians of the time. The monastic gardens kept herbs going through the Dark Ages, both for monastery and public use. Right up to the later years of the nineteenth century, medical use of plant and animal products was much safer, had considerably more practical value, and hence had considerable more impact than surgery. The monks and nuns increasingly included intellectuals, many of whom disdained superstitious, or "magical" science and medicine. The scope can be seen in the collecting, sifting, cataloging, and inventories of illuminated manuscripts and other scholarly works in libraries assembled by nobility and tradesmen with increasing time and money to spend at the end of the Dark Ages and after (such as that of Phillip the Good, 1396–1467, Duke of Bergandy, and charismatic unifier of political divisions and monetary systems). As a point of information technology, many such inventories often included the first rigorous taxonomic systems for knowledge reminiscent of modern classification. A collection of a library catalogued by one Lefèvre d'Etaples in France in 1518 shows twelve subject headings which illustrate both that post-medieval taxonomic thinking and the broad scope of the preceding medieval authors: *theologie, jurs, canonici, juris civilis, philosophies medicine, astrologie, perspective, arithmetice, geometries artis militaris, rei edificatorie, rustice et agriculture, grammatices, logicalium, poesis, eloquentie, historialium* and *grecorum et hebreorum*. The Catholic Church effectively played a role in the development as well as management of medieval medicine, disallowing most "pagan" healing practices even when they might appear more logical. But there was a paradoxical contrast between, on the one hands frequent obsession with rational deduction by the medieval monastic mind and, on the other, the blurring of the natural and supernatural.

COMPUTING IN THE DARK AGES!

What kept a strong rational element alive was that monastic intellectuals were very often applied deductive logic. This included the binary 1/0, yes/no, true/false system of arithmetic, and logical relationships that today form the basis of digital computing. The discipline of logic was originally pioneered by the ancient Greeks, but reduced (or expanded, according to your taste) to an elaborate intellectual pastime in the monasteries of the Middle Ages.

Medieval scholars spent endless hours in constructing logic-based algorithms that would succinctly allow deduction of the 256 variously true, untrue, and irrelevant syllogisms. The classic syllogism example of Aristotelian origin is "Aristotle is a man. All Men are mortal. Aristotle is mortal." Only from some of the 256 syllogisms does the third statement, the conclusion, necessarily follow. Otherwise, it can not be concluded or it is simply wrong. A syllogism is a pretty formally structured set of three statements such as "I am a mammal. Not all mammals are humans. Therefore I am a human." That one is good human speach, bad robot speach, and bad logic. The number 256 arises from the number of different syllogisms when expressed in general form such as "A is B, not all B are C, A is C" (which does not necessarily follow) or "All A are B, all B are C, all A are C" (which always follows), and so on, for the other 254 examples. Syllogisms could be written down, 2 choices at a time, with 8 rearrangements, giving 256 combinations ($2^8 = 256$). The mediaeval scholars constructed, by calculation, truth tables. They developed elaborate proofs for the existence of God. In particular, like the 256 forms of syllogism, logic could be applied to anything. Such combinatorial mathematics underlies much of modern data analysis, theoretical physics, and many other things besides. The endless hours medieval scholars spent in constructing proofs that were rarely wrong, if often solving things that seem trivial to modern mathematics, gave a new method of exhaustively describing problems in the physical world. Applications of medieval logic constrained the wildness of the world; even if a problem wasn't solved, logic bound its scope. Astronomic numbers of rules can be deduced from N nonrepeating parameters, like $2^N - N - 1$ potential rules for the relations between columns on a medieval fact collector's spreadsheet.

The medieval combinatorial approach applied equally to medicine. The most sophisticated efforts required that the combinatorics had to embrace both the spritual and material knowledge too, where relevant to medicine. These two aspects were sometimes called the *devotio* or *affective power* (warm and compassionate spiritual process) and the *scientia* or *intellective power* (colder, harder processes of the mind based on observation and deduction). The thoughts and teaching of Jean Gerson (1363–1429) about these "powers" have been seen by several critics as representing the best unifying presentation of them. His *mystical theology* has also been seen by many as anti-scientific, and certainly he wanted to restore the "warmth" of spirituality against the progressive increase in colder intellectual thinking, including a more physical approach to medicine. However, he actually sought a mutually supporting relation between *devotio* and *scienta*, one that might be seen as a combinatorial arrangement of aspects of correlating and complementing character. From the point of view of religion as a discipline of well-being and relevant to psychiatry, he could perhaps be classified as an early existentialist and phenomenologist (Chapter 7).

Before and apart from Jean Gerson, however, the medieval "mix and match principles" in medicine, although retaining a sense of disease as evil, settled down to emphasize the more physical aspects, and hence rather closely resembled the oriental approach. The underlying principles of medieval medicine were four humors: black bile, yellow bile, phlegm, and blood, and as in Chinese medicine, the balance of these allowed for the well-being of a person. Equally reminiscent of Chinese medicine was the desire to set up conditions describing the body, the environment, and so on, and then to explore the significance of all the combinations and permutations. However, in many matters Western medieval scholars seem to have, on occasion at least, raised the bar for combinatorial computing to a higher level of elaboration than the ancient East.

To aid in combinational computing, there seems to have been not infrequent use of hand calculators, though few have survived. The Voynich manuscript, considered "the most mysterious manuscript in the world," suggests these to have been sliding sheets of parchment or forms of circular slide rule in which disks could be rotated to keep track of the combinations, for example, involving the syllogisms, incantations, mixes of herbs, and even appropriate therapies. There is throughout the Voynich manuscript a continuing interest in generating combinations for magical incantations: 230 pages written in an unknown script and even language that appears to have been generated by combinatorial means, possibly for the purpose of magical incantations (Emperor Rudolph II of Bohemia (1552–1612) probably paid the modern equivalent of $50,000 for it). There was an increasing interest as well in tools for unbreakable ciphers and codes for military messages, espionage, and security. This trend increased in intensity right up to the end of the Middle Ages and beyond. A coding tool known as the Cardan Grille is well documented, and it has been conjectured to be the source of the content of the Voynich manuscript.

But did any medieval monk ever actually build a real, life size computer on any significant scale? Yes, indeed—at least once. Ramon Lull, Spanish theologian and visionary and of the lay Franciscan order, was blessed by a religious vision in 1274 to write a specification for a programming language and computer, whence he retired to the monastery and fully devoted himself to completing the *Ars magna*, the first of about forty treatises on this idea. While Dominican monks have long been associated with herbs and medicine, Franciscans on the whole seem to have taken a mathematical and scientific approach, emphasizing how models of human affairs, including those as material and pragmatic as economics, might be linked to models of the world. In England there was a specifically scientific branch of the Franciscan order. One of the most famous Franciscans associated with it was a contemporary of Ramon Lull, Roger Bacon (1214–1294). He was also a Master at Oxford, lecturing on Aristotle and placing considerable emphasis on empiricism, to the extent of being seen as one of the earliest advocates of the modern scientific method in the West. He was not against mysticism and mysteries: because of his studies in the fields of alchemy, astrology, and languages he is considered by some to be the author of the Voynich manuscript, so one wonders whether the Voynich manuscript was influenced by Lull's computer, or perhaps the reverse. In fact, many of the illustrations of the Voynich manuscript seem to be computer flow charts drawn as trees, elements relating to humans combining flows of work and acting as decision points, and algorithms relating to grids of characters and numbers. In 2007, Claude Martin claimed that the Voynich manuscript is a hoax because it is based on a convoluted anagramming algorithm for numbers that would be inappropriate to the methods of the Middle Ages. But then so was Lull's machine in some respects. Perhaps the Voynich manuscript was the manual and program listing for Lull's machine, or at least reflected some larger Franciscan secret computer project of which Lull's machine was a "tip of the iceberg" as an early experiment or proof of concept!

In *Gulliver's Travels* (pt. III, ch. 5) Swift is thought to be describing Lull's computer: it was contrived as a 20-foot square frame holding hundreds of small cubes linked together by wires. Although Franciscan leaders marveled at it, a rival group, the Dominicans, tended to regard Lull as a shining example of a Franciscan madness, disparaging him as Lull the lunatic. Many centuries later the eminent mathematician Gottfried Leibniz, in his *Dissertio de arte combinatoria* (1666) extolled Lull's work as the basis of a universal algebra by which all knowledge, ethics, metaphysics, medicine, and all else could be shoehorned into a single deductive system. As far as we know Lull's work was the earliest attempt in calculation to employ geometrical diagrams for the purpose of discovering truths, and it could have been the first to use a mechanical logic machine to facilitate the logic calculations.

So first computers make their formal appearance, and medicine makes some, if sluggish, progress. While there were already in medieval times weak links to logic and medicine, computers and medicine won't meet up properly until the twentieth century. A definite link occurs in Lull's vision, for his machine seems to have come from his having used or stared at an herb so hard that mathematical symbols began to appear on it. Whatever else he had in mind for the longer term, much else had to take place before medicine and computers could come together. The final formalization of medical practice in Europe was motivated by the Black Death as no effective doctor was to be found. The same as guilds were created to allow crafts to thrive, and maintain essential wisdom and skills, an education system was refined and extended to teach medicine to the willing and able. Logic became a stronger feature when printed books made proven practice available, when practitioners became competitive and had to succeed in their medical practices to survive, and when physicians had to answer to their colleagues.

OTHER LIGHTS IN THE DARK AGES: EUROPEAN MILITARY MEDICINE, ARABIA, AND CHINA

The medical spirit of the medieval period went on well into the 1500s, and the rise of surgery went well back into the 1200s. Wars were rampant generally, and the battlefield was the school for surgery. Toward the end of medieval medicine, there were a number of developments arising. In the 1400s, treatises and charts and "cautery" (a medical term describing the burning of the body to remove or close a part of it) or cauterization of wounds were common. Gui de Chauliac's 1363 *Grand Chiurgie* described surgical procedures and techniques for avoiding production of pus in wounds, an innovation at that time (though Henri de Mondeville—born 1260—had previously mentioned in his treatise the idea of keeping wounds dry and pus free). Chauliac's book endured to the mid-1500s.

The Arab power of healing appears in many tales of medieval times and in Sir Walter Scott's classic novel *The Talisman*. The Arab world and the Asian world had been significantly more advanced in several respects. As early as the ninth century, when Paris and London were places of mud streets and hovels, Islamic medical practice had hospitals with clean and spacious wards, and cool fountains. There was sophisticated medical terminology. Physicians and pharmacists became licensed professionals with a legally enforced system of ethics. Notable among the dominant figures of Arabian medicine was the Andalusian physician Albucasis, an Arab born in near Córdoba Spain, in the tenth century, who was hailed as an outstanding surgeon. With special instruments he invented, he removed polyps and tonsils. He also described obstetric instruments. He used branding iron and cautery in his practice.

The quest for expansion of trade, which likely started even earlier than the entrepreneurial voyages of Marco Polo in the 1200s, must have brought back information about herbs and medical methods from the East. China continued to make sophisticated progress often based on pulling together and rationalizing the experiences of past ages. Li Shezan was highly influential in Chinese medicine, and he authored the revered text *Bencao Gangmu* (Great Compendium of Herbs), one of the most frequently mentioned books (completed in AD 1578, published in 1596) in the Chinese herbal tradition. Li Shezan's father, Li Yenwen, is known to this day for writing the first monograph on ginseng. He also wrote books on the four diagnostic techniques, on smallpox, on pulse diagnosis, and other techiqnes. Li Shezan was born in AD 1518, at the height of the Ming dynasty (1368–1644), which was a time when neo-Confucianism gained many adherents. This doctrine emphasized the importance of personal behavior, morality, self-cultivation, study, meditation, and careful thought while it downplayed the value of crafts and technology, including the practice of medicine. Neo-Confucianism was to have a significant influence on Li Shezan's life.

The *Bencao Gangmu* presented a huge number of diverse materials: 1,892 medicinal substances (1,094 from plants; 444 from animals, and 275 from mineral sources), including 374 new items. The name *Bencao Gangmu* is derived from the title of the book by the Song dynasty neo-Confucian scholar Zhu Xi (AD 1130–1200), *Tongjian Gangmu*. *Bencao* simply means materia medica (literally: *ben* = plant root; *cao* = plant top; hence: the various parts of plants), but *Gangmu* has special meaning. Shezan called each of his herb monographs *gang* (literally: key link, essential points, subject), while the technical criteria for arranging the herb descriptions were called *mu* (literally: details, indexing, observing). The monographs contained up to 10 points of information about each medicinal material:

- Previously false classification;
- Secondary names, including the sources of the names;
- Collected explanations, commentaries, and quotes in chronological order, including origin of the material, appearance, time of collection, medicinally useful parts, and similarities with other medicinal materials;
- Preparation of the material;
- Explanation of doubtful points;
- Correction of mistakes;
- Taste and nature;
- Enumeration of main indications;
- Explanation of the effects; and
- Enumeration of prescriptions in which the material is used, including form and dosage of the prescriptions.

Li Shezan was able to categorize the medicinal materials into more logical groupings than had been achieved ever before. The groupings come close to the binomial system introduced by Carl Linnaeus during the eighteenth Century (his main books being *Genera plantarum*, 1737, and *Species plantarum*, 1753). Charles Darwin (author of *The Origin of Species*, 1859), in working out his theory of evolution, is reported to have quoted from the *Bencao Gangmu*, which had such detailed information about the variations of plants and animals that it helped flesh out the theory.

MEDICINE IN THE DAWNING AGE OF ENLIGHTENMENT

In medical and several other matters the period from the mid-1500s to the late 1600s could be considered the dawn of the European Enlightenment. Medicine even if not perfect seemed to do good on average. In the medical field this period gave intellectual birth to Andreas Versalius (1514–1564) who wrote the great anatomical work *De Fabrica Corpus* in 1542 and Ambrose Paré (born 1510) who translated it into French in 1561. Paré's own treatise *Method of Treating Wounds* (1545) used a mix of egg yolk, rose oil, and turpentine to close wounds instead of by cauterization—it was essentially a "chemical cauterization"—and it worked. But invasive surgery outside the military setting was still limited. Samuel Pepys (1633–1703), an English writer, had a gall stone removed in 1660, which was something of an event. There were advances nonetheless in basic medical science. Around 1628 William Harvey (1578–1657), an English physician, was the first to describe accurately how blood was pumped around the body by the heart. Still in the 1600s, the next generation of researchers such as Richard Lower (1631–1691), Robert Boyle (1627–1691), and Robert Hooke (1635–1703) made great contributions to basic biology in regard to heart, lungs, and respiration. There were pharmaceutical developments also. Thomas Sydenham (1624–1689), the so-called English Hippocrates, popularized the simple but powerful concept that each disease seemed to require a "specific" plant extract factor or "simples." Paracelsus (1493–1541) had already promoted mercury for syphilis. Jesuits in the new world discovered quinine in Peruvian bark, though a form was also known to the ancient Egyptians as wormwood. Auroleus Phillipus Theostratus Bombastus von Hohenheim, immortalized as "Paracelsus," was born in 1493. He was the son of a well-known physician and Grand Master of the Teutonic Order. It was from his father that Paracelsus took his first instruction in medicine. Andreas Vesalius was a Flemish-born anatomist whose dissections of the human body helped correct misconceptions dating from ancient times.

In the 1700s, Europe's *Age of Enlightenment*, fresh currents of thought were overthrowing medieval-based traditions long due for disassembly. The principal names that roll from the tongue are Descartes, Pascal, Bayle, Montesquieu, Voltaire, and Diderot. The main themes, as expressed by Voltaire, were autonomy of reason, pursuit of perfection and progress, the drive to discover causes of things, principles governing nature, humans, and society, rejection of mindless authority, disgust with nationalism, and solidarity of enlightened intellectuals worldwide. There were others, the intellectual adversaries, who departed somewhat from enlightenment philosophy but who are no less known to us: Jean-Jacques Rousseau (1712—1778) whose political philosophy influenced the French Revolution, John Wesley (1703–1791) whose ministry split the Anglican church and led the Methodist movement, and David Hume (1711–1776) whose works of philosophy, economics, and history had a great impact on Western ideas and were behind the Scottish Enlightenment.

Although the intellectual revolutionary movement of the 1200s was healthy for the mind, the full glare of the Enlightenment did not help health care as much. True advances were made by the great physicians and researchers, but these were mostly theoretical. For example, this was the age when Luigi

Galvani (1737–1798), an Italian anatomist discovered that the muscles of dead frogs twitched when struck by a spark and thus galvanized the world by demonstrating what electricity did for nerves. *Practical* medical advances were somewhat limited. For example, until the invention of anesthesia in the 1840s, invasive surgery was constrained, and surgery was going almost as far as it could go with the tools and conditions available. Recall that thanks to Chauliac, the practice of keeping wounds pus free was not so alien at the time, although substantial improvements in detail would be needed to make this reliable.

But among several success that deserve to be mentioned, one oft neglected is that several discoveries of herbal remedies in the Enlightenment perpetuated the above mentioned useful doctrine of "simples" developed by Thomas Sydenham. Notably, the Reverent Edmund Stone (1702–1768) announced that willow bark (containing aspirin) was a "febrifuge" (fever remedy). These simple factors or "simples" went under study for repeated purification and extraction. Purer extracts of simples and other prominent biological contents such as the molecules of albumin of eggs were to become the objects of scrutiny in the nineteenth century and the first medicinal chemistry, and the basis of molecular medicine in the midtwentieth century.

NINETEENTH-CENTURY MEDICINE: ANALYTICAL COMPUTERS, MOLECULES OF NATURAL PRODUCTS, AND ORGANIC MOLECULES THAT AREN'T

Nineteenth-century medicine is characterized by investigations at the cellular level (including microbial level), the molecular level, and by even more ruthless combination of observation and hypothetical reasoning. Rational, logical methods were notably a feature by the time of late Victorian medicine. For example, Sir Arthur Conan Doyle's medical school teacher taught the system of observation and deduction that is vividly expressed in Doyle's Sherlock Holmes stories.

At the microbial level, any list of great medical research giants of the nineteenth century includes Louis Pasteur (1822–1895), who while deep at work for the brewing and wine industry observed the effectiveness of what we now call pasteurization in destroying microorganisms. At the molecular level Justus von Liebig (1803–1873) helped found modern chemistry. Since space does not permit for too much history, we will focus on two directly relevant developments: early efforts at real computing and the discovery of biological molecules.

Even though computers could not get to work at the time, accounts of nineteenth century attempts to build large mechanical computers reveal a more widespread knowledge of scientific calculation, the appearance of small mechanical calculating aids, and the need to do very challenging calculations. The first device that might be considered to be a computer in the truly modern sense of the word was conceived in 1822 by the eccentric British inventor Charles Babbage. At that time mathematical tables (e.g., logs for navigation) were generated by teams of mathematicians working day and night. Babbage never built his so-called difference engine because he was distracted by an idea for an even more powerful and general *analytical engine*; the difference engine would eventually be constructed from original drawings by a team at London's Science Museum. Cast iron, bronze, and steel were used for its construction. In all there were 4,000 components. The analytical engine ended up weighing three tons, and it was 10 feet wide and 6½ feet tall. But this was a significant miniaturization compared with Lull's 20-foot square frame containing hundreds of small cubes linked together by wires, thought it was basically of the same order of impressiveness.

The next century would introduce electronics, over mechanics, as the way forward in computing. So the enduring force in preparation of a successful machine was in terms of the first true computer programming. It is a remarkable, kind of "small world," story. Augusta Ada Byron was born on December 10, 1815, as the daughter of the poet Lord Byron (Ada, in 1843, married and became Lady Lovelace). Five weeks after Ada was born, her mother Lady Byron asked for a separation from Lord Byron. Going in the reverse direction to the exasperated wives of many crazed scientists to come, Lady Byron was terrified that Ada might end up being a poet like her father, so she pursued and was awarded sole custody of Ada, whom she brought up to be a mathematician and scientist. At a dinner party in 1834, Ada heard of Babbage's ideas for a new calculating engine, the analytical engine. She later conjectured that the machine might be used to generate interesting numbers from number theory, compose complex music, and to produce graphics, as well as serve many practical and scientific purposes. Ada suggested to Babbage a plan for how the engine might calculate integers known as Bernoulli numbers. This is now regarded as the first "computer program." In 1979, a programming language developed by the US Department of Defense was named "Ada" in her honor.

There was also revolution on the biological molecule front. The complex molecules making up the fabric of our bodies are also those we tend to think of (reasonably enough) as key features of our diets. Carbohydrate and fat were early characterized. In 1811 Claude Louis de Bertholet had shown that *albuminous* material, as that from the white of an egg, was different from carbohydrate and fat because it contained not only hydrogen, oxygen, and carbon but also nitrogen. Gerrit Mulder, a Dutch physician, extended this in 1820 to show the presence of sulfur, which is not universally present in proteins. Henri Braconnet, a French naturalist, was making the first step to show in 1820 that these various atoms were focused into smaller units of roughly 20 to 40 atoms, called *amino acids*, that join together in chains to make up proteins. In 1828 Friederich Wohler synthesized urea in his laboratory. Urea had until then been considered a real biological molecule, and to contain hydrogen, oxygen, carbon, and nitrogen the protein, so as a life product it was considered to be totally in the domain of biological systems. Historically this is now seen as the point at which nineteenth century scientists overthrew the notion of life as a special entity or force.

In a hugely formative short period of 1831 to 1840, Gerrit Mulder extracted and studied a ubiquitous material of life which he (or possibly Jöns Jakob Berzelius) called "protein" (from the Greek *proteios*, meaning of the first rank), Berzelius coined the term "catalyst," Matthias Jakob Schleiden (a German botanist) and Theodor Schwann (a German physiologist, histologist and cytologist) established their "cell theory," Hugo von Mohl suggested the name "protoplasm" for the special complex material of these cells, and Charles Darwin laid the groundwork for his theory of evolution. This work formed the bedrock of modern molecular, information-based medicine.

Charles Darwin (1809–1882) deserves special comment not only because of the enormous importance of the concept of evolution to medicine, but because of the (then very difficult) matter of linking this to the "life force" or the chemical basis of life, depending on one's philosophy at that time. Darwin built his ideas on three foundations: (1) the biological classification system of Carl Linnaeus's *Systema Natura* (1735) which hinted that all life was a part of a family tree, (2) Charles Lyell's *Principles* of *Geology* (1830) which demonstrated that the geographic world had evolved, and (3) his worldwide biological studies traveling on the mission of HMS *Beagle* (1831–1836). These ideas led to his *On the Origin of Species* (1859), which was an immediate and controversial sell out, and his *The Descent of Man* (1871), which addressed the controversy of human origins arising from primates in greater detail. Darwin was lost as to the molecular mechanism by which variation might arise and be passed on, conjecturing that microscopic *gemules* from each tissue passed to the sex organs where copies were made for human offspring. It is not a stupid idea: mitochondrion-like extra-chromosomal inheritance factors called *bacteriods* pass from the liver cells of the cockroach (where they provide processing of vitamins) to the sex cells, and are so passed on to descendants, but it just wasn't the universal mechanism. Darwin had the information flow (i.e., tissue to sex cells) wrong, and nothing in his studies would correct it: in theory, evolution could still work either way.

Between the publication of Darwin's two books, in 1865, an Austrian Augustinian Monk called Gregor Mendel published his research on plant inheritance. It should have been a fourth foundation for Darwin's theory, but it did not impact Darwin's second work because these plant breeding studies were to go unnoticed for more than 35 years. That is unfortunate, because they revealed not only how some physical or chemical entity could be responsible for genetics, but more subtly how natural selection, in acting like Mendel picking seeds (peas) from specific plants for selective breeding, could affect evolution without the need of gemules from tissues. We now see that there is, in Darwin's language, a kind of gemule in the human seed and ultimately fertilized egg which *gives rise* to the tissues and organism as a whole, such that if the organism as a whole was at a disadvantage, the seeds would never be selected. They were never selected because they would perish with the organism or their sex cells would fail to be mated with other sex cells, not because the gemules from tissues were required to inform them that the organism was surviving or perishing.

That Darwin missed this subtle difference of mechanism is remarkable because he spent a great deal of time on the details of animal and plant breeding, visiting agricultural markets, and reading seed catalogues. What seemed to divert him from following this direction was two things. First there was his growing feeling that animal and plant breeding as *unnatural* selection was completely irrelevant to *natural* selection as a random progress, as design lacking a designer. This turned out to be true and was a brilliant perception. Unfortunately in discarding his older interests, he "threw a baby out with the bathwater." Second, there is the lack of clarity of thinking that arises when much prevailing opinion saw protoplasm and tissue as a complex interactive medium expressing some vital force in which almost any explanatory mechanism, including Darwin's direction of information flow by gemules, seems equally possible. Again in defense of Darwin, years later, Barry Commoner (b. 1917) would foster a philosophy of highly integrated protoplasm, tissue, and organisms that would be of great value in many areas of biology and ecology. It gave rise to the notion, for a time, that it was the complex system of interactions *per se* that encoded the genetic information, not a molecule, and this was after the discovery of the genetic importance of DNA.

For the US, the *The Descent of Man* controversy was to come to a head much later in 1925 as the Butler Act of the State of Tennessee that made it illegal to teach any theory contesting divine creation. In the "Scopes Monkey Trial" the State of Tennessee tried a biology teacher in regard to that law. It was a matter only finally resolved in 1968 when the Supreme Court ruled in the case of *Epperson v. Arkansas* that any law banning teaching of evolution on creationist grounds was unconstitutional. Specifically, such a law was one *"respecting an establishment of religion; or prohibiting the free exercise thereof; or abridging freedom of speech"* which is in the Bill of Rights of the Congress of the United States.

The pharmaceutical industry today is essentially seen as a primarily an information industry, and that idea partly rests on the notion that nature's solution makes great use of specific information-carrying molecules. DNA carries information about proteins, which in turn in their shape and interatomic forces carry information about the biological molecules and artificial drugs that will bind to them. It also rests on the fact that despite the great complexity of such molecules, they are not fundamentally different from simpler molecules, and so are amenable to the laws of chemistry, and chemical analysis and synthesis. Yet despite the early synthesis of urea, which was relatively very simple (eight atoms), nineteenth-century scientists still hung onto the notion of "life force" in regard to the more complex molecules now known to contain hundreds and even thousands of atoms. Frequently chemists were struck by the slimy, wobbly, flowing form of bodily secretions and extracts, which did not always look so different from the form and motion of an amoeba under the microscope. Mucous, which is primarily a polysaccharide, but also protein, which was often obtained in a colloidal viscous or wobbly jelly forms (e.g., from the white of an egg), often appeared to have lives all their own. Not least, the colloidal viscous or jelly properties became apparently lost on exposure to acid, alkaline, heat, or organic solvents, suggesting that the protein could be killed. Hence as late as 1861 Graham wrote: "The colloid possesses ENERGIA. It may be looked upon as the probable primary source of the force appearing in phenomena of vitality."

Of the nineteenth-century's applied-medicine contributions, rational explanation of infectious disease and hence clean practice, and chemistry, were probably the most notable contributions, including extraction, purification, and even chemical synthesis. Nineteenth- (and twentieth-) century chemistry was preoccupied with discovery and characterization of small molecules of natural origin that were therefore almost always carbon based (as well as later flexing its muscles at some synthesis or simply modification of these natural carbon compounds). In the later nineteenth century, chemistry allowed the development of stains for the specimens on microscopic slides, disinfectants like phenol, and anesthetics like chloroform. Above all, however, it was the development of the roots of pharmaceutical chemistry in which nineteenth-century chemistry revealed its most sophisticated hand, even though the actual application to making real drugs was not really to materialize fully until the twentieth century.

The developments in twentieth-century medicinal chemistry arose, in particular, from the *organic chemistry* introduced in the nineteenth century. The term "organic" needs explanation because it can be confusing to nonchemists even today. In chemistry, "organic" simply means any molecule containing carbon. Unlike "inorganic chemistry," products are obtained from living systems. As the organic chemists flexed their muscle and demonstrated their skills, molecules were synthesized rather than simply extracted and purified. Many natural molecules were chemically modified, and even new types of molecules, not encountered in nature, were made by such modification or even by a completely nonorganic route. More confusing still, there persists to this day the implication that an "organic compound" is specifically *not* of natural origin, that it is synthetic, and further that it is likely to be of low molecular weight. For example, a twentieth-century biotechnology company could partner with a pharmaceutical company in which the former agreed to study the binding of proteins to DNA, and the other the binding of organic compounds as low molecular weight, synthetic carbon-containing compounds.

The ability to "make, not take," such molecules, even without identifying them first in nature, was an important nineteenth-century development that was needed for the medicine of the future. Its effect on the twentieth century was to raise the bulk of medicine from a hunter-gatherer mode to "growing" (in the synthesis sense) and even engineering molecules on demand. But there was still at the end of the nineteenth century a fundamental limitation, which highlights that plants and certain animal, bacterial, and fungal products were nature's great gift of pharmaceuticals to the world right up to the twentieth century. Despite the growing ability of chemists to synthesize novel molecules, the odds of succeeding to make a drug out of the synthesized molecules were vastly against them if their chemical formula drifted too far from the examples given by nature. Hence the discovery of drugs until very recently still depended on serendipity or broad screening (as with the ancient Chinese) to discovering new medicines. This practice still continues, with penicillin from the mold *pencillium* as the famous twentieth-century example.

Could reseach go further and bring computers, medicine, and molecules together? The last part of the nineteenth century was not short of a vision of science fact and fiction. H. G. Wells was in the process of writing just about every science fictional theme in existence today, with quite a bit of fact. But before even thinking about medicine, molecules, and machine, there was a need for a conceptual model for the action of pharmaceutical molecules, and such a model was just beginning to be formulated as the nineteenth century closed.

THE FIRST HALF OF THE TWENTIETH CENTURY: MAGIC BULLETS AND IMAGINARY MOLECULES

It is in the midtwentieth century that computers and molecules first meet up. But at the dawn of the twentieth century there was little understanding of what the interaction between a drug molecule and the body would like in detail, much less how to calculate it.

The important concept that was needed, but missing to establish the rational molecular basis of modern and future medicine, was the concept of the "magic bullet." Its basis was already being developed during the transition from the nineteenth to the twentieth century. The concept had been glimpsed by Thomas Sydenham and others, who noted that each disease seemed to require a "specific" plant extract factor but had no concept of a specific molecular target in the body, for molecules in that extract.

Paul Ehrlich was a young scientist when he joined the research team of Robert Koch. He, along with Emi Behring, developed an interest in the antibodies, sophisticated proteins produced by the human body that interact specifically and strongly with certain molecules against which the body ranges defense, including those at the surface of bacteria, viruses, parasites, and other pathogens. By analogy, this led him to believe that a chemical substance could be produced to work alongside these antibodies, killing specific bacteria without harming the rest of the body. The "magic bullet" was the name given to the much sought after compound that would counteract the spread of infection.

On this basis Ehrlich formed his own research institute, to search for the magic bullet. There he found dyes that attacked malaria and sleeping sickness. Unfortunately, he had picked what remain, even today, hard targets. The big success was in 1906 where the detection by Hoffman of the microbes that caused syphilis—a sexually transmitted disease caused by the bacterium *Treponema pallidum* and also often referred to "the great imitator" because so many of the signs and symptoms are indistinguishable from those of other diseases—opened up a new line of research. Ehrlich's team tested over hundreds of potential antisyphilitic chemical compounds. In 1909 a new boy on the team was given the potentially unrewarding and ignominious task of retesting all of the discarded chemicals that had previously been shown to fail. The 606th compound selected worked, and in 1911 *Salvarsan 606* was used for the first time on humans. Later Ehrlich's work with Behring also led to a cure for diphtheria. Ehrlich was awarded the Nobel Prize for Medicine in 1908 for research in the field of chemotherapy.

By the way, these days nanoscientists are trying to develop a different kind of magic bullet. They are exploiting the unique properties of nanotechnology for self-replication and self-assembly in a living cell, by planning nanoscale robots, nanobots, or nanoparticles to selectively destroy bacteria, cancer cells, and viruses.

In regard to the larger and primary molecules of life, like proteins, the analytic techniques of chemistry revealed very great complexity that did little to dispel the earlier nineteenth-century mystique surrounding them, such as Graham's 1861 assertion that proteins could hold "the force appearing in the phenomena of vitality." Proteins can have thousands, sometimes many thousands, of atoms compared with urea, which has only eight. These thousands of atoms are held together chemically and in space in very specific ways. But around 1902 analytical techniques were not sufficiently reliable. They seemed to reveal complex mixes, even giving the impression that proteins had no specific structure. This difficulty persisted for some 40 years. A review article of the mid-1950s (J. R. Colvin, D. B. Smith, and W. H. Cook, "The microheterogeneity of proteins," *Chem. Rev.* 54 (1954): 687) is the last known publication to argue seriously that a unique chemical and spatial structure for any protein is unlikely, a statement we now know to be quite untrue.

But such major conceptual obstacles to progress were progressively eroded, and by 1943 Richard L. M. Synge (1914–1994), who received the Nobel Prize in chemistry 1952 for the invention of the analytic technique partition chromotagraphy, was at least able to state that "it seems that the main obstacle to progress in the chemistry of protein structure by methods of organic chemistry is inadequacy of technique rather than any theoretical difficulty." Already by 1945, however, Frederick Sanger (b. 1918), the only scientist so far to receive the Nobel Prize in chemistry twice (1958, 1980), was showing specific chemical orders for the amino acid residues in specific proteins, namely that proteins have a specific chemical formula. By the 1950s, protein fragments and small proteins were being analyzed, and even synthesized, quite routinely in laboratories. By 1965, the first automatic laboratory machines for synthesizing proteins were being built by Robert Bruce Merrifield (b. 1921), who received his Nobel Prize for this in 1984. During this period there were of course substantial advances in macroscopic medicine too. For example, heart-lung transplantation became possible in 1953, when the heart-lung machine allowed both organs to be replaced within the time taken to repair disorders of the heart chambers and cardiac vessels. Still in many other areas health care depended on continuing research at the biomolecular level. Notably there was the problem of transplant rejection by the proteins of the immune system, which had yet to be resolved.

The nineteenth century's emerging ability to synthesize small molecules from basic constituents, and the twentieth century's ability to apply this potential to examples drawn from *all* the classes of molecules found in living things, had profound implications. The several millennia of use of chemical products found by serendipity or screening is an era from which Eastern and Western humankind only emerged in the twentieth century, with the design of novel synthetic "organic compounds" *not found in nature*. They were initially imaginary. The molecule being designed did not exist, and the relevant technology and discipline was one of *theoretical* chemistry. In the early twentieth century this discipline emerged particularly in the hand of Paul A. M. Dirac (1902–1984), Nobel Laureate for physics in 1933, who tied up the field of quantum mechanics and laid the basis for modern quantum mechanical calculations.

In 1929 Dirac had stated: "The underlying physical laws necessary for the mathematical theory of a large part of physics and the whole of chemistry are thus completely known, and the difficulty is only that the exact application of these laws leads to equations much too complicated to handle." Computers now began to play that key role: the calculations for designing drugs, based on principles of theoretical chemistry, are far too complex to perform by hand.

THE COMPUTER ERA: BASE 2

Life, as we will explain, runs on base 4: the DNA bases A, G, C, and T. Computers (except analog computers, now rarely used) run on base 2. That is, they are digital and use binary logic for digits, based on two symbols typically expressed as 0 and 1. Deep down, the work in binary logic, such as 1 = true, 0 = false, and binary arithmetic on binary numbers $0 = 0, 1 = 1, 10 = 2, 11 = 3, 110 = 6, 111 = 7, \ldots$, blocks of 8 bits a time (e.g., a byte), could also represent a machine code instruction such as "add" or "jump to another part of the calculation."

IBM computers were in the 1950s the first to be applied extensively to chemical calculations. The new chemists became "quantum chemists," and the keyboard replaced the test tube. By using, as then, relatively slow machines, a famous quantum chemist, Samuel F. Boys (1911–1972), stated: "It has been established that the only factor limiting calculation … is the amount of computing necessary."

With the rise of powerful computers in the 1970s another famous quantum chemist, Enrico Clementi (b. 1931), enthusiastically stated: "We can calculate everything." Well, perhaps one should say—overstated! This was far-fetched for all but the simplest molecules, and Clementi was quick to join IBM to gain access to a high level of computer power not generally available to the average academic researcher. However, his statement reflected the dawning of a new enthusiasm for the power of the union of the science of molecules and of computers. In a sense, as these computers began to be applied to medicinal chemistry and molecular science, they became, the first true *engines of Hippocrates*.

After the 1970s, computers were routinely applied to study and design molecules and increasingly those molecules of importance to the pharmaceutical industry. Eli Lilly, for example, increased the value of its stock by purchasing a Cray supercomputer. Computers in the late twentieth century were also used in medical record keeping, though the full actual patient medical record itself was rarely kept on the computer except the information required for billing.

Computers were soon nonetheless used very extensively in medical image analysis, occasionally of X-ray pictures but especially after the invention of other medically important electronic devices, including (nuclear) magnetic resonance imaging and positron emission tomography. Magnetic resonance imaging (MRI) uses radiofrequency waves and a strong magnetic field to provide remarkably clearer and more detailed pictures of internal organs and tissues in comparison with X rays. The technique has proved valuable for the diagnosis of a broad range of conditions in all parts of the body, including heart and vascular disease and stroke, joint and muscular disorders, and cancer. MRI allows evaluation of some body structures that may not be as visible with other imaging methods. It is widely used to diagnose sports-related injuries, especially those affecting the knee, shoulder, hip, elbow, and wrist. The images allow the physician to see even minute changes and injuries of ligaments and muscles. Imaging methods made a huge impact in some areas of research and raised the level of competition among healthcare providers.

THE GENOMIC ERA: BASE 4

In the 1940s and early 1950s, biological chemsists already knew about DNA's G, C, A, and T parts, and that DNA was a sugar-phosphate–sugar-phosphate polymer with one of each A, G, C, and T nitrogenous bases on the sugar. So one would think that the idea that life is base-4 would be self-evident. However, there were quantitative observations by Erwin Chargaff (1905–2002), and colleagues that made that less obvious. Those readers interested in the history of science, sushi, and exotic seafood will find it interesting to go back to Chargaff's papers and catch the spirit of that:

- D. Elson and E. Chargaff. 1952. On the desoxyribonucleic acid content of sea urchin gametes. *Experientia* 8(4):143–145;

- E. Chargaff, R. Lipshitz, and C. Green. 1952. Composition of the des-oxypentose nucleic acids of four genera of sea-urchin. *J. Biol. Chem.* 195(1):155–160;
- E. Chargaff, R. Lipshitz, C. Green, and M.E. Hodes. 1951. The composition of the deoxyribonucleic acid of salmon sperm. *J. Biol. Chem.* 192(1): 223–230.

What these studies showed is that in DNA the number of G equaled the number of C, and A equaled the number of T. It looks like the information carried by G is that by C, and vice versa, and A by T, and vice versa. While these clues show life to be base 2, generally, the clues were confusing.

Molecular modelers thus put such quantitative work aside for a while. These *molecular modelers* were a new breed of theoretical chemist specializing in large biological molecules, especially proteins and nucleic acids. They worked at first with non-digital calculators. Such calculators would be used up to the early 1960s in laboratories like that of Gopalasamudram Ramachandran in India, who founded a major school of protein molecular modeling and eluci-dated the basic principles of stereochemistry about how proteins adopt their shapes.

In the United States the "wiz kid" of theoretical chemistry in general and biological molecular modeling in particular was Linus C. Pauling (1901–1994), who won the Nobel Prize in chemistry in 1954 and the Nobel Peace Prize in 1962. He had established the α-helical structure of proteins in hair and the β-pleated sheet structure of proteins in silk, and it was becoming apparent that shorter versions of these structures would play important roles as segments of the folded chain of globular proteins such as enzymes and receptors. It was easier to study and verify, by the X-ray crystallography of the time, the stereo-regular periodic structures like α-helix and β-sheet, which are general classes of helix (a staircase-like spiral), with the pitch and other detailed geometric factors yet to be determined. It is no surprise that in the race to understand the DNA structure, Pauling turned to the idea that DNA was some kind of helix. However, the heat of the race seemed to cause Pauling to forget the very chemical laws that he had himself helped establish. He placed the negatively charged phosphate groups on the inside, and the G, C, A, T bases on the outside. It was as if the sense that the message DNA had to be read from the surface (presumably by proteins) overwhelmed his sense of the electrostatic repulsive force. (What good would a good old gramophone record of the time be, if the grooves were somehow buried inside the record, not accessible to the gramophone needle?)

The so-called Human Genome Project (actually "projects") was made pos-sible by the work of Francis Crick (1916–2004) and James D. Watson (b. 1928) in 1953, who got the correct structure. Using individually ambiguous data from X-ray crystallography, chemistry, and biology, they were able to deduce that DNA was a double helix of two chains of nucleotides running in opposite directions. Each nucleotide is a sugar-phosphate molecule with a side chain, so the two strands of the DNA helix were polymeric chains of nucleotides:

again, a sugar-phosphate–sugar-phosphate–sugar- ... backbone with side chains on each sugar. The side chains are nitrogenous bases. Importantly, the bases of four types A (adenine), G (guanine), C (cytosine), and T (thymine), formed the cross links of the double helix, or rungs of the DNA ladder, by each A pairing with T, and each G with C. Since each strand is a complementary copy of the other, either sequence alone defines the genetic information contained. Going up the helix shows a sequence, for example, G–C, C–G, A–T, C–G, T–A, T–A, and so forth, until we have genetic information, which can be represented as GCACTT ... , on one strand, or by AAGTGC ... , on the other. (Remember, the two strands run in opposite direction, so replace A by T, T by A, C by G, and G by C, and write the second derived sequence backwards!) Because the bases really come in pairs (e.g., C–G) as rungs of the ladder, scientists tend to speak of *base pairs* (bp for short) even if they only mention just one letter in the sequence on one strand. So, GATTACAGATTACA is said to be a specific section of sequence of 14 base pairs.

Note again the subtlety of the code for DNA. Where one strand has a G, the other has C, and vice versa, and where one has an A, the other has T, and vice versa. What could previously have misled is that the almost digital-like coding half suspected for DNA, and hence genetics and inheritance, seemed to suggest that in replication of DNA the simplest mechanism would be to have G as a copy of G, C of C, A of A, and T of T, yet G carries *the same information* as C *on the other strand*, C as G, A as T, and T as A. At the same time the double helix model shows that G and C *on the same strand* carry *distinct, nondegenerate, information*, and so do A and T. Even though at first glance it might look like base 2, it is truly base 4! Perhaps the clue should have been that life, love, and sex are based on complementary couples, like G with C and A with T.

But what of the need to read the DNA from the surface, if the A–T and G–C pairs are tiled up with each in the interior? The strands would have to unwind to be read and replicate! And so they do. It looked almost as if Pauling had dismissed something in the clue (but certainly would have thought about it) that cells divide to replicate, and so it makes a kind of intuitive sense if their DNA molecules do too, with each strand going to each cell and forming the template for formation of double-stranded DNA again, in each daughter cell. That is, the G–C and A–T pairs are also the basis of which DNA, and all living things, replicate. The strands separate, and then the complementary copy is built on each, yielding two new DNA molecules. With the crucially important caveat that mutations and exchanges of genetic material are bases of evolution, these DNA molecules are otherwise identical to the original. Incidentally, however, Pauling's gut sensed that the DNA should be read from the outside is not entirely wrong. Many proteins and some anticancer drugs bind to DNA and read what is there through the "cracks" or more properly grooves. The proteins will act on that information, in many control processes. But this is a very local reading, a glance through a crack.

The internal G–C, A–T pairing is the true machine code of the living organism, with one copy per cell, disposed in several archives called chromosomes.

Again, it is a base 4 code, since there are four types of symbol, compared with just 0 and 1 for a base 2 code. Each base, A, G, C, or T can be represented by at least two bits of information (e.g., 0 or 1). It is not the code throughout the process, however. It is the same essentially for RNA, which carries out from the chromosomes and the nucleus copies of each active gene in the cell. These are messages, faxes from the nucleus, and instructions for how proteins will be constructed from the joining together of amino acids. Three RNA (and hence originally three DNA) bases code for each amino acid, making it potentially a base $4 \times 4 \times 4 = 64$ code. For example, GAC codes for the amino acid aspartate. So protein can be built in the cell by the sequence of these triplets such as GAC, which put the appropriate amino acids into an appropriate order. However, because of degeneracy in the mechanism (refined by evolution), some of these triplets code for same amino acid, and some for nothing, which are the "stop codons" saying where the instruction for assembly of a protein stops. In consequence there are only 20 types of amino acid in protein (at least, before metabolic or "posttranslational" modification) that determine how proteins fold up and function. So the next layer of the code is effectively base 20.

And with 20 types of amino acid, so is the mysterious code of how that sequence can determine how proteins fold up more or less in seconds into their functional form. That is the notorious *protein folding problem*. In other words, it is a code not yet fully cracked. We can make any DNA and hence any protein. So if that code could be cracked, we could, like billions of years of evolution, make new proteins to order. But we can at least read and to a good extent understand, if not exactly yet write exquisite new essays!

In a nutshell, armed with these understandings, the reader and scientists worldwide are now in the same position, imperfect but promising, as archeologists who have just recently penetrated the mysteries of an ancient language.

READING THE BOOK OF AGES

Effectively, by seeing the DNA double helix, Crick and Watson had opened a book some three billion years old and cracked the alphabet. The very structure of the book, once glimpsed, spelled *that* out. But the "seeing tools" of the time, both physical and chemical, were not powerful enough magnifying glasses to read the stories therein. That is obviously important to do: after all, the primary aim of deciphering the Rosetta Stone and cracking the secret of Egyptian writing was to gain new information about history that could subsequently be read from a huge number of stone and papyrus sources. Now through the genome projects billions of years of prehistory were transformed into history, written down in molecular structure, and that history also included encyclopedias of what makes us human. Better still, as for the translation of ancient Egyptian medical papyri, much medical wisdom lay therein.

As some DNA sequences began to be determined chemically, much as protein sequence had been sequenced before, the role of *bioinformatics* to manage and analyze the data became important. The twentieth century also brought the requisite computational discipline of bioinformatics, as a term first defined by the European Commission in 1984 in response to a Whitehouse memo that Europe was falling behind the United States and Japan in biotcehnology. The definition has gone through several variations, but it has always been forward-looking and comprehensive in relating the complex information inherent in living systems to the storage and analysis of data. DNA and protein sequences (the essential chemical formula of our most important macromolecules) have always been a key theme, and this is beginning to be extended to the DNA of individual patients. Some conservative definitions of bioinformatics used in industry concentrated only on analysis of the sequence of bases in DNA. Related to genomics and also requiring bioinformatics is the emergence of the study of the proteins and their interactions within living organisms, and the "expression arrays" that read the transcriptome (i.e., detect what mRNA is being expressed as messages from DNA in the cell nucleus, and hence what proteins are being made).

At first bioinformatics had relatively "small" DNA databases to deal with, and pieces of DNA telling just a fragment of the story. Soon arose the genome projects to sequence the whole DNA of various species of organism, benefiting from the fact that the tools of bioinformatics were in position. Notably the Smith–Waterman procedure, and BLAST (Basic Local Alignment Search Tool), were available to identify DNA sequences as related by parts of sequence in common. This is effectively the only way of "looking up" any DNA sequence in a database, unless the sequence is already categorized by species, genes, functions, intercommunication mechanisms, disease consequences, and so on. To get some sense of the acceleration of progress, remember that since each base A, G, C, or T on one strand of DNA matches T, C, G, or A on the other, it is paired, and somewhat confusingly are called *base pairs* or bp. The first billion bp of human DNA were sequenced in four years, ending in November 1999, and the second billion bp just in four months, ending in March 2000. The first chromosome, number 22 in the human cell, was published in December 1999. In addition to chromosome 22, sequencing of human chromosomes 21, 19, 16, and 5 was soon completed.

The twentieth century did not see the fuller culmination of these technologies, however. The completion of the first draft of the Human Genome was announced on June 26, 2000, from Washington. At the close of the twentieth century there was very much an awareness of the formidable amount of DNA, protein, image and other data still to be processed. The noted "bioinformatician" Temple Smith of Boston University (and of the Smith–Waterman bioinformatics tool mentioned above) described the case of late-twentieth-century bioinformaticians as "children playing with delight with pebbles on the beach, unaware of the coming Tsunami."

For the Human Genome Project some 16 international centers participated, with the Whitehead Institute at MIT in Cambridge, Massachusetts, taking a strong role in the United States. But it was freelancer J. Craig Venter, the "wild boy" of the genomics world, who probably did most. He founded Celera to map the human genome in detail using a technique called "shotgun" in which the DNA is fragmented at random, and then the short fragments are sequenced. This drew criticisms of the quality of the result, namely the correctness of the sequence, but the technique worked. Since many DNA molecules are actually fragmented, there will be lots of duplicated overlapping sections between the fragments. If this is done extensively enough, there will be overlaps at the ends of most fragments, so most of the entire DNA sequence can be deduced rather like the full picture in a jig saw puzzle nearing completion. If you do the math, even just a section 10 base pairs long can be unique. To ensure enough overlap, there was typically 10-fold coverage, then assembly by overlaps, and then "finishing" by correcting errors and resolving ambiguities. If just 10 base pairs can be unique, why 10 times? Well, to be sure, the exact degree of uniqueness depends on exactly what the sequence is, and also the laws of probability imply that overlaps will not be found some of the time, so the fragmentation is repeated until that probability becomes very small. But one of the main reasons that such extensive coverage is required is that outside the region of DNA that represents genes, and there is a lot of that outside in human DNA, the sequence has a lot of repeating patterns. That makes it difficult to know that a larger sequence is being deduced from overlapping sections, since the apparent duplication might only reflect a common repeating section.

Advances in computation greatly contributed to the above-mentioned burst in efficiency in reading the genome. While many thanks are due to the fully automatic capillary sequencers, micro-electrophoresis chips, and their flat-out efforts, sequencing 24 hours a day, 7 days a week, much more is due to improvements in downstream processing power, real-time process control, databases with 6 terabytes of storage, as well as, in the laboratory, automated quality control with data-driven process control.

A general approach for genomics, once the sequencing of genome is complete, is to (1) identify genes(s) of interest, (2) characterize genes and the SNPs, and (3) test polymorphisms (i.e., SNPs or SNiPs). There are small differences between the sequences of individuals in a species; they relate to the now popular term genomic *biomarkers* (as mentioned in Chapter 2). The next major step once the genes are found is to discover the function, an activity known as functional genomics. These approaches require significant computing power, storage, and analytical software. Determining the three-dimensional structure of genome is also computationally intensive, even if it is basically experimental in using X-ray crystallography, the diffraction of X rays to work out where all the atoms are.

Recall that the official "completion" of the human genome was on June 26, 2000. According to Jill Mesirov at the Whitehead Institute, a major center for the project, the working draft at that time was estimated to have 99.9% accuracy with 97% assembled mapped clones and 85% assembled DNA sequences, a total of 2.6 billion base pairs sequenced. About 90% of known genes was found in the first draft. More completion took place in 2003 with repeated coverage done about 7 times, yielding 99.99% accuracy. According to Ed Uberbacher at the Department of Energy, we had as of June 26, 2000, some 5,805 cloned sections, 2,649 overlapping or contiguous sections, 596.88 megabases, 20,792 hits on known marker sequences called STSs, and 3,414 genes were archived in the major data bank Genbank of National Center for Biotechnology Information (NCBI). Exactly 24,773 genes were at that time suspected by a neural network program called GRAIL, trained to spot genes in DNA.

There were two main surprises from the sequencing of a whole human genome. The first was that the DNA used was Craig Venter's own DNA. Another surprise was that programs like GRAIL seemed to be finding only about 30,000 genes in the human genome. How little of the human genome is actually taken up by genes? Only 1.1% to 1.4% of our DNA actually codes for proteins, through an intermediate step called RNA (ribonucleic acid). Another 2% codes for RNA but is never converted into protein. More like 80,000 to 120,000 genes were expected, based on the number of proteins that could be made in the body. In the period 1985 to 1999 everyone quoted the number of distinct genes in the human genome (3 billion base pairs) as in that kind of range. However, that number has been revised downward significantly (by most geneticists), first as a result of the completion of chromosomes 21 and 22, where the distribution of genes was found to be somewhat less dense than expected. What makes numbers of genes around 30,000 seem particularly remarkable is that we have only a few more genes than fruit flies (13,000), worms (19,000), or even a plant (25,000). In fact humans have only 300 genes not present in the mouse.

In 2000 there were lotteries being organized to predict exactly how many genes there were in humans. One was organized by David Stewart, director of the Conference at the Cold Spring Harbor Laboratory on Long Island, New York. The winner was to be declared in 2003, by which time the scientific community was expected to reach a consensus and the person closest would be declared the winner. The winner was to take all, with ties dividing the pot equally. By the time the lottery got underway, 38,000 genes had been identified, so any betting less must be of the opinion that some of these "found" genes would ultimately be taken back as being in error.

Was the number of genes surprisingly small because GRAIL failed to spot some genes? GRAIL was not alone. Approaches for gene recognition could also be done by sequence homology (BLASTX, TBLASTX, FLASH, ...), and by statistical analysis of the nucleotide sequences (FGENEH, GenLang, ...). Spotting a gene is not a trivial matter. One has to define the genomic organization: exons/introns from the RNA, and regulatory elements or motifs. Nothing suggested that the number of genes was much larger, however.

Several have felt that up to about 50,000 genes in humans is still a reasonable figure for protein coding genes (RNA-making genes are usually counted separately). However, the reason for this estimate may turn out to be an intellectual bias, perhaps an anthropocentric bias, on the reasonable expectation that a complex organism like a human should have many more. However, if the following latest data is correct, and if the number of genes is a measure of complexity, then we are only some 22 times more complex than the largest known viruses (these are the mimiviruses with about 911 protein-coding genes). The US Department of Energy is a recognized authority in DNA research (and originally largely because of the mutating effects of radiation). Its web page http://www.ornl.gov/sci/techresources/Human_Genome/faq/genenumber.shtml gives updated information about the number of genes in a human. As of September 19, 2008, it stated that the International Human Genome Sequencing Consortium, led in the United States by the National Human Genome Research Institute (NHGRI) and the Department of Energy (DOE), reduced the number from 35,000 to only 20,000–25,000. The consortium researchers confirmed the existence of 19,599 protein-coding genes in the human genome and identified another 2,188 DNA segments that are predicted to be protein-coding genes.

The ability to do a quick estimate of the number of genes in the genome of any organism arises because of a lucky break in biology (confirmation will require evidence that the gene is potentially active, that is, that the information in the gene is at some time and in some tissues expressed). Some 94 of the 1,278 protein families (groups of proteins sharing similar structures and usually similar functions) are unique to vertebrates (though that still means that we humans share 93% of our protein heritage with flies and snails!). Within the vertebrates the corresponding genes are recognizably similar between species, but the surrounding DNA differs quite extensively, highlighting the difference between gene and non-gene nucleotides. So, for example, comparison between human and mouse DNA by computer could identify the genes as regions of similarity, and the surrounding DNA as regions of enhanced variation. This surrounding DNA accounts for 96.6% of human genome and is the so-called junk DNA, consisting largely short and long repeating sequences, like a stuttering message, which had been thought to be without function. The repeated sequences are nonrandomly distributed in the genome, with some found in gene-rich regions and others found in gene-poor regions. Is all this stuttering junk unimportant to life? The puffer fish, a bony fish known for its potent neurotoxin, has very few repeats in its genome, and yet that creature lives pretty well. There is evidently some difference in sophistication between a puffer fish and a human. Maybe the "junk" regions are more than space fillers and not as useless as first thought. In any event, the puffer fish with its near-absence of junk DNA helped highlight the genes. It suggested that there were 28,000 to 34,000 human genes, which in the same ballpark as the surprising new estimates.

It turns out that the huge variety of proteins is actually due largely to "alternative splicing." The DNA does not make proteins directly: each gene is first copied into RNA, a molecule similar to DNA but that codes in turn for the proteins directly. Since RNA sequences can be shuffled in various ways, this generates a variety of proteins, say four types, from each master gene. In billions of years of evolution the shuffled RNA molecules and resulting protein mostly do not represent random nonsense; they do something useful in the living cell. Some 90% of genes discovered were publicly released. However, how many proteins are there? The number does seem to go up and down. Contrary to the first form of the "central dogma" (one gene makes one RNA molecule makes one protein), we now see that one gene can make many proteins because they can be subsequently modified in different ways. Since some proteins live pretty dynamic life cycles with much modification anyway, this phenomenon begs the question of whether many proteins are really just the same with "plastic surgery," or fundamentally different. Proteins are a "fuzzy set," and not so countable!

READING DNA JUNK MAIL

Let us go back to the junk DNA, which occupies 96.6% of human genome but are not used in the process of protein synthesis. The scientists are just beginning to figure out why they are there and what they do to us. That is why it was previously called junk DNA. Almost right up to this day, it has seemed a distraction to the pharmaceutical industry. "Willst du immer weiter schweifen? Sieh, das Gute liegt so nah. Lerne nur das Glueck ergreifen, Denn das Gulueck ist immer da," claimed the famous German writer, Johann Wolfgang von Goethe (1749–1832). That is, "Wilst thou always wander farther? See the good doth dwell so near. Learn this one lesson, to pluck the flower of happiness, for it is ever by thy side." The good in the case of DNA is that while there are many tedious repetitive regions, just like junk mail and TV commercials, the so-called junk regions are worth the wander. They are rich in processes controlled by RNA. Recent work gives for some regions not a picture of a static ancient junk yard, but of a boiling sea of DNA-to-RNA and RNA-to-DNA backcopying reminiscent of the physicists' "quantum foam" in the fine structure of space and time. Such quantum foam may be the origin of the viruses. It may be vital for evolution, with multiple copies and silent genes waking to be awoken. Its more immediate role in cell control, however, is already indicated by the fact that mutations in the junk regions can cause cancers. Clearly, the so-called junk cannot be ignored.

But how much does the DNA "junk" matter for biomedicine, compared with the genes and their well-known controlling regions elsewhere? Overall genome size, and so the amount of junk DNA, are correlated with organism complexity. But the rule is often broken. The genome of the unicellular *Amoeba dubia* appears to contain more than 200 times the amount of DNA in humans, while the pufferfish *Takifugu rubripes* genome is only about one-tenth the size of the human genome, and seems to have a comparable number of genes. That is, the difference between this ameoba, the pufferfish, and us appears to lie in what is now known largely as junk DNA, and the correlation graph of amount of junk DNA with the axis of amoeba–pufferfish–

human of increasing organsim complexity has a nasty great kink in it. It is a mystery.

The answer may lie in one or more of a variety of types of non-coding RNA (ncRNA) that have recently been discovered, mainly in the "junk" regions. ncRNA is defined as a functional RNA molecule that is not translated into a protein, or, more precisely, one that is suspected not to do so. Non-coding RNA genes of relatitively short length include highly abundant and functionally important RNAs such as transfer RNA (tRNA) and ribosomal RNA (rRNA), as well as RNAs such as snoRNAs, microRNAs or miRNAs, siRNAs, and piRNAs. There is also a class of long ncRNAs that include examples with less descriptive names such as Xist and HOTAIR. The number of ncRNAs encoded within the human genome is unknown, but thousands are expected. Many have not been validated for their function, and so it remains possible that some are non-functional.

However, the miRNA are a form of single-stranded RNA which is typically 20–25 nucleotides long, and known to regulate the expression of other genes. Though small, the laws of combinatorial mathematics and information theory are such that this number of bases is enough to recognize one or relatively few sites in a genome or a nucleic acid made from such sites. Control is indeed known to be by base pairing to a complementary DNA or most often RNA sequence. Of course the DNA coding for it contains such complementary sites. Possibly to stop it interfering by such complementary binding with its own production, the processing steps for maturing an miRNA are quite complicated. The DNA sequence that codes for an miRNA gene is longer than the miRNA, including the miRNA sequence and an approximate reverse complement. When this DNA sequence is transcribed into a single-stranded RNA molecule, the miRNA sequence and its reverse-complement base pair region do indeed pair up, the RNA chain overall folding back on itself to form a double-stranded RNA hairpin loop. Drosha, a nuclear enzyme, cleaves the base of the hairpin to form pre-miRNA. The pre-miRNA molecule is then actively transported into the nucleus by Exportin 5, a carrier protein. The Dicer enzyme then cuts 20–25 nucleotides from the base of the hairpin to release the mature miRNA. An miRNA is complementary to a part of one or more messenger RNAs (mRNAs), usually at a site in the region called the 3′ UTR. This binding neutralizes the messenger RNA and so inhibits its translation into a protein amino acid sequence. In some cases, it is believed that the formation of the double-stranded RNA through the binding of the miRNA triggers the degradation of the mRNA transcript through a process which can be induced artificially, by inhibitory RNAs of potential pharmaceutical value. In other cases it is believed that the miRNA complex blocks the protein translation machinery in some way, without causing the mRNA to be degraded.

Complexity of an organism may be more correlated to the number and/or complexity of as yet unidentified functional ncRNA genes than to the number of genes coding for proteins. All this carefully evolved RNA system may be a glimpse of other more complex systems in "junk" DNA, and a living fossil of an "RNA world" of life that existed in the early primordial sea before the ability to make proteins appeared. In this world without proteins, RNA folded up in a way to have (a fairly limited set of) enzymatic functions, and even DNA had not yet appeared as a sophisticated central archive of information. New findings may continue to place proteins in the same relation to nucleic acids as vitamins are placed in relation to proteins. Vitamins are a rather small number of essential small molecules that proteins require in order to help them do certain sophisticated tasks (typically, specific types of catalysis), chemical tricks that are difficult or impossible for proteins to accomplish alone. Similarly proteins may be products of a relatively small number of genes in an organism, and certainly represent more elaborate folding and functional chains of 20 types of chemical unit, not the four units of nucleic acids. They can certainly do many sophisticated chemical things that nucleic acids cannot do alone. So we see that at each stage of life at the fundamental level, the density of chemical information in any small volume of space, and the chemical repertoire (essentially quantum mechanical tricks), increases as we go from nucleic acid to protein and from protein to protein-plus-vitamin. However, the minimal set of sophisticated chemical tricks needed for amoeba, puffer fish, and human was settled long ago, and has little to do with complexity, which resides in sophisticated control.

These are recent perceptions, so it is useful to consider what it will mean for the biopharmaceutical industries. So far with the exception of certain anti-cancer drugs, and some research into synthetic inhibitory RNA molecules, proteins remain the primary targets, and will remain of great importance. The drug molecules will bind to and inhibit or activate their natural functions. But there may be an increasing use of nucleic-acid-like molecules as targets to other natural nucleic acid models, which is for example the aim of Asuragen Inc. in Austin, Texas. In addition, there is now the possibility to keep the bases A, G, C, and T responsible for recognition, and to create new drugs, diagnostics, and biotechnological tools, and maybe ultimately even new life forms, by replacing the backbone by another chemistry, say peptide-like (see Peter E. Nielsen, "A new molecule of life," *Scientific American* 2006;299(6):64–71).

INTO THE "POST–GENOMIC ERA"

Pulled along by the Human Genome Project and its commercial counterparts, the pharmaceutical industry quickly developed new approaches for the identification of genes related to complex high-incidence diseases and tests to qualify users of a particular drug. During the earliest days of the post–genomic era, 10% to 25% of SmithKline Beecham and 10% of Glaxo drug leads were already genomic, causing them to reasonably expect genomic-based entities to represent at least 25% pre annum of the "new chemical entities" (NCEs), which are basically new drugs. It was presumed that this percentage would increase dramatically, say to 75%. In just six years the market for the genomics products and services used in the pharmaceutical industry's R&D efforts was worth many tens of millions, even soon hundreds of millions, of dollars.

The historical phase following the announcement of the completion of the first draft of the human genome in Washington is called, somewhat misleadingly, the post–genomic era. Why exactly is that? Technologies using the DNA data directly most often fall into the class of diagnostics. Although this is very beneficial, it is the next layer on top of genomics, and it is laying the groundwork for the most sophisticated medicine of the future. This layer includes proteomics, comprising protein expression research and the understanding of protein interactions (though based on genomics). Proteomics and RNA detection arrays are concerned with how protein production is regulated by demand, and proteomics in its broadest definition is concerned with how proteins fold up to achieve their structure and function, too. These aspects are *downstream* of the genomic code as represented in the DNA. So it is not so much that we are in a post *genomic-era*, but a *post–genomic* era, that is, in the (PG)E not P(GE), to highlight the grammatical structure of the term algebraically. It is being after the genomics, not after the era, to which the term does, or ideally should, refer.

With microarrays chipsets the DNA expression levels can be monitored for thousands of different genes, and their correlated expression can lead to their function and their pathways of interrelationships. In studying biochemical pathways and disease, it is noted that there are many genes in each pathway and many pathways for each disease (e.g., the biological hypotheses for diabetes). Surprising benefits for humans come from the use of model (non-human) systems, such as drosophila yeast and *Caenorhabditis elegans*, that are beginning to lead us to a better understanding of the functions of genes, such as by genes identified based on homology in the insulin signaling pathway in *C. elegans*. One important tool in all this involves devices that in future forms will doubtlessly play an important role in doctor's office scenarios where, with micro-array chip sets, expression levels for thousands of different genes would be monitored, and their correlated expression, to aid the diagnosis of disease.

By current definition, proteome means simply the internal protein-world of the organism while genome represents its internal DNA world. This definition invokes the all-important issue of three-dimensional structures of proteins, which are in turn the basis of the rational design of drugs. It also invokes many other aspects of protein function, such as protein–protein and protein–drug interactions. Within such broad definition, many companies are now active in areas that can reasonably be described as proteomics.

Thanks to genomics, it is now much easier to deduce the amino acid sequence of a protein than by the older method of direct chemical analysis ("protein sequencing"). It is much harder to get a protein's three-dimensional structure than to get its sequence (i.e., essentially its chemical formula). The latter can be simply be deduced from the sequence of DNA, while the former is a major topic in other grand projects that will impact considerably on both current medicine and future personalized medicine. The most important protein structure data bank (the Protein Data Bank, PDB) was established in October 1971 at Brookhaven following a community discussion about how to establish an archive of protein structures following the Cold Spring Harbor meeting in protein crystallography. By this activity, most folding patterns for proteins may have been discovered, and much of the world of protein structure may be known. That is good news, because while it is much harder to get the three-dimensional structure of a protein than to get its sequence, it is also much harder to predict a protein's three dimensional structure than it is to experimentally determine it. Unfortunately, by "much of the world of protein structure may be known" relates to recurrent themes in parts of the protein structure, called domains, not so much whole proteins. Predicting protein structure, and indeed designing new protein structure, at present mainly consists of trying to recognize these domains as hinted by the sequence, and putting together these three-dimensional pieces into an overall model. It all feels a bit like building cottages in the Dark Ages by scavenging building blocks from more sophisticated Roman structures.

To truly enable high efficacy of personalized medicine, however, requires us to go beyond the molecular players and understand the whole play. It demands a deep and biologically holistic understanding of how interactions of therapeutics with one or more proteins of the patient will affect the patient overall and the patients disease state. We must obtain very highly detailed and unified views of all data relating to each gene and pathway: interactions, pathway biology, linkage, and gene expression, linked to an understanding of drug consequences not only at the proteomic level but also the cytomic and physiomic levels. Through extensive collaborations the first steps are being made in this enormously computationally intensive undertaking, by way of the complete virtual human (homo *in silico*) projects. The rapidly accumulating data about interhuman genomic diversity are suggesting pragmatic solutions on how to identify and treat disease even though a fully detailed understanding has yet to come.

THE RISE OF PERSONALIZED MOLECULAR MEDICINE

The genome projects have given us a story significantly more refined than we ever learned from the school biology of the present generation of researchers. From such a qualitative and quantitative understanding of the basis of our individuality, we have learned that approximately one in a thousand nucleotides distinguishes each of us: this corresponds to very roughly one amino acid residue difference per protein. Recently this estimate has practically doubled. Recall that differences due to one base pair (or few) constitute *genotypes* or single nucleotide polymorphisms (SNP, SNiP, or occasionally simple nucleotide polymorphisms). About 1 million SNPs were discovered by the year end of 2000 and 2 million by the end of summer in 2001. It has subsequently been almost impossible to keep track, noting again that if we all differ by about two base pairs A, G, C, or T in every thousand of the human genome, the theoretical upper limit is huge. Some might even say that almost every base in our DNA could be different in one or few people, and yet ultimately still be shown as relevant to medicine. What matters perhaps more for medical purposes is the number that become officially recognized biomarkers for clinical use. For each disease state there are relatively few at present but the number is constantly growing, enhanced by the capability to use mass spectrometry to look at the protein products of genes directly. For example, protein products called prolactin (PRL), p53, Bcl-2, c-erb B2, Ki-67, CD44, and factor VIII-related antigen (FVIII-RA) are being researched for suitability in identification of primary tumors of stage II and stage III breast cancer and its correlation with disease prognostication. That has been until recently the typical "mere handful" per disease state. Even so, the rapid rise and application of proteomic technologies has still resulted in an exponential increase in the number of proteins (including "normal" proteins abnormally expressed, in the wrong tissue at the wrong time as well as protein variants) that have been proposed for consideration as clinically useful biomarkers. The number approved for use by the Food and Drug Administration has *not* similarly risen in likewise manner, indicating the perceived need to validate their effectiveness as clinical diagnostics.

But there is also awareness that the biomarkers becoming known for each disease are not just optional choices as diagnostics for a particular disease, but interact with each other and others in such a way such that their pattern that becomes important. In fact, simple determinates such as those for eye color are the exception, not the rule. It is a complex issue in advanced combinatorial and logical analytics: a mere handful is more than enough to worry about. Consider, for example, that the reality to be discovered and proven might be that biomarker A will indicate a disease if B and C are present (though B and C themselves do not indicate the disease), but the appearance of D and E together, providing F is not present, will cancel the appearance of the disease. And by the way, perhaps that rule switches to a completely different one if G is present! Considering up to about G, that is, up to about seven players, may be reasonable. On average, the logic that biology uses must in worst cases reflect that the number of protein–protein interactions in which a particular protein is involved is about five, and more precisely three to four for proteins of about 200 amino acid residues or less, and six to seven for those of about 800 amino acid or more (see J. Warringer and A. Blomberg, *BMC Evol. Biol.* 2006; 6: 61 published at http://www.pubmedcentral.nih.gov/articlerender.fcgi). On the other hand, one may conclude from the above that very roughly 100 amino acids represents a recognition domain for protein-to-protein signaling, and many proteins are much larger than that 1,000. There are also more interactions through metabolites and in some cases binding to DNA and RNA, though if one takes 100 as the size of a typical recognition element of a protein, not just for protein binding, that gives some sense of the complexity.

The sequence diversity in the human population appears limited when compared to the difference between chimpanzee and human 1 in just 100 nucleotides. Still the roughly one-to-one correspondence of polymorphism and protein has highly significant consequences. The present routine-use technology of course is not error-free, and likely by an error of 1 in 1,000 nucleotides, which is about the same frequency as the polymorphisms. Hence a major goal is to achieve 1 error in 10,000.

Roughly half the diseases that we present our doctors are due to pathogens; the rest are genetic. How do our genes relate to our diseases? Typically a loss of gene function is responsible. In any event, in molecular-disease studies the general approach used is (1) identify the gene or genes of interest, (2) correlate with a disease, and (3) study it in a population. The candidate genes can be found from gene expression analysis, linkage, and model systems. Linkage analysis, which gives positional candidates for genes, involves building a genetic tree, and it yields better results when two individuals in family share disease. The procedure is relatively straightforward for monogenetic traits, but it becomes ambiguous for polygenetic traits. The follow-up to genomewide linkage scan (i.e., finding variant in genes in candidate regions and interdependencies between them) is considered difficult although ultimately tractable.

What are these consequences, or having roughly one amino acid difference per protein? There is no such thing as a fraction of an amino acid coded for by a base-pair triplet. Thus this is the minimal quantum of variation that we can expect to have to allow two otherwise identical proteins to express or function differently, or interact differently with other proteins and molecules, including therapeutic drugs. Of course, some effects will be neutral, and others lethal. Also the interaction is not uniformly one to one between polymorphism and protein: many of our proteins will be identical, and some will vary by two or more residues. Yet we can still safely speculate that this quantum of variation representing the minimal possible effective individual variation within the species is remarkable, and no mere coincidence but of important evolutionary benefit. Be that as it may, we can be sure that within the individual human lifetime it poses powerful challenges, since our variation effectively demands that health care be tackled on a personal basis cognizant of the differences in our genomes and the proteins structures for which they code.

There is an assumption or two here that should be dealt with; in particular, can we expect changes with effects on health, and in responses to drugs, from just one amino acid within the human species? Certainly examples are abundant of loss of function due to one amino acid change: this is the most common interpretation of what happens when one inherits a recessive gene. Considering, however, proteins that have survived the natural selection process, nature often seems to resist changes in the relevant functional regions despite considerable other variation. That is, the binding and catalytic sites are frequently the most conserved part of the structure. Even distantly related proteins can have very similar geometries. Examples considered by Arthur M. Lesk include

YabJ (*Bac*) and YigF (*E. coli*); both are trimetric complexes of proteins with similar active sites. In another example, a Japanese team led by Nobuhoro Go examined a data set of 491 phosphate binding sites with a common functional step, the binding of a phosphate group. They found that one local atomic configuration is retained throughout each superfamily, which between families showed considerable variation. Hence we might conclude from such examples that it is hard to qualitatively affect the role of a protein, provided that the function is retained at all.

Equally well, we can sooner or later expect to find many examples of variations in function, qualitative as well as quantitative, when an amino acid residue changes and the gross function is retained. A long known example discussed earlier is sickle cell anaemia where the differential response to oxygen might be described as more significant than quantitative difference, since it confers resistance to blood parasites in the original homeland of the population. Further there are examples of functional changes even with changes in conditions around the protein that is otherwise chemically identical. Therefore something as drastic as a change to the chemical constitution could be reasonably expected to be important. For example, *E. coli* HtrA (DegP) is a chaperone at low temperature and a protease at high temperature. Last but by no means the least, there are examples in comparing proteins where the differential action of a potential drug is different due to a change in one or few amino acid residues. For one example, inhibitors of blood clotting bind differently to human and bovine thrombin because of a change in a charged residue in the protein.

There are many processes that affect proteins and can modify or transform them, and these too can differ by genomics, often with serious consequences for the function of the protein modified. Posttranslational modification involves enzymes that can add chemical susbstances such as sugars and lipids to modify the protein. A protease is any enzyme that conducts proteolysis, meaning begins or ends protein metabolism by hydrolysis of the peptide bonds that link amino acids together in the polypeptide chain. Some proteins can have complex life histories, functioning both as hormone-like signallers and receptors at different stages of their life cycles, with each stage marked by a chemical modification or proteolytic cleavage. There is a growing appreciation that some of the more complex proteins, such as the *sonic hedgehog* protein associated with embryological development, and prion protein associated with memory and mad cow disease, can have complex life styles involving several modifications of proteins, spending part of their time as receptors that receive signals to cells and ligands that carry the signal information to receptors. The structure of some such proteins can even contain parts with enzymic function so that such proteins can perform these modifications on themselves, on the fly.

In molecular biology, chaperones are not kindly old ladies but proteins that assist the noncovalent folding or unfolding and the assembly or disassembly of other macromolecular structures. Chaperones, however, do not usually occur in relation to these structures when the latter are performing their normal biological functions. The common perception that chaperones are primarily concerned with protein folding is incorrect, and transportation and more complex roles in the lives of proteins have been indicated.

In the effects of single amino acid changes resulting from genomic changes we may expect to see the whole spectrum, from lethal to qualitative change to quantitative change to neutral. These molecular individuality issues are already of contemporary concern. On one hand, medical treatment is a significant killer in the United States due to the classical approach to catch all rather than personalized treatment. On the other hand, a breast cancer medication specific to an individual genetic variation is already available. It is interesting that with roughly only one-third of the population carrying this gene, previous classical trials and analyses, unmindful of genomic differences, almost certainly missed this agent, classifying it as not significantly effective.

There were 500,000 SNPs discovered by end of 2000, all placed in public domain in an integrated SNP map, and due to new methods the numbers are now in many millions. In centuries or even just decades to come, practically every base pair in our DNA might be found to be a genomic biomarker for something. Yet we still neither can explain what proportion of the SNPs alter function nor figure out how best we can distinguish between what is genetic disease and what is genetic individuality. We don't know completely what are the causes or reasons for the 10 major diseases in the United States, a significant dearth in our knowledge.

THE THOUSAND-DOLLAR GENOME

The path ahead for SNPs is not without significant financial cost. Likely the 2,000 individuals for the so far discovered 500,000 SNPs will equate to 1 billion genotypes. If there was full possible variation, it would be 500,000 raised to the power 2,000, which is trans-astronomic. With conventional technologies in the genome projects, about 100,000 genotypes can be processed in a day. The price of having one's whole genome done cheaply and rapidly is dropping dramatically. On May 31, 2007, James Watson of double-helix fame received the DNA sequence of his own full genome in a ceremony at the Baylor College of Medicine in Houston, Texas. A biotech company in Branford, Connecticut, specializing in DNA sequencing, 454 Life Sciences, generated the data from a blood sample given by Watson. Compared with the many years and billions of the human genome projects, this took just two months and a sum said to be considerably less than one million US dollars.

There have been active searches for cheaper, nonconventional technologies to process allotypes in a considerably reduced time. For example, a technique called mass spectra high-throughput technology has been developed for determining SNPs accomplished with fully automated SNPs assay design. The technology has unlimited assay development capability using inexpensive reagents.

Ultra-high throughput can be obtained by pooling and multiplexing. Other methods are being developed. The goal is that every one of us with a reasonable salary should be able to have our entire DNA sequence done. The goal is the thousand dollar genome, and at the time of writing there are constant steps forward to that vision. Watson's genome (see above) possibly took about $100,000–$500,000 in 2007, and there are indications that by the end of 2008 it was taking roughly a mere $60,000 to sequence a human genome (http://www.futurepundit.com/archives/005150.html). It is difficult to say because you get what you pay for: it really depends on the quality (lack of errors) and on how much of the genome you consider interesting. In late 2007, deCODE genetics in Iceland announced the launch of their $985 personal genotyping product, deCODEme. This product did not do the whole genome, but some million sites, to assess a patient's risk for common diseases, along with providing information about ancestry, physical traits, and genealogical relationships. In the not-so-far future, your whole DNA sequence could easily appear on your digital medical record.

A GROWING PLETHORA OF "OMES"

Genomes and proteomes are not the only "omes." At the close of the twentieth century a number of methods for capturing data (e.g., mass spectroscopy and expression arrays) and a growing interest in systems biology emerged as a plethora of "omes." These and other "omes" important to the medical record will be discussed in Chapter 4.

SOME KEY "OMES"

Genome Essentially genetics in molecular detail, base pair by base pair, the internal world of the genetic data, primarily the full sequence of nuclear and mitochondrial DNA (an extra DNA outside the nucleus inherited from the mother), but arguably to some related issues (modifications of DNA, e.g., methylation, a chemical modification made by the cell to its DNA that controls DNA action). Strictly speaking, we need not confine the genome to what is inherited, but the variations in DNA that occur in different cells and tissues, that is, *somatic* variation. A "deliberate" mutation occurs as part of the response of immune cells to memorize invading molecules, for example (the basis of immunization). There are hundreds of copies of mitochondrial DNA per cell, and these can show variation in health and particularly disease. A retrovirus (e.g., HIV) entering the DNA also effectively modifies the sequence.

Transcriptome The internal world of the RNA molecules of which the most interesting addition through new discovery are the regulatory micro-RNAs (miRNA) discussed above. But even the traditionally previously known RNA world was rich and complex. RNA are copies of just part of the DNA that are sent out from the chromosomes to make special RNA structure concerned with protein synthesis, or messenger RNA (mRNA) with direct instructions to make proteins themselves. The code is very similar except that U (uracil) replaces T (thymine), and the molecules are double stranded. The transcriptome is quite a rich world because, at the dawn of life, RNA appears to have played the role of DNA and even of proteins. The reader with an interest in chemistry will recall that the sugar ribose replaces that of deoxyribose in DNA, and this is important as the cell needs to distinguish DNA from RNA for differential breakdown and regulation. The RNA types include not only this mRNA but also rRNA molecules, which are an important part of the little machines that convert the instructions in mRNA to protein sequences, tRNA molecules that carry information about which three bases of mRNA code for which amino acid residue, and small inhibitory iRNA molecules that bind to messenger RNA and regulate its action. There is also some RNA production in the large stretches of DNA outside the genes in what used to be called the "junk DNA," which appears to be a constant buzz of natural virus-like forms. These may help accelerate evolution, but it is also likely to be these proteins that evolve into retroviruses like HIV.

Proteome Essentially the world of protein molecules made by the genome, all the interactions between these proteins, and arguably interactions with smaller molecules. We are essentially what our proteins make us: if we had to say that we were essentially a matter of one kind of molecule above all others, it would be proteins. Unlike the genome, or at least the inheritable part of it, the proteome is in constant change, in response to the environment. Expression arrays show what mRNA and hence proteins are being made by cells—the expression is seen to vary with tissue and factors like gender, age, diet, exercise, and other life style variants. The old idea that one gene makes one protein is a substantial simplification. There are many protein variants that can be produced from one gene by different forms of editing of the mRNA known as "splicing," and by processing after syntheses, known as "posttranslational modification."

Metabolome Everything to do with metabolism, the complex flow of matter in which, for example, A is converted to B, B is converted to C, C is combined with A to make X, and X inhibits the conversion of B to C, except when A and X are in excess. Protein interactions and modifications are not normally considered as metabolism, though this is an artificial distinction to keep proteomists and metabolomists from treading on each other's turf. The conversions, including the joining molecules together, are a chemical process catalyzed by enzymes. Without such catalysis, these processes would likely occur no more significantly than any other infinite variety of chemical transformations that go on at a very slow rate all the time, and all regarded as noise. Enzymes are, of course, proteins, so the genome defines the metabolome, but this is sensitive to the environment, especially molecules coming in from the environment.

Cytome Everything to do with the cell. This includes the processes discussed above but also aspects of structure, such as closed compartments with the cell that separate metabolic processes, cytoskeletal (molecular scaffolding) organization, and cellular movement and behavior.

Physiome Everything to do with your physiology, typically focusing on skeletal systems and the organ of the heart. Hence the specialist areas have names like "cardiome" and "neurome."

Psychome Aspects of psychology and behavior not covered, including a possible "cerebrome."

Phenome The overall human as shaped by genetics and the environment. Phenotype is an obvious origin of the word. Bear in mind that genotype equates with genome and phenotype equates with environment.

Ethome First coined by the authors of this book, this "ome" covers ethical, spiritual, religious, and cultural factors, the patient's wishes under the Patient Bill of Rights (discussed later), patient privacy requirements and any fine grained consent for research, and so on.

Holome The nature of one's environment, holistically comprising life style, hobbies, workout regime, role and work, and interacting with all the other human players.

There have been "ome" wars, a friendly kind of dispute between genomic and proteomic scientists. The proteomic side emphasizes that humans are a walking, talking stack of proteins, not of DNA; that DNA is merely the "magnetic tape"; that different levels of different proteins are made in different tissues; and that our proteins change throughout our lives, including in disease, and relate most directly to health. The genomic side maintains and emphasizes that it is easy to detect individual differences such as a G where it is usually a C in the DNA, that these differences correlate fundamentally (sometimes in a complex way) with inherited disease, so the ability to detect, for example, the more appropriate chemotherapies by genetic differences is beginning to save much time and unnecessary suffering.

THE RISE OF SYSTEMS BIOLOGY

A computational discipline known as "systems biology" has recently arisen, or at least awakened from an ongoing semiconscious state in 1940s. This discipline seeks to delineate biological functions much the same way as electronic functions are used to analyze biology, by mapping molecular signals to electronic signals, biochemical processes to electronic processes, and biochemical (metabolic) pathways to electronic pathways. In the late twentieth-century systems biology began to be reasonably described as the simulation part of bioinformatics, namely in the running of computational models with some degree of intended physical reality to fit, interpolate, and extrapolate from the available data. Applying systems biology should be distinguished from "simply" fitting statistical parameters or using statistical models: statistics has its role in system biology, but then it does not matter much if the system is a black box. Systems biology is instead a "glass box" approach as it allows the scientist to observe the biochemical, physiological, or neurological processes going on inside it, and to perform "what if" experiments.

An early precomputing attempt from the twentieth century at formulating a systems biology was a work on the brain by the British psychiatrist W. Ross Ashby that related the electronic and mechanical devices being built and studied to certain aspects of animal behavior, especially the behavior related to maintaining various kinds of behavioral stability. Studies of cellular automata and neural networks were studied on some of the earliest digital computers, and certain classes of genetic algorithms appeared not long after. These disciplines are named after the biological areas they sought to emulate. A desire to simulate metabolism similarly inspired Russian and US efforts at a fairly early stage, though they were held back by lack of data, which is still somewhat problematic today: knowledge of all the rate constants for the individual metabolic and chemical steps. (A note for chemists: recall that if these are known in full, equilibrium constants and excitatory and inhibitory constants can be deduced from them). A typical modern example is simulation of interaction of signaling and gene regulation networks inside the cell, to help interpret gene expression data.

Systems biology will be important to medicine because data such as expression arrays may need to be interpreted in order to understand internal processes in the patient. Electronic simulation applies whenever the physician must model what cannot be easily seen. This is a general statement that holds for simulation in general. Models of the body with elasticity, plasticity, and coefficients of friction applied to nerves, muscles and organs might be needed to interpret magnetic resonance image movies for osteopathic and sports medicine.

To be useful to medicine, and to help *you* as a patient, all these "omes" have to be associated in some way with your clinical history and accessible to the physician. This brings us to the point of the next chapter: the patient record in digital form, and augmented by the "omes." But with all this power placed in the hands of the physicians, a vital "ome" is missing. This is the "ethome" that encapsulates all your wishes and rights, and is as important as any other data on record. Ethical, spiritual, religions, and cultural factors are considered in the subsequent chapter.

BACKTRACK: THE RISE OF THE INTERNET

Clearly, the Internet is a key communications player. It also has undergone progressive transformations. In some disasters only the server computers and communications stay up, and the Internet is almost the only means of communication, as during hurricane Ivan in the Cayman Islands (Chapter 9).

Almost everything has a history. There was once the so-called Victorian Internet of chains of towers with mechanical signaling arms viewed by a telescope. Then came the electrical telegraph and the Morse code, the telegram, the land line telephones, and more recently mobile phones and text messaging. All these communications means have developed codes for brevity, efficiency, and secrecy. They all have laid the foundations of, or extended, modern information and communication theory. In 1948 Shannon published *A Mathematical Theory of Communication* in which he considered the problem of how best to encode the information a sender wants to transmit, and this formed the basis of modern computer communications. As important, Shannon introduced the idea of information being negative entropy, which is an occasional theme in this book in various guises as a basis of data mining and analytics, engineering and thermodynamics, drug design calculations, and even the philosophy of medical health, and potentially of unifying all these. Shannon sadly could not appreciate the emergence of these principles and many others of his in computing and artificial intelligence because he developed Alzheimer's disease.

The Internet was first developed for communication among scientists, atomic physicists, in particular, and in 1972 as a means of communication between American military and universities. It is the desk top computer that brought communications to its modern form. At roughly the same time came the start of the human genome projects, home computers, and hence a people's network, the Internet as we now know it, arose. The genome projects and bioinformatics critically depended on it: the disciplines were essentially run on the Internet. The Internet is now a global network connecting millions of computers in more than 100 countries and, for many purposes, exchanging data, news, and opinions. Unlike centrally controlled online services, each participating computer, sometimes called a *host*, is independent and of equal rank.

The Internet was very rapidly adapted for general use. Before home computers, scientists had already established the basic protocols, search, and "surfing" methods that allowed big mainframe computers far apart to be joined to process information together as a vast global communication system, so the system was made more easily accessible. The Internet quickly became an important tool in medicine, and especially in the medical researcher's office.

The production of affordable home microcomputers in the early 1980s made it possible for many nonscientists to join in from home, with medical and health-related queries representing some 34% to 46% of Internet use by 1998. What a difference half a century makes! The first computer introduced in 1946 weighed 30 tons and was 100 feet long, although its computing power was limited merely to 14 calculations of 10-digit numbers in a second. A laptop computer in 2000 cost less than one thousand dollars albeit its computing power was equivalent to more than thirteen times of the then-fastest IBM mainframe in 1970 which cost almost five million dollars. The processing power of a computer has been continually doubled in every 18 months and at the same time its cost of ownership has been cut in half. Today, merely 50 years since the first computer was introduced, the computing capability has grown to tens of trillions of calculations per second, and yet not for simple calculations of 10-digit numbers but for complex floating-point operations involving very large numbers (e.g., 2^{128} or 10^{38}). IBM has developed a supercomputer, referred to as Blue Gene, which will perform more than a quadrillion floating-point operations per second (10^{15} complex mathematical calculations per second) and it is commercially available.

The Internet is a *decentralized* network of connected computers. That is, the "Internet" does not exist in any one central location, and no location is, except in the cases discussed below, any more important than any other. The term *host* is typically applied to any participating computer with an address recognized by the Internet, which could be a home computer, so allowing other computers to access it. The more heavy duty computers specializing in Internet activities and providing services are called *servers*. Servers providing for really high numbers of computers requesting access, like those providing minute-by-minute news from the Olympic Games or the popular lady's underwear company Victoria's Secret, need to be particularly heavy duty servers. Just because you can access the Internet and hence any host computer doesn't mean that you have a host machine with information that you can let any Internet user see, but you could allow somebody else's machine to "host" your information to make it generally available. Early "Internet providers" like Telusplanet and Compusmart were specialists with a room full of computers where they store their clients' *websites*. A website sends information in a standard format such as HTML (hypertext markup language) or XML (extended markup language) and displays a screens-worth page at a time, with means of being able to respond. This is an aspect of the so-called *client–server model*. Each time you access a website, you retrieve information from the appropriate computer, wherever in the world that computer might be, the computer of the retrieving person (typically at home or office) is called a *client*. The corresponding software deployed at the server end used to be the *common gateway interface* (CGI), which was strictly a protocol standard that communication software had to meet, not a specific piece of universal software. The CGI is now almost obsolete and is being replaced with Java "servlets," and most of the newly developed software is based on the Java technology and the Web Services technology (e.g., SOAP[1], UDDI[2]). The software on the client, by

---

[1] Simple Object Access Protocol for intersystem interface for Web Services.
[2] Universal description, discovery, and integration for the directory of objects for Web Services.

which the Internet can be observed and explored, is called a *browser*. Marc Andreseen and colleagues invented the first true browser *Mosaic*, and current browsers include Firefox and Microsoft's Internet Explorer. The simplest kind of browsing requires entering an Internet address called the uniform resource locator (URL), which actually goes to a specific web page on a specific machine, or more correctly to whatever machine the relevant web page is currently registered with.

To move through a network of computers at the speed of thought, you had better know where you are going. The Internet is very much a matter of URLs. An example URL is that for the Houston Medical Archive URL, which is http://dean.med.uth.temc.edu. The suffix .edu means an educational establishment, as opposed to .com (commercial organization) or .org (noncommercial organization), or .gov (government) or .net (associated with the Internet administration in some way). Most computer-literate readers will recognize these and other elements of an URL; often the original meaning of such acronyms is long forgotten, however. Although there were important contributions to the development of the Internet from European physicists, in recognition of the US contribution, a country suffix such as .uk in the Internet addresses is required by other countries, but not by the United States. However, there are now many sites outside the United States that are not particularly interested in advertising their national location, and there is nothing to stop them using the US notation. As an example of a non–US URL, the European Bioinformatics Institute is based now in the UK (it was in Germany) and thus has the URL http://www.ebi.ac.uk. Note another odd change for historical reasons, that .ac. replaces .edu, .co. replaces .com, and so on, outside the United States. The prefix http:// means *hypertext transfer protocol* (see below) and is the most common form of data transfer; others include ftp (file transfer protocol), file, gopher, mailto, and news. These information exchange protocols, are exactly those with which a server in the Internet must be able to cope. Thus ftp://ftp.ebi.ac.uk is an address for digital file transfers between clients and a server at the European Bioinformatics Institute in the United Kingdom.

THE WORLD WIDE WEB

The World Wide Web is not the same of the Internet, but a later development of it, and within it. The www in the http address http://www.ebi.ac.uk for the same institution is an indication that it is set up for participating in the World Wide Web, the significance of which will now be described; however, most websites are similarly set up for such participation even if they do not include www. URLs can be invoked automatically based on what the user wants to know. The Internet today is not only an actual network of computers with pages that you can get to by entering a specific address, but also has a virtual network of knowledge inside it, independent of where the physical machines are. This *World Wide Web* of knowledge is particularly associated with a concept put forward by Vanevar Bush as long ago as in 1945. Ted Nelson in 1965 invoked the term hypertext to describe the similar chaining of text in the Internet: activating one item would allow access to adjacent relevant concepts in a network of knowledge, which would be arbitrarily placed on different machines across the Internet. Tim Berners-Lee in 1989 described the hypertext method used today. A web page is not sent as it is seen, rather it is currently encoded in Hypertext Markup Language (HTML) or in XML (eXtended Markup Language) derived from the ISO Standard Generalized Markup Language (SGML, ISO 8876:1986). This is based on the idea of a markup language long used by editors and proofreaders, conveying such things as "put this in italics" or "center this text" or "insert the picture here." The system uses entities known as marker brackets or *tags* of general form <...> something </...>; for example, <i> something </i> indicates that the text between should be in italics. When a server in the World Wide Web sends "Do you <i> really </i> want to do that?" and the browser will display "Do you *really* want to do that?" However, HTML can do much more than that, including determining which pieces of text or picture you can click on, and where you will go if you do. These hotspots of communication on a web page are called *hyperlinks*. Clicking by mouse on such a piece of text or picture which is at a hyperlink point may take you to a different web page on a very different server, probably with many of its own pieces of text or picture that you can click on. The hyperlink that you click on not only initiates transfer, but contains the address of the server to which you will be connected: this is the URL again.

INTERNET GROWTH OF POWER

Already by the mid-1990s the Internet represented most computer-to-computer communication, supporting email and mailing lists, real-time communication programs (IRC, ICQ, chat), newsgroups, multi-user games, the above-mentioned protocols like http and ftp, the browser gopher and the WAIS system (like the web but without graphics), and the World Wide Web. In addition the computer language Java was used to add executable content to a web page, introducing motion and liveliness such as (most commonly) moving cartoons. However, it might also be a little program that the server sends to initiate a customized database search, for example. At first HotJava was a special browser introduced to show off Java's capabilities. Today almost all browsers support Java "applets" (i.e., small Java programs that are downloaded from a web server and run on a client machine).

Another emerging technology is Web 2.0, which is anticipated to enable a business revolution by using the Internet as a platform to help online collaboration among the people, which is referred to as social computing, through the Internet. Small companies with specific domain expertise became the driving force for the niche market enabled by the Internet. The first evidence of the information age was the rising .com companies that were appearing like budding bamboo shoots after a heavy rain. Those .com companies were trying to exploit the global infrastructure, the Internet, and the World Wide Web for selling information and knowledge on a global basis (see next the section).

Before long the end-users began to get hungrier for more processing power, random access memory, and mass storage because of the ever-growing volume of multidimensional heterogeneous data (e.g., multimedia data) and of the processing power to manage and analyze the data. Digital media, life sciences, weather predictions, and simulation of behaviors of nanosystems, among other things, began driving the ever-increasing demand of the processing power, random access memory, and mass storage. In terms of the telecommunications, in early 1970s, the highest communication bandwidth was 56,000 bits per second for a local connection or 300 bits per second for a remote connection over a wide area network. Today, a fiberoptic communication link can transmit about 1.6 trillion bits per second over a single optical fiber line that is thinner than one-tenth of a human hair. When the 1.6 trillion bits or 200 billion bytes are put in a context, the data volume is more than the aggregate of all conversations among all Americans during the peak hour on a peak day.

For the readers who are not familiar with those large numbers like petabytes and exabytes, the definitions provided by University of California at Berkeley are shared here to help the readers to put those large numbers in a context,: *1 megabyte is 1,024 kilobytes and represents the length of a short novel or the storage available on an average floppy disk* (which is no longer used with the introduction of the CD, or compact disk); *1 gigabyte is 1,024 megabytes and represents roughly 100 minutes of CD-quality stereo sound; 1 terabyte is 1,024 gigabytes and represents roughly half the content in an academic research library; 1 petabyte is 1,024 terabytes and represents roughly half the content in all US academic research libraries; and 1 exabyte is 1,024 petabytes and represents roughly a half of all the information generated in 1999.*

In addition to the revolutionary advancement of computers and telecommunications, the Internet and the World Wide Web revolutionized our daily lives and led us into the new Information Age. Computers connected to the Internet are often referred to as the "Internet appliances." An appliance, by a colloquial definition, is an essential equipment or machinery for our daily living and is usually part of a furnished apartment in many Western countries. The typical appliances include refrigerator, conventional oven, microwave oven, washing machine and clothes dryer, and wall-mounted television set.

With rapid expansion of the Internet in the Information Age, the Internet is becoming a part of our social space and becoming a foundation for a global virtual community. In other words, the Internet is becoming part of the infrastructure of the global socioeconomy. One of the IBM vice presidents responsible for the corporate technology and strategy, who also took the role of the scientific advisor to a president of the United States, made an assertion that one million businesses, one billion people, and one trillion devices will be connected to the Internet in a foreseeable future. Predictions by a famous economic foresight group, the Gartner Group, support the assertion.

It was predicted that one billion Internet users will be willing to afford to be on the Internet by sometime between 2005 and 2010 and that most will be willing to pay for a health and lifestyle query service enabled by reference to personal clinical and biomedical data. As it happens, there have been considerable ups and downs, with the romancing of eHealth to venture capitalists recently somewhat in decline. It is actually a pleasing sign for potential revival that in China, a major source of Internet activity, investment in the Internet by 2008 had declined after saturation and maturation of the investment marketplace, but eHealth may be one area as yet insufficiently exploited. Because of recent (2008) $16.6 billion revenues of Google, $14.8 billion of Amazon. com, and large sums in the range of $2.7 billion to $9.5 billion being made by LibertyMedia, eBay, Yahoo, and Expedia, respectively, quite a lot of spending is believed to be medically related. Much health-related spending may however be indirectly related or leveraged, with users interested in healthcare issues attracted by advertising to other products. Health information is already the most sought-after information on the Internet. According to Deloitte Touche LLP and VHA, Inc., among others, variously 34% to 43% of people who access the Internet use it for gathering health-care information. Roughly 50% of these people seek information on specific diseases, while many others are interested in educational services, prescription drug information, fitness, and alternative medicine. Some 20% of any large group of users have some manifest form of illness or disorder at any one time. More people are willing to share their medical information in the hope that it will help them get a better care through higher accuracy of diagnosis and more effective treatment. The global market issues are humane: for every person in the poorer regions of the world who can afford to be on the Internet, there will be more of his/her neighbors willing to make health and lifestyle queries, and the Internet may provide a more economic, practical, and less hazardous access to health advice than travel and consultation.

As we observe already today, (1) people meet, become friends, fall in love, and develop relationships over the Internet; (2) people search the World Wide Web to find the information for which they used to consult dictionaries, encyclopedia, atlas, or telephone books; and (3) people buy and sell things over the Internet. Some people even seem to go as far as arguing that it is safe to assume a certain thing does not exist at all if it cannot be found in the Internet. One of the key value propositions the Internet provides is overcoming the physical distance, with virtually no cost and time for travel and yet with potential anonymity where gender, age, race, and physical attributes are not exposed at all. There is a saying that no one knows you are a dog on the Internet.

It needs no qualification to say that kids have been a significant force in using computers and the Internet. But a significant force at the other end of humankind's lot of years is frequently neglected. Many "baby boomers" (born after the return of troops from the Second World War), who would have been seeking early retirement, want to remain active and productive. For many, this means doing unpaid research in their own interest areas, or writing articles or books. For many others, this means doing salaried work on home computers and via the Internet. (Yet most corporate policies and government's labor laws are still based on the norm of the industrial age where older workers could not continue to handle the same loads of physical labor, and so decreased in productivity.) In this new information age with an emerging knowledge economy and with globalization of the socioeconomics and geopolitics based on the wide adoption of the Internet as well as the rapid advancement of technologies, the opposite is true. If expertise and insight, which is referred to as know-how, are a key factor in the knowledge era, older and experienced workers who have kept pace with change may be the most valuable and reliable sources of expertise. Based on relationships established over the years and intimate domain knowledge as well as profound industry experiences, these experienced workers could make significant contributions well past their retirement age, even if they choose to devote less time to work, and consequently bring competitive advantages to their companies. Large corporations and governments in North America and Europe are becoming aware that the traditional corporate cultures that pressure knowledge workers to leave at a set age with no accommodation for an ongoing association may be wasting their best assets. Consequently some countries such as Canada are in the process of amending the labor laws to remove the mandatory retirement age. In fact many professionals go back to work after their retirement.

The Internet means that we have entered a world of information-access, products, and services *on demand*. But routine *ongoing* health care and health vigilance does have a further special need, however, if we are to use the Internet as the medium: continuous access to high-speed constant Internet access in the home. The major first steps of this have, of course, already been achieved by high-speed Internet connections over telephone line or television cables. How many readers connect with and disconnect from the Internet, and turn computers on and off, on a daily basis?

Consider also the issue of paying for service. If we are to be permanently connected, it is of concern how much we pay. But it has already become noticeable that the Internet services are becoming more extensively free of charge to access. Remember those days when we actually had to pay subscription fees for radio programs and TV programs? We do not pay for listening to radio stations or viewing many TV stations. The advertisers pay for the services on our behalf: while many of us still pay the Internet service providers (ISPs) for access to the Internet, some Internet service providers, such as Google, already provide free access to the Internet and also provide free email IDs.

Indeed, as foreseen by many people, among them John Patrick at IBM, the Internet is becoming as ubiquitous, free, and easy to use as the air we breathe. John Patrick was the vice president for Internet technology at IBM as well as chief strategist for the next-generation Internet (besides serving as chairman of the Global Internet Project, which is a group of executives from international companies seeking to ensure that private-sector leadership guides the Internet's development). He envisions a world where information appliances are be connected to the Internet so that there will be no more logging on. John Patrick recently left IBM to found Attitude LLC and develop many other affiliations. What is interesting is that, while his interests and web pages were previously "officially" much more general, the blogging (public exchange of views) on his website http://patrickweb.com/index.php is (as of the end of 2008), totally medical.

John Patrick's vision is rapidly becoming historical fact. There are today extensive attachment of other devices *other* than computers alone to the Internet, an auspicious development for the continuous bio-monitoring of our health. By this means we can navigate around our home computers as much of the intelligence of computers will be placed in very small portable devices. Soon information appliances will be everywhere, and consequently in such a *pervasive* (or "ubiquitous") *computing environment* our experiencing the Internet from the PC is going to drop from 90% of user time to less than 50%. In the next few years people will turn to PDAs (personal digital assistants), pagers, mobile phones, and new wireless devices as their preferred information appliances. Already with the recent mingling of home computers and phone technology we can send text or even voice to a mobile computer, and conversely we can trawl the Internet on our mobile devices. If we wanted to pay for them, devices in our homes can communicate via our home computers to our mobiles, alerting us to burst pipes, fires, freezer failure, or simply drying-out house plants when we are away from our homes. On the desk of one of us as he first typed this manuscript, there was a Newsweek magazine of July 24, 2005. The front page reads "Phone of the Future: How Internet Calling will Revolutionize the Way We Communicate." At the time of revision, he is already wearing headphones plugged into his laptop while awaiting a call via the Skype system, and the "land line" on the desk is really an Internet phone operating via the local server. To find a true good, old-fashioned traditional line would require a 15 minute walk to a coin-operated public phone, and in a short while public phones will become obsolete.

As the above comments illustrate, futurology concerning predictions for the social impact of IT has in recent years become an extraordinarily difficult task for the short term, and the situation is no less for eHealth. At the start of the new millennium, many ambitious visions were described for Internet-based healthcare by 2005–2010. The terrorist attack of September 11, 2001, and the global market crash of 2008 has rocked many prediction boats. Yet the need for healthcare creates a relentless juggernaut, or more correctly an unstoppable force for good, that we shall examine more closely in the next chapter. The British Health Minister Enoch Powell is credited with stating around 1962 that "there is virtually no limit to the amount of healthcare an individual is capable of absorbing." It was a more subtle statement than the just the moaning of a government obliged to fund a welfare system supported by taxes. It is a comment on the fact that healthcare rests on very different market laws bound only by the limits of available technology and personal or collective social wealth to buy application of that technology. And yet, even the technology available now does not seem to have reached its exploitation limit in satisfying the healthcare demand. The situation has not yet come to rest at equilibrium. In continued development of the market, institutional intranets and the public Internet will increasingly serve as a low-cost rapidly deployable platform for disseminating medical information between authorized players. And even the institution of US-managed healthcare will further increase the urgency and diversity of the medical information spread. To add to the force of those changes, even the attractor point of existing resources may shift: there is the possibility of a new Internet, as follows.

SPECIALIZATIONS OF THE GLOBAL NERVOUS SYSTEM: DEDICATED MEDICAL INTERNETS AND GRIDS

From time to time there have been fears of saturation of the Internet, and speculation on the need for a second Internet specializing in medical communication and even research. So far that need has not been critical, but its architecture will doubtless mirror the main Internet. Closely related to the Internet and in some respects to the idea of a specialized medical second Internet is the notion of a grid, a collection of computers that can be global or local but characteristically share computation and storage as if they were all one machine. Such a dedicated network of computers does not prohibit, of course, its communication with the Internet. Rather it is often depicted as a local "nerve ring" handling localizable functions.

INCREASING NEEDS AND SOLUTIONS FOR COMMUNICATION BANDWIDTH AND PROCESSING

Global sharing of anonymous data for the common good has been proceeding at alarming speed, especially in medical imaging. The standard Internet works at about 0.1 to 10 megabytes per second but doubles roughly every year. There are thousands of medical imaging devices round the world. Whole body 4D surgical projection imaging in real-time data processing pumps out 100 to 200 megabytes per second per machine. The new computed tomography scanner from General Electric is expected to generate 13 gigabytes per second. Imminently it amounts to 1 to 4 gigabytes per second in 256 to 512 local channels. The Massachusetts General Hospital will have 256 (growing to 512) parallel channels attached to their Siemens 7T MRI scanner. A new "optical pathway" will transfer data from the scanner to the server using 16 (growing to 32) PCI (personal computer interface) cards, each supporting 16 channels. Other commercial, clinical machines at the Massachusetts General Hospital will probably have 32- or 64-channels attaches to 3T or 4.5T MRI scanners.

General Electric (GE) and other imaging device manufacturers take the view that much useful data can be shared without transmitting every byte, on an "only as needed" philosophy. But to share, it may be not unreasonable to routinely lay 256 to 512 fiber channels for a 100-mile stretch between participating medical centers. The High-Energy Physics project team was able to transmit data at 7.6 gigabytes per second from CERN in Geneva to Tokyo, and at 1010 gigabyte per second from Pittsburgh to Los Angeles, in November 2004. It is difficult to say if such records have been broken, because it depends on distance, and how many parallel optical fiber cables one allows. For example, scientists at the Fraunhofer Institute 2006 claimed a new world record for data transmission by transferring a data rate of 2.56 terabits per second over a glass-fiber link of 160 km in length. That is the equivalent to the contents of 60 DVDs, and at least 50 times faster than typical Internet transmission at the time. There is also plenty of opportunity for improvement. Channels with 30 strands of fiber could theoretically support 3,000 gigabytes per second.

Giving all medical centers such enormous bandwidth may not be feasible in the near future. But finally and not least, why do we have to bring the data somewhere to analyze it? Analytical software that can roam around and self-adapt to various systems could go out and perform the analyses for physician decisions support systems. One of the authors (OKB) has developed such system, as discussed later in this book.

ARRIVED AT LAST! THE EARLY DAWN OF INFORMATION-BASED MEDICINE

So we have come to the point where modern molecular medicine and IT are poised for a transition in medicine that is greater than anything in human history. But we will not leave our history entirely behind; we will look back from time to time to consider more specific aspects like the managed health-care and health insurance, alternative medicine, all the while as nanotechnology is shaped by contemporary medical information technologies.

To summarize, twentieth and early twenty-first century medical research have provided the medical technology for the new healthcare, and home computers and the Internet, as well as powerful computers partly motivated by these opportunities. The Internet is becoming the nervous system of the global conglomeration of computers supporting healthcare that we call the Engines of Hippocrates. At the same time there are many other driving forces. In particular, the rapidly enlarging aging population has made escalating demands for accurate diagnostics, for safer and more effective medicines, for higher efficacy and quality treatments, and this has leveraged rapid advances in molecular biology and biochemistry and in IT, and even a visionary desire to exploit rapidly emerging technologies such as robotics and nanotechnology.

The long road to scientific medicine, innovation, and entrepreneurship that is leading to the new healthcare systems began with the inventive and entrepreneurial Galen. The road in some form is older than Galen, of course. Hippocrates had laid the foundations of the first stretch. Nonetheless, the section of road built by Galen had a surprisingly modern outlook.

The road via Galen has been the road that we call mainstream medicine, meaning primarily the state-approved, analytic medicine of the Western world (for many centuries). As we will describe later, it is not the only road that will impact the new medicine. Other roads of origin more ancient than Galen are converging rapidly and are likely to transform the road ahead in a fundamental way. These are the roads of Eastern, folk, natural, alternative, and mystical medicine, emphasizing the philosophy of a personalized and holistic approach, and these, as we will argue, will regain their rightful place in medicine precisely because of the information-gathering and communication power of information-based medicine that can restore the personalized, holistic approach.

4

THE IMMINENT CHALLENGE: MEDICINE AS AN INDUSTRY

In the middle of difficulty lies great opportunity.

—Albert Einstein

INDUSTRY ON THE BRINK OF THE POST–GENOMIC ERA

It is important to move and implement change at the right time. As in surfing timeliness is the wait for the right wave. The challenge for the new medicine, as it is arising now, is an essentially economic industrial one. The history of the world's economy is turbulent, full of ups and downs, and successes and failures. Nevertheless, economists agree that on the larger time scale the world economy follows the industry-driven pattern despite many fluctuations. All things have their time. Alvin Toffler has been much heralded in business circles as promoting the notion of industry occurring in waves, and by his definitions and numbering, healthcare may be the fourth such next big wave (that is, after agriculture, the industrial revolution, and the Internet; for his works, see the bibliography at end of this book). But now can the burgeoning healthcare costs for employers, government agencies, and taxpayers (that Jonathan Gruber, a prominent healthcare economist at the Massachusetts Institute of Technology, and others have considered greatest fiscal threat facing the United States) be seen as the start of any such beneficial wave? Wealth will come, but healthcare is an industry that is driven by the *need* for health, not simply wealth, and that

The Engines of Hippocrates: From the Dawn of Medicine to Medical and Pharmaceutical Informatics, by Barry Robson and O.K. Baek
Copyright © 2009 by John Wiley & Sons, Inc.

buys a huge number of jobs. According to the US Bureau of Labor Statistics, healthcare employment grew 26% by nearly 3.2 million jobs in this decade, to 13.9 percent of all US jobs by 2008, *excluding* pharmaceutical, medical device, and equipment industries (considered separately, as manufacturing). When in the global economic downtown of 2008 nearly 600,000 US jobs were lost, healthcare took on 52,100 in November alone. Many would wish to curb cost increases without sacrificing the quality of care, and as discussed below, $30 billion expected to be spent by the United States on IT in 2009 should help solve this. But the *net* effect of IT is not to save money by replacing jobs for humans. Indeed, an additional $10 billion well spent on health IT for one year could create as many as 212,000 new US jobs, many IT jobs to be sure, but also high-tech healthcare jobs. And many traditional healthcare jobs will become high-tech. "It's been a fabulous journey from physicians being reluctant to now being unable to live without this technology," observed Dr. Karl J. Ulrich, Executive Officer of Marshfield Clinic, Wisconsin, according to *New York Times* correspondent Steve Lohr in "Health Care That Puts a Computer on the Team" (*New York Times*, December 27, 2008). Marshfield is one of many large medical organizations aggressively embracing IT, spanning providers and insurers with thousands of physicians, such as Kaiser Permanente and the US Department of Veterans Affairs, to those with hundreds, like Marshfield and Geisinger Health Systems. An early recognized challenge for the Obama presidency is to link electronic medical islands into a network, one that begins to approach on a national scale what organizations like those above have achieved regionally. Here too, the special nature of the health industry deemphasizes return on investment. John W. Melski, medical director of clinical informatics at Marshfield, in interview with Lohr, noted that it required "the usual leap of faith that knowledge will yield good things—better care, doing things smarter and, yes, saving money in the long run. ... We have to restructure our medical culture ... we have to promote a culture that believes in the evidence and is trained in analyzing the evidence."

Incidentally, he then added: "It's the only long-run answer to the challenges we face in health care—evidence-based medicine." In wave-of-industry talk, this appearance of "evidence-based medicine" is an interesting one. It has long been encouraged irrespective of IT, indeed before the rise of the Internet, and it has been exciting to see it come into widely accepted use in IT, press, and government speech. It is essentially nothing more than the discarding by the physician of subjective judgment, and making use of the best, latest, and worldwide collated medical knowledge based on sound evidence. It was until recently paid only lip-service by physicians, and grudgingly, if acknowledged at all. It is not hard to see why. Without computers and the Internet, it would effectively require the physician to have magical omniscience and telepathy to keep up. It is a best practice, as described later, that has only really become possible with IT.

The primary force behind the growth in the world's economy has been large corporations, powerhouses in the knowledge-based economy wave. Over the last century their niche markets and diversity revolutionized the economic structure. This is the underlying force that has shaped our genome-based economy, bringing us to the brink of a new era of personalized medicine based on the individual's genetic profiles and environmental parameters and variances in lifestyle.

Notably for medicine, significant use of patent genomic data for diagnosis and therapy selection raises the issue of a very basic principle of economics called "the tragedy of the commons." In the English countryside of the fifteenth century, the majority of towns held the local grazing lands in common. It was in everyone's interest to maintain the common land. If anyone owned more sheep than another, it would make him rich but over-graze the land for everyone else. Thus there was a strong pressure for everyone to be fair. A closely related economic problem is the issue of "moral hazard." In the insurance business, the person who fails to reduce risk and hence claims for his or her own property compromises all the other persons insured. In biology, these considerations form an important basis for explaining how animal and human behavior can be altruistic. In medicine, there is additionally the special case of an important principle usually applied to the benefits of sharing of personal medical data (albeit anonymously) to enhance medical knowledge, namely the principle of solidarity (common interest) versus autonomy (self-interest). However, the traditional economic aspect of this, as a money issue, has had a major effect on healthcare, especially in the United States.

Ambitions for medicine as an advanced industry are not new. Galen had bragged that he had done as much for medicine as Trajan (Marcus Ulpius Trajanus, AD 52–117) did for the Roman empire when he built bridges and roads through Italy. He clearly considered himself to be the mogul of the medicine industry. Yet he was already wealthy enough and more interested in impact than in enhancing his assets. He beseeched his physician coworkers to renounce the pursuit of wealth. Galen's double view of eschewing wealth and yet promoting an industry brings us back to the "tragedy of the commons." It is good for all if medicine is not driven by lust for wealth. But how can an aspiring industry mogul eschew the benefits of wealth? Of course, Galen was right: there is more to life than money, and there should certainly be more to health than money. His comments seem incongruous only because our minds tend to mix up money, commerce, and industry. "Industry" does not necessarily imply pursuit of wealth, nor commerce. The dictionaries typically define industry in terms of collective endeavor, and there is a hint of grandeur, respectability, and quality about such endeavors. Academics often work not only on abstract research but cooperate to produce "industrial strength" products and services without a motive in pursuit of wealth. The human genome projects and the Internet are modern examples of such grand collective endeavors. To be sure, many companies spin off from universities, and the human genome projects had great opportunities for wealth creation. But many academics commercialize to get better financial support for their work, to gain greater recognition, or to have bigger impact on society. For most scientists, there is no more horrible specter at their shoulders than the fear that the knowledge that they commit their lives to uncover is of no interest or consequence to the rest of the world.

Still the traditional tensions continue, between pure academic science and the daily concerns of applied engineering and competition for wealth. One of the authors (BR) once ran a series of bioinformatics industrialization workshops. The first was cosponsored by IBM, in collaboration with the Whitehead Institute, the International Union of Pure and Applied Biophysics, and the US Department of Energy, and opened at the Whitehead Institute at MIT in Cambridge, Massachusetts, one of the leading institutions in the human genome project. The workshop happened to open on the same day as the completion of the first draft human genome project was announced from Washington. While there was much excitement, many academic attendees expressed worry over the emphasis on engineering and industry at the expense of experimental science. They were troubled by the business accent given it.

However, biological and medical research, and the healthcare industry, are not just about money, and certainly not just about profit. The healthcare industry has evolved because of a huge, common, collective effort, just like the human genome project. Fundamentally the healthcare industry developed with a humanitarian objective. Folk medicine, alternative medicine, and other nonmainstream disciplines typically disavow the profiteering, or at least money-pinching, aspects of national medicine, yet their patient-centric, personalized, and holistic philosophies will have an enhanced role to play in the new medicine.

That said, an individual, organization, or nation needs money first in order to create and promote an industry. If an industry is big enough to merit the name, both in extent of product success and importance, commerce provides both a push and a pull. In any event, at this point in history, the issue of healthcare cannot be separated from money, even if we think of healthcare finance as no more than the convenient shuffle around of virtual quantities by which a nation tries to manage its health issues, quantitatively assess its efficiencies or inefficiencies, and allocate priorities. Even in a social healthcare system we need tokens of barter between the healthcare industry and the state, and the dispensers of resources. And it remains true that the state of industry has increasingly become a barometer to the economy as it drives it. There is, we may add in defense of capitalism, an inherent tendency of modern humans to participate in commerce. There is increasing conviction among historical anthropologists and population genomicists that the out-of-Africa diaspora (see Chapter 2) that displaced all modern humans and Neanderthals did so because of the capabilities of the new humans in trade.

We can expect the same to be true of medicine empowered by IT. One rapidly growing trend of medical IT is telemedicine, normally considered as the transmission of sound and pictures between patient and physician as opposed to both being physically in the same place. But some industry analysts have used the term to indicate any transmission of medical information between institutions or homes and institutions (e.g., see Virtual Medical Worlds monthly http://www.hoise.com/vmw/00/articles/vmw/LV-VM-01-00-1.html). The market prediction is that telemedicine will represent 15% of future worldwide health expenditures. Because of varying definitions of telemedicine, it is impossible to know whether this is being achieved. A recent review indicates a very cautious optimism (Ronald C. Merrell and Charles R. Doarn, "Telemedicine and e-Health: is it time for a telemedicine breakthrough? *Telemedicine and e-Health* 2008; 14(6):505–506). More than $2,000 billion is the health expenditure of countries technologically advanced enough to have extensive IT. The fraction of healthcare in IT-enabled nations, however, is estimated at 80% of health expenditure on just 20% of population. A much larger fraction than 15% will likely represent some form of IT in medicine. Basic medical IT appears to be moving in the direction of computer-based patient records *controlled by the patient* from home, and in the hands of the physician to manage consent on whether patient information can be used in studies on effectiveness of certain treatments and drugs. It was estimated that while home-health related matters would be slowing to small levels of growth by mid-2008, in 2008 home-health IT would be growing at about 33% per annum and data mining at about 300%.

> There is a critical need to push healthcare into the information age. Our nation faces an aging population, a rising tide of consumerism, escalating healthcare costs, medical safety lapses, and the increased complexity that advances such as genetic discoveries will introduce into clinical data analysis and application. In the face of such challenges, however, healthcare is not taking full advantage of the information and communications technologies that have revolutionized other industries. Enabling timely and efficient access to information can improve both the quality and cost-effectiveness of care and strengthen the efforts of consumers, patients, and caregivers.
>
> —Markle Foundation, USA

ETERNALIZATION: GLOBALIZATION IN TIME AND SPACE

The catalytic effect of globalization of the economy means that the impact of telemedicine will reach emerging player nations such as India, China, Brazil, and Russia. It is a sobering thought for wealthy nations, to remember with compassion that *we are all third-worlders to the future.* All the sick of the world today are separated from physical redemption by space or by time. In space, our poorer neighbors lose out in medical care because industry and the economy is not evenly distributed across the Earth's surface. In time, even the sick of rich nations lose out. They lose out because science, industry and the economy are not static but evolve in time. If only we could have lived at the time of our great-grandchildren, perhaps things would have been so much better. As noted early in this book, from the future perspective, medicine today might look like something from the Dark Ages.

REGULARIZATION: FROM GLITTERING PRIZES TO PRODUCTION-LINE SCIENCE?

In the first quarter of the twenty-first century humankind will have succeeded in routinely decoding the human genome, learned the programming code for major diseases, developed miraculous drug treatments, transformed surgery to one of minimally invasive methods, and elevated the dignity of patients by tailoring diagnosis and therapy on an individual basis. In effect this period will mark the convergence of the life sciences, healthcare, and IT. This convergence is expected to dramatically improve the healthcare delivery system, diagnosis and treatments, the quality of care, and consequently longevity and the quality of life. Healthcare will realize the goal of personalized healthcare. Throughout IT will play a profound labor-saving role. It will provide the principal tool to bond medical knowledge to medical practice and to disseminate healthcare advancements to the healthcare processes.

Do these accomplishments mean that at a time in the near future all discoveries will be made and there will be nothing more to do? That would be nice to know, since if the big discoveries crop up sooner than we foresee them, there might be at very least golden investment opportunities! Otherwise, entrepreneurialism might need to take a different tack. Indeed, while we might not expect revolutionary insights comparable to Crick and Watson's DNA structure, we are steadily moving into an era of high-throughput *translational research*. In the case of new genomic biomarkers for diagnosis and therapy selection, new data arrive daily by a feed that will soon need to be better automated. It will be "regular": routine and organized.

Regularization means that a science has come of age. Unless we are cautious and support one-off endeavors, regularization could in principle have a deleterious economic effect. While regularization and predictability are not so good for the solo entrepreneur looking for gold dust in the steady streams of academic research, they are not a bad thing for an industry that is in the process of establishing itself. A growing industry cannot but benefit from discarding the element of serendipity and be able to guarantee a steady stream of useful data. The results of genomics so far have been realized in two main ways: predictive diagnostics and pharmaceuticals. The genomics healthcare industry up until around 2000 was often considered primarily a "diagnostic" one. Most experts continued to believe that testing would migrate to the site that will enable results to be available most quickly, and that will one day include the home. At the beginning of 2000 one biotechnology firm began offering a home DNA kit that would allow consumers to test their blood for SNPs that herald adverse drug reactions. Pharmaceutical companies are of course acutely aware that every disease, in fact every state of the human body, is either the result of or affected by gene action. Even in the case of infection, gene action still determines susceptibility, defense, and recovery. Some genes make proteins, some genes suppress other genes, and some modify proteins made by other genes. The picture will always be complex and interconnected, but eventually understanding by biomedical researchers will tell us what actually is happening in our bodies on the molecular scale. This should allow them to design better drugs, and a steady stream of new genomic biomarkers drugs relevant to drug selection and design is beginning to appear. We are starting to take for granted that advances in imaging due to progress in applied physics and other science areas, and other technique developments toward being able to do each whole patent genome for a $1,000, are proceeding at close to a production line rate.

But what of scientific revolutions that we have come to expect? Many thinkers at the end of the nineteenth century, and even shortly before Einstein's theory of relativity, and the rise of quantum theory on which modern electronics, IT, and computational medicinal chemistry depend, were predicting the end of scientific surprises. But *it is in the nature of surprises that they are not to be expected.* The world of biology may still hold many fundamental surprises, and still unveils one to us every so often. It was only recently that a new world of RNA control emerged in molecular biology, catching many by surprise (remember the basic biology—DNA makes RNA makes proteins).

Apart from the biological surprises there are some *known* mysteries and grand challenges yet to face. Predicting how proteins fold to achieve functional three-dimensional structures from the chemical formula alone (amino acid sequence) remains elusive even to the world's most powerful supercomputers such as IBM's BlueGene, unless there is help from examining related proteins of known three-dimensional structure. Understanding the mystery of human consciousness, and how to handle and describe the complex interacting systems with as much ease as we apply formulas for enzyme reactions now, may elude humans for some time. In *mathematical biology* we know about the steps of description from point attractor to equilibrium to periodic behavior to quasi-periodic behavior to chaotic attractors, and some like the Edinburgh Group have described higher Telandic or goal-seeking behavior of systems reminiscent of the thesis of W. Ross Ashby's classic book *Design for a Brain* (1960, Wiley). But what is beyond, and what have scientists properly understood up to the level of the basics of Chaos theory anyway?

Quantum mechanics shocked the industrial world and seemed a complete system with incredible quantitative and predictive capability (though no modern theory ever seems to be able to go beyond twenty decimal digits) but is not without its mysteries. Some researchers think that quantum mechanics might have something to do with a theory of everything (TOE), consciousness, and maybe even protein folding! There is a deep physical mystery of why quantum mechanics applies to the world of the very small and of the entire cosmos and yet seems to behave very differently at the scale of biology. Some like Roger Penrose link quantum mechanical behavior to mysteries like consciousness, and others to other real and sometimes hoped-for properties of biology. What behooves us to pay attention that something may be in the wind is that many in mainstream science reject this notion of consciousness.

Part of the problem seems to be that Penrose picked on the microtubules of the neurons as a key player for *physical* reasons, whereas to biomedical scientists, these structural cytoskeletal components do not come foremost to mind as *biological* key players in the mysterious, which they would prefer to consider as emerging from the staggering complexity of interneuron connections (our some hundred billion neurons each have some 7,000 synaptic connections!). And where, if anywhere, hide telepathy, clairvoyance, ghosts, and the immortality of the human soul? In some cases we simply have no way to judge right now whether innovative thinkers are wiser, or nuttier, than the rest of us.

Once a revolutionary period is over, it is in practice proactive entrepreneurs who drive future development. If they do not, even a rich nation might stagnate in a competitive global field. Hence, for example, the reason for the Council for Competitiveness in Washington, DC, and their whitepaper "Innovate America." Entrepreneurs and venture capitalists will only act if they can *make* money, and the government, largely speaking, when it can *save* money or lives. What a government can do is create the right fertile environment, by earmarking finances for new scientific and entrepreneurial efforts. Unfortunately, as for research in any corporation, these tend not to be a priority and innovation is first to go in a phase of declining market. Even when money or other assets have been made available, it puts pressure to make short-term goals, as often management tends to view short term today as precursor of long term tomorrow. Governments and big corporations do not hold to the scientist's dogma that "without the long term today, there is no short term tomorrow." Unfortunately, with the pace of scientific progress that survives even the most jaded cynics, that tomorrow can be months away, not decades.

Unexpected discoveries are a natural part of our ecosystem. Fundamental progress in molecular biology and biochemistry are still a persistent and significant industry driver behind the healthcare reformation. But there are *other* forces that drive industry, that push from behind or pull from the front. Even with a useful financial injection from individual innovators or government, market and industry still does not develop unless "driving forces" have resulted in some clearly defined industry trends. There are many technical advances external to biology and medicine but driving it. These are technical aspects such as IT, medical imaging, the Internet, and robotics. IT is already a catalyst in healthcare. IT is helping providers, and players, medical researchers and pharmaceutical companies in their efforts to transform the healthcare system. The leveraging of IT to enable personalized medicine and preventative medicine (with considerations of individual susceptibility to diseases and drug responses, based on genetic and environmental variants) is a demonstrable industry trend. IT also assists basic research on all those "omes": genomics, proteomics, metabolomics, pharmacogenetics, pharmacogenomics, chemical genomics, toxicogenomics, clinical genomics, physiological genomics, and nutrigenomics.

"NEGATIVE PRESSURE": THE SICKLY
US HEALTH INDUSTRY TODAY?

One of the biggest forces to revolution of the healthcare system is a negative one. Revolution to achieve any new system to take account of many wonderful scientific and technological discoveries can be a painful process. It is thus a big help for change if the existing system is urgently in need of a cure. The business-based US system of "managed healthcare" has been the brunt of much criticism. US healthcare as an industry has suffered criticisms regarding matters of fairness, efficiency, overmanagement, quality, and poor safety record. Efficiency is suspect as well. There are continuing calls for cost reduction in the United States and even countries providing public healthcare such as Canada and United Kingdom. The spending on prescription drugs rose from 5.8% in 1990 to 9.4% in 2000, while the hospital and provider cost increased from 4% in 1996 to 6% in 2000. By 2005 the US national healthcare expenditures exceeded $2 trillion, which is approximately 16% of the gross domestic product, according the National Coalition on Healthcare in United States (www.nchc.org). In addition in recent years healthcare cost has been growing with a double-digit inflation. US payers and insurers in, and the governments that provide public healthcare such as Canada and United Kingdom are beginning to adopt new economic strategies based on outcome-driven funding allocation.

The US Institute of Medicine carries out studies on the quality of medicine. In its Forum on the Science of Health Care Quality Improvement and Implementation in 2007, it noted that there were even deficiencies in methods for assessing healthcare quality. This remark is relatively politic compared with those of some other critics. Criticizing healthcare has now become a popular sport and entertainment industry. Search entries like "healthcare is sick" get thousands of Internet hits. Not least, Michael Moore's 2007 film "SICKO" is a compendium of horrors about Americans suffering at the hands of private insurers. At the premiere in Sacramento, hundreds of unionized nurses embraced Moore like a rock star.

HOW DID IT HAPPEN?

But how did the healthcare mess come about? After the prehistoric phase of the wise village Shaman, many physicians likely worked for money rather than rely on voluntary donations like a great guru or Buddhist philosopher. Chaucer's physician in *Canterbury Tales*, written at the end of the fourteenth century, clearly had his eye on the big money: "But yet in spending money he seemed meager, To keep the fees he earned most eager; For gold's a sovereign tonic; so in short, Great Stores of Gold were what he chiefly sought." However, a smaller group of earlier classical great physicians like Galen did have their own money, so they practiced medicine only because they wanted to do so.

Much later, for much of the nineteenth century the practice of medicine was a way for men of means to keep their minds alive, and give purpose to their lives. Physicians and medical scientists, like other scientists, were highly respected, besides being rich and at least adequately well-off. Eighteen-year-old Mary Shelley wrote the first great medical thriller *Frankenstein* as her entry in an informal horror-writing competition with her husband, poet Percy Shelley, Lord Byron and Dr. John Polidori. Dr. Victor Frankenstein creates a living being from body parts, but the tortured creature returns and demands a mate for companionship. As with Galen, Dr Frankenstein's money was inherited. He was a baron. Physicians and scientists not born into money worked second jobs that provided subsistence, as did Charles Darwin. Not least was the cost of medical schooling needed to obtain universally recognized medical qualification, so any aspiring physician had to have at least some financial means to getting to the state of being a physician in the first place.

The situation changed economically in the late nineteenth and early twentieth century. With the rise of industry moguls came the concept of scholarships from the mega-rich and generally broader accessibility of higher education to the poorer classes. Medicine became viewed as a profession and a good source of wealth, although on average the doctor was in worse financial shape than his Victorian and Edwardian Age predecessors. Before the Second World War the industrial nations, including the United States, had a relatively social system of medicine in which city hospitals paid physicians low stipends to care for the poor, and private physicians lived a relatively low-income middle-class life, accepting endless delays in payment, and often giving up and accepting chickens instead.

Things soon changed again, out with increasing rapidity in the alternating waves of well-meaning intention and economic and administrative failure. In the second half of twentieth-century, medicine, with its low ratio of physicians to patients, gained much in the way of scientifically based technology but lost much of the personalized, holistic approach of medicine of earlier life. While it may not be fair to say that the desire and vision for holistic and preventative approach was lost, it just didn't get very far despite the enthusiasm of its visionaries. The US system at the time of writing often seems far from a social, public welfare, caring system, yet in several waves in the last century, the medical profession flirted with a more caring, preventative, and personal system of medicine before each time getting sucked into the undertow of commercialism.

Prepaid medical care of any kind is when physicians and hospitals are paid a set amount to care for a group. The first well-intentioned efforts related to provision of care for employees by big companies on a somewhat feudal but paternal basis. Large-scale engineering, construction, railroad, and mining companies provided company doctors and hospital facilities, but rapidly began to favor free choice and externally provided service plans. Because neither employer nor employee benefits from lacking the appropriate best physicians for appropriate cases, there was a move to insurance and choice regarding care. Today, for example, the top three US automotive companies have some hundred billion dollars in healthcare obligations. Private fee-for-service and healthcare insurance schemes blossomed in the 1930s. The Kaiser Company set up provision to provide for war workers based on the model of the Garfield clinic set up for construction of the Grand Coulee Dam. In 1942 Henry J. Kaiser set up several centers on the West Coast, employing physicians and running company-owned hospitals.

A similar flowering of healthcare was taking place in most industrial nations, though on a different, more socialized basis. As Western Europe and Canada recovered from war and in the late 1940s and 1950s moved to a new postwar prosperity, a variety of medical state-supported healthcare schemes were developed. Despite the travails of the British National Health Service, for example, a concept of "population health" was promoted in Canada and the United Kingdom by politicians such as T. K. Young. There was a search for understanding why some people are healthier than others as well as the policy development, research agenda, and the resource allocations that come with it. This came close to basic "personalized medicine" without computer technology. The structured, administrative approach to the first ripples of a revolution for personal medicine won adherents even among the conservatives.

Around that time too, Kaiser's vision for healthcare was flowering. About 200,000 people were enrolled, but the system needed to be thrown open to the public to survive. Kaiser genuinely regarded his experiment as a healthy financial success justified by a major public benefit. To some extent the economic history and justification mirrored that of the railway and telephone systems. Nonetheless, although grounded in well-meaning intention, the United States was becoming trapped by its health insurance view of the world. The United States was being penalized by being first to start a nationwide facility, and it became stuck with a subsequently antiquated and hard-to-overhaul system. A clear "green field" is usually the easiest way to build a new system, and indeed by losing the war Germany and Japan had their fields cleared for them, and rapidly became even stronger industrial nations. In effect, the basic ideas from the private fee-for-service and healthcare insurance schemes from the 1930s had become *entrenched*. Competing for customers, service became ever more competitive and demanded high technology, and risk-management by the healthcare industry, in general, was perceived to be over-oriented, patient-selective, and penny-pinching at patients' expense. Coverage was frequently denied for reason of prior illness, which may not have occurred for some time but might, or might not, recur or worsen. Costs and profits soared in a way suggesting financial self-interest. There was certainly some conflict of interest with socialized healthcare by definition, in the sense that when President Harry Truman proposed a national health program in 1948, the American Medical Association campaigned *against* it, and won. However, there was at least significant US government input in terms of funding to the

Armed Service and Veterans Administration, the Public Health Service, Medicare, and Medicaid social security benefit.

This is not to say that the US insurance-based vision could not claim success. Relieved of funding a great deal of national healthcare, the government was able to invest in substantial medical research via the National Institutes of Health, achieving technical superiority in many areas. The "thrown open" insurance companies appeared to thrive. By 1960 the Californian Kaiser Foundation Health Plan supported some half a million subscribers; some 30 years later it dominated healthcare in California and controlled access to medicine in some 80 clinics and hospitals. Nonetheless, many patients could not afford the new medical technologies, and many more who could not afford to pay at all fell between the cracks. There was still no provision for the aged and unemployed until the Kerr-Mills Act of 1960 founded the predecessor of the US system of Medicare. In 1964 President Lyndon Johnson made Medicare a priority of his "Great Society" program.

Other undercurrents had their effect. Up to as late as the 1970s, it is amazing, in retrospect, to realize that many American general practitioners still performed their own surgery at least for minor cases. As the practice became increasingly outsourced to experts, the GP was still listed as performing the surgery, collected the fee directly, and then reimbursed the surgeon, often on a "split fee" basis. This arrangement began to escalate to a profitable business in the United States for surgeons and other medical specialists. The surgeons soon became more central and began to hire GP's to provide primary care and pass on patients to for surgical treatment. Surgeons soon established the major group centers such as the Mayo and Cleveland clinics. The move to specialization by experts was undoubtedly a good thing. Who today would want their local friendly GP performing major surgery on them, however well intentioned?

But profitability, and medicine as a business, grew still more in the United States. It made the "pressure selling" of medical services when less justified somewhat akin to many other everyday commercial practices. For example, there is the common US "commercial nutrition care" practice of selling double-sized portions in restaurants, and providing "doggy bags" to take the second half of the meal home to eat next day … a clear case of "needless overnutritioning." If there were not common occurrences of deliberately needless tests, surgery, or other treatments, there were nonetheless frequent excuses of lack of evidence, so that it was always easier to "test again," "look and see," or "operate just in case." This still happens at the time of writing in the United States: many tests are ordered that have been performed before, relatively recently. If performed before in another country, the fact is dismissed by the U.S. GP as if the patient had just emerged from a grueling medical experience in some subhuman community of which the ability to obtain valid clinical data barely surpasses its mastery of fire (even if its economic index of technological innovation now exceeds that of the United States).

Happily in the 1970s there was escalating evidence from studies by epidemiologist by John Wennberg and others. Doctors were making decisions and having surgery performed to spend healthcare dollars with little scientific justification. Wenberg spoke of "provider-induced demand" as the phenomenon of the pressure to sell unjustified medical services. A system of "outcomes-based" and then "evidence-based" medicine was increasingly promoted. It favored using scientific evidence and results of clinical and other trials. This objective met pressure from physicians who could have been profit motivated but could also argue that the evidence could not be obtained quick enough for practical application in many cases, was non-standardized, and open to interpretation. In the absence of any significant IT infrastructure, that had to be solved in the interim by some administrative, local organizational structure.

By 1986 influential Minneapolis physician Paul Ellwood, proposed the HMO (health maintenance organization) to funnel medical knowledge to where it was needed, and to devote resources to promote health instead of marketing services to cure preventable ills. In the views of many this well-motivated initiative was also inevitably doomed. Ellwood himself had assumed a Kaiser-like, not-for-profit basis for HMOs. But several years later, for-profit HMOs appeared on the New York Stock Exchange, and the downward spiral into the obsession with profitability began again. Preventative medicine remained a motivation for a while, until it began to be realized that a short patient access due to a constantly moving, job-changing population, and conversely the long time per patient required for preventative medicine to be economically viable, required another model. Like the GPs earlier, the HMOs began to contract out, to other doctors and hospitals, and often becoming little more than brokers. Entrepreneurial physicians hired colleagues into Independent Practice Associations (IPA) to meet the outsourcing demand. Poorly regulated, the IPA administrators seemed often to put economy and profit above patient's interest and put heavy pressure on the well-meaning IPA physicians. John Wenberg's "provider-induced demand" was back again in a new guise as if it had never gone away. The system of interaction between HMOs and IPAs was economically unstable, and also healthcare costs were rising rapidly. As a result many IPAs went bust by 1998, and even the major insurance schemes could not keep up. A national health plan began to look relatively attractive. Today, often the health insurance is still a benefit provided by the employer, who pays on a monthly basis. The insurance company is "reduced" to processing claims and handling other administrative details. The physician, in submitting a claim, is in effect acting indirectly as the employer's agent. These considerations are affected by the Employee Retirement Income Securities Act (ERISA) of 1974, which makes the employer exempt from state law concerning the benefit plans. Even here already, there are good intentions that have gone awry. The good intention was to stop every state in the United States from meddling with management of these matters by a large national or global corporation, and so the risk of bringing things to a grinding halt.

However, the negative consequence this time is that while a physician may remain liable, a HMO is immune to malpractice suites if it denies care, except in the case where the patient is a government employee.

As mentioned above, there were successes, and up to the 1970s medicine looked to be in relatively good shape, at least technologically. The United States had an exceptional high standard of living, and the baby boom had not yet begun to bite in terms of a large aging population. Major infectious diseases like tuberculosis and polio had been defeated toward the end of the twentieth century, but there were yet the disaster of the birth defects caused by Thalidomide in the 1960s, AIDS (acquired immunodeficiency syndrome) that struck in the 1980s and whose cure proved and continues to prove incredibly difficult, and more recently SARS in the 2000s and other new epidemics such as Avian flu fueled by the specter of terrorist biothreat and the post-9/11 anthrax letters. Feminists campaigned for rights to decide regarding their own bodies. Humanitarians campaigned, and large mental hospitals, serving as little more than dumping grounds for the medically ill and socially unacceptable, were shut down. Animal rights protestors in the United Kingdom harassed the pharmaceutical industry and their suppliers (while less vocal in the United States, there are still protests against animal research). And above all, US healthcare costs continued to spiral.

Yet the need for a revolution in healthcare was too long overlooked, and healthcare as a knowledge industry has been the biggest laggard in the use of IT. Patients are dying everyday because of preventable medical errors. Errors are not new to medicine, and earlier medics, such as William Osler writing in 1892, had rather stoic views about medical errors due to error in judgment or the art of balancing probabilities of a curable case: "Start out with the conviction that absolute truth is hard to reach in matters relating to our fellow creatures, healthy or diseased, that slips in observation are inevitable even with the best trained faculties. ... You will draw from your errors the very lessons which may enable you to avoid their repetition."

The issue of errors is aggravated further by the special challenges faced by doctors today. The patients doctors see every day generate hundreds of pages of paperwork and phone calls. The demographic projections of a growing aging population present an urgent need for a stable system that can ensure the availability of the high quality medical services.

In fairness, not everyone shares the critical view of the US healthcare system, although most medical practitioners agree that it needs fixing. Dr. Jerome H. Grossman, who was the head of the New England Medical Center, Boston, and the healthcare industry's guru, developed one of the first automated medical records systems for HMOs, called COSTAR, in Massachusetts. His attitude was basically this: if something is broken, don't keep whining about it, just fix it. The White Paper Grossman composed from the Boston-based Pioneer Institute for Public Policy Research offers an overall view of what went wrong with healthcare in Massachusetts, and what to avoid doing in the future. In his view, a watershed event was the decline of the system starting in 1988 when Massachusetts attempted to be the first state in the country to provide universal health insurance and ending with the state's taking temporary control of Harvard Pilgrim Health Care late 1999. Grossman calls the HPHC receivership a "classic failed merger" that could happen to any group at any time. Anyone sick was taken care of by a doctor, no matter what the cost was. The doctors and hospitals did not have any fiscal responsibility, said Grossman. Then the Balanced Budget Act was passed in 1997, and suddenly the spending had to be curbed in because Medicare reimbursements were cut. Hospitals balanced their books, and doctors were forced to manage the cost under the direction of their HMOs.

In his White Paper Grossman makes two suggestions. (1) Control of one's care should be returned to the doctor and patient; that is essentially basic personalized medicine. (2) Every HMO should offer healthcare plans and prices for the "consumer" to choose from; that is in accord with bringing the healthcare system into the twenty-first century with information technology. Although healthcare industry has been slow to catch on, IT applications are expected to cut costs and improve efficiency by automating workflows for clinical practice as well as financial management.

MEDICAL ERRORS IN MORE DETAIL

Medical errors are a big driver for change. Still it would be unfair to put medical errors among the deficiencies of any healthcare system. Rather than an example of "what went wrong," we could imagine that the situation might have been just as bad at this moment in history and industrial development prior to the saving effects of medical IT and pharmacogenomics. Nowhere else in the world is the track record as good as in the United States. Yet the US healthcare industry appears to have had the worst safety record of any other US industry. According to a report by the Agency for Health Care Research and Quality in the United States, medical errors injure 1 out of every 25 hospital patients, and medical errors by 700,000 physicians in United States killed approximately 119,000 patients in the United States in 2001. Medical errors in the United States claim 44,000 to 98,000 lives yearly in hospitals alone (more than motor vehicle accidents, breast cancer, or AIDS) at a cost of $37.6 billion, of which $17 billion are preventable costs. Adverse drug reactions (ADRs) are believed to be the fourth leading cause of death today in the United States. The American Medical Association concludes that a large percentage of ADRs are unavoidable because the doctors lack critical data and analysis tools.

It is, of course, tempting to give many nerve-wracking anecdotes about medical errors. Newspapers reveal bizarre cases almost daily. More prevalent are wrong diagnoses, wrong prescriptions, and wrong dosages. A recurrent theme of what may be considered continuing incompetence, without even the benefit of ignorance or slip of the pen, is the sorry state of hospital hygiene, where "superbugs" put patients more at risk of serious infection than at large in the outside world. However, some things are easier to criticize than fix, and while a case could be made using the new generation of microorganism detector chips, for example, IT is probably not the prime cure in outsourcing of cleaning duties.

Other apparent bloomers seem, on face of the evidence, more in the nature of injudicious advice or the patients not heeding advice. A flight attendant delivered a baby on a flight. After the woman's waters broke, it seemed that she would get coverage of costs for her premature baby by flying to another country. Someone wryly stated that healthcare costs are more manageable on the airline, and the service is better too. IT could have helped a lot in this circumstance. Physician decision support systems could include not only inference for diagnosis and best therapy choice, but also for governance, compliance, and accountability, and best practice generally. Advice to patients is not the only big error where IT can help.

Another error is the prescription that goes wrong for the patient even when, from the classical medical perspective, the prescription should have been fine. To put things in perspective, medical errors claim 44 thousand to 98 thousand lives in hospitals alone, and this makes hospitals a more dangerous killer than motor vehicle accidents. Even more disturbing is the fact that out of the 119,000 deaths caused by fatal mistakes by 700,000 US physicians in 2001, a large percentage of these deaths were unavoidable because the doctors lacked critical data and analysis tools.

TWO OTHER PRESSURES ON THE HEALTHCARE SYSTEM REFLECT ITS CURRENT PLACE IN HISTORY OF WORLD AFFAIRS

Soldiers returning home after the Second World War contributed to the birthrate explosion that is the major reason for the growing demands on US healthcare today. The growing and aging baby boomer population are a major driving force for safer and more effective medicines to treat their numerous ailments and illnesses. The demand is for a proactive, patient-centered, outcome-driven, wellness-oriented continuum of healthcare service to ensure diagnosis with high accuracy and treatment with high efficacy and safety in consideration of individual patient's genotypic and phenotypic variances. With the fastest growing segment of the US population consisting of retirees (over 65 years old), it is projected that a quarter of all Americans older than 65 in 2050 will utilize three to five times more health services than today's senior over 86 years old.

"Homeland security" is a significant driver in the United States and elsewhere presently. Thought of biological warfare strikes terror in the minds of most people. It is in the nature of terrorist warfare that new methods of destruction are constantly evolving. Governments have developed security measures to deal with the unimaginable horror that biological warfare could inflict. The United States has led the way in the areas of defense and security. The United States Homeland Security Act and the US Public Health Security and Bioterrorism Preparedness and Response Act are two major actions taken by the Bush administration government to protect the American people. The US Department of Defense has applauded the idea of the installation of automated generation of nucleic acid biosensors for biothreat agents, and the application of real-time fluorogenic polymerase chain reactions to enable nucleic acid-based detection biothreat agents. The US commitment to this plan is steady—it has granted $1.7 billion a year to NIH biological defense, and has allowed a US federal budget of $4.5 billion (in 2003) for fighting bioterrorism.

ARE THEY SPENDING ON IT TO FIX THE PROBLEMS?

The market for the most basic electronic health records in the United States is poised to top only about $5 billion in 2015, according to a 2007 study from Kalorama Information. Others say that to reduce US healthcare expenditure, well over $200 billion will need to be spent over the next 10 years on replacing patient records for use by physicians' offices and hospitals, of which about a quarter might be quickly recuperated by money saved in comparison to a paper-based office. To get a sense of the market, it may be noted that there are almost 900,000 physicians in the United States according to American Medical Association studies (somewhat more than usually quoted), and we know that physicians who are already spending on the medical record IT are paying over $37,000 for a system and at least $10,000 maintenance per annum. Smart additions with text analytic software could very soon add some $4 billion at current rates of acceptance. Recent studies from Minnesota University and other institutions put current acceptance rates by physicians at 18% to 33% for solo physicians and small practices and 36% to 39% for large practices. Obviously the systems are expensive for small practices. Medicare, which says the lack of digital patient records is one of the biggest bottlenecks in improving healthcare, has decided to intervene in an unprecedented move, to offer doctors free electronic records systems. Medicare is provided to doctors free of charge—software to computerize their medical practices. An office with five doctors might make a saving of more than $100,000 if they choose the Medicare software rather than buy software from a private company.

Bigger practices tend to go for the industrial strength, all bells and whistles, versions of medical information technology built round the digital record. The full potential expenditure on IT of very large practices like the Mayo clinic is significant. The editorial board of the *Minneapolis Star-Tribune* recently (2007) praised the Allina Hospitals and Clinics for putting a quarter of a billion dollars into computerizing its 8 hospitals and 65 clinics. The federal government believes the adoption of IT systems by all healthcare providers could save $140 billion annually. In consequence the Senate Health, Education, Labor and Pensions Committee passed the Wired for Health Care Quality Act of 2007 (S.1693) on June 27, 2008. A bill was approved to modernize the US healthcare system through increasing the use of IT systems. The bipartisan bill was sponsored by Senators Edward Kennedy (MA), Michael Enzi (WY), Hillary Clinton (NY), and Orrin Hatch (UT). Electronic records systems are expected to save lives and money by reducing errors and duplicate paperwork and also give easy access to medical records for physicians and other healthcare providers.

There is more to the use of electronic systems than for medical record keeping, of course. When all IT applications for X ray, MRI, CT, PET, SPECT, gamma, nuclear medicine, ultrasound, infrared, mammography, microscopes and digital pathology, catheter optics, MI-guided robot surgery, molecular imaging, and relevant IT inside and outside the increasing programmable, increasingly computer-like image capture devices were added up, a further $25 billion were saved in 2007. Then there are the projected uses of data-analytics and support for evidence-based medicine, clinical bioinformatics, genomic and proteomic analysis, the insurance and payer software, workflow control, governance and accountability software, with compliance coming potentially from the patient's fine-grained wishes expressed as consent, epidemiological, public health, and biothreat vigilance, as well the use of supercomputers for data mining, in silico simulation and drug design, and so forth, for personalized medicine, medical R&D, and pharmaceutical R&D. In the very near future wireless, RFID chips are expected to be used to identify patients by physician hand-held devices and voice recognition, optical fibre cables, security and standards implementation, and so on. Naturally difficulties of market assessment remain and these include, on the one hand, scope, meaning what is actually included in clinical IT or healthcare generally, and on the other, market demand, which is likely to rise steeply over the next few years.

THE BUSINESS CASE FOR IT IN HEALTHCARE

In pursuing investment to start a business, one needs a business plan, ideally in a nice glossy brochure, with revenue projections. When the "promised" revenues look enticingly large, some qualitative justification may suffice in the form of a succinct lists of driving factors, the "value propositions," and the key benefits of the particular approach taken. With that in mind, let us review the business case for information technology based medicine.

First, the key business drivers for a new healthcare system are as follows:

- Reduction of the cost of healthcare services through sharing critical personal health information in a near real-time basis (government perspective)

- Timely quality services (patient's perspective)
- Lower operation cost by minimizing duplicate lab tests (government's perspective)
- Fewer repeated time-consuming and expensive lab tests (patient's perspective)
- Universal healthcare services including rural areas and the handicapped (government perspective)
- Increased competitiveness in the private healthcare market through timely quality services (hospital's perspective)
- Provision of cost-effective after-services (hospitals' perspective)

The anticipated value propositions of the information technology are as follows:

- Increased automation of shared information, increasing productivity and helping providers make informed decisions
- Identification and eligibility checking done on a real-time basis
- Patients' health records dynamically assembled on demand and shared in real-time across providers
- Paper use minimized or eliminated
- Different levels of authorization for access based on role, purpose, and logical location (e.g., ER), including full access (physician), or to simply validate identity and add information (test locations)
- Electronic communication and status indicators available throughout the system on a real-time basis
- System support of workflow by automating work where warranted
- Complete historical record provided on demand and on a real-time basis
- Capability of laboratories and pharmacies to pick up the work order on demand
- Availability of consistent patient information
- Decision support on drug interaction at multiple points using the same patient record and drug information sources
- Reference and educational information is readily available online to providers and patients
- Email communication available within and across organizations
- Calendars and meetings automatically synchronized and scheduled
- Executive information system to alert abnormal indicators throughout the system
- Convenience
- Secure information sharing on a "need to know" basis
- Drug safety

- Faster service
- Duplication of information across providers so that no information is lost
- Paperless and filmless where feasible
- Timely comprehensive advice from service providers
- Better access to educational and reference information

The following list summarizes key benefits provided for healthcare service providers:

- Optimization of resources and time
- Added value of event status indicators
- Reduced administrative process overhead
- Efficiency and accuracy of record keeping
- Comprehensive health records
- Reduced duplicate testing
- More efficient and effective collaboration among service providers
- More timely access to results
- Reduced risk of adverse patient reaction to drug
- Information available for outcome measurement
- Just-in-time research and medical education
- Operational efficiency in reduced cost of purchases

CONTRAINDICATIONS: THE CHALLENGES FOR HEALTHCARE IT

Any fair brochure seeking to raise capital for a new business should consider the downside. Projecting the scope and impact of a new development is a challenge particularly when administrators must avoid treading on more conservative toes. Thus adoption of healthcare IT is hindered by problems associated with deeply ingrained practices and issues embedded in the healthcare system. Ingrained practices could be the biggest barrier of all. Change is a risk. But no change keeps the patient at risk, as the key issue driving change is the huge number of medical errors.

Another big challenge is creation of a working system of interdisciplinary communication and collaboration across the business and scientific domains. Information sharing among multidisciplinary professionals entails also that different segments of the business and science worlds cooperate and pool their resources toward achieving a common goal. Institution-wide data integration requires, of course, transparent access to diverse, heterogeneous data at various sources. Further, to protect the patient, there should be regulatory-driven standardization for compliance to emerging statutory requirements by organizations as represented by privacy laws and regulations (e.g., HIPAA, FIPPA, PIPEDA, PHIPA, EU Privacy Directive, FDA CFR 21 Part 11).

An obstacle in this requirement is the well-known reluctance of professionals to share their information and resources. Another problem in achieving communication and collaboration lies in the dispersed heterogeneous nature of the data sources, and their diverse ownership and custodianship. For effective information sharing all the data across many domains must be readily accessible as needs arise. Data sources may be ever increasing their already vast amounts, but the range is deceiving: information may be spread out on a multidimensional level but sparse in each dimension, rendering the comprehensiveness of the data an illusion. Then, besides the incomplete, uncertain, and inconsistent nature of the data sources, there is the challenge to information sharing across the multiple disciplines of the complex structures of data sources that keep on changing.

Key to the development of a biomedical informatics architecture is the ethics and privacy issues inherent in any healthcare endeavor. Even though the IT industry sees this as an opportunity not a contraindication, the handling of genotypic and phenotypic data requires a high level of security to protect its highly sensitive and personal nature. Conformity to the statutory requirements for the protection of privacy will require the biomedical informatics field to be developed with the issues of privacy and security in mind.

Practical problems in research and development based on translating the extremely complex relationships between genotype and phenotype into drug targets have been aggravated by the complexity of emerging disease targets. The biomedical informatics strategy should be to first understand the molecular mechanisms of the diseases involved, and next to discover the individual's predisposition for a disease. From this information optimal therapies can be selected and the outcomes monitored. By the informatics approach it is anticipated that diagnoses will be more accurate and treatment safer and more effective.

MORE ON ADVERSE DRUG REACTIONS: WRONG PRESCRIPTION, BUT WHO COULD EVER KNOW?

As we noted above, adverse drug events are prominent among medical accidents. But this is not always the fault of the physician armed only with current knowledge. People differ in various previously unpredictable ways in their responses to the same medication. Many errors relate to wrong doses, or even wrong drug, but much of what is wrong with the drug, and indeed the dose, pertains to what is thought, on average, to be the right drug in right dosage. Unfortunately, patients have their own genetic and immunological issues that govern their responses to a drug. Previously there was no way to tell and no reason to suspect any problem, save by prior experience. That is why the paramedics in the United States often ask about "any allergies?" The "allergies" part is effectively a euphemism for any adverse drug reactions. In the well-known case of the sensitivity to penicillin, the problem is an autoimmune effect brought on by strong binding of the penicillin to serum albumin, and indeed a response of the immune system in some patients is because the drug complex looks like an alien invader. However, the matter usually lies deeper, in our individual DNA.

If DNA held a mere 30 genetic factors that could be categorized as simply as yes/no for each patient (as in male/female), that could potentially distinguish 2^{30} individuals, much larger than the US population. Cardiovascular diseases and many cancers may involve not 30 but up to 100 or more critical (and often not two-valued) factors that may not be fully reduced into simpler guidelines. It is easy to see why every patient is a special case, and no single patient can very be considered average. The significance of the new genomic technologies is that they can lead to hundreds or thousands of patient descriptors, which implies trans-astronomic numbers of potentially interesting combinations: for a 1,000 factors there are almost exactly 2^{1000}, meaning 10^{301} combinations including all the combinations in the different possible size sets of 1, 2, 3, ... , 1,000 factors).

Approximately 100,000 patients die due to ADR (adverse drug reactions) each year in the United States. ADRs and ADEs (adverse drug events) are universally acknowledged problems that need to be solved. A drug that does not work is also serious, since it delays treatment. Many drugs are effective for only approximately 60 percent of the people who take them (e.g., antidepressants). Genomics may not only remove guess-work from the process of finding the correct drug and dosage but also speed recovery time and increase safety by minimizing and eventually eliminating the likelihood of adverse reactions. Quick genomic tests are already being used for the best choice of antidepressant. From a business perspective, *pharmacogenomics*, with IT to support it, holds promise of less contraindication for a new medicine besides the opportunity for the science of genomic diagnosis to predict patient–drug response. Pharmacogenomics could potentially dramatically reduce deaths and two million unnecessary hospitalizations that occur each year in the United States as a result of ADRs (see below).

Paradoxically the acronym ADR, which, as noted above, can mean great suffering from drug reactions, also refers to a kind of legal or sub-legal dispute. So the clinical use of ADR should not be confused with a possible consequence, the well-meaning effort to reduce legal hassling over compensation by *alternative dispute resolutions*—also called ADRs. Disputes with health insurers or managed health care organizations can be bitter and prolonged. A trained arbitrator presides over the debate and gives a final, binding decision. Mediation, in contrast, is an alternative less bitter process. A mediator, chosen by the disputing parties, facilitates discussion and approach to a resolution. The training and skills of a mediator are more facilitative than those of an arbitrator, whose task is to preside, and help the players reach the final conclusion. Even so, recall that in the United States legal and other reactive costs arising from medical errors cost about $40 billion a year, of which $17 billion are considered avoidable costs.

FDA AMENDMENTS: GREAT SOCIAL PROGRESS, DISRUPTIVE MARKET FORCE?

Regarding feedback from patient–physician interactions about drugs in the market and other medical products and procedures, Janet Woodcock, director of the Center for Drug Evaluation and Research for the FDA, cautions "The science is not developed yet. … We get all this data, but what does it mean?"[1]

Her comment is in regard to drug regulation takes on new significance as a consequence of the 2007 FDA Amendments Act (FDAAA) discussed below. The IT-based solutions that it behests the FDA to organize will release massive amounts of data visible to analysis by the public and hence all players, and thus increase the detection and reporting of adverse drug events. The ability to rapidly extract data could unleash a new interactive dynamics of healthcare and pharmaceutical players at the global level, and trigger a discontinuity in market opportunity in all three sectors.

While IT-based healthcare has been slow in the United States, in the Britain, despite the absence as yet of a nationally distributed *detailed* digital patient record, the NHS (National Health Services) has had access for several years to patient data from the General Practice Research Database (GPRD) and IMS Disease Analyzer. The UK Prescribing Support Unit and other agencies have routinely used patient-level source data. The GPRD and IMS have jointly a comprehensive source of longitudinal patient level data, which is the largest in Europe. The GPRD, a nonprofit unit under the Medicines and Healthcare Products Regulatory Agency (MHRA), has for many years helped government and pharmaceutical industry with information for epidemiology and R&D applications. The GPRD group has highlighted the potential use of observational data for pharmacovigilance data based on the concept of absolute risk.

In 2004 the US Food and Drug Administration introduced the Critical Path Initiative (CPI), to advance safer drug development by incorporating recent scientific advances, such as genomics and advanced imaging technologies, into the process. The motivation was that the pharmaceutical industry has had the perceived reputation of not being a responsible driver and being a "closed shop" in monitoring safety of marketed drugs. The FDA had previously estimated that only 1 out of 10 adverse events is actually reported. At the same time the FDA had not been perceived as particularly strong in embracing stratified medicine and genomics, limiting itself to recommendation for a few handfuls of drugs, nor in advanced data analytic methods to monitor patient

---

[1] Source: Murray Aitken, SVP, *Healthcare Insight*, for IMS HEALTH, Norwalk, CT, 2008.

therapy, which would be required for more serious effort in this regard, on the basis of evidence. The data analysis problem is nontrivial, especially when genomics is included because of the high-dimensional, multiparameter nature of the data.

The critical path planned for *public–private* partnerships and consortia is to accomplish the needed research. The CPI plan for such a partnership, OMOP (Observational Medical Outcomes Partnership), may lead the way in determining the feasibility and value of using observational data to identify and evaluate the safety and benefits of prescribed drugs. This partnership will be governed by the FDA, led by the NIH through the Foundation of the NIH, and funded by PhRMA. OMOP planned to have results to report by the end of 2008, including a report on scientific and technical findings, peer-reviewed articles on pilot experiments, and a "lessons-learned" white paper.

The early phases of these efforts laid both the intellectual basis for the signing of the Drug Safety Law, namely the FDA Amendments Act (FDAAA), by President Bush on September 27, 2007, and the timing requirements for implementation under that Act. On March 4, 2008, Senate Finance Committee member, Chuck Grassley (R-Iowa), called for a General Accountability Office investigation into how the FDA monitors safety and efficacy of approved drugs.

The Drug Safety Act, by force of law, moves postmarketing data collection and analysis out of the grasp of pharmaceutical industry and into the public domain as a transparent but regulated system. The data will be accessible to the public, academic researchers, patient advocacy groups, health insurers, academic centers, and employers, and not least pharmaceutical companies, all of which will have access and all bodies with diverse and often conflicting interests. The worthy aim should allow patterns of adverse events and safety issues to be recognized and pharmacovigilance (detection, evaluation, comprehension, and risk prediction), risk management, meta-analysis, and postmarketing data to be integrated with clinical trials, a federation of heterogeneous sources, adverse event detection, and reporting. From these data it will be possible to identify associations and correlations of disease incidence and therapy in a stratified, population-specific way on the relative efficacy of treatments.

By this legislation, the FDA gains more authority and can strengthen its focus on drug safety and drug efficacy. The FDA is responsible for the postmarket risk identification and analysis system (Section 905 of the FDAAA). The FDA was granted $125 million, spread over five years (until 2012), to develop methods for obtaining postmarket patient information and establish a means of collaboration for the public and private sectors to create the necessary public–private partnership. The main objective, as set forth in Section 905, is to create a current and accessible surveillance system for 100 million people by the year 2012 (25 million patients by 2010). The FDA is under pressure to find a way to meet the 2010 and 2012 objectives laid out in the legislation. It must submit a report to Congress by 2011 on how it is *using* the system.

Currently accessible US data sources include claims, transactional, and billing data, Medicare data and data from the Department of Veterans Affairs. The FDA cannot control these data sources without a distributed data network. This distributed network will be developed and managed in collaboration with a nonprofit private partner, the Reagan-Udall Foundation that remains to be founded for that purpose. The foundation will coordinate adverse event reporting with the NIH and FDA. The US Department of Health and Human Services will be involved to develop methods of collecting and sharing data under HIPAA compliance, integrating diverse sources, alerting about adverse events, and exporting the data for statistical and epidemiological analysis.

Because the FDA has the authority and funding, competition among competing IT organizations will stimulate new software developments. Further, with the growing participation of NIH, the pre- and postregulatory arena will become complex. Pharmaceutical companies are encouraged to participate and be seen to "clean up their act," but increased transparency poses huge risk for them. There is likely to be a huge increase in the number of adverse events *reported*, which is exactly the intent of the original Critical Path Initiative and the FDAAA legislature, so the pharmaceutical industry will need to find more efficient ways of working to keep up with the additional analyses.

Pharmaceutical companies will need to scan the databases themselves for adverse events using the very best data analytics for high-dimensional and multiparameter data, so that they can take appropriate corrective actions, limit damage, or preempt the FDA with a suitable genuine defense, where possible, for false positive alerts and as appropriate for genomic targeting (i.e., identification of the correct genomic "strata" of patients). Wyeth and GlaxoSmithKline have already begun to build on the Observational Medical Outcomes Partnership (OMOP) data, which is key to the plan.

PHARMACOGENOMICS: TROUBLEMAKER, AND WHITE KNIGHT TO THE RESCUE

Although pharmacogenomic diversity is the cause of many adverse drug effects, a scientific discipline that, with IT, has the potential to create drugs that fight disease without dangerous trial and error. At its fullest, pharmacogenomics includes or relates to toxicogenomics, clinical genomics, physiological genomics, chemical genomics, nutrigenomics, and psychogenomics. Additionally pharmacogenomic studies of immunological and environmental variants can impact drug behavior in patients. Genetic variation in the activities of enzymes and transporters responsible for the absorption, distribution, metabolism, toxicity, and excretion of drugs underlies many examples of individual differences in drug response. Rapid metabolism and clearance makes a drug ineffective faster, whereas slow metabolism leads to excess levels and potential accumulation, often associated with adverse events and toxicity.

The case of Voriconazole (an orally administered antifungal drug) illustrates several points. In vivo studies indicate that an enzyme involved in the metabolism of Voriconazole exhibits genetic polymorphism, a common phenomenon in which several forms of the same enzyme or other protein can exist within or between patients differing in amino acid sequence and enzymological or other properties. It is convenient that the percentage of patients carrying specific biomarkers often tend to vary significantly with the ethnicity, or more precisely the scientifically determined genomic constitution. Among Asian populations, 15% to 20% may be expected to be poor metabolizers of Voriconazole, whereas among Caucasians and African Americans, the prevalence of poor metabolizers is just 3% to 5%. However, the indications for administration of Voriconazole can be made precise by testing the patient for the genomic feature associated with poor metabolizers. Making biomarkers diagnostics on a chip that could be applied in a physician's office would allow for individual, rapid, and safe treatment.

Big pharmaceutical companies have begun to seek another path. Their objective is to find a gene or haplotype through genome polymorphism or SNP mapping and then identify its connection to a disease and so ascertain the susceptibility of the patient. The idea is that a molecule will bind the encoded protein selectively to block its action, thereby putting a halt to its adverse effects, in theory at least.

The performance goal set by the leading pharmaceutical companies is triple the number of new drugs developed in a year. Adverse reactions are prominent factors in the pharmaceutical economic ecosystem. Putting together data from many sources, it appears that the number of US drug approvals is rising from about 134 in 2006 to about 273 in 2013. The global pharmaceutical drug market is estimated at rising from $596 to $957 billion for this period, putting the worth of each new pharmaceutical compound currently at between 800 million and 2 billion. To attain this, the estimated pre-clinical research expenditure by the pharmaceutical industry in this period is correspondingly estimated at $56 and $86 billion worldwide, again meaning for 2006 and 2013, respectively, plus, importantly, $62 and $82 billion, respectively, for "research" in the clinical trial and post-clinical phase. The latter is needed because there were 2,178 product and batch recalls for the year 2006, and will be 3,037 in 2013 by projection of current trends, and the cost of morbidity and fatality is estimated at $150–260 billion worldwide (in 2008). Spending in the drug regulatory and surveillance industry is thus justifiably huge and expected to rise at an AAGR of 10% to reach $265 billion by 2010 (http://www.bccresearch.com/report/PHM047A.html).

CURRENT ECONOMIC DRIVERS OF PHARMACOGENOMICS

Pharmaceutical companies not only need to increase output (in terms of new chemical entities, or NCEs) each year to stay solvent, the new medicine demands that drugs be available that differ with disease and patient too. This may seem like fantasy, but the chemical and microfluidic (tiny pipe and pump) elements, for a microlab-on-card technology, may some day be available to allow new drugs to be designed and assembled for each patient on demand, even on the spot. However, right now it takes on average (at time of writing) $1.2 billion and 14.7 years to develop one drug, and on average the top 15 pharmaceutical companies have been developing one new drug a year.

While on-the-spot drug development is envisioned for the future, the growth of pharmaceuticals in 2007 raised the estimated global market to $712 billion, an increase of $178 billion, or a market growth of 6.4%. That sounds healthy. But despite a strong year in 2006, the 2007 figures actually reflect a slowdown in global growth that began in 2003, when the market grew by 10.3%. From large R&D-based multi-national companies to small biotech companies, the general positive 2006 trend was replaced by a rise or fall according to corporate innovation and business acumen. Overall, the United States, Japan, and the aggregate of European five big markets grew less than 5% in 2007. Causes include the production of generic drugs ("drug copies") in major therapy areas, and their stultifying effect on NCEs (again, new chemical entities, i.e., basically new drug candidates). There was also increased scrutiny of drug efficacy and pricing levels, and increased access to medicines, especially in poorer countries. Emerging drug markets (China, India, Brazil, Mexico, Turkey, Russia, and India) grew in excess of 14%. Things were good for NCEs for cancer drugs angiotensin-II antagonists, antidiabetes, and antipsychotics, which all grew by more than 10%, with new products reaching more patients. But lipid regulators and antidepressants declined by 7% with declines in exclusivity, safety confidence, and new offerings.[2]

Innovation now critically depends on pharmacogenomics. Many diseases that appear as single clinical conditions have a number of underlying causes and an enhanced understanding of the genetic basis of such diseases will provide information about drugs that might be effective in the different classes of the disease. In a number of cases, notably cancers, diseased cells have different genotypes and expression proteomics from those in normal tissue. This is seen in the case of breast cancer, where a particularly aggressive form of the disease is characterized by overexpression of the protein Her2.[3] High levels of Her2 expression are associated with a good response to the drug trastuzumab (Herceptin) but this agent is essentially ineffective against other breast tumors.[4]

Already there is evidence that genomic diagnosis can lead to fairly detailed guidance on administration and on contraindications. For example, some patients have a genetic defect leading to reduced levels of activity of a P450

[2] Murray Aitken, SVP, *Healthcare Insight*, for IMS HEALTH, Norwalk, CT, 2008.
[3] Mokbel K, Hassanally D, From HER2 to herceptin, *Curr Med Res Opin* 2001;17:51–9.
[4] Harries M, Smith I, The development and clinical use of trastuzumab (Herceptin), *Endocr Relat Cancer* 2002;9:75–85.

cytochrome, namely P4502D6. Fluoxetine, like other agents that are metabolized by P450 IID6, inhibits the activity of this enzyme form. The FDA thus recommends that therapy with other medications that are predominantly metabolized by the P450 IID6 system, and that have a relatively narrow therapeutic index, should be initiated at the low end of the dose range if a patient is receiving fluoxetine or has received it in the previous five weeks.

What technical bottlenecks does the industry need to tackle in order to realize the benefits of pharmacogenomics? They are several, but automation of workflow for efficiency, reproducibility, compliance, and best practice; integration of diverse information to knowledge; better data mining and inference from it; and better solvent calculations in drug design can all be traced back to the importance of our old enemy *entropy* as negative information. The pharmaceutical industry is in essence, through the discovery and refinement process, an *information industry*, and so it is becoming increasingly dependent on IT.

WHAT IS PHARMACOGENOMICS ANYWAY?

The term "pharmacogenetics" was originally defined in 1959 as "clinically important hereditary variation in response to drugs" by Frederich Vogel.[5] A discipline by that name was established by Werner Kalow's monograph *Pharmacogenetics* in 1962.[6] A small number of further examples accrued from the 1950s onward, generally involving a small number of related individuals showing aberrant responses to a number of specific agents.[7] In the late 1960s, there had been showed remarkable similarity of response to several drugs in identical twins who share 100% of their genes as contrasted to fraternal twins who only share 50%.

The early working definition of pharmacogenetics is still used in academic circles to refer to the study of variability in drug responses attributable to hereditary factors. This is also more or less the definition that we use for the term *pharmacogenomics* throughout this book. For others who prefer the older word, the term *pharmacogenomics* is reserved for the analysis of genomes and genomic expression as they relate to drug responses. Of course, however these two fields are defined, they inevitably overlap, especially in terms of the technologies that they both employ. Nonetheless, pharmacogenomics offers different properties from pharmacogenetics, and stands to offer some very different results. A quick summary of its scope is that it is the field of study of associations and linkage disequilibria between aetiology of diseases and SNPs (simple nucleotide polymorphisms) and other genetic variants in the DNA

[5] Vogel F, Moderne probleme der Humangenetik. *Ergeb Inn Med Kinderheilkd* 1959;12:52–125.
[6] Kalow W, *Pharmacogenetics: Heredity and Response to Drugs*, Philadelphia: Saunders, 1962.
[7] E. S. Vesell, Pharmacogenetics: multiple interactions between genes and environment as determinants of drug response. *Am J Med* 1979;66:183–7.

sequence affecting drug response. In simple terms, pharmacogenetics allows for patient stratification based on responses to drugs, by studying the association between diseases and their corresponding alleles and SNPs. Also involved are the drug responses based on genetic variances, resulting in the one drug for a multiple genomes approach. This includes complex genetic issues with terms like *monogenic defects, multifactorial complex disorders, chromosomal imbalances*, and *mitochondrial mutations*.

Be that as it may, let's use *pharmacogenomics* as the broader term, including the notion of the development of more effective drugs, by keeping in mind associations between diseases and proteins, enzymes, and RNA. Pharmacogenomics aims to develop personalized medicine, adapted to each person's genetic makeup and environment. Environmental factors are important because features such as diet, age, lifestyle, and state of health can influence an individual's response to a drug. However, understanding an individual's genetic makeup is considered to be key to creating personalized medicine with greater efficacy and safety, and ultimately safer drugs. By basing the best available treatment on genetic profiles, speedy recovery, and preventing adverse drug reactions, dosages will be administered accurately in ways unimaginable until now. Instead of basing dosages on weight and age, practitioners will be able to rely on genetic profiles, to dose each drug amount to the individual patient at hand. Genetic profiles will enable advanced screening for assessing which diseases are likely to occur. This knowledge can be used to advance knowledge of a patient's susceptibility to a disease and increase wellness through an appropriate lifestyle and diet. Other benefits include more effective vaccines, reduced time and cost for drug discovery, and reduced cost of health care.

CRYSTALLIZING THE BENEFITS OF PHARMACOGENOMICS

"Change your ways or have them changed for you" is effectively the message from the US government to drug R&D as much as to clinical practice. But the pharmaceutical industry has already taken a positive view of the value proposition of pharmacogenomics. So what is the value proposition, more exactly? We may summarize the potential benefits of increased understanding of all this as follows:[8]

1. *Improving drug safety.* If a specific genotypic variant is found to be associated with an adverse reaction, doctors could avoid prescribing the medicine to patients with this genotype.
2. *Adjusting dosage.* Knowledge of genotypes with specific pharmacokinetic characteristics could be used to adjust the dosage of affected drugs,

[8] Wolf CR, Smith G, Smith RL, Science, medicine and the future: Pharmacogenetics. *BMJ* 2000;320:987–90; Evans WE, Pharmacogenomics: marshalling the human genome to individualize drug therapy. *Gut* 2003;52(suppl 2):ii10–8.

reducing the trial-and-error approach of prescriptions to determine the most effective dosage.

3. *Enhancing efficacy.* Many widely used treatments for major diseases, such as diabetes, depression, and asthma, are reported to be effective in only half the population. Rather than using trial and error with all its attendant problems, pharmacogenetics may identify responsive and non-responsive patients or offer new medicines designed on the basis of the genetics of the disease.

4. *Drug pricing.* Improving the pricing or sale worth of drugs could be according to their worthiness for specific genomic strata of the population.

The primary anticipated benefit of genomic insight is that more powerful medicine will be provided *appropriately* to patients. As a result pharmaceutical companies should be able to create drugs based on proteins, enzymes, and RNA molecules associated with genes and disease. Drug discovery will thus proceed with drug makers producing therapies that are targeted to specific diseases, and tailored for specific genetic characteristics. Such accuracy will not only maximize therapeutic effects but also decrease damage to nearby healthy cells, thereby minimizing the toxicity of side effects. In sum, pharmacogenomics will enable more accurate drug dosages to be determined, as there will be provision for advanced screening for diseases. Our knowledge of our genetic code will allow us to make adequate lifestyle, environmental, and/or diet changes at an early age and avoid or lessen the severity of potential genetic diseases. The priori knowledge of our susceptibility to a particular disease will allow our doctors to carefully monitor us, and introduce treatment at the most beneficial stage to maximize therapy.

With the improvements in the drug discovery and approval process due to pharmacogenomics, pharmaceutical companies will be discovering potential therapies with greater ease via genomic targets based on genetic markers. Drug pricing will be profoundly affected as a result because of the genomically defined markets. Older drugs or drugs in the pharmaceutical pipeline intended for other purposes might, like Viagra, have new applications that will depend on genomics. Previously failed drug candidates or drugs like thalidomide can often be "repurposed" or retargeted as they are matched with a niche population. The drug approval process will be facilitated as trials are targeted for specific genetic population groups, providing a greater likelihood for success. Moreover, the cost and risk of clinical trials will be reduced, since only persons capable of responding to a particular drug will be targeted.

Still another anticipated benefit of pharmacogenomics is superior vaccines, also personalized on a genomic basis (see Chapter 9). Vaccines made of peptides by laboratory chemistry and mimicking parts of dangerous organisms will keep all the benefits of existing vaccines without the connected risks. These vaccines will be designed to activate the immune system and to be inexpensive, stable, easy to store, and capable of being engineered to carry several strains of pathogens at once but unable to cause infections, a key negative factor associated with current vaccines.

Therefore pharmacogenomics should bring about reduction in the overall cost of healthcare, which is especially relevant for governments that provide public funded healthcare such as in Canada, the United Kingdom, Australia, Belgium, and Germany. Pharmacogenomics will decrease the number of ADRs, the number of failed drug trials, the time it takes to get a drug approved, the length of time a patient is on medication, the number of medications that a patient must take to find an effective therapy, the negative effects of disease on the body through early detection, and, most important, the number of sick days of productive workers, and thus increase a country's gross domestic product.

That's the good news. Despite these anticipated benefits pharmacogenomics has still scientific and mathematical barriers to its progress. A few factors like eye color depend on very few genomic factors, but that is not the rule. One barrier is the complexity of finding gene variants that come together to affect drug response. Data mining discussed in later chapters will be a key IT tool in helping sort out such knowledge, and systems biology, also frequently mentioned, in interpreting it. SNPs affect roughy one in every 300 amino acids in the proteins made by each gene. Multiplied for a three billion base human genome results in millions of SNPs to be identified and analyzed to determine their involvement in drug responses. So the first difficulty is that since many different genes are likely to influence the response, obtaining the big picture on the impact on gene variation is labor intensive, time-consuming and very complicated. Another obstacle is that there are limited drug alternatives; only one or two approved drugs may be available for the treatment of a particular condition. Patients with gene variations that prevent them from using these drugs will have no alternatives for treatment. A further difficulty is that there is little incentive for pharmaceutical companies to produce multiple pharmaceutical products as pharmaceutical companies have so far been successful with their one-size-fits-all approach to drug development. In the face of an average cost of over $1 billion for development and a time commitment of 15 years to bring one drug to the market, how will pharmacogenomics motivate pharmaceutical companies to develop alternative drugs intended to serve only a small population percentage? The last barrier is the requirement of healthcare providers to recommend multiple pharmaceutical products, in the treatment of the same condition for different subsets of populations with a multitude of different drugs. The unavoidable effect of personalized medicine, tailored to individuals and targeted for specific genes, complicating the process of prescribing and dispensing drugs will call for ongoing education on procedures and protocols for physicians and pharmacists to resolve the problem.

Yet, despite the challenges and barriers listed above, the general consensus of the industry is that the anticipated benefits of pharmacogenomics will render rapid growth in drug discovery and development. This growth area is increasingly viewed in terms of a biomarker market, but also in terms of how to deliver drugs to their target. In the recent past advanced drug delivery accounted for 6% of the global pharmaceutical market, and this figure increased to approximately 25% from 2003 to 2008. The global market for drug delivery technologies, in conjunction with the leveraging of pharmacogenomics and IT, was about $80 billion in 2005. In the United States alone, the market for drug delivery technologies was about $41 billion with an annual compound growth rate of 11% in 2007. Biotech companies and IT companies, anxious to secure a share of the global market in new drug discovery and development, are tripping over themselves to get onto the bandwagon. But will the biotech companies suffer the fate of the dotcom explosion, or will pharmacogenomics fulfill its promises and build a permanent and sustainable existence for the biotech companies?

From the anticipated the ability of pharmacogenomics to perform patient–specific drug selection and personalize drug dosages based on one's genetic and phenotypic variances, doctors will be able to make preventative diagnoses and present patients with a selection of specific lifestyles based on diet, potential allergies, drinking, exercise, sports, travel, risks, and education. Besides enhancing genetic, diet, lifestyle, marriage, and pregnancy counseling, targeted gene therapy promises a solution to the prevalent problem of autoimmune disorders. As more personalized synthetic vaccines are developed and tailored to each patient's immune system, some autoimmune disorders will be a thing of the past.

Unlike "clinical genomics," which is *genomics* applied in the clinic, *pharmacogenomics* pertains to research trials and pharmaceutical development of drugs targeted for the particular genetic and phenotypic characteristics of each individual. Essentially clinical genomics is the rational application and evaluation of *treatments*, and clinical genomics and pharmacogenomics both aim to increase the efficacy of drugs and treatments while reducing the number of ADR. Like pharmacogenomics, clinical genomics was derived from the fields of genetic polymorphism and SNP mapping, as it became evident that some people react well to certain drugs, some get no benefits, and some unfortunate ones respond adversely to the medication. One explanation is that the drug is sensitive to the target but is only slowly inactivated as it is cleared from the bloodstream, making the drug effective at lower frequencies and doses. Alternatively the drug is sensitive to the target but is rapidly inactivated metabolically and cleared from the bloodstream, making it more favorable at higher frequencies and doses. In a few cases, an immunological reaction can neutralize the drug. Yet another scenario is that the drug is not sensitive to the target at all, resulting in no benefits to the patient. A final possibility is that the drug is sensitive to only a particular form of the disease, and maybe even produces a toxic effect without finer diagnosis.

In sum, clinical genomics and pharmacogenomics will astound us with the research possibilities for the discovery and improvement of new therapeutic tailor-made agents. The vast amount of multi-patient data will provide the core material for medical research and medical training and will enable the CDC (Center for Disease Control and Prevention), FDA (Food and Drug

Administration), and WHO (World Health Organization), insurance providers and nursing and social services to make informed decisions in their areas of competency without breaching individual patient privacy. In addition multiple-patient pharmacogenomics data will provide raw material for medical research and medical training.

OTHER PLAYERS: MAKING INTERNET E-MONEY AROUND MEDICINE

The Internet has proved to be a major force in the world economy. Growth in Internet physician–office and Internet home medicine is a natural tendency combined with general consumer use of the Internet. The Internet as a channel for health information and communications is well suited to fulfill consumer expectations. It is readily accessible and available anytime and anywhere, is inexpensive, easy to use, provides a diversity of rich information, and opens its uses to a global network of people with common interests. The Internet will offer a low-cost, rapidly deployable platform for disseminating information across vertically and horizontally integrated health care organizations. Managed care increases the diversity and urgency of information flow.

Consumers spent an estimated $8 billion (out of roughly $2 trillion in overall consumer spending) online, and over $100 billion in 2002, and the trend to online purchases has continued. The total effect of this trend is that many millions or even trillions of dollars worldwide must surely be being spent via the Internet at the time of reading this book, with a significant fraction on medical matters. The online healthcare business-to-business medical market was projected to grow to $348 billion by 2004. Past projections make it likely that soon at least 24% of hospitals, and 12% of physician practices, will buy the majority of their healthcare products online. Routine observation and anecdotal evidence suggests that will rapidly draw closer to 100%. The Internet will be an important means of communication between healthcare services. Not least, doubtless the Internet will be a major medium through which the home user will access the healthcare services described below, and thus it remains of great personal interest to the public. Some sources will be central to your health, and some will be paid for as additional enhancements of your well-being much as you would order a book from Amazon.com.

Whether healthcare is run as a business or as state or social medicine, the business aspects of the Internet have been important for establishing and demonstrating the potential of the Internet as a powerful tool for healthcare and medical practice. Patient record aspects of the medical business will be discussed in the next chapter. Developments in other businesses on the Internet have helped drive new technologies, the widening reach of the Internet with a rise in the number and power of servers (Internet–service–provider computers), improved security, and wide home acceptance of the Internet.

Whereas the e-business approach is flourishing in many industries—high-tech, finance, brokerage securities, manufacturing, distribution, transportation, and retail and paradoxically the communications industry the very backbone of the Internet—is still having difficulty in making a successful transition to online business. With increasing market challenges from new players such as utilities and cable companies, traditional communications service providers must now foster exceptional customer relationships in order to acquire and retain their most profitable customers. e-Commerce, customers expect a sophisticated web purchasing and self-service channel, so the communication service providers must not only construct customer-centric web interfaces that help customers easily pick and choose among bundled offerings but also develop e-business solutions that integrate with their operations support systems infrastructures. Providers need to offer a single point at which customers can order and maintain communications services, regardless of the organizational silos and operations support systems complexity behind the fulfillment of those services.

The communications industry has been slower to adopt e-business than the manufacturing, distribution, transportation, and retail sectors largely because of an inability to visualize what such a system would look like, given the industry's complex products, operational infrastructures, intricate carrier relationships, disparate vendors, and confusing logistical issues. In the early 1990s, when people talked about online book selling, people just couldn't conceive of it. Would customers walk through a virtual bookstore and "flip" through the pages of a book? Then Amazon.com had people nodding their heads in a chorus of, "Now I get it." To overcome these conceptual barriers, providers must assemble teams that combine both telecom and e-business experience. While there are many folks with expertise in one discipline or the other, finding the experts in multiple disciplines is a challenge. They are rare at best. The second barrier is a technological one. In their initial thinking about e-business solutions, providers must realize they have to integrate and manage data across internal operations support system infrastructures, billing systems, partner networks, and supplier systems. Tying together silos for marketing, sales, ordering, billing, complaints, and so forth, is a formidable challenge. In all this, who it really is or who wants what, is an issue. On the Internet no one knows that Web server they are dealing with. No one knows it is really you they are doing business with. With the impossibility of bringing all these disparate systems into the Internet age, providers must instead build an integration layer that ties together e-business solutions with their existing operations support system infrastructures and business processes. The financial services industry can serve as a reference point. For over a period of decades it has built a series of complex legacy systems. When it comes to e-business, the financial industry didn't replace the systems; they built user-centric interfaces that covered the mess of their existing systems, in effect hiding customers from their internal business processes while still allowing for the necessary level of interaction.

There are some developments nonetheless that can help with the security issue. Digital identifiers will soon be introduced in the Internet so that individuals can be identified and validated for authentication and authorization. With a digital identifier you will no longer have to send your log-in and password over the Internet. A digital identifier will be issued by a Certificate Authority, who can certify that you are who you claim to be. The Certificate Authority can be a bank, an insurance company, a government, or any trusted third party. They will then issue a digital identifier to each individual to be stored in a smart card, perhaps in the mobile phone, or maybe in something that is attached to a keychain. The digital identifier will be biometrically activated by a thumbprint, iris pattern, retina pattern, voice-pattern, fingerprint, or face geometry. Used in tandem, these will ensure that no one can impersonate someone else on the web. The digital identifier will be a key ingredient in enabling each individual to protect his/her privacy, medical records, and the integrity and confidentiality of financial transactions. Also despite hypertext markup language (HTML) that allows display and surfing the Internet to be highly structured (see Chapter 9), the data on the Internet today are mostly unstructured. The XML (eXtensible markup language) is going to transform the Internet by providing an underlying structure for web pages so that they don't just show what they look like but what they mean. For example, when people search on William Shakespeare, they will find things by him, about him, and also someone's web page of favorite authors. XML will add context to web pages so that people can find wanted information, and applications can communicate with each other.

To access the Internet, it is increasingly becoming possible to use a variety of different computers, from hand-held mobile phones and Blackberry-type devices up to supercomputers. Accessing the Internet will get easier still because the type of operating system will soon be universal. Operating systems manage use of your computer and run the application programs such as word processors, spreadsheets, camera image editing, games, and interactive language courses. Microsoft Windows is an example of an operating system. The operating system Linux is spreading like wildfire because people are finding it easier to work with a common platform. More people can concentrate their efforts on key business issues when there are not so many incompatible platforms that create unnecessary problems. Because of this, Linux over time is going to have a profound impact on the future of the Internet. In May 2004, Red Hat Inc. announced the availability of an early release of the Red Hat Linux source code for the upcoming Intel Itanium (Intel's first implementation of the IA-64 architecture) microprocessor. Red Hat Inc. placed a free download version of the code on its corporate website for anonymous download. This software plus Intel's recently released *Itanium Processor Microarchitecture Reference*[9] are meant to allow developers to create programs that will be 64-bit Linux ready.

---

[9] A guide for software developers that details the functional behavior of Intel's Itanium microprocessor.

The aggressive push by Linux software vendors to make the early release of the development environment available for Intel's Itanium microprocessor illustrated the industry's interest in leveraging the increasingly capable hardware that is still under development by systems vendors. Additionally this move demonstrates that Linux will be an important operating environment for systems based on the new microprocessor. Another dynamics that could help promote the growth of 64-bit applications on Linux is that many companies developing next-generation Internet and e-commerce applications are still in the early stages of construction and have less momentum and smaller install bases to drag over to 64-bit compiles of their products. This relative lack of baggage sped the movement to full use of the 64-bit Linux environment. IDC (International Data Corporation) predicted that Linux on IA-64 will succeed as an operating environment for servers, especially those supporting web infrastructure functions, high-performance technical computing, and digital content creation. Linux on IA-64 is also likely to be successful on workstations for researchers, scientists, and academicians. Making the Linux software available at no charge may win over Unix developers who are considering Linux but have not yet taken action.

Considering how the subdivisions or the business partners are located around the world, the enterprise information portal (EIP) must be provided to meet real-time access to the most current data around the clock. In addition the performance of the enterprise information portal is critical, and yet these systems are not designed to provide rapid reporting response to thousands of customers or partners. Therefore, for the next generation Internet, the server systems must provide high performance, reliability, fault-tolerance, and scalability, among other properties.

Today, substantial numbers of physicians leverage the Internet for consultation with colleagues and specialists and for e-health and other issues. Quite a few medical companies have emerged on the Internet too. Recall that health information is the most sought-after information on the Internet, averaging 34% to 43% or more of Internet time. There are presently more than 1,500 healthcare Web sites on the Internet, and e-health retailers were expected to take in $300 to $400 billion. Currently however the global market for eHealth is estimated to have a potential value of roughly only $60 billion. Europe is progressive here and represents one third of this; eHealth can be considered the third largest European health industry, after pharmaceuticals. As noted by eHealthNews, the problem is that eHealth businesses must overcome many barriers preventing them from re-selling products developed for one healthcare institution. This is largely due to the lack of the famous interoperability: the ability of one system to work with or "talk to" another (http://www.ehealthnews.eu/content/view/1386/37/).

It is estimated that more than 200 million US and Canadian consumers spend $500 to $1,000 or more annually on Internet-accessed health, of which $200 per annum might reasonably be "routine" inquiries, representing revenues of $40 billion. Patients are sometimes declining physicians who do not use digital imaging technology to send images by Internet to expert analysts, and who are not able to communicate with patients by email.

Telemedicine—or the use of computers to interact with patients, physicians, and specialists who are separated in space—has been predicted by conservative professional analysts to grow yearly by 40% to markets worth several tens to hundreds of billions of dollars. Waterford Telemedicine Partners of NY has taken a geographically and technologically broader view and projected the curves into the future to a market of $300 billion or more. As noted previously, it is difficult to know whether these projections are being realized because of the question of what the definition of telemedicine is, that is, its scope (see, however, Ronald C. Merrell and Charles R. Doarn. "Telemedicine and e-Health: Is it time for a telemedicine breakthrough? *Telemedicine and e-Health* 2008;14(6):505–506). Their broader definitions include, besides patient–doctor interactions, all other health-professional interactions with insurance, FDA, CDC, and WHO, inquiries with specialists, and consultation with research universities, all of which could benefit from access to clinical records.

The incentives for businesses to conduct medicine-related activity on the Internet has changed a bit. Because of this new economic trend where technical information has become an important asset, many organizations are being fragmented in diversity and targeting niche markets. Information sharing among the fragmented subdivisions and with business partners is critical to business success. The Internet is at the center of not only established information but transmits alerts and messages on portable electronic devices carried on the street.

New information and observations on clinical and biological research can save a life or make the sick well. But mining vast amounts of information on databases and the Internet to discover new combinations represents new facts and rules. This will be discussed in later chapters. Vast and complex assemblies of raw data are not much better than no data at all, so it is not necessarily new data but the knowledge, wisdom, insight, and action based on them that is the core of new medicine, as in any business.

NEW BUSINESS PRACTICE FOR MEDICINE: IT AND BUSINESS TRANSACTION MANAGEMENT

Of course other forces than high-flying science and the Internet, and much more familiar to down-to-earth healthcare administrators, have driven innovations to healthcare. There have been issues of poor safety records and extensive litigation, and of paper-based bureaucratic inefficiency, that information the new medicine can and must fix. Today's healthcare industry contends with a common set of challenges: the pressure to contain and reduce the cost of patient care; an aging population and the commensurate increase in the demand for healthcare; the desire to maintain or improve the current quality of patient care; organizational mergers, acquisitions, and consolidations; and the need to comply with statutory requirements for protection of privacy. Tremendous amelioration of these difficulties is anticipated as healthcare moves to a system based on advances in biology and biomolecular science, and IT. In fact the benefits of IT are thought to be so considerable that government pressure for change by physicians and healthcare organizations is escalating as we write. But that it not to say that it will be an easy road. For one thing, whatever the huge power of the engine "under the hood," providing a user-friendly and intuitive interface to a health informatics or biomedical informatics solution is critical. The vast majority of the healthcare professionals or medical researchers are not necessarily savvy technology users.

Under the hood, the engine must provide means of trouble-free linking of all work in a physician's clinical or hospital setting. Everyday practice of healthcare business is linked to the notion of workflow, meaning you do something A first, then B, then C if X is the case; otherwise, D, and so on. Workflow management, as well as a good user interface, is one of the key unmet industry needs and will be one of the critical success factors for the health informatics or biomedical informatics to be widely adopted by the healthcare and life sciences industry. These approaches also apply to clinical activity in emerging more high-tech areas, like clinical genomics.

Many of the workflow management offered by IT vendors provide comprehensive functionality and are robust. However, these products were developed for the nonmedical business world and are thus modeled on the assumption of a mature and stable business process such as in the financial or retail industry. It is hard to see what is the imminent worldwide commercial cost and market is for healthcare IT, but it is some measure that during his campaign for presidency, Mr. Obama vowed to spend $50 billion of government money over five years to spur the adoption of electronic health records and said recently that a program to accelerate their use would be part of his stimulus package (*New York Times*, December 28, 2008). The currently available products have required a team of IT specialists to set them up because of the complexity of the underlying technology and lack user-friendly and intuitive human interfaces. So those products require also a team of IT specialists to make any changes after the initial setup.

The healthcare and life sciences industry would benefit from a lightweight and flexible workflow management solution to assist the healthcare providers and the biomedical researchers. It should be highly customizable to be easily changed by non-IT people, namely by the healthcare providers or the biomedical researchers. In addition the workflow management solution should be adaptive to changes so that it can improve itself through machine learning and ultimately grow smart enough to function with minimal human intervention. For example, the workflow management solution may be configured with default parameters initially, and then continue to reconfigure itself based on the changes through ongoing monitoring of scenarios and usage patterns.

However, there are problems in simply adapting current business IT to medicine. The traditional or current distributed computing model has an

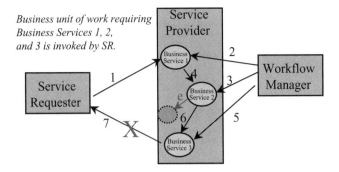

When an unanticipated business event or condition is detected by
Business Services 2, the entire business unit of work will
be aborted and thus the results provided by Business Services
1 and 2 are completely lost.

Figure 4.1 Conventional business transaction model

assumption ingrained in it that all the necessary business service components
are available, on the selected set of service providers, to complete the business
service request or business unit of work. This seems to be a harmless enough
assumption, but it can lead to some unfortunate results. If a required business
service component is not available on the service provider system, then the
whole business service request or transaction request is aborted. Consequently
the entire transaction or business unit of work must be restarted all over again.
In the healthcare and life sciences industry this could mean losing weeks, if
not months, of work, and maybe occasionally a patient too. This is aggravated
further by the fact that the work cannot be complete until the missing application component is developed and integrated with the rest of the application
components, which could take months, if not years. In addition the traditional
(nonmedical) business model mandates that all the possible business events
and conditions are addressed in advance and reflected in the application/
system design. This fact, coupled with the globalization of industries, the
increasing interdependencies in the supply chain, and the increasing number
of stakeholders (people, organizations, etc.) has resulted in business models
that are too complex to analyze in advance all of the possible business events
and conditions (see Figure 4.1). All these glitches in the system cry out for a
new technology, one that has the capability to dynamically handle unanticipated business events and business conditions as they are discovered during
the processing of a business service transaction.

For the unique requirements of the healthcare and life sciences industry,
clearly a "dynamic business unit of work management is required." But what
does this mean? Put simply, it is a mechanism that addresses the medical
informatics requirement for the online collaboration in a distributed environment. In this vision the business flow management system (DBFMS) handles

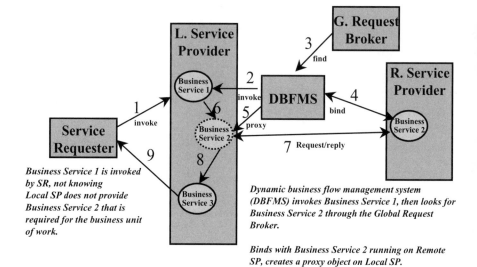

Figure 4.2   Dynamic business transaction model

all of the business service components, or business objects, that are involved in a business unit of work, by finding the business service objects and invoking them in a sequence based on the business rules associated with the business unit of work.

All this type of work is not easy for the non-IT person to follow, but here is an interesting twist. In the experience of the authors, we have become aware that a TODIS (true on-demand innovation system) can provide the infrastructure framework for the challenge of designing drugs automatically. This is a solution one of us proposed for an initially poorly defined workflow that was specified in a special sophisticated human-friendly computer language by a manager. The system could identify the components that were still poorly or ambiguously defined, or not defined at all. So, if the manager could not remove the ambiguity by being more precise, he would attach a specification of what was required to the ambiguous piece, and that would go off automatically to an expert to be defined. As the experts specified the problem more precisely using the same sophisticated computer language, the system would progressively itself gain all the details required, avoiding the need for intervention by experts in the future.

The benefits of this kind of system could be enormous, in particular, for the crucial issue of current business unit of work management, discussed earlier. Instead of aborting the entire request when a business service object that is required to complete the business transaction is not available, the dynamic business flow management system (DBFMS) will globally search the required business service component and dynamically integrate the business service component with the rest of the business service components, and complete, not abort, the specific business unit of work. Another plus: this entire process is accomplished behind the scenes (see Figure 4.2).

STAKEHOLDERS IN THE GAME

In the above discussion, a few new terms such as "stakeholder" could creep in. If you are in healthcare, it wouldn't get you unscathed past your managers and peers if you continually use the wrong term in the wrong context, or the right term in the wrong context! We don't have time nor space to go into the details that these matters deserve. But at least this section and the following will give you enough to get you through a healthcare cocktail party. One of the authors recalls a cocktail party where he spoke to the late great Hans Krebs, elucidator of the Krebs cycle (or citric acid cycle) of metabolism. When he asked what the definition was of molecular biology as opposed to biochemistry, Sir Hans informed him that molecular biology was the interesting part of biochemistry. It is clearly important to get these things right.

The term stakeholders is not new to the healthcare cocktail party or boardroom. Its use in healthcare discussions has increased dramatically with consideration of information-based medicine. It is important at healthcare parties because it means anyone with a stake in the healthcare game. By tacit agreement it includes patients, physicians, other providers of care, payers of care, biomedical researchers, institutions of care, and research organizations. The important thing is not to exclude anyone of these from the stakeholder group. For example, researchers get upset that they are often not considered as having a stake in healthcare. Strictly speaking, support staff too have a stake in the healthcare business, as do, for example, secretarial, legal, maintenance, and cleaning staff, but the stakeholders are probably best confined to the main groups of practitioners, patients, policy makers, and payers. Of course, others with a stake in healthcare might be outside investors, venture capitalists, and entrepreneurs who are interested in the business performance aspects of healthcare and biomedical research, and they most certainly are aware of their stakeholder roles.

The term "stakeholders in patient data access" is in common use. In the future of medicine, all stakeholder classifications and definitions will need to be tightened up for data security purposes. *Clinical messaging systems* will ship patient information only to the stakeholders authorized to have access to that information, the main users, the practitioners, patients, policy makers, and payers who are the target populations for a clinical messaging system, and definitely not the maintenance staff, venture capitalists in healthcare, and outside investors. More specifically, the system would be set up as follows. *Patients* communicate with practitioners about healthcare needs, follow-up of chronic conditions, learning the results of tests, and the like *Practitioners* (nurses, physicians, physiotherapists, psychiatrists, etc.) communicate to seek consultation, share information, educate, discuss professional matters and plan services (e.g., call schedules). *Providers* of health services (laboratory information services, pharmacy information, special interest groups, patient education services, government service agencies) communicate with practitioners and patients. *Policy makers* (hospital administrators, regional health authorities, guideline developers, quality assurance staff, etc.) communicate with practitioners about practice patterns and new guidelines, for example, and with patients about usage of services, for example *Payers* (government, third-party insurers, etc.) communicate with practitioners, patients, providers, and policy makers. However, it will not follow in future that these parties can all access patient data without patient permission even if they sometimes seem to act like they have that right at present. Probably most controversial is the health insurance companies. Insurance providers do have a right to collective anonymous data on patients because they need that for amortization purposes to perform as a business and continue to service patients. However, certain information such as genetic information that is predictive in regard to disease may be withheld.

MORE PARTY CHAT: SOME NEW "OMICS"

Genomics and pharmacogenomics is not the only "omics" of importance. Some we quoted without much explanation above. You will definitely never be fully able to bluff your way through modern healthcare cocktail parties if you do not know the latest precise definitions of the "omics" and other terms that have come up in the news over the past five years or so. We have already discussed the established ones. At the time of writing, recent offerings and some new spins on the old, are as follows:

Toxicogenomics is the study of the toxic potential of drug candidates through the use of gene expression profiles for early tolerability prediction. It focuses on the toxic effect of chemical compounds on the cells. This topic usually crops up at parties in discussion about how to avoid a hangover the morning after, because there is a strong genomic component.

Cytomics and physiomics are as obvious as cytology and physiology perceived as "omes," or a body of information and activity in the cell system, and in the whole body as the system of physiology, respectively. But the occasionally mentioned *physiological genomics* can get you to link two conversations. It acts a bridge, a bridge that links genomics and integrative physiology and clinical medicine. Originally launched by the American Physiological Society in 1999, it started out as a study of an organism's DNA in the full set of chromosomes. This was a radical change from the former practice of simply studying a single gene or a family of functionally or structurally related genes.

Physiological genomics has evolved to encompass a wide range of disciplines, including genomics, proteomics, genetics, clinical research and physiology, and now studies of those mechanisms at the gene and molecular levels that mediate an organism's response to disease, environment, inheritance, and so forth. Essentially this study boils down to microarray expression profiling to identify a particular physiological state.

Metabolomics, was mentioned before, but it is worth throwing it around at the party because of its growing links with *systems biology*, (an "absolute trendy must" that is discussed below and much later). Also a handy party one-upmanship hint, to be really trendy, is to refer to it instead as metabonomics. This is also a study concerned about metabolites, namely identification and quantification of biochemical compounds or small molecules in the human body. It is Jeremy Nicholson at the Imperial College in England, who derived the term from "meta" meaning "change" and "nomics" meaning rules. Cynics have said that this is simply a more global treatment of biochemistry, definitely a "no go" word. If you are a biochemist, introduce yourself to the opposite sex as a metabonomist. Metabolites are small molecules made by proteins. Metabolites, which can be identified and quantified through chromatography (not trendy) or mass spectrometers (e.g., "mass spec," very trendy), provide a more direct readout of physiology and analysis of metabolites, since it is easier to track small molecules than analyze gene transcripts or proteins. Metabolomics is anticipated to speed the drug research and development, help identify biomarkers for more accurate diagnosis, and enable presymptomic testing through metabolic profiling. For example, NMR (nuclear magnetic resonance) comparison of serum metabolites from healthy and atherosclerosis patients provides rapid, noninvasive diagnosis of heart disease.

Nutrigenomics is the consideration of how food and nutrition are influenced by genomics (remember again the fava beans of Chapter 2) and how particular diets can help overcome some consequences of genomic differences. We touch on this "omic" sporadically in this book.

Psychogenomics is the interplay between genomics and psychology. This is a key area undergoing rapid development, for example, in regard to how genes may influence healthy or abhorrent behavior involving choices in many different areas. On August 6, 2008, a team of researchers from Massachusetts General Hospital (MGH), Boston, described how they used brain imaging, genomics, and psychology to identify relationships between "brain reward circuitry, a behavioral measurement of preference and a gene variant that appears to influence both." The August 4 issue of *Archives of General Psychiatry* described how polymorphisms in a gene involved with the brain's reward function are associated with the activity of a particular brain structure and with the effort study participants make in viewing pictures of emotion-laden faces.

MORE PARTY CHAT: SOME OTHER INFORMATICS

Here is a party chat survival hint: Don't confuse biomedical informatics, medical informatics, and health informatics. While saying "something informatics" is still not at present as trendy as saying "something-omics," that will come. It even goes down very well now in speaking with healthcare gurus. More important, if they do come up in conversation, it is a *faux pas* if you get them confused. The term "biomedical informatics" (as opposed to "medical informatics") is often intended to convey an emphasis on biomedical matters, namely the overlap of biology and medicine with a stronger, purer research connotation. If the more clinical aspects are indicated, then "clinical informatics" is indeed a respectable term. "Health informatics" can be used for the healthcare system as a whole, but the term is often seen as embracing all the above-noted aspects. Nonetheless, definitions of medical informatics by many authoritative sources also include all the scientific aspects from the outset, namely the whole range of healthcare and biomedical practices of acquiring, representing, processing, and managing knowledge and data.

Medical informatics differs slightly in its popular definitions. According to Dr. Edward Shortliffe, chair of the Department of Medical Informatics at the College of Physicians and Surgeons at Columbia University in New York, and an early guru of medical expert systems, medical informatics deals with the storage, retrieval, sharing, and optical use of biomedical information, data, and knowledge for problem solving and decision making. It is a version of biomedical sciences that uses modern information technologies to compute and communicate, namely as applied in medical informatics based on bioinformatics (at molecular and cellular levels), imaging (of tissues and organs), and clinical (on patients and individuals) and public health (on populations).

The broad scope of medical informatics reflects the vision of healthcare decision makers who see the cutting edge currently reserved for the research elite eventually being available in routine clinical practice. It is not far-fetched that someday the computer will tell us whether a certain protein involved in a pathway is related to a CNS disorder, and give also its 3D structure, elucidate the level of expression in all brain cell types, and list all the known chemical compounds that bind to the protein, including the toxicological profiles of these compounds. This is the direction in which biomedical informatics is heading, and this is the ultimate practical application of personalized healthcare.

There is much we still don't know or don't understand. Scientists don't always come up with tools and then do the experiments; often it is instead that tools evolve with the experiments. So it is with the current challenges in medical informatics. The vision of researchers is broadening. Imagine yourself fifty years from now taking a leisurely stroll in the New York's Central Park on a sunny Sunday afternoon. Suddenly a large noise startles you. Your intake of breath catches sharply in your chest, and your weak heart, unable to cope with sudden stress, begins to struggle. Whirring into action, the automatic cardiac monitor embedded in your wristwatch detects the irregular heartbeats of your besieged heart. It immediately alerts the implanted defibrillator, that temporarily stabilizes your heart. The automatic cardiac monitor assures you that help is on the way and tells you to stay put as it deftly calls 911. The call, transferred to the health emergency response system (HERS) at Mt. Sinai Hospital springs the hospital to action. You are located using GPS (global positioning system) and an ambulance is dispatched to assist you. As the ambulance speeds to your aid, HERS alerts a heart surgeon on duty of the situation, and links your cardiac monitor to the surgeon's workstation. Using this system, the surgeon is able to monitor your heart's condition on line and perform combinatorial analysis using your health record on line, all before the you even set foot into the hospital.

MORE PARTY CHAT: HOW TO HANDLE SYSTEMS BIOLOGY

Systems biology is one of the most rapidly spreading terms these days in the academic medical research community, the biotechnology industry, and the pharmaceutical industry. The general consensus across academic, biotechnology, and pharmaceutical industry sectors is that systems biology will "revolutionize" our understanding of specific diseases and radically improve treatment of such diseases, and subsequently prevent illness and help us realize the concept of preventative medicine for wellness-oriented healthcare. So it is worth ensuring that, in party chat, you get it right. Be cautious, though, as there is no consensus in the industry about the exact definition of systems biology, and some people get quite heated about the precise definition. Dr. Leroy Hood, who is a co-founder of the Institute for Systems Biology (ISB), and is widely regarded as a founding pioneer of modern systems biology, has defined systems biology as "the study of all the elements in a biological system (all genes, mRNAs, proteins, etc.) and their relationships one to another in response to perturbations." Other definitions of systems biology are much more encompassing than what is defined by Dr. Hood. Assorted definitions are captured in the following amalgam: "systems biology is the science of integrating genetic, genomic, biochemical, cellular, physiological and clinical data to create a system network that can be used to predictively model a biological event(s)." Part of the difficulty in defining systems biology is the fact that systems biology is more appropriately a process rather than a new subdiscipline of modern biology. As noted previously, it is the integration of "omic" (genomic, proteomic, etc.) as well as clinical, physiological, and imaging measurements that is central to the paradigm shift of systems biology.

So what is the consensus? According to the survey conducted by *Genome Technology* in May 2004, some 90% of respondents listed the following requirements as critical to realizing the practical concept of a systems biology:

- Data cleansing/curation for high-quality data for modeling
- Behavioral and cultural changes in the way scientists interact and work together
- Innovative tools and algorithms to fully leverage IT

In terms of the required tools and algorithms, (1) data visualization and management, (2) modeling and simulation, (3) microarray assays and analyses, and (4) gene and protein profiling are all listed as critical for the advancement of systems biology.

If all else fails in the cocktail chat on a specific healthcare or biomedical movement or discipline, one can always wax lyrical or bluff by discussing the diversity of definitions. But in bluffing, you should at least know the foundations of the idea, movement, or discipline. If at the cocktail party you mention enjoying "The Seven Pillars of Wisdom" by T. E. Lawrence ("Lawrence of Arabia"), it is wise to be prepared to remember what the seven pillars are. Likewise it is so in regard to the actual practice of systems biology. It is a tricky party topic because although in broad definition it has been multiply defined, consistent with the doctrines of any systems thinking, the pillars have been systematically formalized. Unfortunately, the pillars of the practice of systems biology number ten or more, relating to eight different data input processes and a minimum of two data output processes, all of which, should you feel up to it, you should memorize as follows:

1. *Biological question and experimental design.* The biological system (body fluid, organelle, cell type, tissue, organ, or organism) to be studied needs to be selected, along with the appropriate hypothesis or discovery-driven question to be answered. The necessary controls (normal vs. diseased), sample histories, and outcomes as well as statistically significant sample numbers to be analyzed also need to be determined.

2. *Data acquisition.* "Omic," clinical, physiological, and imaging data are acquired on a variety of analytic platforms. Data sets are obtained on both control and perturbed (e.g., diseased, drug or toxin treated, and knockout animal) cohorts of samples. Modules of systems biology involve a process consisting of numerous interchangeable modules. The order of the process is determined by the biological question being investigated.

3. *Data preprocessing and integration data.* Files are smoothed, aligned, normalized, and ultimately merged into composite files.

4. *Data correlation and causality-merged data files.* These files are compared, and ultimately correlation and causal networks are produced. Tools for data visualization are applied at this juncture.

5. *Component identification and knowledge.* Assembly–statistically significant components differing between control and perturbed cohorts are identified. Ultimately correlation or causal networks are interro-

gated against all known knowledge using a variety of tools, from simple text mining to semantic web protocols.

6. *Biological validation.* Correlation or causal networks must have biological relevance, so findings must be related back to the biology of the system being investigated. Strategies such as RNA interference, high-throughput cellular bioassays, and knock-in or knockout organisms can all be used to provide a biofocusing of data back to the relevance of the biological question posed originally.

7. *Modeling and simulation.* Data and correlation networks are used as a framework for further modeling and simulation studies of the biological processes being investigated.

8. *Biological engineering.* Once a system is modeled and understood, the pathway or network can be reengineered to produce a better outcome (e.g., disease-resistant crop) or to identify the optimal therapeutic agent.

9. *Biological knowledge.* This output is produced to answer, in part or completely, the original question posed.

10. *Predictive understanding.* Modeling and simulation studies of the biological system being investigated should make it now possible to predict the outcome of specific changes in the pathway or network.

Note that the specific process flow and the connectivity of the modules are determined by the initial biological question posed. For example, a discovery-driven question may require the aforementioned modular flow. However, a hypothesis-focused question may necessitate a restructuring of modules, such as knowledge assembly, to be is carried out before data acquisition. In any event, the systems biology process attempts to capture and portray the staggering complexity and interconnectivity of cellular and organism events that occur on the microsecond time scale. This unique modular approach with its combination of tools, technologies, and resulting systems knowledge potentially holds the key to dissecting disease onset, progression, and treatment as well as accelerating the bottlenecks of the therapeutic drug discovery and development process.

MORE PARTY CHAT: SOME NEW "MEDICINES"

Patient-centric medicine is essentially *personalized medicine*, but with the accent only slightly taken off the pharmacogenomics and placed on the broader picture that essentially corresponds to *holistic medicine* to be discussed later. These distinctions are subtle and fragile, and it is perhaps clearer and truer to say that patient-centric medicine is a corporate strategy in the IT industry. But this is good: it reflects the deep recognition by the IT industry of the kinds of principles discussed in this book.

Preventative medicine is a popular theme at parties because there even the non–medical party-goer wakes up, whereas in discussing systems biology, the uninitiated probably moved off already. If you can move fast and catch them as they show first signs of wandering, you can say "… which brings us to preventative medicine." That phrase can be just about thrown in anywhere, because it is a major goal of most or all of the themes discussed above. You already know it by now, because preventative medicine is a central aspiration behind information-based medicine, and a goal of stratified, personalized, patient-centric, and holistic medicine.

However, there is potential learning needed here for some of the principles of *alternative medicine* and *nature medicine* (see Chapter 7 for accounts), and you can certainly use these concepts fruitfully, when conversing with the non-scientists, within the topic of preventative medicine. Much more difficult is to not sound like a hippy or food-faddist or naturist when talking to scientists (unless you want to, or are one of these). In spanning the cultures, be trendy *and* well-armed, and really make sure that you read Chapter 7. In mainstream medical thinking, however, the key theme of preventative medicine is a focus on the prevention and treatment of more complex diseases as a new drug target. With the bulk of society growing older and older, attention must be turned toward those chronic degenerative diseases associated with an aging population. Another major aspect is the development of a personalized diet and lifestyle, which is what brings the approach into direct continuity with holistic medicine. Still many practitioners are seen as "faddists" or "cranks" by orthodox medical thinkers. As R. J. Williams has argued, the vacuum created by the abandonment of nutrition by orthodox medicine is directly responsible for nutrition becoming an *alternative* therapy.[10] Nonetheless, some in the medical community regard nutrition as the primary method of prevention. After all, we would all like that fewer people take drugs less often, but everyone likes to be able to eat more than once a day (most people eat three times a day in one way or another).

Evidence-based medicine (EBM) is an established term that has recently risen in popularity, as explained in the last chapter. Here is roughly its story. EBM has epidemiological roots. Archie Chochrane, a Scottish epidemiologist, through his book *Effectiveness and Efficiency: Random Reflections on Health Services* (1972) and subsequent advocacy caused increasing acceptance of the concepts behind evidence-based practice. Epidemiologists are, of course, not just concerned with epidemics but any factors adversely affecting public health. As discussed elsewhere in this book, the more recent epidemiological findings appear to confirm Chochrane's earlier concerns. The top three of the ranked concerns in healthcare are cardiovascular disease, cancers, and *doctors* (e.g., Human Rights Report on the United States, 2004), based on the kinds of medical errors and accidents discussed in Chapter 3. The idea of EBM is to avoid personal experience and anecdotal experience, even so-called expert

---

[10] See R. J. Williams, *Nutrition against Disease*, New York: Pitman, 1971.

opinion, and certainly old medical training, and get the latest facts as "best evidence." That brings in *translational research* also discussed elsewhere in this book. The term *evidence-based medicine* first appeared in the medical literature in 1992 in a paper by Guyatt et al., and explicit methodologies used to determine "best evidence" were largely established by the McMaster University research group led by David Sackett and Gordan Guyatt. David Sackett moved on to help run the National Health Service R&D Centre and at Oxford, England, a major force in EBM.

Because it is hard to imagine practicing best use of all available and latest data without IT, there is a strong case with few complaints that *EBM + IT = Information-based medicine*, and plus genomics it is stratified medicine (medicines for genomic groups) and even better personalized medicine. Information-based medicine should be slightly distinguished from info-medicine, which appears in some medical school curricula, and although the word is a contraction of information-based medicine, it emphasizes also to the students the importance of library work, biostatistics and epidemiology, and personal physician research. The ultimate goal of information-based medicine is to leverage IT particularly for a high accuracy of diagnoses and increased efficacy of treatments. This goal would be achieved by considering an individual's genotypic and phenotypic variances, and by the provision of predictive and preventative healthcare. The term is also intended to emphasize the information-integration aspect for transparent access independently of the geographical locations, of data types, of data formats, of databases or file systems managing the data, of operating platforms, and of network protocols, among others. In that sense it comes close to the subject matter of the next chapter. Perhaps more than any of the closely related informatics disciplines, we listed above, information-based medicine is a systems architecture capable of converting medical information in text form (unstructured data) into a more structured form, and then converting that to sets of rules to facilitate decisions by researchers and physicians alike.

More specifically, information-based medicine describes the process of improving existing pharmaceutical and medical practices with knowledge generated from the integration of diverse clinical and biomedical research data. Information-based medicine could help healthcare and life sciences stakeholders in the diagnosis and treatment of diseases by accelerating the industry trend toward targeted therapies and personalized healthcare.

CONCLUDING THOUGHTS: CHANGE OR BE CHANGED

Business is business, and some is good business. Potentially and ultimately, all good things are possible for humankind, but all of the sick of the world today are separated from redemption either by space or by time. Today, the sick of nonindustrial, poor, or emerging nations could benefit from technologies and products available in more industrial nations, but logistics, ignorance, insularism, indifference, callousness, greed, or some combination of deterents prevents delivery. People get sick in the richer, industrial nations, but the spectrum of diseases is different.

Enough IT is available today, but aspects of it remain imperfect in all industries. The underlying *mathematics* need as yet to be properly solved. Algorithms still need to be fine-tuned for the system to be able to obtain fluid access to patient records and perform undirected and directed data mining against very high-dimensional data from diverse sources. This work involves combinatorial analyses for associations and correlations among multidimensional heterogeneous (diverse) data based on statistical tools called multivariate analysis and association analysis. In addition the industry needs a three-dimensional medical visual analysis and four-dimensional (three-dimensional plus time) simulation environment for disease modeling and predictive toxicity analysis, but this is as yet a long way from being met. Yet another requirement of clinical and biomedical informatics that has to be fulfilled is effective integration of tools and applications from various sources for plug and play.

None of such problems and their solutions are relevant to the public until there *is* a universal adoption of the patient digital medical record. And there are more immediate pressures. For example, lack of a proper information database denies rapid access to patients in a street accident. Practitioners instead must rely on their memory for not only the diagnosis but also for the treatment and prognosis. The dangers are evident: practitioners must make quick opinion-based diagnoses and prognoses, and thus treatment is reduced to an empirical trial-and-error approach. Without a suitable method for handling health information, authorized persons unable to access information are hindered in the effectiveness of their treatments. But once if an effective method of sharing information and preventing medical accidents is introduced, this attitude could be reversed.

IT is also needed to provide a continuum of services. The initial stages of diagnosis, to treatment, to prognosis are presently interconnected in a haphazard way. The three services are not linked appropriately, resulting in a dangerous gap between primary care and tertiary care. IT could even alleviate the looming burden of a growing and aging Baby Boomer population and of a rising demand for safer and more effective medicines to treat the numerous ailments and illnesses of the aged. However, these issues pale in comparison with the pressing concern of the danger that healthcare today poses to patient safety in general. For example, the beneficial results of healthcare and treatment are countered by the ever-increasing high rate of ADR. To help counter that, IT could access rapidly all of an individual's genetic, or somatic mutation, physical trauma, immunological, and toxicity history.

Health administration organizations (e.g., managed care organizations) would like to have medical information available for questions about eligibility for treatment. Delivery networks (e.g., hospitals) would like it to be available to the services within the system (clinical, administrative, and financial). Individual healthcare providers would like the record to be available as the patient enters their practice. This scope extends far beyond the walls of the facility where a patient is usually seen. For example, a patient with haemophilia who is involved in a car accident and is taken by ambulance to the nearest hospital would need his records to be available there. Moreover citizens in rural locations are requesting the same level of healthcare and experts that are available in the metropolis, and therefore the pressure on enabling tele-medicine for patient–doctor interaction is critical. All the above will not be possible without providing access to the medical records. An XML-based standard (IHE) that combines the hospital/clinical information standard (HL7) and medical imaging standard (DICOM) is being evolved and is tar-geted to address the need of healthcare organizations. IHE stands for inte-grated health environment; HL7 stands for health level 7, in reference to the OSI seven-layer architecture, which is a messaging standard for exchange of clinical data. DICOM stands for digital imaging and communications in medicine, and this standard is used for centralized and digitized management diagnostic images.

At a 2005 Dallas convention, sponsored by the Healthcare Information and Management Systems Society and attended by more than 23,000 people, Dr. David J. Brailer, a federal official dedicated to dragging the nation's healthcare system into the computer age, delivered a warning to the healthcare industry: *Take steps soon to make it happen, or government may impose a solution.* This threat may be the historic first step needed for the development of informa-tion-based holistic medicine, and it is discussed further in Chapter 7. In brief, Dr. Brailer told everyone to come up with agreed-upon standards for elec-tronic health records. The approach, he said, must include a method to certify that the records can be opened and read by doctors and specialists, as autho-rized by the patient, even when different clinics and hospitals have different computer systems. In most markets, technical standards have enabled the growth of markets and industries that are built on those public standards. Once a basic standard for electronic health records is in place, Dr. Brailer says, it will be less risky to invest in digital records for doctors or hospitals that now worry that the software they purchase today, and struggle to learn to use, may become obsolete sometime later. The industry group that is supposed to develop the electronic health record standard, the Certification Commission for Healthcare IT, was formed in 2004. Of crucial importance is the establish-ment of the capability of transparent access to diverse data from diverse sources.

The relatively simple position is for the capture, storage, analysis, and move-ment of patient data, but that is not the only aspect required. The data must be converted to clinical decision intelligence. Clinical decision intelligence is the application of IT to enable evidence-based clinical practice and medical research, and to encourage best practices in them by utilization of all available data. The two main aims are (1) to improve the quality of patient care and safety by enhancing speed and efficiency, and by reducing safety risks and needless costs, in clinical diagnosis, treatment and healthcare management, and (2) to facilitate biomedical research and pharmaceutical development wherever it is based on inclusion of clinical and related data. By such means the implementation of IT to the business of medicine must go hand in hand with a more holistic philosophy of practice, or else it simply will not make any sense. The practitioner must be able to delve into the patient's life and into the core and underlying cause of the problems because all attention and effort must be focused on the emergency problem at hand. These aspects are discussed in the next chapters.

5

THE NEXT DECADE: PERSONALIZED MEDICINE AND THE DIGITAL PATIENT RECORD

You are the one!

—The movie *The Matrix*

So far we have followed the development of medicine up to the present day and immediate future. Now we will follow it over the next decade. What is the single most important unit of information that will be manipulated in the imminent future information-based personalized medicine? From this chapter's title it is clear that we think the answer is the electronic patient record (EPR), sometimes called the digital patient record (DPR), the electronic medical record (EMR), the electronic health record (EHR), the longitudinal health record (LHR), the integrated medical record (IMR), and a few other things besides. *Information-based personalized medicine*, we may recall, is *information based* (i.e., run on computers), *personalized* (i.e., taking account of our individual lives, our individual DNA, proteins, and other molecules, or the way we differ from other people), and *preventive* (i.e., not just a means of cure but prevention, well-being, fitness, and excellence). The digital patient record will be central to this weighty objective.

When we first planned this book, a widespread abundance of digital patient records seemed just a science fiction dream, and companies keeping them were pioneers. Now, however, companies like Cerner and General Electric vie for acquisitions and mergers, and critique each other's philosophies. But the status at this time is still mixed. One of the authors can go to his local government

The Engines of Hippocrates: From the Dawn of Medicine to Medical and Pharmaceutical Informatics, by Barry Robson and O.K. Baek
Copyright © 2009 by John Wiley & Sons, Inc.

health services authority and submit his data to a Cerner system. But even if he did, it may have little impact right now on the system used by his physician, a quite separate "institution" who keeps paper records along with minimal computer entries on a very basic general record system. This dual paper-digital system, one notes, has at last time of reference got that author in twice as two patients of same name and birth date, but with distinct subsets of basic medical information. This kind of so-called Doppelganger error (where a patient, bureaucratically speaking, has a mythical extra self) could be almost as disastrous in an emergency as if another patient's record is accessed by mistake, because either version is incomplete. It also risks breach of privacy if the patient is asked whether the suspected duplicate record is likely to be that patient's or not. These are just two tips of an iceberg of problems resulting from the fact that there is still no universal patient identifier, no communication between the centers even if there were, and the patient, not the healthcare system, is considered the ultimate reliable source if a glitch occurs. It arises, notably, when the patient is believed to be new to a medical center and the paper file is not available at the time, whence he or she is asked to fill out again a form with personal and medical details. The chances of this Doppelganger error seem to be increased if a patient switches health insurance companies; this may reflect the enthusiasm of primary physician organizations to ensure that the seemingly often most important parameter of a patient from the managed healthcare perspective, the currently valid healthcare insurance coverage, is captured, even at risk of creating an extra record.

Usually records collect very dry data. But the patient's record of the future could be fairly elaborate and capture the essence of the patient. Over the long term, the record the future patient will be associated with software that can help interpret and give advice. The patient's record will be not just about disease. Remember, we ideally want to record not just reaction to treatment of disease but prevention and well-being. So, in this sense the record in the world of IT would represent a kind of guardian, an ancient Egyptian shadow soul or *Ka* perhaps.

There are some types of medical records that have a related but somewhat different and sometimes less elaborate purpose. A medical *event* record, for example, is more concerned with recording things about transactions or events that occur between the patient and a hospital. Some medical event records are different but still elaborate, of course. The Clinical Data Recorder Group at St. Mary's Hospital, Imperial College London, is more concerned with recording, for legal and medical training purposes, a complete account of an operation in second-by-second detail. Other records might be about prescription drugs in a pharmacy, and some of the entries might be the references to patients who have been given those drugs. Of course, using computers, records in digital format can be brought together so that a single large record is built for every patient: this process is called, reasonably enough, *joining.*

In late 1999 we began to set up a research unit to study what it would take to have a digital patient record that includes details about the patient's DNA. It was then considered unique to think about the patient record in digital form although several centers around the world, varying from an institute in Indiana to a group in the Greek island of Crete, had been building digital records. By 2002 the iCapture team, a large and highly successful academic group at the University of Columbia, Vancouver, led by Bruce and Janet McManus, began working with the authors. They assembled at first just a few example records, but in great detail, including detailed traces of molecule physiology, such as the rate at which calcium ions crossed the membranes of the patient's heart muscle cells. By 2003 Bill Knaus at Virginia University had assembled the order of a million patient records for the authors to process and analyze by computer. For actual clinical practice, right now the Mayo Clinic and Kaiser Permanente are among those leading the way.

It should be obvious that if a physician can pull down a patient's record from a computer very rapidly, that is a good thing; but what is the point of analyzing all the patient record's together, millions of them? What possible *collective* value can patient records have? Data mining tools enable statistical risk management for patients, insurers, CDC, pharma companies, and the FDA, and let physicians find similar patients with similar symptoms in order to find out what was the best diagnosis and therapy. The job of data mining is to ask the computer to find interesting correlations between things that essentially represent medical information. Information–based medicine, with evidence drawn from a patient population database (including patients in clinical trials), will provide high-quality care for the next 10 and maybe 20 years. Indeed that will likely continue until the individual patient's record is so detailed, even down to the atomic level, that it can be used to perform simulations from first principles.

THE DIGITAL PATIENT RECORD AND THE CASE OF THE VENOMOUS NORWEGIAN BLUE PARROT

Consider the following scenario: Imagine that a Norwegian male has embellished his prudent life savings by a financial killing on the stock market, and wants to retire. He has one green and one brown eye. He has two interesting polymorphisms (i.e., SNPs or SNiPs) that we will call XB45T7 and YBM79. In his youth he was bitten by the venomous Norwegian blue parrot (*Parrotus norvegicus*). He loves drinking green tea. His digital medical record shows all this. He lives in Norway, but he would like to retire to the tropics. He asks the computer, "Should I retire to the Caribbean?" The computer replies. "You have a bite from venomous Norwegian blue in your record. Patients who have a history of this and move to the tropics die within one month of drinking green tea." Clearly, unless the patient is suicidal, and with the caveat of certain statistical matters discussed below, he has two choices.

Fictition perhaps, but this prognosis scenario (based loosely on a couple of Monty Python comedy sketches) is one that has been used in medical teaching because it validly illustrates several things. Records save lives. Information-based medicine is preventative medicine. Medical information is a matter of everyday life guidance. It can be consulted at home if there is no need for a doctor to immediately ratify the decision. Both patient and physician need a computer. The patient needs his or her medical record in digital form. Indeed many patients have contributed their records, though mostly anonymously for the common good. The Norwegian did not have to contribute his record to obtain the prognosis, but if he did not, he might soon die in the sun. Information-based medicine is effectively an issue of patient *autonomy* versus *solidarity* (or *cooperativity*).

There are no venomous Norwegian blue parrots. A more tangible example already suspected by medical science is the following (confirmation will require the assembly of many patient records for analysis). We pick this example because it was one of the areas in which one of the authors found new insight by using the tools of information-based medicine, especially by data-mining the patient data and medical literature. If you were once bitten by a scorpion, then avoid hypothermia (as opposed to the tropics!), alcohol, oxidative stress, a job on board an airplane, intensive dieting, insecticides, prolonged use of antibiotics, and so forth. If you do not follow this advice, your chances of developing pancreatitis would be extremely high. Pancreatitis is a painful and dangerous inflammation of the pancreas that is extremely common in some countries and of enhanced risk in certain professions. If you have an acute pancreatic attack, your risk of death, at least until recently, was about 5%. The origins of a disease are its *aetiology*.

The following is a list of the factors that are considered aetiologies of pancreatitis, obtained through data mining of medical records and literature. The number in front roughly reflects the risk factor, or at least medical sciences' belief in that factor. Note that some are genetic, some environmental.

Risk Level	Causes
4	Gallstones
3	Scorpion bite
3	Malnutrition due to restricted tropical diets
3	Cystic fibrosis
1	HIV
2	Alcohol
2	Oxidative stress due selenium/carotene/vitamin a, c, or e deficiency
1	Porphyria
1	Chronic renal failure
1	Hyperglycaemia
1	Insecticides
1	Inflammatory bowel disease
1	Duodenal obstruction or infection
1	Anorexia nervosa
1	Hydrophobic agents (e.g., aliphatic/hydrogenated)

Risk Level	Causes
1	Essential fatty acid deficiency
1	Hydrocarbons (aviation fuel) anesthetics
1	Hepatitis B
1	Mumps
1	Rye's syndrome
1	Cardiovascular bypass surgery
1	Haemolytic uraemic syndrome
1	Diazinon
1	Long-term antibiotics
1	Fasting
1	Hypothermia
1	Cardiopulmonary bypass
1	Trans-lumbar aortography
1	Serum triglycerides >20 mm/L
1	Vasculitis
1	Surfeit after fasting
1	Mumps
1	Post–renal bypass/transplant
1	Trauma

Note that these factors are not necessarily additive in their effect. In the case of our retiring Norwegian, it may be that some or all the factors, not just the venomous Norwegian Blue Parrot, had to be present for green tea in the tropics to have a high risk of fatality. When factors come together to have such devastating effect, we use the term "combination effect." Good data mining and statistics will sort these issues out, and if every patient with the same correlations died after drinking green tea in the tropics, and no others, there is huge room for concern. It is basically a matter of *pattern recognition*. Still patterns need to be tested to see whether all the variables show up on a chance basis, as this is a quantitative way of testing the combination effect (which is actually a matter of degree, not simply combination effect vs. no combination effect). Fortunately, such task is easy for a computer to perform repeatedly, from the same record archive.

Pancreatitis and venomous Norwegian Blue Parrots are not likely to be high among most peoples' personal risk factors, statistically speaking. Of more general interest are diseases that cause death, and how they might be avoided. While everyone dies sooner or later, up until now few people died of old age. Several medical thinkers, like Ray Kurzel and Terry Grossman in their book *Fantastic Voyage*, argue that if we can just keep going, medical technology will constantly evolve to keep us going a bit longer (see Chapter 10). There is good reason to believe that even right now, your potential life span is about 121 years, because Frenchwoman Jeanne Calment lived to that age. Perhaps almost all of us die because of disease or accident.

In the United States according to the National Vital Statistics Report (2005), the biggest killers by far are heart disease (652,091 deaths, 26.6% of the total deaths) and cancer (559,312 deaths, 22.8% of the total deaths), which account for 49.4% of the total deaths. The notorious cardiovascular disease called stroke (interruption of blood supply to the brain) follows as the third leading cause death at a "mere" 143,579 deaths, or 5.9% of the total deaths. The very latest update according to the *Wall Street Journal's* "Market Watch" web page (http://blogs.marketwatch.com/healthmatters/2008/06/11/us-deaths-from-many-of-the-biggest-killers-drop-in-2006/) is positive for the United States. Deaths from eight of the 10 leading causes dropped significantly between 2005 and 2006, and life expectancy hit a new record of more than 78 years. This report concerned the preliminary data from the National Center for Health Statistics in 2008. Deaths from influenza and pneumonia dropped nearly 13% from 2005 to 2006, deaths caused by chronic lower respiratory diseases dropped 6.5% in that time, while those from heart disease fell 5.5% and fatalities from cancer slid 1.6%.

The details depend, of course, very much on the age group 1–4, 5–14, 15–24, 25–44, 45–64, 65–74, and 75– ... 121? In the United States the age group of 25 to 44 (all races and both sexes combined) will most likely die of accidents (27,182 deaths—but including medical accidents; see below), cancer (20,436 deaths), heart disease (16,139 deaths), suicide (11,354 deaths), HIV (8,356 deaths), homicide (7,383 deaths), chronic liver disease (3,786 deaths), cerebrovascular diseases (3,201 deaths), diabetes mellitus (2,549 deaths), and pneumonia and influenza (1,068 deaths). At 1 to 4 years old, accidents (1,826 deaths) still dominate, but this is followed by congenital defects (495), cancer (420), homicide (356), heart disease (181), pneumonia and influenza (103), septicemia (99), prenatal conditions (79), so-called Benign neoplasm (i.e., simply meaning that they don't spread) (53), and lower respiratory diseases (51). For age 75 and up, it will be heart disease (471,302), cancer (242,235), cerebrovascular diseases (124,396), lower respiratory diseases (75,218), pneumonia and influenza (51,368), Alzheimer's disease (45,462), diabetic mellitus (35,470), nephritis (24,235), accidents (23,353), and septicemia (19,082).

Again, an important aspect of personalized medicine is personalized drugs and treatment in consideration of the individual patient's hereditary traits. In the early postgenomic era, massive genotyping experiments promised to generate new, higher quality targets for drug discovery and novel diagnostic assays to target drugs to an individual's genetic predisposition. All the examples above, of the preceding paragraph, depend at least partially on genomic factors and are affected by differences among our individual genetic constitutions. Therapies can be fine-tuned if the relevant genomic aspects are known and understood. Well-known examples include that typical cancer chemotherapy will not work if you have a certain polymorphism and that your chances of the anti–breast cancer drug Herceptin working are very high (and poor otherwise) if you have a certain other polymorphism.

Not all genomics address such serious proclivities. Some homely examples come out of data-mining records too. For example, individuals tending to have dandruff in response to certain shampoos might avoid eating fatty duck. This is probably due to a sensitivity to lanolin, in which duck fat is rich. Another example is a certain polymorphism common in roughly half of all Caucasian males that causes males over the age of 50 to experience discomfort after drinking red wine. Because this discomfort is not huge, it went unnoticed until the genomic era and the beginning of good keeping of patient data.

The ethical case for a more personal medicine markets, namely for drugs affecting only a fraction of the genome pool, was already promoted in 1994. Writing in 1997, Classen found that between $1.6 billion and $4.2 billion were being spent each year in the United States for additional treatments to deal with adverse reactions (Classen, 1997), and later Lazarou estimated adverse reactions to have caused over 100,000 deaths during 1994 (Lazarou, 1998). Genetic tests would enable the physician to avoid some of these risks and so treat patients more effectively.

Because bringing a new drug to the market at that time cost approximately $500 million, it seemed at first economically impossible to personalize medicine and target small patient populations. The brunt of the implicit costs of nonefficacy, and up to some $4 billion per annum, for adverse interactions was instead allowed to be borne elsewhere. However, research into personalized medicine proved to enhance the drug discovery process in general, and genomic subpopulations were a natural spin-off. The market experience with the more personalized drug Herceptin suggested an imminent worthy market of $200 million per product (new chemical entity, NCE). Based on Smith Kline Beecham and Glaxo percentages, $10 billion to $20 billion for personal drug revenue suggested a reasonably attractive target for the smaller company. Further the personal drug market responded with an increase in the number of anticancer drugs, stemming from newly discovered and protein targets and the introduction of high-priced biologic agents. Merrill Lynch analysts predicts the global market opportunity of $15 billion for therapeutic protein and $8 billion for antibody products based on personal genomics. The Cambridge Healthtech Institute predicted their personal genomics-based cancer market potentially to be $12 billion.

The early research on Herceptin demonstrated the importance of correlating combinations of drugs with genomics-based treatment. Women with metastatic cancer got better results when they took Herceptin together with the chemotherapy drugs Taxol or Adriamycin (doxorubicin) plus Cytoxan (cyclophosphamide). These drug combinations reduced the tumors of 45% of women treated, while only 29% who received chemotherapy alone had a similar response. When Herceptin plus chemotherapy was used, it boosted survival, by an average of 5 months.

A particularly noteworthy illustration of "combination effects" was that a small number of the women taking the combination of Herceptin and Adriamycin developed heart problems, including congestive heart failure. However, studies suggest that this was not a hugely strong "combination effect," and the problem only arose when the two drugs were used together. Herceptin on its own rarely causes heart damage; Adriamycin was blamed for most of this effect. Nonetheless, careful statistics showed that the two drugs given together created more heart damage than could be anticipated. For this reason the combination of Herceptin and Adriamycin is no longer recommended.

It is well known that certain combinations of drugs can have interactions with other drugs, "cross-reactions" as described on the sheet of warnings that, in the United States at least, comes with the drugs obtained at a pharmacy. Data mining to find these combinations is therefore an important application of data mining medical records; another important area is finding new relations between diseases and laboratory results, such as based on the blood triglyceride level. However, the goal of information-based personalized medicine is for patients to be made aware of their personal genomic factors, or any other factors that can reasonably be cited on their record. For example, there is a real sense in which immunological factors change one's molecular constitution, and this is not solely a matter of inheritance, as in the case of sensitivity to penicillin, which in some patients is due to an adverse immune reaction to penicillin bound to serum albumin. Still, because different genes of the immune system such as HLA genes are inherited, there is always a chance of a genomic factor having an influence even in immunological matters.

As in the bizarre story of the Norwegian Blue Parrot, in the diagnosis, therapy selection, and prognosis, and in all the other manipulations of data that take place to ensure your health and well being, your digital patient record will be frequently manipulated. The issues, benefits, and risks that genomics-based profiles will entail are described in the rest of this chapter and the chapter following.

PATIENT DATA NOW

Currently accessible US data sources include claims, transactional, and billing data, Medicare data and data from the Department of Veterans Affairs, as well as significantly large local collections in the Mayo Clinic, Kaiser, and the State of Virginia, to name a few. As we noted in Chapter 4, in the United Kingdom, despite the absence as yet of a nationally distributed *detailed* digital patient record, the NHS accesses patient data from the General Practice Research Database (GPRD) and IMS Disease Analyzer, and the Prescribing Support Unit and other agencies have for several years routinely used patient level source data. The GPRD and IMS have comprehensive longitudinal patient level data, the largest in Europe.

CURRENT BILLING RECORDS WITH DISEASE AND TREATMENT CODES

Not surprisingly, in the US Managed Healthcare system, patient billing has been the first process to be highly automated, with digital patient data. Medical (bill) coding is vital to every US healthcare provider today: healthcare providers get paid for their services by filing a claim with the patient's health insurance provider or managed care organization. Overall, medical coding must translate all types of encounters into a defined classification scheme, including services, tests, treatments, and procedures provided in a medical office, clinic, or hospital.

It should be noted from the outset that the current systems related to billing are rather weak on outcomes data. In reduced structured data from such sources for analysis of outcomes research, it is not always possible to deduce directly whether the patient died or got better, which are startily different outcomes. All that can then be learned with assurance is that the patient has currently passed beyond the concerns of healthcare insurers. So for this reason alone, aside from other omissions, these data are not a replacement for the digital patient record, but only a good first step and supplement.

Still, billing-related records carry well-worked out classification codes for diseases and treatments represented in standards, such as ICD-9-CM volume 1 and 2 as the code set for diagnosis codes, ICD-9-CM volume 3 for inpatient hospital services, CDT for dental services, and NDC codes for drugs. This is enough form to obtain knowledge for the common good on analysis of patient data. Pharmaceutical companies, FDA, and medical researchers have already started to access and analyze the anonymized form of these data.

The development of medical codes has in fact been an international and US success story that shows bureaucracy at its best. The use of medical codes dates as far back as 1893, when a French physician, Jacques Bertillon, introduced the Bertillon Classification of Causes of Death at the International Statistical Institute in Chicago. A number of countries quickly adopted Dr. Bertillon's system, and in 1898, the American Public Health Association (APHA) recommended that the registrars of Canada, Mexico, and the United States also adopt it. The APHA also recommended revising the system every 10 years to ensure that the system remained current with medical practice advances. As a result the first international conference to revise the International Classification of Causes of Death convened in 1900, with revisions occurring every 10 years thereafter. The sixth revision, included morbidity (serious disease) and mortality (fatality) conditions, and its title was modified, to reflect the changes, to *Manual of International Statistical Classification of Diseases, Injuries and Causes of Death (ICD)*.

A kind of (mostly) friendly game of tennis between the WHO and US health authorities evolved the system dramatically. By the ninth revision the ICD manual expanded to three volumes and used five-digit subclassification! Prior to the sixth revision, responsibility for ICD revisions fell to a mixed commission, but in 1948 the World Health Organization (WHO) assumed responsibility for preparing and publishing the revisions to the ICD every 10 years, and sponsored revisions. They served the ball for the main game, but the US Public Health Service took it and kept it in the air for a while (1959–

1962). In that time it revised and extended ICD as ICDA, adapted for Indexing of Hospital Records and Operation Classification, and later published the eighth revision, referred to as ICDA-8, to code diagnostic and operative procedural data for official morbidity and mortality statistics in the United States. The WHO then got the ball back and in turn kept the ball in the air a while until they published the ninth revision of ICD (ICD-9) in 1978. Then the United States took back the ball again modified it to meet the needs of American hospitals.

From this ball game the ICD has become the most widely used statistical classification system in the world. With ICD well in position it became very natural to develop a coding for therapies and other medical diagnostic procedures. Although some countries found ICD sufficient for hospital indexing purposes, many others already felt that it did not provide adequate detail for diagnostic indexing. The original revisions of ICD did not provide for classification of operative or diagnostic procedures, and in general, more focus needed to be on each patient rather than be used only for statistical groupings and trend analysis. The *Clinical Modification*, or CM system, was thus developed and implemented in order to better describe the clinical picture of the patient. The diagnosis component, at least, of ICD-9-CM is completely consistent with ICD-9 codes. Hospitals and other healthcare facilities currently index healthcare data by referring and adhering to ICD-9-CM as published by the US Department of Health and Human Services. The new version ICD-10 was adopted in 1999 for reporting mortality, but the ICD-9-CM remains the data standard for reporting morbidity.

Fluid working among many authorities and bodies went beyond ICD to the procedural issues mentioned above. In billing, the diagnosis (ICD) codes have to match up in some way with the services rendered to justify medical necessity. One cannot normally claim insurance for a foot X ray when reporting a head injury, for example. The Health Care Procedure Coding System (HCPCS) of 1978 is based on the American Medical Association's *Current Procedural Terminology* (CPT) published in 1966. The first edition contained primarily surgical procedures, with limited sections on medicine, radiology, and laboratory procedures. The second edition was published in 1970, and presented an expanded system of terms and codes to designate diagnostic and therapeutic procedures in surgery, medicine, and the specialties. At that time a five-digit coding system was introduced, replacing the former four-digit classification. Another significant change was a listing of procedures relating to internal medicine. The fourth edition, published in 1977, represented significant updates in medical technology and allowed for periodic updating to keep pace with the rapidly accelerating medical environment.

In parallel there have been other developments requiring good interaction among authorities. Revisions of the ICD-10 have also made progress to incorporate both clinical code (ICD-10-CM) and procedure code (ICD-10-PCS) with the revisions completed in 2003. Other parallel developments have been the Patient's Bill of Rights, and the Health Insurance Portability and

Accountability Act HIPAA, which impact the above. HIPAA 1996 actually requires the Department of Health and Human Services to name national standards for electronic transaction of healthcare information. This includes not only national provider identifier, national employer identifier, security, and other tools of privacy but also the transactions and code sets. To be used at all, a coding system in the United States *must* now be a HIPAA-mandated coding system. HIPAA 1996 made the HCPCS mandatory for Medicare and Medicaid billings and prescribed the healthcare information standards noted above. The so-called final rule of 2000 names CPT (including codes and modifiers) and HCPCS as the procedure code set for physician services, physical and occupational therapy services, radiological procedures, clinical laboratory tests, other medical diagnostic procedures, hearing and vision services, and even transportation services including ambulance. Also in parallel Medicare and Medicade have been well impacted since 1983 when CPT was adopted as part of the Centers for Medicare and Medicaid Services (CMS), and with this adoption, CMS mandated the use of HCPCS to report services for Part B of the Medicare Program.

However, while these classification systems per se are wonderful, the alphanumeric and numerical codes representing them are tedious, diverse, and, to the uninitiated, enigmatic. Level I CPT is *numeric*. Level II codes are *alphanumeric* and primarily include nonphysician services such as ambulance services and prosthetic devices. Level III consists of *local codes* for state Medicaid agencies. The current version of CPT is the CPT-4 is divided into three sections with further codes, two for performance measurement and one for emerging technology.

The best that can be said for all these codes, again *per se*, is that they keep a job market going for billing specialists called "coders." The codes must be increasingly "under the hood" of IT. At least it is helpful to this end that the first AMA edition not only helped encourage the use of standard terms and descriptors to document procedures in the medical record but also provided the basis for a computer-oriented system to evaluate operative procedures, as well as contributed basic information for actuarial and statistical purposes.

Still, even well-trained billing coders have problems as long as the bare bones codes of the classification systems are manipulated. The status on billing errors seems almost as bad as the current medical errors whose avoidance or reduction was one of the early purposes of these code systems. The frequency of rejections, denials, and underpayments is said to be high (often reaching 50%), mainly because of high complexity of claims and data entry errors. The current medical coder must chose from a combination of three coding systems totaling over 10,000 codes. These systems change annually. Worse, in terms of difficulty of transition for current coders, is the transition to the rather different ICD-10 mentioned above. The "straight through billing" technology, procedures, and training help manage the billing process to receive all payments on time but fall short of a fluid translation from physician vocabulary into the billing, or any patient data, system.

IN INFORMATION-BASED PERSONALIZED MEDICINE, THE TRUE DIGITAL PATIENT RECORD RULES

Although the preventative aspect of medicine was emphasized in the previous section, the following discussions make it very hard to imagine any personalized medical system that isn't based on a collection of medical data about each individual, namely a personal medical record. If in the vision of a future information-based personalized medicine there is one concept more central to any other, it is the concept of the digital patient record enhanced by genetic and other biological information about us. As noted above, example applications include helping physicians make decisions regarding diagnosis and prognosis, helping patients make lifestyle choices, and of course, helping institutions make decisions for medical research (the latter raises many issues discussed in the next chapter).

Here is an example of how we see such a patient record. The term HALO (heterogeneous archival life object) is a terrible acronym in some respects but natural to the IT industry, or at least its researchers, who talk that way. In any event the concept and term HALO became popular in the Internet and was reported in WIRED magazine.

The concept of an integrated medical record (from womb to tomb) or heterogeneous archival life object (HALO), shown in the Figure 5.1, goes back

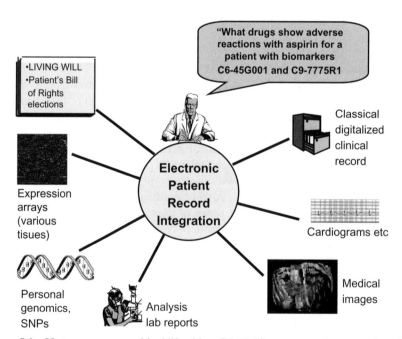

Figure 5.1 Heterogeneous archival life object (HALO) as a type of integrated medical record (IMR)

to late 1999. Its form was not very well understood at that time, but a few countries such as Canada, Belgium, the United Kingdom, and Malaysia had already experimented along this line. For example, the Province of Alberta launched in 1996 the e-health initiative called "Alberta wellnet" for province-wide e-health infrastructure to enable online sharing of personal health record (PHR) data among healthcare professionals to provide outcome-driven patient care with an assurance of continuum of patient care. Malaysia launched in 1998 a national e-health initiative dubbed "Malaysia On-Line" to establish a nationwide infrastructure for sharing its Personal Life-time Health Plan among the healthcare professionals, policy makers, and the general population. Nevertheless, even putting aside the question of including genomic data, the notion of a digital patient record having *massive healthcare significance* was relatively novel at that time. This is despite a small number of interested research groups around the world, including some places that might not spring to mind as obvious such as in Alabama and in Crete.

Talk of using computers extensively in US healthcare, and of maintaining some kind of digital patient record, came around the early 1990s. In 1992 Kaiser Permanente in Colorado made the breakthrough, hooking up with IBM to create an electronic patient record for Kaiser's use in their ambulatory setting. That application Clinical Information System (CIS) was completed and implemented in 1998. There were 27 physical locations (including clinics, emergency centers, and a call center), 350,000 active patients (with a 1,000,000 record base), 3,500 workstations (located in exam rooms, nurses stations, hospital floors, etc.), and 2,700 clinicians. The paper charts were retired in 1999 and 99.9% of all patient visit charting was done with CIS. The system included order and results messaging for pharmacy, laboratory, and radiology; results messaging from an EKG tracemaster; messages for the dictation system from CIS and the resulting transcription to CIS; messaging for provider identification and patient demographics information exchange; and messages for appointment data display in CIS from the appointment system.

Even earlier, in 1990, the first Bush administration called a group of health-care industry leaders together to discuss how healthcare administrative costs could be reduced. This group concluded that this could be done best by increasing the use of electronic data interchange (EDI) within the industry. The subsequent exploration of digitalization, and initially in regard to health insurance, created growing public concern about privacy. Regulation relating to privacy was not issued until August 17, 2000, however, with the Standards for Electronic Transactions. The US Federal Act for protection of personal privacy associated with the patient records, known as the Health Insurance Portability and Accountability Act (HIPAA), followed and was published in the Federal Register on December 28, 2000. The US privacy law was initially intended for the healthcare industry but today is being applied to other industries dealing with personal information. The US statutory requirements for protection of personal privacy (i.e., HIPAA) took effect on April 14, 2003. European countries were more concerned about the protection of personal information and started legislating the policies and compliance guidelines much earlier. The European Parliament and the Council of European Union published a directive for protection of individuals with regard to the processing of personal data and on the free movement of such data on October 24, 1995.[1] This privacy law, which is referred to as the *European Union Privacy Directive* or as the *EU Data Protection Directive*, took effect the next day, on October 25, 1998. All fifteen EU member states were obliged to enact comprehensive privacy legislation for organizations to use in implementing personal data policies to include the statutory requirements.

Recent history has been fraught with similar public concerns about patient data. The US government issued draft guidelines in the summer of 1998 that recommended the adoption of a unique patient identifier, a necessary step to the universal digital patient record, though still a far cry from it. The ensuing firestorm of public criticism took the policy community by surprise. As a result the US system is without a universal identifier, and medical information on patients today remains largely distributed and fragmented. Because medical records cannot currently be accessed in an integrated way, it is not clear without a lot of work what data belong to which patient. Within the medical environment there is a tendency for patients and populations to migrate across various points of care. Similarly medical records are maintained only at points of treatment. The problem is assembling and making available information at the point where it is needed, as the patient's record must first be identified and located within and between organizations. This formidable chore remains undone, and so remains the main obstacle to creating an integrated medical record that can be used by Healthcare providers, by patients, or by research institutes that can leverage this information to work toward personalized-drug delivery and other research areas. There is, however, a promising solution. The Healthcare Information Locator Service (HILS) is an effort initiated by an international, open membership, not-for-profit computer industry consortium called *The Object Management Group* (OMG). OMG is working to identify locations of information across a distributed organization without actually using a publicly accessible identifier. A bonus of this joint effort may be that the medical information would pertain to a population with a defined set of characteristics, and not just an individual.

Lack of public confidence in public and private institutions' ability to prevent health information from being disclosed to employers, courts, and law enforcement agencies, or to protect consumers from inappropriate use by healthcare providers was a major point in the public opposition to the use of unique identifiers. Janlori Goldman recently reported that 27% of respondents to a Louis Harris poll believed that their personal medical information would be improperly disclosed. Of this group, more than 30% felt

---

[1] *Directive 95/46/EC of the European Parliament and of the Council of 24 October 1995 on the Protection of Individuals with Regard to the Processing of Personal Data and on the Free Movement of Such Data.*

that they would be adversely affected by the disclosure. The significant numbers of Americans who pay for healthcare outside of insurance plans do so to seek care for sensitive problems and thus to avoid creating a record of the problem.

Solomon Appavu, who leads the ANSI Healthcare Informatics Standards Board's Unique Health Identifier task force, wrote a 180-page White Paper explaining the unique health identifier for patients. He stated that the biggest obstacle to implementing this unique ID is assuring patients and physicians that every computer system used in the healthcare industry is secure, and that only individuals authorized to gain access will be able to do so. He blamed the news media for focusing on information coming from the group opposed to the unique patient identifier. Citing the public hearing in July by the National Committee on Vital and Health Statistics (NCVHS), an advisory group to the secretary of HHS, Appavu claims: "Most of the people that testified said they would like to have the unique patient ID." Indeed many US patients today seem to have little concern about using their social security numbers as their universal identifier on medical forms and records.

Many of the less desirable features of US Managed Healthcare that are at the root of public concerns about privacy may be driven out by IT. Advanced IT privacy mechanisms include good security measures that the patient can control, and so dissipate the privacy concerns.

Since the anthrax attacks in the wake of 9/11, the public has shown acceptance of a national, computer-based medical defense system, which the Clinton administration had envisaged to have profound effect on twenty-first century medicine and defense. Well before 9/11, a White House web page gave a justification for such a medical defense system by reporting that Bin Laden was preparing for *anthrax attacks* on the United States. More recent continued appearances of new human epidemics of animal origin, including severe acute respiratory syndrome (SARS) and "bird flu," present just as disturbing natural biothreats, and with far more catastrophic consequences than terrorist biothreats. SARS has been relatively quiet of late, but fears remain ("5 years after SARS, Hong Kong chooses caution, closing schools amid flu outbreak" (*International Herald Tribune*, March 17, 2008)).

MORE VOICES AGAINST

We need to be fair. Not everyone likes patient identifier codes, digital patient records, nor particularly the idea of sharing them. To be sure, matters have not been helped by clumsy government phrasing that gives license for rather liberal interpretation. Both sides raised issues that need careful attention. That is the nature of bioethics. For example, in 1999 the *Washington Post* "exposed" an Outcome and Assessment Information System (OASIS) that came with a congressional mandate to the Health Care Financing Administration to create a prospective payment system for home healthcare services provided to participants in government healthcare programs. The final federal rule on collection was published January 25, 1999. There is still a degree of resistance to a simple code, and moves to instead to use fingerprints, records scans, and DNA as identifiers (D. D. C. Leonard, A. A. Pons, and S. S. Asfour, "Realization of a Universal Patient Identifier for Electronic Medical Records Through Biometric Technology," *IEEE Transactions on Information Technology in Biomedicine*, ePub ahead of print May 30, 2008). The Citizens' Council on Health Care released 10 objections to the OASIS home health data collection system (http://www.cchconline.org/).

1. Patients must choose between privacy and healthcare. At a time in their life when they are at their most vulnerable, patients must decide whether healthcare or privacy is more important to them. For the first time, the federal government has said they will not be allowed to have both—unless they can find a non–Medicare certified home health agency, of which there are few. Providers must collect the data with or without consent.

2. Federal officials overstep bounds of authority. Although HCFA's role is as an insurer for a defined population, OASIS (Outcome and Assessment Information System) demonstrates HCFA's desire to be the overseer of the entire American healthcare system. The Balanced Budget Act mandated a prospective-capitated-payment system (PPS) for those insured under the federal government. While government officials, acting as a payer, have historically been able to access medical information through claims data, the OASIS assessment intrudes into areas not necessary or statutorily required for development of PPS. In addition HCFA has not received authority to collect and register data on all patients using home health services. OASIS establishes new state and national healthcare databases without congressional authority. Note: OASIS exempts data collection on children 0 to 18 years and pregnant women.

3. OASIS permits coerced unconsented research. OASIS represents an attempt to coerce fragile patients into unconsented research. Since little of the data collected in the 19-page, 105-data-element assessment collection form (quality of life, life expectancy, schooling, financial status, quality of housing, behavioral risk factors, behaviors indicative of depression or anxiety, and living arrangements) are relevant to development of a PPS, this qualifies as unconsented research against those who are vulnerable and in need of care. According to federal research regulations, unless certain conditions are met (minimal risk, no harm to patient welfare, no violation of rights, impracticable to get consent), fully informed consent must be obtained prior to research.

4. Family privacy rights violated. Patients and family members are required to open their doors for a state and federal inspection of their home in return for access to healthcare services. Data collected is not limited to

the patient. Information on family members, including financial status and home environment, is collected and registered as well. This is a violation of the Fourth Amendment rights of families. OASIS creates government reporters out of home health providers.

5. Fourth Amendment rights violated. The Fourth Amendment states: "The right of the people to be secure in their persons, houses, papers, and effects, against unreasonable searches and seizures, shall not be violated, and no Warrants shall issue, but upon probable cause, supported by Oath or affirmation, and particularly describing the place to be searched and the persons or things to be seized." The public understood this right in the outcry against the national medical ID number.

6. Public resistance verified. In a report to the government, a researcher studying the impact of the questionnaire in a 90-agency pilot study, writes that the most significant problem in implementing the system was patient and family resistance. In particular, patients resisted or refused due to the intrusiveness of the questionnaire (schooling, finances) and the length of time it took (20–60 min).

7. Federal explanation less than forthright. Federal officials claim OASIS is required for fraud prevention and standards of care development. Yet the 1997 Balanced Budget Act only requires a PPS for home healthcare within government healthcare programs. Federal rationale attempts to lead the public into acceptance of government intrusion in all medical records and the creation of national patient databases. Ironically, OASIS may invite fraud by encouraging inflated—potentially discriminatory—patient assessments to increase federal funding for home health services.

8. Federal Privacy Act violated. By requiring collection of social security numbers in the Outcome and Assessment Information System (OASIS) without congressional authority, the Healthcare Financing Administration violates the Federal Privacy Act of 1974 which states "It shall be unlawful for any Federal, State, or local government agency to deny to any individual any right, benefit, or privilege provided by law because of such individual's refusal to disclose his social security account number … [unless] … any disclosure … is required by Federal statute. …"

9. Privacy rights superseded by new "national priority." Never before has the federal government claimed a right to medical data on all patients within one type of healthcare setting. If allowed to proceed, this presumed right coupled with the battle cry of fraud prevention, will permit the federal government to take away the citizens' right to privacy in all healthcare settings. All doctors, all hospitals, all clinics—and all their patients–will be monitored for the national agenda of fraud prevention in all public and private programs.

10. Privacy rights of all patients in jeopardy. OASIS, along with the four new healthcare enumeration systems (National Provider ID, Unique Patient

Identifier, Employer ID and Payer ID) and Secretary Shalala's "privacy" recommendations—to be enforced if Congress fails to pass privacy legislation by August 1999—jeopardize medical privacy for all. Her recommendations include the "public['s] responsibility" to allow government access to medical records without consent, for four national priorities: healthcare system oversight, public health, medical research, law enforcement—and state health databases."

Countries with a more social medicine approach have fewer concerns about digitalization of the patient record and related matters than the above. The United Kingdom is well advanced in exploring transcription and digitalization of the patient record, and is in the process of establishing a national DNA databank. Also, for example, according to the Canadian Institute for Health Information, healthcare in Canada is the largest single sector of the economy and over $150 billion business, accounting for approximately one-tenth of the country's GDP. Canada and the United Kingdom therefore feel that there are relatively few concerns as their current environment is witnessing an investment in healthcare and IT, specifically moving to meet the growing appetite for unified, accurate, timely, and comparative health information.

OTHER BARRIERS

Another perceived problem of the late twentieth century was that physicians would be slow to adopt computers. Historically the physician has been the principal integrator of knowledge in healthcare. It was appreciated that it would take a great deal of persuading to convince skeptical, busy clinicians that after all the broken promises of the past two decades, that computers can simplify and strengthen their practices. The lack of trust is even more a problem with physicians than with patients. IT has sometimes been imposed on physicians by hospitals, health systems, or health plans. Vendors and information managers frequently encountered physicians' fear that information systems will be used to profile them, gather information about their practices, discipline them, or deprive them of income.

But this is already history. For most clinicians under age 35, using network computing to acquire information and to communicate is as natural as breathing. In at least one school, medical students were banned from using the Internet for a while because they spent so much time on it. The issue is not of physician's dislike, but the fact that they are constantly on the move. A different form of input and output, like voice recognition, is required.

The difficulty will not be in the novelty of computers, but the novelty and variety of the options it reveals. Enabled by the digital patient record and the Internet, there will soon be a bewildering number of diagnostic and treatment options to choose from. While new, innovative technologies can be confusing and difficult to assimilate by physicians and patients, as Moses and

Matheson (2005) note in the *Journal of the American Medical Association* (http://www.informatics-review.com/thoughts/next.html), physicians still need to have and maintain comprehensive knowledge and understanding of progression and innovations in medicine. To help the physician to make sense of the influx of data, decision-support tools are required. To help attain that, there is a need for a publicly accessible database of the results of all treatments, which could simply be archives of anonymous forms of the patients and data-mining and decision-support tools that help the doctors (and the patients) select the most appropriate diagnostic tests and therapies on a highly personalized basis.

BUSINESS OPPORTUNITIES

The medical business potential of the application of patient digital records has attracted many entrepreneurs, but the task ahead is daunting. This following summary is abstracted from *The Future of the Internet: A Five-Year Forecast*, written for the California HealthCare Foundation by Mary Cain and Robert Mittman:

> By 2005, more than half of US consumers will have high household incomes, some college education, and access to a computer at home or at work. Healthcare consumers of the future will be more actively involved in making decisions about the healthcare they receive. They will expect high levels of choice, control, customer service, interaction with their healthcare providers, and access to information. They will use the Internet to help meet those expectations market forces in healthcare. Market forces have been at work in healthcare for a decade, in the form of managed care, employer purchasing coalitions assertive government payers and regulators, and consumer organizations. Web technologies—intranets, extranets, and the Internet—will serve as a low-cost, rapidly deployable platform for disseminating information across vertically and horizontally integrated healthcare organizations. Managed care increases the diversity and urgency of information flow; more of that communication will move to the Internet. Competitive healthcare organizations will use the web as a channel to promote their services. (http://www.informatics-review.com/thoughts/future.html)

As medicine moves from reactive to preventive, and preventive to enhancement and physical excellence, it will be perfectly respectful to speak of the "patient" as "consumer." As David Collin, MPH, of the American Cancer Society, Oakland, California, has noted: "The line between illness and other treatments for cosmetic and enhancement purposes will continue to blur with enhancement becoming the objective of more people and of treatment entrepreneurs. As severe conditions become more manageable the health care market will continue to move toward removing limits and enabling optimum performance. More billions will be spent on troubling, but not life-threatening, conditions. Public acceptance of genetic interventions will follow this trend.

The professions of health will become less about disease and death and more about marketing, and their education will reflect that. More interaction with patients will be conducted by high-bandwidth multi-media and supported by heavy information processing to improve precision and lower professional time spent. Although physician/patient face-to-face interaction will be reduced, physicians will get live, rich telemetric data." (http://www.informatics-review. com/thoughts/next.html)

Against the background of these trends, extensive use of the digital patient record seems inevitable.

MODELING AND THE PATIENT RECORD

It should be apparent from reading so far that genomic information, both SNPs and as much DNA sequences as possible, will some day be a very important part of the digital patient record. It seems natural and inevitable to most medical thinkers (1) that there will be a healthcare system based *on the fusion of digital patient record with genomic information*, (2) that this will be essential for personal and preventive medicine, (3) that it will have a profound affect on our well-being, (4) that its use will grow to represent a major global endeavor, and (5) that this endeavor will ultimately favorably impact the character of civilization.

In 1999 and early 2000 the authors were involved in architecting one of the first clinical-genomics systems including the digital patient records with genomic data, and security, privacy, and analytics features (http://www.wired. com/medtech/health/news/2001/09/47083).

Things changed rapidly in four years, probably as a consequence of the announcement of the completion of the first draft of the human genome in June 2000. In evidence of our uniqueness of vision at that time, and of what healthcare thinker Ray Kurzweil has called "an acceleration of paradigm shifts," we may quote two key books published in 2001. These are *The Nation's Health* by Philip R. Lee and Carroll L. Estes, an authoritative work for healthcare administrator then in sixth edition, and *E-Health, Telehealth and Telemedicine* by Marlene M. Maheau, Pamela Whitten, and Ace Allen, probably one of the earliest serious extensive works on medical IT. As far as we recall these books make little or no mention of the combination of genomic and related data with a digital patient record. While *The Nation's Health* was likely written for healthcare workers who may take digital patient records for granted, it is hard to imagine a chapter on the future of digital patient records that would miss out the DNA aspect when considering so may other kinds of data, such as medical images, unless it simply was not in the collective mindset at that time.

It was clear that having information about the patient's DNA on the record could one day be vital to the selection of the correct drugs, for example, using the Blue Gene supercomputer to model patient protein–drug interactions in atomic detail. A demonstration was possible in 2000 on a much slower computer because it is not required to model proteins from first principles. That remains extraordinarily difficult feat. Truly rational personalized molecular medicine demands modeling the patient's proteins (with about one polymorphism or SNP, i.e., typically a single amino acid change) against templates represented by master "standard" protein structures, followed by drug design or virtual drug screening against the protein-model's ligand (e.g., drug) binding site. When a very similar template structure with a very similar sequence is established, say with just one or two residues different, this is will be a relatively trivial procedure. New initiatives from the NIH and DOE plan to obtain some 100,000 structures over the next few years, "filling in the white spaces" of known proteins in considerable detail.

The most important protein structure data bank to date (the Protein Data Bank, PDB) was established in October 1971 at Brookhaven following a community discussion about how to establish an archive of protein structures following the Cold Spring Harbor meeting in protein crystallography. The PDB had an exponential growth for many years. The present state of the PDB is one of continued dramatic growth that has included transition of owners (to the Research Collabatory for Structural Bioinformatics), curatorship, structure, and format. Important for drug design is the associated Ligand (HET) dictionary now tidied up to roughly 3,000 files. By this effort, most folding patterns for proteins appear to have been discovered, so much of the world of protein structure may be known. While there may be out-fliers, data on those membrane proteins, including the drug receptors, is as yet extremely sparse. In any event, the new folds represent only 10% of total PDB depositions in 1999, a remarkable achievement in nailing down at least some template "parts" for which protein modeling and drug design can be carried out by pharmaceutical companies. A rare few protein structure motifs may continue to elude protein structure science for some time, simply because that rarity decreases the chances that they will be in a protein of which the structure is being determined experimentally.

The form of patient record that will emerge in the next decade will be a digital representation of each patient's physiology. The records will contain information about specific genomic markers (SNPs), and even extensive records of parts of the DNA sequence, facilitated by fast and inexpensive gene sequencing, and higher resolution PET, CT, and MRI scans. There will be extensive anatomical modeling, adjusted to represent the patient. Researchers have already produced a digital skeletal system, with digital heart and digital lungs. Pharmacogenomic data will be included and allow drugs to be tested in virtual reality on the patient data. Already FDA-approved DNA "wet" chips (i.e., real miniature laboratories, not computer simulations) can predict how a patient will respond to drugs because of pharmacogenomic differences. Other labs-on-a-chip will appear using microfluidics, namely tiny miniaturized piping. Systems biology tools are already available to help researchers analyze massive genetic data sets generated by DNA and microlab chips, and the main aim is to accelerate development of genetic diagnosis and therapy.

DRUG REACTIONS AND THE PATIENT REORD

A science vision as that discussed above has a lot of exciting benefits. But, as noted earlier a major motivator for transition in the industry is that physicians make mistakes; they make mistakes because they do not yet see, or rather they are not able to see, that patients are different from each other at the molecular level as well as anatomically and in appearance. Of course, the broader reason for bringing powerful techniques of computing to bear is that healthcare providers and systems are staggeringly inefficient at assimilating, processing, and applying new scientific information, and at converting it correctly and safely to healing knowledge. According to the 2000 Project HOPE–People-to-People Health Foundation, the core knowledge base of healthcare—biomedical science—is expanding at a geometric rate, driven by $40 billion a year in public and private sector research and development (R&D) spending, while the applied science of healthcare is not.

Still, without doubt, most scary are again those surgical errors, medication errors, and other adverse drug events that currently *kill or injure* 770,000 people in US hospitals each year,[2] or more conservatively kill 180,000 per year.[3] From the perspective of the "accident ratings," the statistics of leading causes of death presented earlier, we find the medical accidents as the biggest killer in the 1 to 44 age groups. Medical accidents kill more Americans than car accidents, AIDS (acquired immunodeficiency syndrome), or breast cancer. It was estimated that between $1.6 billion and $5.2 billion were spent each year in the United States for additional treatments to deal with adverse reaction in the 1990s. The cost may have been underestimated. In any event the total cost to healthcare systems, individuals and industry of morbidities and mortalities may be currently more like $150–$160 billion worldwide by our addition of the figures. It would explain why "spending in the [drug] regulatory and surveillance industry is expected to rise at an AAGR of 10% to reach $265 billion by 2010 with the emphasis on oncology, cardiovascular, hormonal, contraceptive and mental disorder drug markets (www.bccresearch.com/report/PHM047A.html). There is something odd in regard to projected IT spending in pharmaceutical surveillance. If spending is $265 billion by 2010, why is IT spending in this area look like a mere $100B chunk? Does this mean a discontinuous take-off of IT circa 2010? Possibly in part, since several factors will probably change. Fees paid by pharmaceutical companies to physicians to report adverse reactions may vanish: the FDA Amendment Act is moving to *demand* physician input and make analyzed data public. Drug pricing, sales and distribution will be on rational basis of feedback from patients. The effect on marketing of drug quality based on Best Evidence will greatly reduce unjustified "push" marketing, plus lobbying at about $10M per annum in the

---

[2] Source: Federal Agency for Healthcare.
[3] *To Err is Human: Building a Safer health System*, National Academy Press 1999.

United States! Honest reporting of adverse drug reactions will dramatically increase reports, and the pharmaceutical industry will want "first heads up." With standardized electronic health records clinical trial phase will be much less time-consuming and costly to source and enroll participants, and will effectively merge with post-clinical surveillance. There will be accelerated focus on pharmacogenomics and biomarkers to rationalize and avoid adverse reactions. Physicians will be required to practice evidence-based medicine based on latest findings. There will be a massive rise in data mining and data analytics to make sense of data "good and bad": he who best and fastest transforms data to knowledge wins. Forcing drug companies to be very conservative in their drug releases will at least help bring investment stability. Not included are current cost estimates on the longer term value and expenditure of the pharmaceutical company, nor consequences of investor perception. According to Richard D. Marcus, Steve Swidler, and Terry L. Zivney of the University of Wisconsin-Milwaukee, firms suffering drug recalls experience security losses many times larger than any reasonable measure of their direct cost. They found that "the implied standard deviation of stock returns from the Black-Scholes option pricing model significantly increases after a drug recall. ... The higher systematic risk after a product recall must raise the discount rate used by investors. After a recall, stock prices are reduced in line with the lower expected future earnings and are further reduced because of a higher discount rate" (*Managerial and Decision Economics*, 8, no. 4 (2008): 295–300, John Wiley and Sons). It is thought that genetic tests will enable the physician to avoid some of these risks and to treat patients more effectively. It is presumably not a unique experience that the wife of one of the authors was offered 25 mg of a drug instead of 0.25 mg in a hospital recently. But is not just a defect of US Managed Health Care, the UK hospital error record does not do much better. Throughout the West, certain well-known recurrent errors relate to common ways that doctors write prescriptions (their handwriting) that can be misread as a much higher dose. "The pen is the most dangerous, wasteful medical device," once said Neal Patterson, chairman of Cerner, the health-IT veteran company. California was the first to pass a bill requiring hospitals to install technology by 2005 that will help reduce medication errors.

The lowest estimate for medication errors in 1999 was about 7,000 deaths a year in the United States, but that is still 7,000 deaths too many. At another extreme, according to some sources, in the twenty-first century there has already been an incredible fatal accident rate of almost two per thousand physician encounters a year in the United States. There is no reason to expect that accident figures have changed dramatically yet, until at least IT starts to have effect, but there is further information regarding errors in diagnoses. The Kaiser organization in late 2006 (http://www.kaisernetwork.org/Daily_reports/rep_index.cfm) described studies showing that physician errors are a factor in about 60% of medical malpractice claims relating to diagnostic errors. Physician errors included failures in judgment (79%), memory problems (59%), lack of knowledge (48%), patient-related issues (46%) and patient handoffs from other physicians (20%). It is easy to see why IT could help. It may be true (if only because this was used by the US. "gun lobby") to argue that keeping a gun at home is 9,000 times safer than going to see a doctor. In other words, medical accidents bear comparison with the 0.0000188 accidental deaths per annum by US gun owners. There may be a decimal point error here, and we must consider the relatively noble objectives of medicine, and the mixed motives of some gun owners, but it doesn't speak too highly for the safety record of the US healthcare system either.

MOLECULAR PERSONALIZED MEDICINE REVIEWED

A partial solution lies in molecular personalized medicine. A significant fraction of medical errors (it is not clear yet, we await for example the outcome of the FDAA legislation described earlier) has been due to a drug designed for all that is not necessarily good for that one individual at a given place at a given time, and certainly with a given genetic constitution or immunological history. We should hope to understand these figures better as soon as data comes back; in 2008 the FDA awarded about $2.5 billion in contracts to the IT industry, and must have the system working to get feedback from 25 million US patients by 2010. If that is on track, 100 million should be feeding back information on drug responses by 2012. Indeed it is likely that many deaths due to an abreaction, because of a genetic difference, might not be classified as errors. The fraction is also difficult to distinguish at present because environmental effects determine part of our personal constitution and because both genetics and environment also affect our resilience to an *error* in a drug or a drug dose, as well as to the so-called normal prescription. A common very bad reaction to drugs of the penicillin group is immunological, and not directly genetic. It is due to patients becoming auto-immunized against penicillin bound to their own serum algorithm. In other words, their immune system got confused. That said, the extent to which the immune system can get confused is itself governed by genetic factors. Indeed a very high degree of variation among individuals is present in the immune system genes, such as the HLA genes, to ensure that some fraction of a human population has some chance of surviving an epidemic.

Let us recapitulate on the human variations underlying the above, with some more explanation, and dig deeper. Human beings differ for a number of reasons, but they may be classified into two broad groups, nature and nurture—or genetics and environment.

All human beings differ in at least 0.01% of their DNA (see Chapter 2) because of mutations that have occurred to the sperm or ovum while still in the gonads that have not proved fatal. They could have just occurred (about a hundred per new embryo) or have been passed down from an ancestor (the rest). Since the human genome comprises just under 3 billion base pairs, 0.01% is still a few million changes. The mutation distribution is about equal in genes and in the vast tracts between them—only a few percent of our DNA is comprised of the 30,000 or more genes. Most of these genes code for protein molecules (others code for tRNA, rRNA, etc., ultimately involved in helping make proteins). Of the hundred mutations only about four will change the amino acid sequence of a protein; about three of these hits will be a harmful change. This is because proteins are polymer chains, of 20 types of amino acid residue, each residue being coded for by three base pairs in the DNA. An error in a base pair may result in the freshly made polymer chain not folding up properly to a mature, compact protein, or it may impair or alter its function.

Many biomarkers selected for use in prescription may have nothing to do with the SNPs that signify a defect or indeed any change in the gene. They merely "travel with" those SNPs. Mutations have bad press, thus a bad connotation. However, many mutations are harmless, a few are even beneficial, at least at some points in human history, and many others serve as biomarkers without themselves significantly affecting a gene (see Chapter 2). The many differences among us are the "good genes," and these either (1) are the essence of human diversity, giving individuality in terms of skin color, weight, height, looks, temperament, personality, intelligence, and so forth, or (2) are of little or no effect whatsoever but are at least useful markers by which we can study human prehistory and also the likely group of SNPs to which an individual belongs. These groups fall into patterns called "haplotypes" and "haplogroups." They reflect our differing human histories, and so have much to do with "race." Typically races are distinguished not by unique genes (i.e., genes with unique polymorphisms) but by different characteristic proportions of the genes in the population. Arguably race is not the issue. The matter is one of different "molecular ethnicity," which may correlate with what we think of as race. In fact the (0.01% of) differences, among us all, are clustered so that the overall picture is like a tree, on which you and I may belong on the same twig or a very different branch. The notion of race breaks somewhat arbitrarily at some particular level of this branching.

Among those mutations that are at the essence of human diversity, there are some that may not be so good, depending on the circumstances and the point of view. These mutations directly affect propensity to certain diseases, or different responses to different drugs. This may mean that doses need to be varied for certain individuals. Some variants of a dose needed may be so high that the drug is out of question, and a normal dose is an underdose. Genotype frequencies for the so-called "C3435T (7q21.1) MDR1 polymorphism" for the gene that makes P-glycoprotein, differ among groups. HIV infected West Africans and African-Americans with the C/C variant may need higher doses of protease inhibitors.[4] In other instances a drug may just be a very bad prescription and have harmful effect, as we learned from the example of patients

---

[4] J. Fellay et al., Lancet 359, 30–36 (2002) The protease inhibitor in HIV pharmacology is a class of medication that inhibits HIV protease.

suffering from favism in Chapter 1. Then, again, some drugs may have no effect, which can delay treatment, put the patient at risk by delay, and even cause unneeded suffering, as in the case of a gene affecting certain types of chemotherapy.

Some commercial aspects of genomics were discussed in Chapter 3; we look here from a slightly different perspective. The path ahead for including SNPs on the patient record is not without significant cost. It may not be enough to use just a few 100 SNPs. It cost hundreds of dollars per base pair and took years to get the first human genome sequence of three billion base pairs. Ideally for 2005 to 2010 a technology is required so that 5% of a patient's DNA can be sequenced at a thousandth of a cent per base pair, for which the patient can at least contemplate paying $10,000 to get an extensive genomic representation (the cost will be a great deal lower some 5–10 years later). Consequently the search is on for cheaper, nonconventional technologies capable of achieving 100,000 genomic types per day, which is a considerably reduced time. Today, mass spectra high-throughput technology can be used for determining SNPs and accomplished with fully automated SNPs assay design. The technology has unlimited assay development capability using inexpensive reagents. Ultra high throughput can be obtained by pooling and multiplexing. In addition new laser and others methods seem capable of reading through sequences of base pairs very rapidly—and cheaply.

Massive genotyping experiments may hold promise of generating higher quality targets for drug discovery and novel diagnostic assays to target drugs to an individual's genetic predisposition. Because bringing a new drug to the market currently costs approximately $800 million and 15 years on average, it seemed at first economically impossible to personalize medicine and target small patient populations, and rather let the brunt of the implicit costs of nonefficacy, and up to some $4 billion per annum for adverse interactions, be born elsewhere. However, the cost of having an $800 million project drug abandoned because of a death in clinical trials due to unexpected pharma-cogenomic factors is a sobering thought for pharmaceutical companies. They have been turning extensively to providing clinical trials patients with the kind of care, respect, and medical record with molecular detail that every citizen should enjoy in the future. At the turn of the twenty-first century 10% to 25% of SmithKlein Beecham and 10% of Glaxo leads for research were genomic, so we may reasonably now expect that genomic-base entities to represent at least 25% of the new drugs per annum (about 40–70 new drugs per annum). It is presumed this percentage will increase dramatically, say to 75%. The drug companies also think of pharmacogenomics as identifying markets for drugs, meaning the subset of people who can benefit. A bonus may be the ability to see a safe marketplace that allows a new life and new applica-tions for drugs once rejected, or highly constrained, in days of relative genomic ignorance.

The advent of personalized drugs does not mean a sudden leap from one drug for all to a completely individualized treatment regime. Rather, drug companies can home in on finer fractions of a population. This was the case with the first such more "personal" (breast cancer) drug, Herceptin. Based on the SmithKlein Beecham and Glaxo percentages above, an imminent market $10 billion to $20 billion for personal drug revenue seems reasonable. A large chunk of this market would be due to an increase in the number of anticancer drugs, stemming from newly discovered and protein targets, and the introduction of high-priced biological agents. For pharmacogenomic therapeutic protein and antibody products Merrill Lynch analysts expected $15 billion and $8 billion market opportunities for the start of the twenty-first century, and the Cambridge Healthtech Institute expected genomics-based cancer market to be $12 billion. In face, the global biotechnology market, extensively comprising such products, grew by 12.6% in 2006 to reach a value of $153.7 billion. By 2011, the market is forecast to have an annual value of $271.4 billion, an increase of 76.5% since 2006. Medical products account for 62.5% of the global market's biotechnology revenues and the Americas is the largest region, accounting for 58.3% of the global biotechnology market's revenues (http:// www.bioportfolio.com/cgi-bin/acatalog/Biotechnology_Global_Industry_ Guide.html). The unexpected burst is possibly due to the exploding Asia-Pacific biotechnology market, which in 2007 was more than US$41 billion. It may take some hit from the global recession, but on the other hand remains a tempting area for investors when other areas are not delivering.

As with penicillin, not everything is genetics. Scarring, the loss of an appendix, or of a limb, are examples of environmental effects that leave a lasting mark with differing degrees of severity. In addition the environment can affect our molecular constitution, which is not all inherited. We may be exposed to molecules, or in the case of malnutrition, to lack of them, which leave their mark upon us. A variety of tumor promoting and inhibiting agents should be in balance in our diet, else the risk of cancer is increased. The immune system will constantly respond to allergens and pathogens, with lasting effect, and indeed a smart process known as "immune maturation" involves a kind of mini-evolution in which the DNA is actually changed. However, these are somatic mutations, meaning they do not occur in the sex cells and thus cannot be passed on to offspring (i.e., as far as we know, since increased understanding of retroviruses and ongoing retrovirus-like processes, occurring in the vast tracts of DNA between genes, could one day alter the establishment view).

The pharmaceutical industry cannot, in the large, focus on all these aspects yet. To that end, it prefers the term *stratified medicine* to envisage the "molecular ethnicity" of large chunks of the population.

COMPARE THE DAWN

Let us review, also, how it recently was. Compare it with the situation at time of reading this. It is not so long ago that the dreams and visions mentioned in previous sections were not even remotely deemed probable. There was a whole missing computational and relevant bureaucratic infrastructure in healthcare. US managed healthcare seemed particularly poorly poised for such developments. There was until recently the key component, the digital patient record, in such an infrastructure.

Indeed, in contrast to the visions and mighty aspirations above, around AD 2000 even a nice desktop computer record was a big improvement over the bundle of papers tied up with string. But Germany already had smart medical record plastic cards carried by the patient, albeit the information contents were brief. The UK countries were moving into massive endeavor to transfer medical information onto a computer network (significantly, this is paralleled by DNA sampling of a reasonable first sample of the patient population). And, whereas a US medical school might justifiably brag at having some 10 really detailed digital patient records as proof of concept, by 2003 0.7 million fairly elaborate patient records could be analyzed in the state of Virginia for previously unseen correlations between aspects such as clinical lab results and disease. Countries with social medicine, with welfare healthcare, romped ahead. Canada is moving rapidly toward digitalization of the patient records.

There had, of course, been efforts at many universities and medical centers. Recall that, in 1992 Kaiser Permanente in Colorado had embarked on a project with IBM to create an electronic patient record for Kaiser's use in their ambulatory setting. That application (called CIS) was completed and implemented in 1998. There were 27 physical locations (including clinics, emergency centers, and a call center), 350,000 active patients (with a 1,000,000 record base), 3,500 workstations (located in examination rooms, nursing stations, hospital floors, etc.), and 2,700 clinicians. The paper charts were retired in 1999, and 99.9% of all patient visit charting was then done with CIS. The CIS application interfaced with 10 external ancillary department systems and included order/results messaging for pharmacy, laboratory, and radiology, results messaging from an EKG Tracemaster, messages for the dictation system from CIS and the resulting transcription to CIS, messaging for provider identification and patient demographics information exchange, and messages for appointment data display in CIS from the appointment system. (These messages used the standard HL7 message exchange protocol, distinct from the later HL7 CDA XML discussed below, with some modification where standards had not yet been defined.)

DO YOU REALLY NEED TO PUT YOUR DNA ON A COMPUTER?

In the above dawn, the feeling was often that DNA would not go on the record for a long time. DNA is just a digital code, two bits for each of A, G, C, and T. This idea raises the question of "why bother?" Isn't much of the information "digitalized" in your DNA already?

So why even carry all your DNA information on, for example, a little chip in a medallion on a chain around your neck, when the science of molecular biology can directly access the DNA in your cells rather quickly? And hence, why have it in computer storage of any kind if DNA is "the medical record of the human race" and you as one descendent of it? In fact that record was obtained by looking at the DNA record in humans today in different parts of the world, so each sampling is also a snapshot of DNA record of the individual. Molecular biologists can get a partial "readout" of our DNA fairly quickly, and think of our DNA as "constituting libraries as real as any paper or digital library. To make the point about the interchangeability of real DNA sequences or their computer representation, note that it would be possible to store your DNA sequence in digital form on a computer and have it synthesized to clone you long after any physical remains have entirely disappeared, were lost or cremated.

However, the extent to which such a clone on a machine is very different from the real you is in part a reflection of the very argument why we should have further information for any patient record, other than what can be read from the DNA itself, be it either in digital form or a direct readout by laboratory methods. The main argument for a digital record is that DNA is only part of the story. It is not "record enough." The protein aspect, and the clinical history, are major aspects. Experience, trauma, and immunology change us. In addition there are ethical aspects reflecting the patient's religious beliefs and wishes, the same as they reflect other medical treatment or consent for research. The question of ethics is obviously important and is discussed briefly below, and at length in the next chapter.

Arguments for having DNA on the record in digital representation are that the patient or the DNA-reading equipment may not always be accessible in an emergency. Moreover it is expensive and a slow process, inappropriate for an emergency. Of course, "chips," micro-labs of the order of the size of a postage stamp, are designed so that certain key parts of the DNA can be tested, usually in the form of the messenger RNA, which DNA first generates in order to make specific proteins. In spring 2003 Roche brought out a chip for the doctor's office in which the patient could be tested as for what antidepression drugs would be appropriate for his or her genetic constitution, though it still took a day for the test (such tests will ultimately be reduced to seconds, however).

The argument for having full DNA, or at least as much as possible, rather than just a few hundreds of thousands of key SNPs, is that there may be far more than just a few thousand that are relevant. Mutations going back several recent generations might be important. Even as few as three mutations acquired from our parents may be harmful (see above) and put us at risk to certain drugs and therapies.

Another useful concept is that of *annotation*, which generally means the extra information that a curator or specialist can add to an item in a book or physical collection of things. If we were to take a DNA-centric view, it would be possible, and necessary, to think of the further information as a particularly rich form of *annotation* to the DNA coded in digital form. In other words, for a particular gene or mutation we could have a textual account written by the specialist, or have it combined with an X ray, MRI, PET, or other medical image associated with the physical effect, the phenotype, of the mutation. As it happens, we have been involved in pilot systems known as "genomic messaging systems" that take this view, and transmit DNA sequence of collections of fragments or mutations, or mixes of all of these, suitably annotated to the level of a full medical record.

Yet another way of thinking about a medical record is as the *genotype* and the *phenotype* of a patient. In medicine *both* must be available at a quick request. The genotype is that which characterizes the genetic constitution—the DNA. The phenotype adds to the genetic expression all diseases as well as healthy states, including medical images, lab data, and protein and expression array data. Previously we discussed the plethora of "omes" of the twentieth century. These concepts map to the systems perspective of *genome* and *phenome*, and genomic or phenomic information in digital form but on digital patient records. However, because we are unable to deduce a person's worldview from DNA, partly because it is also a matter of environment and life, the ethical aspects have to be added to represent the *ethome*. Ethome represents the beliefs and wishes of the patient, which certainly affect medicine. These include privacy issues, details about what medical research the patient gives for personal data for (if any), and for how long, and so forth, religious beliefs that affect things like blood transfusions, a living will about what to do, for example, if the patient is in an apparently unredeemable coma, various matters to do with the patient's rights under such documents as the US Patient's Bill of Rights.

THE OTHER TYPES OF DATA IN A MEDICAL RECORD

The digital patient record will be the heart of future medicine, and such a record needs to be a little more conceptually structured. It should be a structure to which we can apply statistical methods because, if we can find correlations between things in many patient records, we can use them for diagnosis and prognosis for a specific patient and also for medical research.

Whatever the nature of the digital record's format and data structure used to express it, there are some underlying ideas. An important matter in regard to standards concerns types of structure, called *ontologies*. Ontology is about meaning in a specific context. Of considerable importance is the *metadata*, which is data about data, and that gives it "that touch of class," meaning here as in *classification*. For example, take the headings of columns of a spreadsheet with one row per patient. An entry below the heading "Age", say 40, has no meaning in itself, but Age:=40 does. In addition there can be "metametadata," or data about data about data, and so on. In classification biology, family, genus, and species, are meta-metadata (or "second-order metadata"), metadata, and data, respectively, and (in some broader sense) so in the human family are "grandmother, mother, and me." And note meta-metadata can plough on backward through higher order metadata, like a tree structure (hence the discussion of XML below, which is well suited to trees).

Initially the meta-metadata will be a list of things of current interest to our physicians. They fall into certain sets, namely sets of kinds of things. We can imagine these sets as prefixes to whole groups of data. For example, "Rx:" will be the prefix for any prescription such as in Rx:erythromycine. Our choices extend the set of "Rx" for prescriptions, "Dx" for diagnosis, and the occasionally used "Px" for procedures. These prefixes could change to something more mnemonic as already widely used, but this illustration gives some sense of what is currently being done. A real patient record comprises complex information that can be primarily classified as in Tables 5.1, 5.2, and 5.3. (The classes are more important than the specific names for the classes given, and we have tried to draw from wildly accepted usages.) Many of the sets in the table defined by a prefix could easily comprise 100 distinct factors, such as, in "Lx," hemoglobin, blood glucose levels, triglycerides, and biopsy results. Ethical data (ETHx:) is a little different: it determines rather than becomes involved in the analysis itself. Ethical data represent the wishes of the patient, including informed consent about how the data may be used.

TABLE 5.1 Example Formats

Format	Meaning	Examples
data	Data without metadata	broken_leg
Metadata:=data	Data with metadata	Smoker:=yes
Metadata(count):=data	Metadata with data with event count	Systolic_ BP(20):=140
Metadata(count):=timestamp	Data with event count and metadata with universal timestamp.	Systolic_ BP (20):=1984.64325
Metadata:=>data	Data in range with metadata (equal to or greater than)	Age:=>42
Metadata:=<data	Data in range with metadata (less than)	Age:=<42
L1:Metadata:=data	Data with metadata and level 1 qualifier	Rx:Cyclosporine:=50u
L2:L1:Metadata:=data	Data with metadata and level 1 & 2 qualifiers	INF:Rx:cyclosporine:=50u HEM:Lx:hemoglobin:=normal
L3:(L2:L1:Metadata:=)data	Rule as metadata, data, and prefixes. Parts in bracket optional	KP:: HEM:Lx:hemoglobin:=low, GYN:Dx:=pregnant

TABLE 5.2   Level1 Metadata Prefixes: Data and Physician Input

Root Prefix	Meaning	Examples
PHIx:	Personal health information, identity data	Name, ID, HIPAA sensitive data
IDx:	Identifiers deemed non-PHI	Record code
DMx:	Demographic data deemed non-PHI.	Country of origin, cultural, country of residency, overview of job:
ETHx:	Ethical data, patient wishes	Living will, Patients' Bill of Rights issues.
CONx:	Research consent issues	Scope and purposes
INSx:	Insurance and billing	Insurance company, coverage
LSx	Lifestyle and social history	Smoking, alcohol intake, exercise
SATx:	Patient satisfaction status	Feeling unwell
ATNx:	Attention	Warnings, diabetic, drug abreactions, etc.
TYPx:	Description by typically invariant characteristics	Gender, race, eye color, etc
DESx:	Description by typically variable characteristics	Age, weight, height,
PHSx:	Physiological results	Blood pressure, cardiogram, nerve testing, CNS data
Lx:	Clinical laboratory results	Hematology, biochemistry
HISx:	Histological results	Slide sections, reports
MIx:	Medical imaging data	X ray, MRI, PET, CAT, etc.
Cx:	Condition, status	
REFx:	Referral data	Type of specialist
Dx:	Diagnoses	
PRGx:	Prognosis	
Rx:	Prescriptions	Drugs, ointments, etc.
Px:	Procedures	Surgery, physiotherapy, etc.
Ox:	Outcomes	
Bx:	Biopsies	
PRx:	Proteomic data (including expression aray data)	
FAMx:	Family, genealogical data	
DNAx:	Genomic data	Sequences, SNPs
GENx:	Genetic data	Other genetic information
COMx:	Comment	

The specific entry, the value of the blood pressure, such as 70 represents the *data*. The union of the two PHSx:resting_pulse:=70 represents the *entry*, or the *item* or *data item*, or *qualified data*, or just *data* (though ambiguously, the same as we used it above) for short. In specifically writing PHSx:resting_pulse:=70,

TABLE 5.3 Level2 Metadata Prefixes: Disciplines, Domains, and Systems

Discipline/System	Meaning	Examples
INF:	Infectious disease	
IMM:	Immunology	Immunological disorders, allergies, autoimmune disorders
TOX:	Toxicology, chronic	Long-term accumulative
POI:	Acute poisons, venoms, stings	Sudden critical toxic events, chemical warfare
CVS:	Cardiovascular	
PUL:	Pulmonary	
GI:	Gastrointestinal	
HEP:	Hepatic, biliary	
MET:	Nutritional, metabolic	
END:	Endocrinology	
HEM:	Hematology	
ONC:	Oncology	
LYM:	Lymphatic	
MUS:	Musculoskeletal, connective tissue	
NEU:	Neurological	
PSY:	Psychiatric	
GU:	Genitourinary	
GYN:	Gynecology, obstetrics	
PED:	Pediatrics	
ENT:	Otolaryngology	
EYE:	Ophthalmology	
SKN:	Dermatology	
DEN:	Dental, oral	
PHY:	Matters due to physical agents	Burns, sunburn, heatstroke, hyperthermia, diving bends

PHSx:resting_pulse is also said to be the qualifier, not just metadata. It is further possible to consider the prefix (e.g., PHSx) as a qualifier of whatever is to its right, so in this case it could be considered a qualifier of a qualifier, or metaqualifier. If we use ":=" to represent such qualification, then PHSx:=resting_pulse:=70 is meaningful. In fact, consistent with "meta-metadata" and so discussed above, we could have a long chain of such phrases where in ... :=D:=C:=B:=A, letter A is the data, B is the metadata, C is the meta-metadata or "second-order metadata," D is the meta-meta-metadata or "third-order metadata," and so on. Branched forms are also possible, as in vertebrates:= (mammals:=primates, birds:=finches). This represents a simple case of a graph. Such graphs represent a *hierarchic ontology.*

We mentioned that in Age:=40 the data 40 alone makes no sense. It is, however, possible to have data without any qualifying metadata, as in "broken leg." The converse that metadata makes no sense without data, applies unless it means all items under that metadata (and hence also everything that is branching out from that point in a hierarchic ontology). However, we say "not exactly true" because there are instances in unstructured data where metadata and data are not easily distinguished, and in some cases we could argue that it doesn't have to be. For example, "smoker" could imply smoker:=yes, or habits:=smoker. It is good practice to go for a structured ontology however. For example, encountering "smoker" in a formal setting, and leaping immediately on the habits:=smoker meaning, would be erroneous if smoker:=no was implied. There is some case for arranging things such that the final data is "yes", "no" and even "don't know", which can be converted to number 1,–1, and 0, for example. The advantage of this is that the statistical techniques for analyzing trends between numeric data (e.g., multivariate analysis) can be brought to bear on the data, while otherwise we are confined to techniques merely based on the number of times such an entry occurs (e.g., association analysis).

Classical medical records have material not in any particular order, except for date and maybe time, in which case it is said to be *time-stamped*. Normally, however, e.g., one would create a separate entry such as PHSx:resting_pulse_time=08/03/2004 11:46:00 or even PHSx:resting_pulse:=time:=08/03/2004 11:46:00 to go alongside PHSx:resting_pulse:=time:=70, and similarly for other items, so allowing time series analysis (effectively correlations between time of observation and the observed value). To do this requires conversion to some universal leap-year-free decimal time such as 2009.98666, which is some moment of December 2009 (there are also things called leap-seconds to take into account).

XML AS THE STRUCTURED REPRESENTATION OF THE MEDICAL RECORD

This section is for the more technically minded. That's because it is impossible today to discuss formats and standards for medical records without discussing XML. *Let's face it: standards for describing anything can be boring.* Often even scientists and engineers find such discussions boring, and maybe irritating to some degree. There is good reason for irritation. A standard does not have to be a best technical choice for describing something (it usually isn't); it just has to be the agreed choice. It can make a scientific or engineering perfectionist choke. And to make things worse, standards that are accepted as standards (and agreed on and "legislated" by some authoritative designated body) are rarely agreed on by everybody. But standards are essential to pursue if you don't want to change everything by hand, or import, process, analyze, or display data every time, and more importantly if you want to collaborate with others, especially outside your organization. Like the old chauvinist lament (on whichever other sex was intended), "You can't live with 'em, and you can't live without 'em." But, seriously, *living*, meaning *survival*, is an issue. Standards remove ambiguity, and when there is ambiguity, a patient can die because of a wrong decision, or lack of decision. The kind of ambiguity we are talking about is more or less exemplified by the prescription errors mentioned above. Good standards supported by IT can readily enforce correct dosages and give warnings to drug abreactions, cross-reactions, and the like, and can control doses, ensuring that the correct units are connected to the right numbers—and the right patient. And when a bad response is due to different patient DNA features, it should be in the record as well and properly represented.

More accurately, XML is not itself a standard; it is a means for defining standards that fall into the same general philosophy. That philosophy is the philosophy of hierarchical ontology. Ontology discussed above had data arranged in a hierarchy, types of information within types of information, and kind of structure. XML in general reflects that. XML, or "extensible markup language," hints at its origin in the international standard SGML (standard generalized markup language) for representation of data, their hierarchy, structure, and types in an electronic document. SGML was also the origin of the fixed-form HTML or "hypertext markup language," which controls the format and layout of web pages. Remember that HTML is that text with all those numerous embedded < > </ > that shock you when something goes wrong with your favorite Internet web page, or the wrong software or option is used to display the web page. A famous "computer geek" cartoon shows a user collapsed back in his office chair in a state of near-fatal shock when an error occurs and he is accidentally exposed to the raw HTML behind a friendly looking web page.

The term "markup" comes from the notion of marking proofs of books, papers, and articles for printing and publication, typically as an editor's way of coding elements that call for special treatment by the typesetter. For example, a pencil might be used to show that a certain part of a mathematical equation, or a reference note, should have been a superscript, as in example superscript. In HTML, this is conveyed by example but displayed as example superscript by Internet browser software such as Windows Explorer. The effect of XML is that when converted to HTML, coded data can be easily displayed and in a readable manner.

Still the main role of XML is quite different from that of HTML. It is to break up stored and transmitted data such that the contextual and hierarchical meaning is conveyed. Any particular meaning so portrayed is the ontology. XML is a system of brackets or tags which specify the content. In XML, vertebrates:=(mammals:=primates, birds:=finches) becomes <vertebrates> <mammals>primates</mammals> <birds>finches</birds> </vertebrates>. "Extensible" means that unlike in basic HTML, users can create their own tags (and other elaborate additional data in the tags), as well as specifications of the ontological "language" that they thereby create. In particular, valid tag names and modes of use can be constrained to a more fixed format. It is encouraged that group or project names be included as a kind of prefix to the tag name, such as "smithsonian" in <smithsonian:vertebrates> so that there is no clash with other people's ontology. Some of these ontology "languages" become widely accepted standards, and everyone (ideally) agrees to use those specifications.

Once you know XML a bit, it is easy to write a specific embodiment of it, which has the recognizable < > ... </> bracketing system but is otherwise specialized to your needs. In the case of medical record, the most widely used XML-based ontology is Health Level Seven's "HL7 Clinical Document Architecture." Table 5.4 shows a fragment of a patient record in this ontology. Note that the XML system (and HL7) allows potential new standards to be introduced if the bases of all features are not covered. For example, the HL7 tags contain the string "cda:" (for "Clinical Document Architecture"). At time of creating this document for a bone marrow transplant patient, there was a need for genomic data for which Health Level Seven had not yet established a clear ontology. Hence tags contain the prefix string "gms:" to indicate that they come from the IBM Research project, "Genomic Messaging System."

The power of XML is that it can communicate the knowledge it represents hierarchically, among many different processes. Any one writing a new program needs only to understand how XML works and make relatively little effort to make it work with their program. By XML convention, there are only certain places that you need to look to find what information you need. That is the reason why the emerging and yet rapidly becoming a de facto standard called "web Services" uses XML for representation of data for storing, exchanging messages among systems across the network or components within a system. A pilot clinical GMS (genomic messaging system) technology for processing, annotating, and analyzing the patient record was developed at IBM to be broader than XML, and its primary function is to break down XML and use that information unraveled, or modify the document and rebuild it (or both). In 2004 we showed in a scientific paper that using GMS and XML, patient DNA can be encoded for storage and transmission by computers (B. Robson and R. Mushlin, "Genomic messaging system for information-based personalized medicine with clinical and proteome research applications," *J. Proteome Res.* (Am. Chem. Soc.) 2004;3(5):930–948).

Working with IBM Research team in Haifa, Israel, who had access to appropriate medical data, our demonstration was related to bone marrow transplant patients. One of the major problems in transplantation is determining whether a transplanted organ will, or is, undergoing rejection. Individuals vary in their response to immunosuppressive therapy. Personalized medicine, including diagnosis, prescription, and prognosis based on patient genomics, would not only alleviate patient sampling discomfort and undesirable side effects but reduce the enormous cost of blanket use of currently expensive rather coarse-grained diagnostics and immunosuppressive drugs. The major source of the body's control over rejection of structures carrying alien molecules are the six

TABLE 5.4

```
- <cda:paragraph>
  <cda:content>Follow-up in our out-patient clinic on coming
Sunday.</cda:content>
  </cda:paragraph>
  </cda:section>
  </bmt:Discharge_Plans>
- <bmt:Instructions_To_Patient_And_Family>
  <cda:section />
  </bmt:Instructions_To_Patient_And_Family>
  </bmt:At_Discharge>
  </bmt:BMT_Discharge_Body>
  </cda:section
  <cda:verify_correct_genelab_id patient_code="00hzYw5m.HyAY"
expected_patient_code="test" />
- <cda:section>
  <cda:caption>IBM Genomic Messaging System Data</
cda:caption>
- <cda:paragraph>
- <cda:content>
- <cda:local_markup ignore="markup">
  <gms:annotation>GMS-augmented document created Mon May 13
8:34:59 2002 gms:environment tags allow use of valid xml as
annotation mixed with DNA in ..GATTACCA.. format, and
executable GMSL (Genomic Messaging Stream Language) as
content. The GMSL will activate immediately when program gms
is run with the IBM-Yorktown legacy conversion cartridge
option selected for IBM-Haifa CDA hospital files.</
gms:annotation>
- <gms:genomic_data xmlns:gms="GMS_schemas">
- <gms:dna sequence="1" base="1" locus="1">
- <gms:manual_annotation>
  <gms:gene patient_code="00hzYw5m.HyAY" expected_patient_
code="test" gene="HLA00664" other_name="DRB1*0101"
length="801" checksum="80C9FCB6" />
- <gms:nonsequence_annotation> <gms:t_cell_epitopes
relation = "associated with disorder, peptomimetic lead">
- <gms:protein> pkyvkqn
<gms:pkc_phosphorylation>tlk</gms:pkc_phosphorylation> a
  <gms:protein_feature type="whole_sequence" sequence="1"
context="binding peptide?" readingframe="1" start="1"
stop="12" />
  <gms:protein_feature type="pkc_phosphorylation"
sequence="1" readingframe="1" start="8" stop="10" />
  </gms:protein>
- <gms:protein> gplkaeiaqrle <gms:protein_feature
type="whole_sequence" sequence="1" context="binding peptide?"
readingframe="1" start="1" stop="12" />
  </gms:protein>
  </gms:t_cell_epitopes>
  </gms:nonsequence_annotation>

ATGGTGTGTCTGAAGCTCCCTGGAGGCTCCTGCATGACAGCGCTGACAGTGACACTGATG
GTGCTGAGCTCCCCACTGGCTTTGGCT
  <gms:experimental_start_of_mature_peptide />
  GGGGACACCCGA
  <gms:template_start />
```

key HLA genes, which make HLA protein. These proteins are very highly variable among individuals (i.e., highly polymorphic) because in prehistoric and historic time it enabled at least a small fraction of a population to survive an epidemic. In transplantation healthcare, understanding of the different responses that patients have to immunorejection and to immunosuppressive therapy is crucial.

In our demonstration study sequence information concerning the patient's specific HLA genes, the primary genes responsible for transplant rejection (and illustrating high degree of patient-specific polymorphism), was shipped in the patient's medical record in HL7 clinical record format. The record also contained information regarding epitopes to which that patient had been exposed in his immunological history. The HL7 record illustrates exactly these epitope types. "Epitopes" are short sections of protein sequence, namely peptides that the body has detected in the past and memorized, and these peptides will bind to the HLA proteins that HLA genes make. The source of the original epitopes could be parts of proteins of a bacterial, viral, or other infection or an allergen, on any system to which the patient had been exposed and to which his or her immune system had responded.

The DNA sequences were automatically annotated and translated into a protein sequence (remember that every three base pairs translates to one amino acid residue). The protein sequence was then additionally annotated by special XML tags. "Annotation" means in this case indication of where the mature protein starts and stops, where the sites linking sugar molecules are, and so forth. Such changes, meaning *posttranslation modifications*, occur after a protein is made in the cell but before it is actually used, in this case on the immune cell's surface. In other words, annotation provides a detailed description of how the molecule looks when active in the patient's body, and this varies with the patient. The implication is that the record tells the computer how to model the patient's protein. This kind of calculation would have used the Blue Gene machine. However, Blue Gene was still being planned at that stage, so the calculation used several approximations to allow the sequencing of the proteins to be done on available machines in a short time.

The annotated protein sequence was thus used to model the patient's polymorphic protein, and to design peptidometic compounds that would function as competitive inhibitors at HLA protein binding sites, so potentially enabling the patient to accept a specific transplant. The starting point for this modeling was the epitopes described above. The process was highly automated and very rapid. Although the demonstration was to show only information technology and no drug was synthesized and tested, the principle researchers had achieved earlier success in the application of peptidometics in this area that showed all steps to be feasible. This does not mean, of course, that such a process will become routine within the immediate future, only that no huge quantum leaps will be required to develop such technology.

The trouble with XML is power at the price of bulk. Means of recording medical information in the old days was much much simpler. That is, XML has substantial overhead to process huge complex (with multilevel hierarchical structures) documents. One brief note in a clinical record should ideally unfold to the source data, and include large-memory graphic items such as the X ray. The implementation of just one single routine hospital transaction explodes from a few lines to substantial number of lines in XML, and a large document style declaration. Although a traditional clinical record would typically encode this only once or few times, it takes substantial work to specify the corresponding HL7 record. An example may give a better impression of how the different methods for essentially the same medical information would look like (see also Tables 5.5 and 5.6.) Note that HL7 codes may have changed by time of reading.

Traditional clinical record entry to clinical record

```
Chest X-ray 1960-01-01. Normal.
```

HL7 Messaging (Not real patient data.)
```
Chest X-ray # 1501/71020, patient ID 1234 5 M11 (P8754),
John Doe, (male) born 1960/01/01. Requested by p.o.c.
physician 1987-03-28,15:30 taken 1987-03-29, 08.00. Normal.
MSH|^~\&|XRAY||CDB||||ORU^R01|K172|P<cr>
PID|||PATID1234^5^M11||Doe^John||19600101|M<cr>
OBR||P8754^OE|XR1501^XR|71020^Chest X-ray
PA||198703281530|198703290800<cr>
OBX|1|TX|71020||It is a normal PA Chest X-ray||||||F<cr>
```

Now look at Tables 5.5 plus 5.6 and see how transmitted data grows! However, Table 5.7 could be kept and need not be sent every time. Still, despite the problem of expansion of overheads, XML is great for information on personalized medicine. Like the phenomenon of spreadsheet it has currency for expressing patient records for medical research. Spreadsheets cannot draw together, at least with quite such ease, so complex sets of heterogeneous data, consisting diverse forms of text, medical images, cardiogram traces, DNA sequences, expression arrays, and so on.

TABLE 5.5 (Not Real Patient Data.)

```xml
<?xml version='1.0'?>
<?xml:stylesheet type="text/xsl" href="hl7-2.xsl"?>
<HL7>
<R01>
<MSH>
    <SeAp>XRAY</SeAp>
    <ReAp>CDB</ReAp>
    <MeTy>
        <type>ORU</type>
        <TrEv>R01</TrEv>
    </MeTy>
    <MeCoID>K172</MeCoID>
    <PrID>P</PrID>
</MSH>
```

TABLE 5.5   *Continued*

```
<PID>
     <PaIDIn>
          <IDNum>PATID1234</IDNum>
          <ChDi>5</ChDi>
          <ChDS>M11</ChDS>
     </PaIDIn>
     <PaNa>
     <FaNa>John</FaNa>
          <GiNa>Doe</GiNa>
     </PaNa>
     <DTofBi>
          <date>1960-01-01</date>
     </DTofBi>
     <Sex>M</Sex>
</PID>
<OBR>
     <PlOrNum>
          <EnId>P8754</EnId>
          <Namesp>OE</Namesp>
     </PlOrNum>
     <FiOrNum>
          <EnId>XR1501</EnId>
          <Namesp>XR</Namesp>
     </FiOrNum>
     <UnSeID>
          <Ident>71020</Ident>
          <text>Chest X-ray PA</text>
     </UnSeID>
     <ReqDT>
          <date>1987-03-28</date>
          <time>15:30</time>
     </ReqDT>
     <ObsDT>
          <date>1987-03-29</date>
          <time>08:00</time>
     </ObsDT>
</OBR>
<OBX SetID="1">
     <VaTy>TX</VaTy>
     <ObsId>
          <Ident>71020</Ident>
     </ObsId>
     <ObsVal src="x-ray.gif">It is a normal PA Chest
     X-ray</ObsVal>
     <ObsReSt>F</ObsReSt>
</OBX>
</R01>
</HL7>
```

TABLE 5.6

```
<xsl:template match="/">
<HTML>
<xsl:apply-templates select="HL7/R01/MSH"/>
<xsl:apply-templates select="HL7/R01/PID"/>
<xsl:apply-templates select="HL7/R01/OBR"/>
<xsl:apply-templates select="HL7/R01/OBX"/>
</HTML>
</xsl:template>

<xsl:template match="HL7/R01/MSH">
<DIV STYLE="background-color:red">
    <SPAN STYLE="font-weight:bold; color:white; font-
size:14pt">Message Header
</SPAN>
</DIV>
<xsl:apply-templates select="SeAp"/>
<xsl:apply-templates select="ReAp"/>
</xsl:template>

<xsl:template match="SeAp">
<DIV STYLE=" margin-left:20px">
    <SPAN STYLE=" font-weight:bold; color:black; font-
size:14">From: </SPAN>
<SPAN STYLE=" color:blue; font-size:14">
    <xsl:value-of/>
        </SPAN></DIV>
</xsl:template>

<xsl:template match="ReAp">
<DIV STYLE=" margin-left:20px">
    <SPAN STYLE=" font-weight:bold; color:black; font-
size:14">To: </SPAN>
<SPAN STYLE=" color:blue; font-size:14">
    <xsl:value-of/>
        </SPAN></DIV>
</xsl:template>

<xsl:template match="HL7/R01/PID">
<DIV STYLE="background-color:red">
    <SPAN STYLE="font-weight:bold; color:white; font-
size:14pt">Patient Identification
</SPAN>
</DIV>
<xsl:apply-templates select="PaIDIn"/>
<xsl:apply-templates select="PaNa"/>
<xsl:apply-templates select="DTofBi"/>
<xsl:apply-templates select="Sex"/>
</xsl:template>

<xsl:template match="PaIDIn">
```

TABLE 5.6   *Continued*

```
<DIV STYLE="background-color:white; color:black;
font-size:14pt">
    <SPAN STYLE="font-weight:bold; color:black"> Patient ID
(internal)
        </SPAN></DIV>
<xsl:apply-templates select="IDNum"/>

</xsl:template>

<xsl:template match="IDNum">
<DIV STYLE=" margin-left:20px">
    <SPAN STYLE=" font-weight:bold; color:black; font-
size:14"> ID Number: </SPAN>
<SPAN STYLE=" color:blue; font-size:14">
    <xsl:value-of />
        </SPAN></DIV>
</xsl:template>

<xsl:template match="PaNa">
<DIV STYLE=" background-color:white; color:black;
font-size:14pt">
    <SPAN STYLE=" font-weight:bold; color:black"> Patient
Name
        </SPAN></DIV>
<xsl:apply-templates select="FaNa"/>
<xsl:apply-templates select="GiNa"/>
</xsl:template>

<xsl:template match="FaNa">
<DIV STYLE=" margin-left:20px">
    <SPAN STYLE=" font-weight:bold; color:black; font-
size:14"> Family Name: </SPAN>
<SPAN STYLE=" color:blue; font-size:14">
    <xsl:value-of/>
        </SPAN></DIV>
</xsl:template>

<xsl:template match="GiNa">
<DIV STYLE=" margin-left:20px">
    <SPAN STYLE=" font-weight:bold; color:black; font-
size:14"> Given Name: </SPAN>
<SPAN STYLE=" color:blue; font-size:14">
    <xsl:value-of />
        </SPAN></DIV>
</xsl:template>

<xsl:template match="DTofBi">
<DIV STYLE=" background-color:white; color:black;
font-size:14pt">
    <SPAN STYLE=" font-weight:bold; color:black"> Date of
Birth:
        </SPAN>
<xsl:apply-templates select="date"/>
</DIV>
```

TABLE 5.6 *Continued*

```
</xsl:template>

<xsl:template match="date">
<SPAN STYLE="color:blue; font-size:14">
    <xsl:value-of />

</SPAN>
</xsl:template>

<xsl:template match="Sex">
<DIV STYLE=" background-color:white; color:black;
font-size:14pt">
    <SPAN STYLE=" font-weight:bold; color:black"> Sex: </SPAN>
    <SPAN STYLE=" color:blue; font-size:14">
        <xsl:value-of />
        </SPAN></DIV>

</xsl:template>

<xsl:template match="HL7/R01/OBR">
<DIV STYLE=" background-color:red">
    <SPAN STYLE=" font-weight:bold; color:white;
font-size:14pt">Observation
        </SPAN></DIV>
<xsl:apply-templates select="ReqDT"/>
<xsl:apply-templates select="ObsDT"/>
</xsl:template>

<xsl:template match="ReqDT">
<DIV STYLE=" background-color:white; color:black;
font-size:14pt">
    <SPAN STYLE=" font-weight:bold; color:black"> Observation
Request (Date/Time): </SPAN>
<xsl:apply-templates select="date"/>
<xsl:apply-templates select="time"/>
</DIV>
</xsl:template>

<xsl:template match="time">
<SPAN STYLE=" color:blue; font-size:14">Time
    <xsl:value-of/>

</SPAN>
</xsl:template>

<xsl:template match="ObsDT">
<DIV STYLE=" background-color:white; color:black;
font-size:14pt">
    <SPAN STYLE=" font-weight:bold; color:black">
Observation  (Date/Time):
        </SPAN>
<xsl:apply-templates select="date"/>
<xsl:apply-templates select="time"/>
</DIV>
</xsl:template>

<xsl:template match="HL7/R01/OBX">
```

TABLE 5.6 *Continued*

```
<SPAN STYLE=" font-weight:bold; color:black; font-size:14pt">
Observation Result
        </SPAN>

<xsl:apply-templates select="ObsVal"/>
</xsl:template>
<xsl:template match="ObsVal">
<DIV STYLE=" background-color:navy; margin-left:20px">
    <TABLE><TR>
            <TD STYLE="COLSPAN:2"><IMG><xsl:attribute
name="src"><xsl:value-of select="@src"/></xsl:attribute>
</IMG></TD>
<TD STYLE="padding-left:1em">
<SPAN STYLE=" color:black; font-size:14pt">
    <xsl:value-of/>
        </SPAN></TD></TR></TABLE></DIV>
</xsl:template>

</xsl:stylesheet>
```

TYPES OF ARCHIVES

No doubt most people see benefit to a quickly accessible record that reduces the current toll of errors and gives access to the best technologies for diagnosis, treatment, and prognosis. But all have expressed concerns that this should be a very well-guarded system. Where will the record reside? In some nations, a large fraction of patients prefer to keep records at home. There appears to be a fear that an invading foreign power, as in the days of Nazi Germany, might use medical and ethnic data to their own dark ends. Others like US citizens tend to like the idea of it being handheld by the physician. Countries providing public healthcare services like Canada want the Ministry of Health to keep the health records, although they publicize that technically patients own their health records but government safeguards the health records as the "trusted custodian" (despite the general notion in North America and Europe that governments are not trustworthy and that the word "trust" and politicians do not go together). The reason given is that otherwise family members or prospective employees might more readily put pressure on the patient to expose data. For example, a son might not want his parents to know yet that he is HIV positive, or a husband might not wish his wife to know that he is using Viagra.

While it is essential for the physician at work and the patient at home to access his or her health records with individually identifiable information, there are plenty of organizations that do need to see the records, but only in the collective statistical sense without identifying the individual. They include, most controversially, the health insurance companies, which do have a right to statistically survey the data for amortization purposes. But they also include medical research and teaching institutions, the Center for Disease Control and biothreat monitoring agencies, the Food and Drug Administration, the World Health Organization, pharmaceutical R&D companies, health authorities, local public health and hygiene organizations, nursing and welfare centers, and so on.

For such purpose one might consider an ARC, that is, archive of "anonymous record contributions." Such an archive would essentially mirror contributed records, except for being "anonymized" (see the next chapter). However, fairly sophisticated software would need to be used to serve as gatekeeper between the identified and "anonymized" archives. Moreover such sophistication will need to extend to police the gates between the ARC and the researchers so that no researcher opens a means of threading back to identify the patient. That is, unless a patient required that he or she be warned of freshly identified medical risks, a process that itself can involve complex security so that outsiders cannot intervene in or reproduce the "tracking back" mechanism.

Some health records may need to be archived from the system after a period of time, in order to keep the database system down to manageable size and also to keep the analytical processing manageable. An archive and record-keeping services will be used for management of health records such as visit records, diagnostics, and treatments. The key functions provided by the archive and record-keeping component are generation and capture, maintenance of retention period, retrieval, removal (destruction of content, but retain the tombstone data), and report generation.

Some researchers, of medical scientists or biostatisticians, have maintained that the same record could be used for all purposes: it is merely a matter of what the researcher is allowed to access. There seems to be a general feeling that an ARC should be a distinct archive outside the security firewall, with the identified records held inside. Moreover there are subtleties in statistics that allow certain statistical overviews to nail down detailed data. For example, if a spreadsheet, contains multidimensional data with only averages in the rows and columns, it should not be possible for anyone to work back from the marginal summaries to deduce the interior of the spreadsheet. But in fact a mathematical algorithm is already known to medicine that allows medical images to be constructed—*tomography*.

THE SHAPE OF RECORDS TO COME

A record cannot reside forever in a big computer, however. For support of mobile medical service, selected health records may need to be collectively copied onto a handheld system. All the sensitive information copied or replicated onto a portable system need to be stored encrypted, and the copy/replication event will be digitally signed or logged in the system for nonrepudiation and security audit. As sophistication increases and size decreases, these devices could be worn as digital watches or as medallions around the neck.

But several organizations are looking even further ahead, and developing computer chips the size of a grain of rice that might be inserted under the skin in an arm or wrist. The microchip is referred to as a subdermal microchip or subdermal microelectromechanical system (MEMS). This brings many diverse concepts together (including the question of real DNA and digital DNA as both constituting the genomic record). More important, we need to understand the long-term effect caused by MEMS and ultimately the future nanobots or nanoelectromechanical system (NEMS) that can much more freely roam within the body and penetrate cell membranes MEMS with MEMS our medical records would be secure as part of our identify, ensure our security in buying goods or doing banking transactions, and function as charge cards that would be automatically read at the supermarket checkout. Note that such a chip might also be in communication with other similar chips placed at different body locations. They could ultimately include micro-lab features that read out biochemical and physiological data relating to our current state of health and to our different organs. To prevent terrorists or criminals from excising and using the chip, it could be protected by biometric authentication such as facial geometry, fingerprint data, and DNA data. As nanotechnology, the technical art of making the very small, improves, it might directly report our DNA sequences, or more important, what messenger RNAs and proteins are being made in our blood tissues.

There is a potential continuum from implanted human materials to implanted animal material to implanted artificial material. When we speak of "IT within us," we mean life as a natural information system, and that continuity with artificial intelligence opens up many possibilities. Besides ways of keeping data such as your medical records, there is (in principle) nothing to stop data on genealogy, inheritance, living will, and patient consent, from being converted from its normal representation into a string of base pairs … ATGC … and implanted in your DNA using techniques like those of gene therapy. These data could subsequently be sampled and read out on a gene sequencer as needed. The instructions for a human that we carry in our cells are quite "tight," so the amount of extra information we might insert is probably not huge. While the cells would have to accommodate significantly extended chromosomes, based on a back-of-the–envelope calculation, the equivalent information to a hundred or so digital camera pictures might be possible. And planted in the right cells, any of this information could even be passed to your offspring.

LAST THOUGHTS FOR THE RECORD

Wherever it resides, as the patient record becomes more sophisticated, it will provide computer models of our bodies that can be queried and used to answer "what-if" questions, at many levels from whole limbs and organs down to the molecular level. Certainly, at an early stage, physical simulations including the elasticity, plasticity, and coefficients of friction of nerves, muscles, and organs will be used to interpret dynamic 4D medical imaging, in space (3D) and time for osteopaths, cardiologists, and sports physicians. In some sense, and perhaps ultimately in a very real sense, it will be our shadow, our own Avatar, our guardian angel, our representative in the mind of the computers, that will need to be of enormous power in order to support advanced medicine. It could one day become so detailed that it becomes a total backup of our physical being and our memories and responsibilities, a kind of digital clone plus. This vision raises many concerns and ethical issues, and fears of tampering. Because of social concerns this is precisely why the authors will often increasingly look in this book to mythology, the lessons of history, futurology, and even science fiction. Above all, our humanity calls for there to always be concern for ethics.

6

ENFORCING YOUR RIGHTS: MEDICAL ETHICS, CONSENT, PRIVACY, AND IT

> The patient has the right to considerate and respectful care
> —Article 1 of the US Patient Bill of Rights.

A STEP BACK IN TIME

"They knew how to count time, even within themselves. The moon, the wind, the year, the day, they all move, but also pass on. All blood reaches its place of rest. ..." wrote Chilam Balam of Chumayel, regarding the Mayan civilization of Mesoamerica. In our perusal of history we missed out the civilizations of Mesoamerica and South America—Mayans, Aztecs, Tolmechs, and others—and so almost did Western history. The Yucatan Peninsula was not discovered by the West until Francisco Hernandez da Cordoba in 1517, and even then the culture was largely ignored for study until de Landa, third bishop of the Yucatan, arrived in 1549. Yet these civilizations were some of the most advanced in history. The Mayan civilization, for example, endured from about 1500 BC to about AD 1600, when the Spanish conquistadors brought to its knees by superior weaponry, smallpox and other diseases. Much about the Aztecs and Mayans is known from the records written on stone and wood, and the fact that the Mayans still exist today as forest village cultures, still speaking the old language (though laced with Spanish) and practicing many of the old ways. Similarly midwives in Central America are considered "walking

The Engines of Hippocrates: From the Dawn of Medicine to Medical and Pharmaceutical Informatics, by Barry Robson and O.K. Baek
Copyright © 2009 by John Wiley & Sons, Inc.

encyclopedias" orally preserving the ancient medical knowledge of the Maya passed down from the mother line for many generations. Their knowledge of gynecology, obstetrics, and pediatrics is considered remarkable. In general, such knowledge preserved today includes medical and ritual use of herbs as psycho-active agents. The Balche ceremony is still practiced by the Mayan Lacandon tribe; rites consist of consecrating and offering to the old gods the drink from the Balche tree, fermented with honey. *Sting*, the autobiography of the English pop musician of the same professional name, includes in its opening chapter an excellent account of Sting's participation in a Brazilian old religious ceremony involving a typical presentation of psycho-active brew, although descriptively reported as a brew clearly vastly less flavorsome than the Balche preparation!

As well as an advanced knowledge of basic medical practice and herbs refined over millennia, a core group of these cultures developed a powerful computational system to record and analyze the past and predict propitious times for individuals and nations, fluctuations in public health, agriculture, war, and catastrophe, that last event being, it is said, the Spanish conquest. Whatever its true predictive power was, the system involved computation using symbols on wood and stone and sometimes patterns of knots and beads. Being based on the periodic motions of not only the sun and moon but many stars, it involved combined use of multiple number-base systems, not just our base 10 (or base 2 inside computers). Although operated manually and not comprising electronics or mechanical parts, the system is said to be capable of predicted dates without error up to 90 million years.

These cultures were also knowledgeable on anatomy, a great deal of which came not just from the injuries of war but their apparent preoccupation with sacrifice and torture. It seems that these peoples maintained control by practices of almost unparalleled cruelty. Well that may not be entirely true, but rarely in all history does it seem that it was built so fundamentally into the religious system.

It is tempting to say that these were not *ethical* peoples. That would be unfair: clearly for the most part the Maya believed that sacrifice was essential to the survival of their culture, that it was part of their faith. And in the midst of that, life, love, dedicated parenthood, and friendship went on as usual, as many of their poems testify. However, their official ethical system was not the basis of a system of medical ethics as we have known it from Hippocrates and beyond. They were definitely not a welfare state. The pursuit of perpetuation of life and freedom from pain played little role in that ethics at least for the subservient classes in the eyes of the ruling lords. In the years called *muluc* and in the month called *pax*, the Mayans practiced a warrior dance called the *Holcan okot* or *Batel okot*. In the dance a young man was sacrificed, and the accompanying chant contains the following lines: "Make three fast turns, around the column of painted stone, over there where the virile young man, chaste and immaculate, is bound. Make the first, and on the second turn, lift up your bow, fit the arrow to the string, aim at his breast. It is not necessary to use all your force, when you let fly, so that his flesh will not be too deeply wounded, *so that he may suffer a little, as the Lord God intended"* (Inga Clendinnen, *Ambivalent Conquests: Maya and Spaniard in Yucatan, 1517–1570* (Cambridge University Press, 2003).

Of course civilizations of the West are sullied by cruelty as well. The image invoked by the Maya text inevitably recalls as striking images of the martyr Saint Sebastian, effectively the patron saint of deliverance from the Black Death, shot full of arrows but not directly into the heart. Definitely a representation of the pain element is intended as opposed to a quick death. So oddly enough, this is not entirely a real martyrdom. What Sebastian's hagiography tells us is that he was accused of being a Christian, tied to a tree, shot with arrows, and left to die. But he survived, recovered, and returned to preach, and the emperor then had him beaten to death. During the fourteenth century, when epidemiology was not, to say the least, an exact science, the seemingly random nature of infection with the Black Death caused people to see the plague as if their villages were Saint Sebastian shot by nature's armies of archers. Or at least they prayed for the intercession of an appropriately arrow-associated saint, and so Saint Sebastian became associated with the plague. Likely the Mayan virgin sacrifice of that "virile young man, chaste and immaculate," was similarly a sacrifice in the hope of protection against the "slings and arrows of outrageous fortune" (Shakepeare's *Hamlet*).

In the end, however, substitution of a few sacrificial humans in the spirit of protecting many seems to fall short of the Hippocratic and modern Western ethical ideals. Looking back from the modern comforts of our society we tend to view ancient practices, even in the post-Hippocratic West, as morally tainted and, in the kindest judgment, demonstrating confused views of personal and public healthcare. As it happens, however, this complacency is not justified. In our modern world there has been considerable confusion over respect for the rights of the very few *versus* respect for the rights of the many. When we look for IT to monitor and protect the rights of the patient, we must reflect that we are looking back from a revision of an ethical view that is so recent as to have evolved at the same time as digital computers, even supercomputers. And being so young, it is still so fragile that it needs constant vigilance to maintain it.

MEDICAL ETHICS AND CODE OF CONDUCT BEYOND THE HIPPOCRATIC OATH

In 1993 Eileen Welsome, an investigative reporter from a small local newspaper in New Mexico, published a series of investigations. She claimed that there had been secret experiments conducted by the US government in which unsuspecting hospital patients had been injected with plutonium. Her report spread rapidly to the national press. The accusations extended to claims that there had been experiments involving retarded children, prisoners, and even pregnant women. She was proved right and ultimately won the Pulitzer Prize.

These were very grave accusations against the government and against the American scientific establishment, perhaps as horrific as the (proven) accusations against the Nazis. There were extreme accusations of violations of human rights. President Clinton called for an independent National Commission.

All together the commission collected over 4,000 documents. To its great credit, this process was so thorough it was even responsible for the declassification of literally thousands of documents of the cold war. The commission also interviewed 900 cancer and heart patients about their involvement in this research. The review took 18 months. The final report was 900 pages long and expressed concern that (1) the "human guinea pigs" numbered in tens of thousands, (2) unlike many pharmaceutical trials, the research offered no prospect of medical improvement, (3) the research was also conducted on patients without acknowledgment for consent, and (4) sometimes there was deception about the nature of the research. Horribly, one case study unveiled investigated radiation experiments in which the subjects were children, another radiation experiments in which the subjects were prisoners, and the other four involved cancer patients exposed to total-body radiation. Also investigated were the the "atomic veterans," soldiers who participated in the atomic bomb testing in the 1950s and became radiation victims.

Surprisingly, the commission found that such research was not otherwise unique. Other reprehensible research discovered was that directed to nutrition. Institutionalized, mentally retarded children, abandoned by their parents, were used. They were offered a chance for a trip to the beach and the chance to join in a science club. There was also investigation about something affecting a broader section of the population—the intentional release of radiation into the environment (the purpose was to run tests to try and understand the consequences of what the Russians were believed to be producing). Yet these releases were not only being conducted secretly, they were kept secret for four to five decades.

This whole story is recounted in Ruth R. Haden's "Human Radiation Experiments: Reflection on the Ethics of Biomedical Research" (www. cesil.com/0798/enfade07.htm). She was a leading spokesperson in the commission.

Such recent practice also seems far from what Hippocrates had in mind in advancing medical knowledge. In order to illustrate the value of IT in protecting human rights, it is useful to start with a more detailed review of the twentieth and twenty-first century status of the Hippocratic Oath. Although this Oath governs the practice of physicians, and is less obviously a key matter for medical technology, it was until recently the sole ethical directive.

To be sure, physicians and medical researchers, just like any craftsmen, can make genuine, and sometimes disastrous, mistakes. That doesn't make them evil craftsmen, just inexcusably bad craftsmen. "Of all the clumsy constructions that are part of the florid verbiage used in legal formalities, a candidate for the least felicitous is that painful phrase 'purports and holds himself out to be' when it is used against a craftsman or professional person being sued for an unfortunate outcome of his efforts" (Sherwin B. Nuland, *Biography of Medicine*, page 63). Such "florid verbiage" dominates the nightmares of US physicians today, constantly afraid of being sued. Physicians and medical researchers can, however, make errors of many kinds other than purported incompetence. There have been errors of ethical judgment by groups of medical researchers on massive scales, as in Nazi Germany, and as discussed above. Probably the broadest "catch-all phrase" is to say that most things that we can consider bad medicine are those that would be against the wishes of the patient were he or she aware of the facts available to the physician or researcher and taking into consideration the state of the art (including the wish not to suffer from an avoidable accident!). There are fuzzy boundaries even here: euthanasia, psychological experiments that necessitate deception, psychopathic and masochistic tendencies of patients, and so forth. It is not exhaustive of all possible bioethical issues either: stem cell research does not quite fall into a consideration of this type, for example. But it is not a bad start.

As illustrated by the disturbing incidents mentioned above, a big issue is the *informed consent* by the patient. This now includes consent for use of data (including the digital medical record, which may be the only embodiment of the data) and medical samples, for research purposes. Actually, assuming a basic right to privacy, versions of the Oath do imply the need for soliciting consent because they require the physician to share his experiences, to teach other budding and established physicians, and to enhance the art by adding to the collective pool of medical knowledge. If the entire clinical workflow is well regulated by IT to conform to best practice and patient wishes, it will be extremely difficult for the physician to proceed without compliance, much as IT assists compliance in banking. And while it is difficult to guard against massive stupidity, fatigue, or fraud, it may be that, with the current physician accident rate so high, use of recordings or "black box recorders" may be welcome to help ensure that the primary care, point-of-contact physician does what he promises at the computer. Recording systems linked to IT for such purposes have been developed at many centers including St. Mary's Hospital in London, and are being marketed now at least for surgery. They are actually attractive to many physicians: no physician wants to make mistakes, and in order to reduce spurious unwarranted claims against the physician, they are seen as the lesser of the two "evils." As discussed below, consent can be sufficiently fine grained and complex that detailed coverage has an important place on the digital patient record.

The earliest form of the Hippocratic Oath was not as strong as modern public opinion, on the matter of privacy. Privacy possibly did not matter so much in ancient times when staying alive was the imperative, and everybody in the village knew everyone else's business anyway. When in modern times the issue of privacy does crop up, despite cases of our knowledge of privacy that did thrive in dark deeds behind locked doors, it is in situations where the desire for privacy is, or naturally seems, reasonable. In the United States, it is not hard to accept that the healthcare system with all its glaring errors should at least reside in the hands of the state. Although health insurance companies would love to know our genomics to hedge their bets about our survival chances for risk management of their business, from a statistical viewpoint, they merely want to compute the odds better. But our genetic cards are dealt once, and in a way that is at no personal request of ours. To us, our defects came as un-requested and initially masked data, and on those grounds, so it should be the same for health insurance companies. Further our quality of life, compensation for our loved ones that we leave behind, should not be governed by a healthcare system. And most important, our DNA is our own record no more or no less than any written or digital record. We have rights to keep it confidential, to control its use, and to have access to it when required through the medium of medical science.

In modern times the pressure of the public is such that from the collective view, privacy takes priority over consent. This focus on privacy does not mean that the public does not care if scientific experiments are performed without consent. Rather the view is that no experiments or use of data will be allowed except by occasional one-off agreements on paper. While this "all doors are closed except by special request" is not good for the advancement of science and medicine, to leave science so fallow doesn't help the individual either. So a balance has to be found between individual needs and fears.

For all its faults the Hippocratic Oath is one of the ancient world's most long-lived success stories, standing alongside the religious traditions, great religious texts, and the mathematical and geometry proofs of the Greeks. Yet US medical teaching and managed healthcare issues seem to be at odds with the original Hippocratic Oath. The original Hippocratic Oath calls for free tuition for medical students. In an environment of increasing medical specialization, one single oath for all seems less appropriate. The Oath calls for doctors never to "use the knife" (i.e., conduct surgical procedures), which is obviously out of step with modern surgeons as physicians. Does the ancient Greek flavor of the Oath make it inappropriate to modern physicians? The recent versions of the original Hippocratic Oath, and certainly the practice of medicine, have moved away from the basic tenets of the Oath. For example, according to a survey of 150 US and Canadian medical schools in 1993, only 14% of modern Oaths prohibit euthanasia, 11% hold covenant with a deity, 8% foreswear abortion, and a mere 3% forbid sexual contact with patients. These are all sacred principles of the classical version. And not least, while the classical Oath calls for "the opposite" of pleasure and fame for those who transgress the Oath, fewer than half of Oaths taken today insist the taker be held accountable for keeping the pledge. Further, with governments and healthcare organizations demanding patient information as never before, how can a doctor be responsible for a patient's privacy?

EXTENDING MEDICAL ETHICS AND CODE OF CONDUCT BEYOND THE OATH

Parallel to many technological developments, the twentieth century saw an evolution of medical ethics and medical legislation that went way beyond the content of the Hippocratic Oath. The need for all these considerations was precisely because the Hippocratic Oath provided no guidance to twentieth and early twenty-first century issues, such as the patient's rights, the ethics of experimentation, team care, and a medical researcher's or healthcare practitioner's societal or legal responsibilities.

The matter is one of how these issues are to be handled or monitored in the computer-dominated medicine of the test of the twenty-first century. Paper records locked in a drawer are not safe, and do not ensure that the patient's wishes are respected in remote locations where there is medical need for the patient, that his or her wishes are respected while unconscious, and that the use of his or her data is controlled in medical research in accordance with the patient's wishes. The question is not one of problems *created* by computers, but how, with a potential Tsunami of data of so many patients being processed, *can computers be used* to protect the patient and the public?

The key among almost all patient wishes in modern times, and mentioned many times above, is the wish for *privacy*. This is the assumed wish by default if not otherwise specified, and of no less concern to national security.

In the more recent scene, David Korn, in his presentation "Genetic Privacy and the Use of Archival Patient Materials in Research," ASIP Public Affairs Session at Experimental Biology 1998, put the position as one of genetic technology having "profound effects on individual and societal equanimity."

Indeed typically the strongest of a patient's concerns is vague and ill formed. As also discussed below, if the privacy of health-related information, such as the Protected Health Information (PHI) defined by the Health Insurance Portability and Accountability Act (HIPAA) enacted by the US Congress in 1996, is compromised, we could be talking about a bankruptcy of a financially healthy institution or a prosecution of senior executives of the institution. The biggest challenge with privacy compliance is limiting the use of personal information to the purposes stated at the time of collection.

THE PATIENT'S BILL OF RIGHTS

The Patient's Bill of Rights was promoted by President Clinton in 1997. It is now effectively compulsory reading for all US patients, or at least it is compulsory for the health contact to provide the patient with the relevant text. It is an attempt to ensure that the patient (not in this case a research subject) does not fall through the cracks of the system, and especially that his or her wishes do not. The key rights are the Right to Treatment Information, Right to Privacy and Dignity, Right to Refuse Treatment, the Right to Emergency

Care, and the Right to an Advocate in the case of disputes. We will not explore all these rights in detail, but it is difficult to see how any of them can be implemented properly in a timely manner, without computers to get the data that will provide support for decisions the patient must make. This will sometimes need to be done fast, in an emergency situation.

Examination of present recommendations suggests that IT will not only be consistent with required practices; IT will be required to fully enable each patient's rights. For example, George J Annas's[1] interpretation of a Patient's Bill of Rights, as proclaimed by President Clinton in his last State of the Union Address, comprises the right to all relevant treatment information, including personal risks and any relevant research protocols, the right of the patients to privacy, dignity, and access to their own records, and the right to full information that would enable patients to make decisions in regard to refusal of treatment, demand or decline transfer for treatment to another center, and the right to full access to health plans and insurance, or that of an advocate in case of dispute.

Here's a synopsis. Some sources change the order slightly. A few additions from us, but with *original* source text in quotes:

- "The Right to Treatment Information." The patient has a right to informed participation "in all decisions ... the risks and serious complications ... the diagnosis and prognosis ..." the implications of personal genomic and expression array data, "... the existence of any research protocols which are relevant. ..."
- "The Right to Privacy and Dignity ... and Access." The patient has the right to "all the information in his or her medical record ... ," but data-mined records for research must be anonymous.
- "The Right to Refuse Treatment." The right to "attach and amend a proxy or living will to his or her clinical record" and health care professionals are "obligated to honor these directives."
- "The Right to Emergency Care." The patient has a right to the best emergency care and cannot be transferred "unless it is in the patient's best interests because of superior medical care." The patient must have access to all relevant information and "if the patient does not agree to the transfer, he or she may not be transferred."
- "The Right to an Advocate." No health plan may interfere with or limit communication between the patient and his or her healthcare provider. Health plans must provide "timely access to an independent appeals mechanism," and the patient has a right to access "a copy of the entire contract for his or her insurance or health plan ... to receive an itemized and detailed explanation of all services provided ... a right to timely prior notice of termination of eligibility of coverage or denial of a healthcare benefit with an opportunity to contest the termination or denial in a

[1] See George J. Annas, "A National Bill of Patients' Bill of Rights," pp. 157–165, in *The Nation's Health*, P. R. Lee and C. L. Estes, 6th ed., Sudbury, MA: Jones and Bartlett, 2001.

timely and fair manner before an independent, qualified and neutral decision maker."

The first right makes the IT contribution particularly clear, even though it is not (typically) with regard to an emergency situation. The patient has the right to informed participation in all decisions affecting him or her and to obtain all information about all medical treatments and their alternatives, and the qualitative appraisal of the probabilities of all the risks and benefits, including the success statistics of those medical staff involved in the treatment.

Now let's take what might at first seem the worst-case argument for computers to illustrate the point. The only right that might not, at first, seem to benefit from computer technology is the Right to Privacy and Dignity. How can a computer help there? In fact privacy and computer security issues are so huge that they are protected by US federal laws such as the HIPAA. These topics will be discussed separately below. While computers might present just another risk to privacy, the computer is also an essential tool to protect privacy and dignity. It can sometimes be a tedious, time-consuming, embarrassing, even unnecessarily humbling, ingratiating, and very public matter for a patient in US managed healthcare to make contact with his primary physician (compulsory point-of-contact physician). Yet with IT there doesn't typically have to be physical presence. Cameras, including internal inspection ear-eye cameras, blood pressure devices, and other monitors and probes, could work equally well over the computer line from home. Patients would avoid making the trip to the reception room when they don't need to and when they risk spreading infectious disease. Not least they would avoid dealing with receptionists who typically in loud voice ask "What do you want to see the doctor for then?" and then to your whispered verbal reply, respond with a "How do you spell syphilis?" On the other hand, for progress in medicine to occur patients need to understand that they have an obligation to serve the collective good. Patients should consider giving consent for as much medical detail from their record as they feel comfortable with, although that level of comfort may differ from patient to patient. This information will not be traced to the patient, so the patient should not feel that there is even a remote risk of the medical data being traced back to him or her or the patient ever being identified.

MEDICAL RESEARCH: LEARNING FROM THE MISTAKES OF THE PAST

The modern clinical trial (see section at end of Glossary) is an example of medical research. The two watershed events for the required ethics and structured ethical directives were the Nuremberg Code in response to Nazi experiments and the Helsinki Declaration on Human Rights (1964). These well-publicized events laid out the basic ethical principles for medical researchers to follow. Yet these principles were violated in several other reference cases and these in turn gave rise to the modern US regulations.

A key and oft-quoted unethical study that began before the Nuremberg trials is the Tuskegee Syphilis Study, a research study by the agency that gave rise to the Center for Disease Control. "Unethical" would be to state it mildly. The downright cruelty exercised by the researchers is unbelievable. Before we describe this study, we should try to understand how such errors of judgment are made by intelligent, medically motivated, well-educated people and to understand the pressures, temptations, and misconceptions about "the greater good" and "the end justifies the means" arguments that subsequent legislation sought to correct. To some extent the case was a product of teachings of preceding generations, namely by Jeremy Betham, who preached utilitarianism and neo-utilitarianism to an ethically chaotic world of industrial society. Central to Betham's philosophy was the notion of 'good' as the greatest good for the greatest number of people. While today no one would probably ever dream of yielding to the same pressures and temptations, and mostly due to corrective power of that subsequent legislation, the same issues could pertain in contemporary healthcare. However, with regard to the practice of personalized medicine, the focus is on the individual; any thought of performing horrific experiments on individuals in order to benefit the greater majority of people would be censured by public opinion and the legal courts.

So what was the Tuskegee study about? In 1932 some 250 African-Americans diagnosed with syphilis were enrolled into a long-term study program without being told that they had syphilis. The horror is that they were denied penicillin even when in 1943 it became known, and in 1951 widely accepted, that this was an effective cure. The researchers adopted the greater good argument that the study could not be altered less an opportunity be lost for their research result merely *because* of the recent availability of penicillin. There is a lot of misunderstanding about this study. It is not that the control group was denied treatment. The control group was simply a set of the population that did not have syphilis. The definitive work is said by many to be James H. Jones, *Bad Blood: The Tuskegee Syphilis Experiment* (Free Press; revised ed., 1993). According to the Encyclopedia Britannica (http://www.britannica.com/eb/article?tocId=9002212), "the subjects were not told that they had syphilis or that the disease could be transmitted through sexual intercourse. Instead, they were told that they suffered from 'bad blood,' a local term used to refer to a range of ills. Treatment was initially part of the study, and some patients were administered arsenic, bismuth, and mercury. But after the original study failed to produce any useful data, it was decided to follow the subjects until their deaths, and all treatment was halted. Penicillin was denied to the infected men after that drug became available in the mid-1940s, and it was still being withheld from them 25 years later, in direct violation of government legislation that mandated the treatment of venereal disease. It is estimated that more than 100 of the subjects died of tertiary syphilis."*

---

* Yet "denial" of a new drug is what happens to the control group in a clinical trial. It leads to the idea of *cross over*, in which every patient ultimately takes it.

In 1974, following disclosure by the *Washington Star* in 1972, a class-action suit against the federal government was settled out of court for $10 million, and the US Congress passed the National Research Act (see below). In 1997 President Bill Clinton issued a formal apology for the study. In the public reaction, concerns were in regard to: (a) The fact that the individuals had not been protected from harm, (b) The fact that informed consent had not given, since the subjects were not aware that they had syphilis nor were told the purpose of the study, (c) The study concentrated on a particular ethnic group, and (d) The study concentrated on the poor social class.

Among some other unethical reference cases was the Manhattan Project's plutonium injection experiments running from 1944 to 1974. In this case too the participants were uninformed as to the true nature of the study. More recently a 1999 gene transfer experiment was led by an American university. History does not seem to place this in the same dark class of sins of commission as the Tuskagee incident, but rather to see it more as a serious sin of omission in neglecting aspects of best practice. In September 1999 the clinical experiments in gene transfer research resulted in a tragedy that was a direct consequence of the gene treatment. A 19-year-old male with a metabolic disorder received a high dose of a genetic treatment directly into his liver. He exhibited a systemic inflammatory response to the method used to deliver the new gene, followed by multiorgan failure induced by an adult respiratory distress syndrome, and died. While initial public response to the tragic incident was temperate, as it seemed just a well-intentioned scientific venture with the patient's interests in mind that went wrong, the FDA cited the university investigators in December 1999 following for multiple violations of correct protocol in the trial. Then the NIH revealed that only 6% of all serious adverse events observed in patients during past and current clinical gene transfer studies were reported to the NIH as required. Several federal regulatory agencies, including the FDA and the NIH along with the American Society of Gene Therapy (ASGT), then proceeded to initiate corrective actions. It is unusual for a journal to play a strong direct role in clinical trial regulations, but *Molecular Therapy* has published recommendations regarding protocol and how NIH should fund clinical trials involving gene therapy. Its editor David A. Williams has participated on key committees, notably the ASGT committee appointed by Theodore Friedmann and led by Arthur Nienhuis (see D. A. Williams, Editorial, *Mol. Ther.* 2006; 14: 607).

However, these developments have a broader impact on us. So it is worth going into the processes by which the United States set up a shield, starting in 1974, to protect the individual against such abuses of scientific method. It is not a perfect shield. It is a hard path in medical research to balance the protection of the individual against the benefits of the whole such as may or may not include that individual. The very care, attention, and respect that is given to a clinical trials patient, even down to the genomic level, is the same care, attention, and respect that should be accorded to every patient. The twentieth-century regulations were developed in recognition (1) that even well-intentioned researchers may inadvertently violate ethical norms if they do not identify and examine the ethical assumptions of their actions, and (2) that *in the absence of strong, comprehensive interpretation, guidance, and directive in regard to ethical norms*, researchers can repeat mistakes of the past even those that have been well publicized.

The Belmont Report (1979) contains the ethical principles on which the federal regulations for protection of human subjects are based. The three basic principles are respect for persons, beneficence, and justice. Respect is reflected by the consent process. As a result the term "autonomy" is used in the research and healthcare context. A patient is normally regarded as autonomous if he or she can make his or her own judgments and decisions. In the absence of such ability, for example, as in the case of children, prisoners, and those with mental disorders, the person must be protected. In the Belmont Report and Beneficence, beneficence is the process of minimizing harm (risk) and maximizing possible benefits (usually for the community as a whole). "Justice" is the term used for the criterion that subjects must be fairly drawn from a variety of ethnic, social, and other groups.

THE UBIQUITOUS IRB: A BALANCING ACT WITH BUSINESS, SCIENCE, AND LEGAL IMPLICATIONS

The Belmont Report of 1979 also led to important federal regulations of the Food and Drug Administration (FDA) and the Department of Health and Human Services (DHHS). These 1981 regulations were designed to protect patients in biomedical and behavioral research. Importantly the DHHS introduced the concept of an independent review board, an *Institutional Review Board* (IRB), composed of persons with broad background and reflecting community attitudes to represent reasonable samples of attitudes in regard to "ethical norms." More explicit regulations followed in 1991, whereby seventeen federal agencies agreed to adopt a "Common Rule." The relevant regulations underpinning the Common Rule also looked back to the 1974 National Research Act (emphasizing the need for informed consent). The Common Rule covered:

- the need for informed consent, meaning consent that is informed, understood, and voluntary;
- the need for a first review by an Institutional Review Board (IRB) that seeks to ensure that the *safety* and rights of the subjects are protected; and
- the need for the research institution to file an "Assurance of Compliance," specifically, a federal-wide assurance (FWA) agreeing to abide by federal regulations in the research and to be guided by the Belmont Report.

The FDA stepped in to assist this evolution after the trial monitoring program in 1972 to 1974. The FDA launched its Bioresearch Monitoring Program in

1977, which included inspection of clinical investigators, biopharmaceutical laboratories, toxicology laboratories, and IRBs. The FDA is alerted when a drug (or medical device, or in principle a new food additive, etc.) is involved, and it has set procedures for scheduled or unannounced site visits (effectively, audits) to institutional review boards, clinical investigators, and so on. The FDA can demand correction to anything found deficient: no investigator wants to receive the dreaded form FDA 483!

For example, the FDA must be made aware of tests of new drugs, although getting the required input has been historically bound by the scope of jurisdiction of the FDA. For vigilance in the interest of public health and initially the safety of human experimental subjects in new drug studies, the traditional means by which tests of an investigational new drug (IND) in humans first go on the "radar" of the FDA arises because federal law requires that a drug be the subject of an approved marketing application, before transportation and distribution across state lines. That applies for clinical investigation of new proposed drugs, and unless there is exemption approved by the FDA. The request for exemption constitutes the IND request. Vigilance requires the notion of an *alert*, meaning a red flag that something departs from what we (and specifically here the FDA) would like to be the case. An alert in the most general sense is a departure from an expectation. The first alert to the FDA therefore resides in the concepts that may here call for "expectation of reasonable safety for human administration" (subsequently here called E1) and of departure from that expectation (subsequently here called DE1). The latter DE1 will be inherent in the following submitted "IND data":

1. Animal pharmacology and toxicology studies
2. Previous experience with the drug in humans (often foreign use) if any
3. Manufacturing information
4. Detailed protocols for proposed clinical studies
5. Information on the qualifications of clinical investigators
6. Commitment to obtain informed consent from the research subjects
7. Commitment to obtain review of the study by an institutional review board (IRB)
8. Commitment to adhere to the investigational new drug regulations

Of these, the first item constitutes the most impacting but also the most difficult if we wish to produce comprehensive alert metrics based on DE1. Moreover it is potentially a powerful key to further alerts that may be generated from the ongoing clinical trial process, if it is genuinely believed that the experimental tests on animals are ever to be in any way indicative of safety in humans. Because the genomics and consequent physiology of humans is different from that of animals, the actual performance of the drug in tests on human subjects is subject to what is considered an "expectation of reasonable safety for human administration conditional upon the animal studies and previous data from many other humans" (subsequently here called E2), and departure from that expectation during the clinical trial (subsequently here called DE2).

Drug safety would be hugely empowered by the predictive power of computational chemistry and systems biology. Our level of understanding of the pharmacogenomics and test animals and humans should ideally be included as the state of the art develops, but the solution to the issue resides largely at this time in the analysis of the empirical experimental animal and human data. The IT solution ideally requires (1) data mining of many animal laboratory records not involving the drug and distinguishing healthy and pathological states, (2) data mining of other more classical analyses of the records of the specific test animals comparing those given the drug and controls, (3) data mining of many digital patient records not involving the drug and distinguishing healthy and pathological states, (4) data mining or other more classical analyses of the dynamically updating records of the specific clinical trial subjects comparing those given the drug with those control subjects given the placebo, and (5) inference from all of these to establish a final DE2, or rather a constantly updated one during the course of the clinical trial. Clearly, this inference is complex, but it is tractable by considerations of "best practice" for the process used.

Of course, considerable organization via dialogue between administrators and IT providers would need to be put in place so that the human and animal records have the same data types ("metadata") and format. Moreover, if the fullest informative procedure of the five-step kind described above is to be used, that dialogue must involve many other bodies and source to standardize and provide large bodies of comparative animal and human record data. At present much of the data are available or becoming available or potentially available, but highly dispersed and often in inconsistent metadata and format. So it behooves us to consider getting it and using it.

Getting alerts following the initial approval of an IND request is also a problem for the FDA. It is currently done in the absence of IT by the site visits, announced and unannounced, as audits. There is no way of implementing the "alert issue" of how best to select sites for audits from a large number of trials planned and going on. But note this. IRBs in the United States are governed by Title 45 CFR (Code of Federal Regulations) Part 46. The Research Act of 1974 required IRBs for all research that receives funding, directly or indirectly, from what was the Department of Health, Education, and Welfare at the time, and is now the Department of Health and Human Services (HHS). Typical IRBs are themselves regulated by the Office for Human Research Protections (OHRP) within HHS, not the FDA. The division of labor seems complex. According to the OHRP website: "Some protocols described on clinical trial websites also may be subject to Food and Drug Administration (FDA) regulations. The reader is advised to consult with FDA about its regulatory requirements and guidance in this area." As yet FDA does not require IRB registration, but IRBs that approve studies of FDA-regulated products must be established and operated in compliance with 21 CFR part 56. An "assurance" is a document negotiated between an institution and the Department of Health and Human Services (HHS) in accordance with HHS regulations. Currently FDA regulations do not require an assurance. FDA regulations (21 CFR parts 50 and 56) apply to research involving products regulated by FDA–federal funds and/or support do not need to be involved for the FDA regulations to apply. When research studies involving FDA-regulated products are funded or supported by HHS, the research institution must comply with both the HHS and FDA regulations. There are significant differences in HHS and FDA regulations for the protection of human subjects.

To the uninitiated, an audit may seem complex. An audit of the research subject record is performed by the OHRP's clinical trials auditor (CTA) during the investigator's site research study audit. The purpose is to assess that all required research study documents and protocols are prepared in compliance with federal, state, and local policies. The division of labor now becomes especially tricky to understand, since it appears that both OHRP and the FDA can audit an IRB and a clinical trial site (in theory, the same IRB and same site). Remarkably the OHRP and FDA do not share a common database.

Today, the IRB is rightly a key theme in modern medical research. The primary role of the IRB is to protect the rights and welfare of the research subject. The researcher must adhere to the protocol once deemed final, but the IRB has the authority to approve changes in protocol. However, one may request changes to the protocol that need to be approved by the IRB, such as changes in the consent form. There is allowance for the researcher to depart from protocol. That is, the researcher must take steps to minimize risk to the subject if unexpected severe effects are observed that call for departure from adherence to the protocol. The IRB must, however, be immediately informed.

It must be said that things tend to turn safely out for the best if one takes the highest moral ground in the research subjects' interests and picks away remorselessly at every little thing that seems to have a even a remote chance of being contrary to the expected results. That is, one must act to protect the subject from harm as there is significant room for deep introspection in ethical philosophy and individual judgment. Say a patient's quality of life depends only on a new experimental drug. While the best efforts should be made to predict life expectancy with and without the drug, only the patient can speak for the quality of time in both scenarios, provided that all other factors are equal and all efforts are made to supply the patient with all information.

MISCONDUCT AND CONSEQUENCES

There are many ways in which scientific misconduct can occur. An example that often gets publicized by the press is *scientific* misconduct pertaining to the falsification of results, namely publication of fictitious or altered results claimed to be true. With IT digital records of research, electronically signed and dated by medical researchers and their managers would prevent falsification. IT could also protect the public from "honest error" and "differences in interpretation of data," besides from fabrication, falsification, plagiarism, and departures from other community-accepted practices for proposing, conducting, and reporting research. Funding politics etc. (such as involving funding from biased industrial sources) and delay of publication are not normally considered scientific misconduct but could fall under this rubric. Likewise publication of negative results, in which a hypothesis is not confirmed, is not as common as publication of positive results, but should be encouraged where appropriate.

A lot of responsibility resides not with the researcher but with the researcher's institution. The medical research institutions have to accept responsibility to comply with the DHSS and the FDA (as registering with these agencies is not manditory) and impose safeguards for human subjects (even on research at remote sites). Medical research institutions must provide training to educate researchers in ethics, must investigate scientific misconduct, and enforce a policy on conflict of interest reporting to the Office of Research Integrity (ORI) when there arises need for *in-depth* investigation of an alleged scientific misconduct (but not necessarily every allegation). Research institutions share with their researchers and sponsors (funding agencies) the responsibility to ensure that study subjects are adequately protected and that their institutional review boards (IRB) are in compliance with federal regulations.

Reviews of conflicts of interest must include the investigators' institutions, the IRB, journals, and the FDA. It is important to keep the patient informed of potential conflicts of interest via disclosure on the consent form. Already public concern is bringing about such change of rules, as concerns public safety and the biasing of generated "knowledge."

COMPLEXITIES OF INFORMED CONSENT
FOR COMPLIANCE TO PRIVACY LAWS

The Hippocratic Oath hints at the responsibility of the physician to solicit consent (so that the state of medical art can be advanced). Still physicians and medical researchers should not unfairly focus only on less fortunate economically disadvantaged or impressionable types of patient who would readily consent. Advertisements to recruit subjects for medical research involve consent, and should be reviewed by the IRB. Representative populations drawn from different majority and minority sexes, age groups, and ethnic groups are generally required to meet FDA-regulated studies and are required when funding is obtained from NIH (National Institutes of Health) in the United States. Barriers to minority participation could be reduced by providing study materials in different languages and by including minorities on the research staff, by being flexible in location and business hours, and by providing transport. Community-based qualitative research (CBQR) studies communities as a whole. The assumption is that the community is an authority on its circumstances, strengths, needs, and potential solutions. Also the community may be assumed not to have the cultural biases of an outside research team risk that could skewing the research and its interpretation.

Other issues relate to how consent is obtained. Stigmatizing topics may mean that a patient is cautious about having any link to his or her name that is included on the consent form. Thus only verbal consent may be given. Such fear should decline with a reliable IT proven to guard privacy well. Informed consent in any human research undertaking should be based on information, comprehension, and voluntary agreement, as specified by the Belmont Report. Also, in considering the consent process, the researcher should know not only all the usual "what" elements of consent, but also when, where, how, and by whom the consent process is conducted in consideration of the subject's well-being and provision of the best opportunity for a correct decision by the subject. Factors to avoid in obtaining informed consent are "undue influences," meaning coercion or dependency on the investigator's judgment, as well as any undue influences due to the circumstances and setting, which may be harder to control.

There is a physical kind of record that is as important as the digital record. When materials, tissue samples, DNA, or protein sequences are collected from a subject, the consent process should include what will be collected and how they will be collected, the type of research (including genetic), potential risks of disclosure of the information inherent in the tissue (e.g., to health insurance companies), potential benefits for the subject, confidentiality procedures, the extent of anonymization of the data, whether the sample will be destroyed on request, how long the sample will be kept, and whether there are commercial applications of the research. Keeping track of samples and linking the records to corresponding samples may also be an issue. For example, the Veteran's Hospital in the Bronx, New York, keeps a large bank of brain tissue samples for national research and a digital record system to monitor distribution and ensure that the experimental data relate to the correct patient history.

A MEDICAL RESEARCHER'S HIPPOCRATIC OATH

In consequence of the preceding discussion, we can construct a medical researcher's counterpart of the Hippocratic Oath:

> I must place human rights and welfare above scientific knowledge. I recognize that the greatest concern in regard to human rights and welfare is usually in regard to risk of physical harm.
>
> In behavioral studies, risk of harms must be minimized, namely psychological, social, economic, and legal harms to the subject. However, I recognize that there is also the risk of "wrongs." I recognize that an individual can be wronged even if

not harmed. This is held in regard particularly to privacy (the right of an individual not to disclose) and confidentiality (the obligation of the researcher to keep disclosed information private). Intrusions on privacy are not justified even if confidentiality is maintained.

I will ensure that Certificates of Confidentiality are requested from the [in the United States] National Institutes of Health to protect myself and my institution from being compelled to disclose confidential subject data, at the federal, state, or local level, to a court of law.

When my research is sponsored by a company or agency, a contract will be negotiated, and the contract must be signed by an authorized representative of the institution. Such a contract should include such matters as to protect my right to publish the results of the research (providing it respects confidentiality of the subject), but with the right to publish not being axiomatic.

GENETIC WATCHDOGS

At the time of writing no comprehensive regulations exist that address all issues of genetic research. The need has created a thriving academic "industry." Bodies such as http://www.onlineethics.org/CMS/research/modindex/genres. aspx, and Case Western Reserve University Center for Genetic Research Ethics and Law continue to canvas for well-founded legislation. There is however much progress regarding genetic diagnostics. Senator Edward Kennedy (D-MA) proposed a piece of legislation before the US Senate on March 1, 2007 called the "Laboratory Test Improvement Act." The Act is proposed as a series of amendments to the Federal Food, Drug and Cosmetic Act (FFDCA). "The legislation will mandate that all providers of 'homebrew' laboratory tests provide the FDA with evidence that verifies their analytical and clinical validity. All of the information submitted to the FDA will be compiled into a database, which will subsequently be made available to the public on the Internet. Presently, an overwhelming majority of the laboratory tests employed by health care facilities are homebrew tests that have not been approved by the FDA. In some instances, homebrew tests are used to diagnose Huntington's disease and susceptibility to breast cancer. As such, the results of homebrew tests affect the lives of thousands of Americans and their families each and every year" (http://kennedy.senate.gov/newsroom/press_release. cfm). Recent legislations such as HIPAA are primarily concerned with privacy and protection against discrimination, but the main reason for the lack of comprehensive legislature is that our knowledge about the implications of specific genetic features such as mutations is constantly evolving. Still gene transfer studies must conform to FDA regulations. In addition the Institutional Biosafety Committee (IBC) was founded to protect the public from any effects arising from gene transfer studies. The IBC must be informed of genetic studies along with the IRB, and both institutions must be consulted for a review of the research plan prior to any clinical trials or treatment. In principle, private institutions not receiving NIH funding for recombinant DNA research do not need to follow NIH guidelines (although they may in the opinion of the NIH not be eligible for future NIH support). A further safeguard, known as "Appendix M," is only an obligatory safeguard mandatory for research funded directly or indirectly by NIH. Because the IBC is responsible for ensuring that recombinant research is conducted according to NIH guidelines, it can nevertheless withhold approval. Modifying germ line cells (the DNA of which can be passed on to offspring children) is not expressly forbidden, but there are technical and ethical issues. All these issues are, however, in state of flux and could be changed even by the time of publication. If naught else, it is remarkable how recently legislation on such matters has evolved.

WHAT PRIVACY MEANS IN A NUTSHELL

The IT industry has been preoccupied with security and privacy in healthcare, as it should be. Although the appearance HIPAA regulations gave some disorientation among the grassroots programmers and IT researchers, it was still seen as an opportunity for an industry that had already gained considerable experience, and honed several IT tools regarding security and privacy in supplying IT to the banks and Internet businesses. The meaning of *security* is relatively well understood, but the meaning of *privacy* is not really well comprehended by the general public (and even sometimes the self-claimed security experts). It is critical to distinguish *privacy* that is concerned with personal control of the collection, use, and disclosure of personal information from *security* that is concerned with control of access to assets (information and resources) that are used in a healthcare or business context.

Security is an important part of *privacy* as security is an essential building block for implementation of privacy. If *privacy* of health-related information, such as the protected health information (PHI) defined by HIPAA in the United States, is compromised, we could be talking about bankruptcy of an otherwise healthy organization and criminal prosecution of directors of the organization. One of the biggest challenges with *privacy compliance* is limiting the use of personal information to the purposes stated at the time of collection.

Concerns for medical data hold also for personal data of all kinds, and in many countries medical data are treated within the same set of laws as other personal and business data. In many businesses, data collection, such as the names and addresses, is simply a part of doing business. Other information, such as demographic or personal financial data, is frequently collected to find out as much as possible about consumers and retailers.

Sadly, the potential for exposure of private information to unauthorized persons has increased remarkably. There are huge temptations to use data for other purposes, and for it to be sold to others against the interests of the persons to whom the data relates. At the very least there is the resulting inconvenience of spam (of e-mail, telephone, fax, or letter-box "junk mail"). Also, without any policing or identifiable author held responsible, data can be out of date or erroneous (e.g., erroneous business telephone numbers that might now be those of private residents). At worst, there are issues of identity theft, defamation of character, use of medical or financial data to make decisions about a potential or existing employee, or subscriber to a health insurance scheme, or even blackmail. Good security, meaning primarily protection of privacy, can have indirect as well as direct benefits. Defamatory or alienating medical statements about a person published on the Internet are much less likely to be believed if it was believed that security is good, and that the information is thus unlikely to be genuine.

"Codes of conduct" are the subject of intense negotiation among businesses, consumer groups, and governments. These codes on data collection are compromises between the need to protect the individual privacy and the desire of organizations to collect personal data for marketing and other commercial purposes, including pharmaceutical research and development. The emerging privacy laws require that researchers conduct a data-collection audit. The emerging laws will force researchers to obtain consent before collecting, using, and/or disclosing such personal data.

The US Federal Trade Commission presented a report to Congress in May 2000 on "Privacy Online: Fair Information Practices in the Electronic Marketplace." It is worth mentioning because of the useful way it breaks down components of the overall challenge. The report states that consumer-oriented businesses would be required to comply with four basic information practices, that is *Notice, Choice, Access, and Security*.

- *Notice* requires a disclosure of what information they collect, how they collect it, and how they use it.
- *Choice* requires consumers' ability to choose how information will be used beyond the purpose for which it was collected.
- *Access* requires that consumers have reasonable access to the information collected, including the opportunity to review, correct, or delete that information. This means that each organizational entity needs to allow its clients to access the client registry for viewing, updating, and deleting personal information, in other words, the bank you are dealing with is obligated to provide you with access to its customer information file (CIF, as most of banks call it) so that you may be able to ensure the information the bank has collected about you is accurate and current. Does your bank do this? Another example may be that the IRS (Internal Revenue Service, the US tax agency) needs to provide you with access to their database so that you may ensure the information about you in the IRS database is accurate and current.
- *Security* requires performing reasonable steps to safeguard the information they collect.

It is critical for an institution to conform to the statutory requirements associated with protection of privacy, especially for the profiling data, which may deal with personal information. It is worth repeating that *compromised privacy* can jeopardize the very survival of an organization while *compromised security* can cause financial damage for an individual whose information is stored, and the organization.

THE SECURITY MODEL HAS BEEN CHANGED
TO PROTECT FROM INSIDERS

The traditional IT security model has been focused on physically securing computers and preventing outsiders from accessing application software and the data stored in the computers. The premises behind the traditional IT security model are that selected people within an organization can be fully trusted, that security threats are outside the organization, and that masquerading computer systems is practically impossible and financially unjustified. However, traditional assumptions are no longer valid due to technological advancement, such as powerful portable computers and high-speed global computer networks. In addition, in any office or organization, a significant security threat has so far been from the traditionally trusted people inside the firewall such as the people working in the CIO's office. As a result the traditional security model cannot ensure confidentiality, personal privacy, nor conform to the statutory requirements, especially when transactional services are offered through a public infrastructure such as the Internet.

There are three aspects of security: physical security (e.g., locks for buildings, badge access to secure rooms), logical security (e.g., passwords for computers or networks, smart cards), and operational policies and procedures (e.g., oath of office, management approval). Adequately protecting assets and assuring personal privacy requires attention.

The technology protection is just one aspect of security. Logical security plays a major role in ensuring that proper access and security policies are enforced. At the same time physical security is as important as (if not more important than) logical security for protection of the tangible assets. For example, invaluable samples and expensive instruments such as mass spectrometers in the proteomics research laboratory of a biotechnology company or diagnostic modalities such as MRI (magnetic resonance imaging) or PET (positron emission tomography) scanners in the diagnostic laboratories can be protected through adequate physical security.

Logical security must provision authentication, authorization, confidentiality, and integrity, protection of privacy, nonrepudiation, and availability. Logical IT security services are briefly described below:

- *Authentication* provides an assurance of an identity of an entity (a person, an application or a system) based on what they know (e.g., user identification and associated password), what they have (e.g., access card, badge), or what they are (biometric—finger prints, iris patterns, retina patterns, facial geometry, voice patterns).

- *Authorization* ensures that only the authorized entity accesses information or services, by granting access rights to the authorized entities. Authorization depends on the successful authentication of an entity (e.g., individual, business entity) and applies to granting access privileges.
- *Confidentiality* services prevent unauthorized disclosure.
- *Privacy* prevents disclosure of personal information without consent from the individual.
- *Integrity* prevents unauthorized alteration of information.
- *Nonrepudiation* prevents individuals or business entities from denying their involvement in a transaction.
- *Availability* protects systems from denial-of-service attacks.
- *Audit trail* keeps a chronological record of system activities for the provision of nonrepudiation.

One aspect of security alone does not assure the needed protection. All three aspects of security—physical, logical, and operational security provisions—must be enforced.

PRIVACY AND SECURITY OF THE PATIENT RECORD

Obviously all the sensitive data stored in archives or exchanged over the untrusted public network such as the Internet should be secured against willful or accidental access or tampering, by unauthorized or unidentified parties, through generally available encryption standards. Sensitive and private information should be further encrypted for transmission or for storage in order to provide additional protection. The authorization for access to sensitive services or information needs to be controlled based on the identity of the accessing entity (person, business entity, computer system), the role of the entity at the time of access, the purpose of access, the location where the access is initiated from, and the access channel (e.g., you may want to allow less privileges for the person accessing sensitive information through insecure wireless communication channel than the person accessing the information through a secure private land line). In addition provision of nonrepudiation based on digital signature (or other alternatives) and transaction logs are required for security audit. The PKI standard (public key infrastructure referring to the distributed security based on asymmetric cryptography) can be used for implementation of digital signatures. PKI (public key infrastructure) is an industry standard based on the ISO standard certificate (X.509) and used by large organizations and governments. The conceptual schematic of PKI security infrastructure is depicted in Figure 6.1. Protection of privacy should

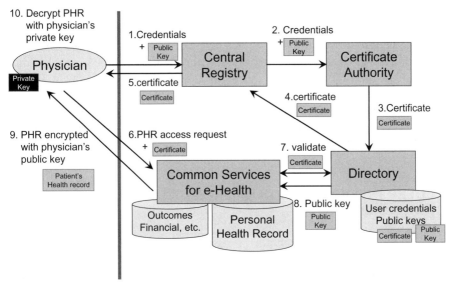

Figure 6.1 Health informatics security infrastructure based on public key infrastructure

be ensured through systematic acquisition of an informed consent from the owner of the personal information before the system grants an access to an individual, or other systems. Two-way authentication is essential for a health-care system, since the accountability lies with an individual, meaning the individual service providers, rather than the organization. This is despite the fact that the legal liability is quite often assumed by an organization, for example, a hospital assuming a legal liability for a physician affiliated with the hospital.

Security services will be provided for applications to apply appropriate business rules for access control of records based on the identity, roles, and purposes (i.e., business functions), in addition to distributed security services for authentication, authorization, confidentiality, integrity and nonrepudiation, to protect the best interests of stakeholders. Later in this book we will discuss the notion of a *stakeholder* in healthcare. It suffices here to say that these are the people legitimately involved in healthcare such as the patient, physician, and emergency medical staff. In some definitions stakeholders are the only people who can access the patient record. There are usually a special provisionings for the emergency care staff to access the patient data without an explicit informed consent in the event that the patient is unconscious.

There are three key requirements for the security services of the new healthcare system in terms of these stakeholders: (1) protection of privacy for individual stakeholders to manage their consent, under their direct control, for other stakeholders' access to their personal information; (2) security that includes identification, authentication, authorization, data confidentiality, data integrity, and nonrepudiation; and (3) auditability. Protection of privacy is assured by the fact that the physician as a service provider has acquired an informed consent from the patient as a service recipient of the personal information. This assurance will be provided through the privacy profiles that contain the proof of acquired informed consent and are managed by the healthcare system. For example, the privacy profile for a physician as a service provider, which will be located based on the physician's personal identifier, contains the list of identifiers of patients whom the physician has acquired informed consent from.

PROPER INTERPRETATION OF PRIVACY LEGISLATION REDUCES RISKS

Several governments throughout the world and various industries are trying to address the issue of privacy through legislation, regulations, and standards. Among others, Australia, Belgium, Canada, France, Germany, Japan, New Zealand, South Africa, Sweden, United Kingdom, and The Netherlands are leading the way to legislate privacy laws, and the federal government agencies are taking responsibilities for governance of compliance to protection of privacy. The statutory requirements for protection of privacy vary country by country. However, there are a common set of themes and principles, which are briefly summarized below:

- Organizational entities are required to obtain an individual's informed consent before collecting or disclosing personal information in any medium.
- Individuals have legally guaranteed access to the personal information collected about them.
- Organizational entities are prohibited from using personal information for any purposes other than for which it was originally collected.

In general, personal data are prohibited from being shared without consent, and typically collection of personal data must be legitimately explained as to its scope and purposes. Here is an example list of well-known and oft-cited privacy laws around the world:

- Health Insurance Portability and Accountability Act (HIPAA), USA
- Directive on the Protection of Individuals with Regard to the Processing of Personal Data and on the Free Movement of Such Data, also known in short form as the EU Privacy Directive, The European Union
- Personal Information Protection and Electronic Documents Act (PIPEDA) and Freedom of Information and Protection of Privacy Act (FIPPA), Canada

The regulations of the US federal privacy law, HIPAA (Health Insurance Portability and Accountability Act) are complex. They comprise hundreds of pages and are very detailed and specific, with close to "zero tolerance" for failure to comply (but not as precise as several other counties; see below). For example, if a researcher's computer is stolen and the patient records on it subsequently appear on the Internet, the researcher may be equally liable. Compliance to the privacy laws means a legal assurance for *protection of personal privacy*, in addition to the traditional security requirements such as authentication, authorization, confidentiality, data privacy, "non-repudiation," and "auditability." HIPAA prohibits anyone from collecting or disclosing an individual's personal information without explicitly stating the purpose(s) of collecting or disclosing the individual's personal information and acquiring an explicit informed consent from the individual.

When first announced, the HIPAA regulations threw some medical researchers and a few designers of medical information systems into a panic mode because of the room for multiple interpretations due to the ambiguity and the absence of best practices. Canadian and European regulations are much more specific and rigid, and they tend to be clearer as to interpretation that suggests "best practices." These privacy laws also cover all the industries, not just healthcare industry.

The statutory requirements for protection of privacy in Canada are governed by two federal laws, among others: FIPPA (Freedom of Information and Protection of Privacy Act), which is targeted for public organizational entities, and PIPEDA (Personal Information Protection and Electronic Document Act), which is targeted for private organizational entities. These two laws confer extensive rights on individuals to control the collection, use, and disclosure of their personal information by any organizational entities. An individual has the right to demand a read/write access to his/her personal information that is collected and administered by an organization, to ensure that it is accurate and current. For example, consumers have the right to audit a financial institution's customer information.

FIPPA and PIPEDA mandate a very rigid fine-grain access control based on the principal's role, the purpose(s) of access to personal information, and the (logical) locations where the access occurs. For instance, access privileges for a physician helping an unconscious patient at an ER (emergency room) are different from the privileges when the physician sees the patient at an office visit. Fine-grain authorization needs to be provided at the record level and at the instance level. An example of an authorization at the *record level* is to prevent a physician from accessing other diagnostic/treatment information that is not required to treat an illness. An example of an authorization at the *instance level* is to prevent a physician from accessing the "whole history" of diagnostics/treatments that are not necessary to treat an illness. For example, to treat a broken leg, the physician may not need to access the patient's genetic information or the patient's 10-year history of medical events.

Canada's FIPPA also permits "sealed records" (i.e., the existence of the record is hidden) and "locked records" (i.e., a special permission is required to reveal the contents but the existence of the record is generally known). PIPEDA requires business entities to offer individuals certain guarantees regarding the collection and use of personal data. For example, an individual's consent must be obtained before data can be shared with affiliates or commercial partners, and also for access to that data for review. The bill, introduced in October 1998, in response to growing public concerns about personal privacy, establishes a series of protections, with the core being the Canadian Standards Association Model Code for the Protection of Personal Information.

In order to comply with the privacy laws, organizations are required, by federal law, to develop an institutional privacy policy. The central obligation under the legislation is that data collectors provide transparent privacy policies so that individuals are accurately informed about (1) what kind of data are collected, (2) who is collecting their data, (3) why the data are collected, (4) how the data will be used, (5) who will be using the data, and (6) what purposes the data will be used for. As such, each organization needs to define a security policy and procedure to accurately inform individuals on the data being collected and for what purpose. The data profiling system must comply with the statutory requirements by providing mechanisms for:

- obtaining an individual's informed consent before collecting or disclosing personal information, and
- allowing individual access to information collected about them.

In addition the policies and procedures should be in place to prohibit employees from using personal information for any purposes other than that for which it was originally collected.

In the European Union data protection is governed by a Data Privacy Directive is officially called Directive on the Protection of Individuals with Regard to the Processing of Personal Data and on the Free Movement of Such Data (or DPIRPPDFMSD for short). This EU Data Privacy Directive was adopted by the European Parliament and the Council of the European Union on October 24, 1995, after five years of deliberation, and it is also very rigid. Its design principle is based on the premise that "data protection must be considered a fundamental human right." There are a few articles published on the EU Data Privacy Directive, and among them is a comprehensive article written by William W Lowrance, "The European Parliament and the Council of the European Union, Directive on the Protection of Individuals with Regard to the Processing of Personal Data and on the Free Movement of Such Data" available at http://aspe.hhs.gov/datacncl/PHR.htm. The following summary is a quote from his article:

1. "Personal data" shall mean any information relating to an identified or identifiable natural person ("data subject"); an identifiable person is one

who can be identified, directly or indirectly, in particular by reference to an identification number or to one or more factors specific to his physical, physiological, mental, economic, cultural, or social identity.

2. "Processing of personal data" ("processing") shall mean any operation or set of operations which is performed upon personal data, whether or not by automatic means, such as collection, recording, organization, storage, adaptation or alteration, retrieval, consultation, use, disclosure by transmission, dissemination or otherwise making available, alignment or combination, blocking, erasure, or destruction.

The EU Data Privacy Directive also has great breadth and intimately entwines matters of privacy and consent and stipulates that *Member States shall provide that personal data may be processed only if*:

1. the data subject has unambiguously given his consent;
2. processing is necessary for the performance of a contract to which the data subject is party or in order to take steps at the request of the data subject prior to entering into a contract;
3. processing is necessary for compliance with a legal obligation to which the controller is subject;
4. processing is necessary for protecting the vital interests of the data subject;
5. processing is necessary for the performance of a task carried out in the public interest or in the exercise of official authority vested in the controller or in a third party to whom the data are disclosed; or
6. [Some other circumstances apply].

In this Directive, the data "controller" is "the natural or legal person, public authority, agency, or any other body that alone or jointly with others determines the purposes and means of the processing of personal data." As for consent, the Directive defines it broadly but firmly: "The data subject's consent" shall mean any freely given specific and informed indication of his wishes by which the data subject signifies his agreement to personal data relating to him being processed." Notice that the consent is to be "specific and informed." If applied literally, for some secondary research this would require solicitation of more focused consent than is now commonly sought.

PERSONAL HEALTH INFORMATION (PHI) TO BE PROTECTED

For research purposes there is no reason why the identity of a patient needs to be known (see previous chapter). However, it should be born in mind that if the researcher finds something of critical importance to the well-being of a patient, it would be useful to have some way of feeding the data back to the patient or the patient's physician. Removal of the key information that can be used to identify an individual constitutes "anonymization." If identity could be replaced by some key (e.g., an irreversible encryption that generates a garbled string of symbols but is still unique to the patient) that allows the patient to be traced, it is "reversible anonymization." As you may imagine, the latter is controversial, but the potential benefits to the patient as medical science accelerates, as noted above, may make that worth considering. Hence this could be considered a matter of consent. A patient could, reasonably enough, then allow their identifying information to be used and disclosed for research with their written permission in the form of an authorization. Similar considerations may allow two sets of medical data that are anonymous to be combined, and yet preserve identities of the two different patients. These and related aspects are discussed in the following sections.

In any event, the problem of encoding key identification remains the same, whatever we do with them. The US statutory law for protection of personal privacy, namely HIPAA defines 17 specific personal information items as *protected health information* (PHI). "Protected," by the federal law, has a catch-all "other" categories of information as protected health information (PHI 18) to prevent an individual from being re-identified based on "other" nonpersonal information that can be used as a link to a particular person. The 17 PHI must be de-identified to comply with the federal law, which came into effect on April 1, 2003. HIPAA, in general, was not enforced until April 15, 2005, and calls for compliance by all healthcare organizational entities in the United States.

Compliance with HIPAA is challenging on two counts. First, the rules are too broad and open-ended, and there are no best practice guidelines. For example, as noted above, the eighteenth PHI (protect health information) is referred to as "other" information that can be used to identify a specific individual. To make things even worse, there is no general consensus on the interpretation of the law in the legal community, and no standard measures exist in the healthcare industry. Each IRB makes its own business decisions, and sometimes not necessarily legally correct decisions. Second, there is the challenging issue of whether medical information such as genomic and proteomic information, or a detailed medical image of brain-wave readouts, might inevitably nail down a person given other data, or a sample from, or test on that person. Good information security is required so that this cannot happen. On the other hand, the issue of keeping one's DNA sequences, on the computer, is not really the problem. In the future it will be easier than penetrating security to, for example, obtain a sample of DNA from a person, say from a drop of blood from a smear on his or her desk, and use bioinformatics to nail down the patient's genetic risks. Legislation is required to address this conundrum too. But it can still arise even if DNA and proteomics are never added to the patient record.

With an attempt to address at least the former problem, URAC (Utilization Review Accreditation Commission, a nonprofit accreditation agency for the US healthcare industry charged with a mission "to promote continuous improvement in the quality and efficiency of healthcare delivery by achieving a common understanding of excellence among purchasers, providers, and patients through the establishment of standards, programs of education and communication, and a process of accreditation") and the NIST (National Institute of Standards and Technology) along with the Workgroup for Electronic Data Interchange are developing guidelines for HIPAA compliance based on best practices, case studies, and other standard efforts by various organizations like the Healthcare Information and Management Systems Society. Institutions are expected to adopt such guidelines for HIPAA compliance for their IRB policy. (As noted earlier, privacy laws in Europe and Canada are similar to HIPAA but they cover cross-industries and are more rigid.)

The HIPAA rules require someone to de-identify data by removing all 18 elements that could be used to identify the individual or the individual's relatives, employers, or household members. The authorized person also must ensure that the remaining information could not be used alone or in combination with other information to identify the individual who is the subject of the information. They may also use statistical methods to establish de-identification instead of removing all 18 identifiers. The authorized person may obtain certification by "a person with appropriate knowledge of and experience with generally accepted statistical and scientific principles and methods for rendering information not individually identifiable" so that there is a "very small" risk that the information could be used by the recipient to identify the subject of the information, alone or in combination with other reasonably available information.

General rules for anonymization of the Protected Health Information defined by HIPAA are described below to give you a sense of the 18 PHI elements and how they can be anonymized for de-identification process. The term *de-identification* is a legal term to indicate that provisions have been made to prevent someone from being identified. Therefore any information directly attributed to a specific individual needs to be removed or obfuscated, as well as any other information that can be used to identify the individual, even if the information is *not* a personal information (this is precisely what the PHI element 18, "other," is all about):

1. Names should be removed or replaced with an alias.
2. Addresses of all geographic subdivisions smaller than a state, including street address, city, county, precinct, zip code, and their equivalent geographical codes should be removed. The safe harbor provision does not allow the institution to keep city/town, especially for towns with small and maybe skewed populations. If the institution is outside the safe harbor provision, a statistical expert may declare the risk of re-identification through linkages with external data (e.g., town records). For example, if there are only 3 people in the town born in the year 1900 and one of those 3 has a medical record then there is a significant

risk of identification. An exception for the initial three digits of a zip code applies if, according to the current publicly available data from the Bureau of the Census:

    a. the geographic unit formed by combining all zip codes with the same three initial digits contains more than 20,000 people; and

    b. the initial three digits of a zip code for all such geographic units containing 20,000 or fewer people are changed to 000.

3. All elements of dates (except year) directly related to an individual, including birth date, admission date, discharge date, and date of death should be removed. In addition all ages over 89 and all elements of dates (including year) indicative of such age should be removed, except that such ages and elements may be aggregated into a single category of age 89 or older. Year and month can be added through an IRB approval and also based on assessment of re-identification risk.

4. Certificate/license numbers should be removed.

5. Diagnostic device ID and serial numbers should be removed.

6. Biometric identifiers (e.g., voice, finger print, iris, retina) should be removed.

7. Full face photo or comparable image should be removed.

8. SSN should be removed.

9. Telephone numbers should be removed. Area code and prefix can be kept only if geographical information is missing and also based on assessment of re-identification risk.

10. Fax numbers should be removed.

11. Electronic mail addresses should be removed.

12. URLs should be removed.

13. IP addresses should be removed.

14. Medical record numbers should be removed.

15. Health plan numbers should be removed.

16. Account numbers should be removed.

17. Vehicle ID, serial number, and license plate number should be removed.

18. "Other" information that can be used for re-identification of a particular individual also should be removed.

The HIPAA rules require a data use agreement to contain the following provisions:

- Specific permitted uses and disclosures of the limited data set by the recipient consistent with the purpose for which it was disclosed (a data use agreement cannot authorize the recipient to use or further disclose the information in a way that, if done by the covered entity, would violate the privacy rule).

- Identify who is permitted to use or receive the limited data set.

- Stipulations that the recipient will:
  - not use or disclose the information other than permitted by the agreement or otherwise required by law;
  - use appropriate safeguards to prevent the use or disclosure of the information, except as provided for in the agreement, and require the recipient to report to the covered entity any uses or disclosures in violation of the agreement of which the recipient becomes aware;
  - hold any agent of the recipient (including subcontractors) to the standards, restrictions, and conditions stated in the data use agreement with respect to the information; and
  - not identify the information or contact the individuals.

THE NOTION OF THE COVERED ENTITY, LIMITED DATA SET, AND DATA USE AGREEMENT

Surprisingly, HIPAA rule permits a "covered entity" (a person) to have access to health information for research purposes, without obtaining an authorization or documentation of a waiver or an alteration of authorization, to use and disclose PHI included in a limited data set. A covered entity may use and disclose a limited data set for research activities conducted by the covered entity itself, another covered entity, or a researcher who is not a covered entity if the disclosing covered entity and the limited data set recipient enter into a data use agreement. Limited data sets may be used or disclosed only for purposes of research, public health, or healthcare operations. Should the patient find this objectionable, it may be possible to formulate reform such that a patient still contribute anonymized records to an archive of Anonymous Record Contributions (see Chapter 5):

- A *Data Use Agreement* refers to an agreement into which the covered entity enters with the intended recipient of a limited data set that establishes the ways in which the information in the limited data set may be used, and how it will be protected.
- A *limited data set* is described as health information that excludes certain, listed direct identifiers as shown below but that may include city, state, zip code, elements of date, and other numbers, characteristics, or codes not listed as direct identifiers. The direct identifiers listed in the privacy rule's limited data set provisions apply both to information about the individual and to information about the individual's relatives, employers, or household members.

THE RISK OF RE-IDENTIFICATION TO BE MITIGATED

In addition to 17 fairly obvious items, HIPAA also defines the eighteenth PHI element, called "other," as designed to prevent a potential re-identification when other non-PHI is so unique or rare that a particular individual can be identified using one or more non-PHI. "Other" information may need to be removed based on assessment of re-identification risk. Examples of potential re-identification of a specific individual based on non-PHI include (1) a patient suffering from a serious leopard bite acquired at a DeMoins Zoo fire incident, (2) one's disorder traced back to grandfather named Thomas Zeus Jones, and (3) a descriptive free text "Her Majesty felt unwell" that appears in a patient record, referral letter, and so forth. It can't be too hard to track down the particular individual in this case even if all of the PHI elements have been removed.

HOW TO LINK DE-IDENTIFIED HEALTH RECORDS FROM MULTIPLE INSTITUTIONS?

Removing identifying data, or avoiding use of a universal identifier, has its price: how can we link the health records gathered from various sources to an individual when the all personal information from the health records has been removed? Not only that we need a method ensuring that two records belonging to different individuals are not linked to one individual. This is because it can be more harmful to link two records that belonged to different individuals than to miss linking two records that belonged to the same individual, since tolerating any false links will lead to an incorrect result of association/correlation studies. Hospitals and diagnostic laboratories collect full name, date of birth, address, phone number, gender, and health insurance information as a minimum. An alphanumeric person identifier that uniquely identifies an individual can be generated with reference to full name, date of birth, gender, and postal code in addition to other personal data attributes such as social security number (with legal clearance), residential address, previous last name (maiden name), driver's license number, hospital identifier, patient identifier, health insurer name, and health insurance number and residential phone number, to be used to link health records retrieved from multiple institutions. We call the alphanumeric person identifier that can be used to uniquely identify an individual the anonymous global person identifier (AGPI). Think of AGPI as an anonymized MPI that cannot be used to re-identify an individual. Its use is shown in Fig 6.2.

AGPI is unique in time and space and is used for integrating, on an individual basis, the "de-identified" health records gathered from multiple institutions in different jurisdictions and at different times. AGPI is an opaque alphanumeric structure to be used as the primary key to associate (one-way longitudinal integration of personal health records) de-identified health records from various sources to construct personal EHR (electronic health record) as depicted in figure 6.2.

AGPI is generated based on selected PHI during the de-identification process. The PHI candidates to be used for generation of AGPI are listed below with implications:

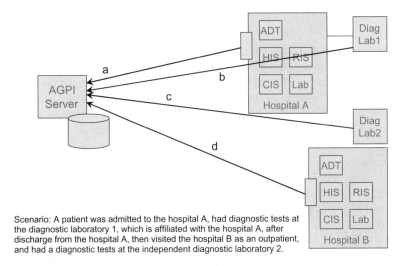

Scenario: A patient was admitted to the hospital A, had diagnostic tests at the diagnostic laboratory 1, which is affiliated with the hospital A, after discharge from the hospital A, then visited the hospital B as an outpatient, and had a diagnostic tests at the independent diagnostic laboratory 2.

The health records [a] and [b] will have the same hospital ID and patient ID, but the diagnostic data [c] or the health record [d] will have different patient IDs. In this case we need to assign an AGPI based on demographic data.

Figure 6.2 AGPI for longitudinal integration of health records

1. Name. Fuzzy search is required because of potential variances, such as Robert A. Smith, Bob Smith, Robert Ashley Smith, Rob Smith, Robert A. Smith Jr., and Robert A Smith III. Also last names of females change upon marriage.
2. Date of birth.
3. Gender.
4. Race. The statutory laws in some countries prohibit collecting this information, although this information is commonly used in the United States.
5. SSN. SSN itself can assure a unique identifier for an individual, but it may not be available and also requires a legal clearance to be used for deriving a system internal key.
6. Study ID and Institution ID. These are not reliable.
7. Patient number and hospital ID. These are not reliable because quite often a patient has several hospital cards. The patient numbers are not shared by diagnostics labs.

Key concerns about use of name as the primary means of identification of an individual is that it can have many variations that are difficult to be computationally analyzed so as to declare that two or more records belong to the same individual. Fuzzy logic can be used for searching to increase the matching threshold.

DATA OWNERSHIP COMPLIANCE: A TIME OF TURMOIL

You can get your financial information from a bank, but are you sure you even own copies and processed forms of your own medical data? Are these even yours to worry about? It was probably hard enough getting a copy of your medical record from your US physician before, and now there may be a payment to get it. We must leave this all by repeating that we are at the time of incredible transition and evolution, and much will change even before this book gets into print. At any formative time there is opportunity for discontinuity between guidelines on patient data and federal, state, institutional, and IRB requirements. Hopefully such issues will soon be resolved. The fact that regulations are not always clear-cut and often conflict makes them uncertain rules, and suggests that guidance could be by essentially the same clinical decision support systems that take account of uncertainty in making medical decisions.

To recap, federal ruling seeks to promote research through privacy. But in effect ruling 45CFR46.102.f reads that a de-identified human being is not a human being, and thus the patient has no rights over medical data. But that is not the end of the matter. A key issue on whether patients can have rights over their data depends on the definition of a human subject. Again, a de-identified human subject, or a dead one, may not necessarily have such rights. A startling differences between the federal definition of a human subject and the state definition, notably federal ruling 45CFR46.102.f is: *"Human subject means a living individual about ..."* (emphasis added in italic). NY State (Article 24A, section 2441): "Human subject shall mean *any* individual ..." (emphasis added in italic). So, whereas federal law overrides in cases of doubt, the state law conflicts, and many extenuating circumstances may be allowed according to weight. The North Shore Long Island Jewish Healthcare System extrapolates that in New York research regulations apply to both the living and the deceased. However, New York State rules exclude epidemiological studies, whereas the federal requirements do not. HIPAA does not apply to the information of the deceased, except that New York State does not create that distinction. Federal law regarding legally authorized representatives defers to state law, and state law makes no mention of research. Adding to this cocktail is probably the expectation that there will emerge, sooner or later, a landmark case that limits who can provide consent and the fact that most IRBs have structured policies relating to the above walk the line and await a day of legal challenge.

With many such apparent inconsistencies still awaiting resolution at the time of writing, we turn in the next chapter to an area that seems entirely different from the complex bureaucracy of mainstream healthcare in transition. Yet several thinkers believe it embroils issues as fundamentally ethical as those discussed in this chapter.

7

HOLISTIC MEDICINE AND IT

Health is a state of complete physical, mental and social well-being, and does not consist only of the absence of disease or infirmity
—World Health Organization's definition of health

THE NEW IT-BASED MEDICINE: SOME BETTER PRINCIPLES OF ANCIENT AND ALTERNATIVE MEDICINE

A unifying river runs through alternative medicine and doctrines, folk medicine, ancient Indian, homeopathy, and nature medicines, life energies, mystical medicine, and the modernity of Zen. It is the river of well-being. Do we want to be known to the guardians of our health only through our diseases, or through the state of our well-being? The World Health Organization's definition of health as "complete physical, mental and social well-being," is useful and accurate, but many people would consider it unrealistic. That is because using the WHO definition classifies 70% to 95% of people as unhealthy. So in the WHO view, there is massive room for improvement for almost all of us.

The WHO, in other words, emphasizes health as well-being in its broadest sense, in terms of mental state and social interactions with the rest of society. The results might have been less effective in the absence of modern biomedical science, but the ability to offer care and counsel within this larger holistic picture, we have noted, was easier for the ancient village shaman and physicians prior to the twentieth century. Then there was a smaller patient to physician ratio, little delegation to specialists, and far less influx of new biomedical science to try and take into account. Attention to wellness matters sometimes bordered on the spiritual, complementing the priests, and often times the shaman *was* also the spiritual guide of the village. In contrast, the industrial and biomedical revolutions brought on an "assembly line" treatment of patients of the late twentieth century. Who in the United States has not felt processed by waiting in the examination room for referral or for further processing by diagnostic labs and specialists? Clearly, IT, with its ability to reach out and integrate, and process vast amounts of information into digestible knowledge for point of contact and family physicians, opens the opportunity to restore the better parts of the older, as well as introduce modern alternative, methods.

A PRAGMATIC VIEW

The definition of history, as opposed to prehistory, leaves us with continuing written information. From the view point of modern mainstream medicine, who should ignore data at best interpreted as "clinical trials" that have involved millions of people for thousands of years, and at worst as a "marketing survey" that shows what satisfied millions of people over thousands of years? There is a rise of popularity of evidence-based medicine (see especially Chapter 10) with epidemiological origins that eschew anecdotal evidence, "common knowledge," personal experience, and so-called expert opinion in favor of hard facts and gathered statistics. But where anything is wrong, we can put it right by our deeper molecular understanding today, in conjunction with the emerging ability to analyze the lifestyles, therapies, and health outcomes of millions of patients in real time. The ancient holistic shaman would love it!

In a sense, then, it is proper to dig into a little more history and consider ancient and alternative approaches with holistic aspects, within the same chapter as a discussion of how IT can restore their time-honored values. Those who believe in an alternative, and perhaps more spiritual side, deserve respect for many reasons. Not least, a preference for medicine that reflects such world views, and practice of it at least as a supplement to modern medicine, are a considerable and enduring part of our population. Sympathy with those of that disposition is not hard for the present authors. We take the view that oral prehistory and written history represent a greater chunk of time than that in which modern medicine resides. Yet even these seeming great vistas are nothing to the grand long play of evolution. Indeed our ancestors in those periods were not significantly smarter, nor more foolish, than we are today, and much turns out to have a basis there as judged by our discoveries and new thought.

But why should the pharmaceutical industry care about ancient science, "old wives' tales," and fringe beliefs? Again, it is reasonable to suppose that therapies that are believed by many and often go back hundreds or thousands of years must confer some benefit. Accepting for the moment that they do, then the therapies must basically, almost like opposing armies, fall into two camps:

- those that work, and we don't know why, but we should do so
- those that work, but should not do so, and we don't know why they do.

Consideration of these two aspects will hopefully stimulate the interest of even the most materialistic reader in the rest of this chapter, because of the following considerations.

In the first camp lie, of course, the opportunities to discover new drugs in herbs, and perhaps discover the leads to a potential wonder drug. It is a marvelous *sequitur* (almost a tautology) that biology provides wonderful leads as to molecules that are biologically active. So far, other drug discovery techniques based on wholly nonbiological entities have been less perfect. There is also a general sense held by the public that natural products, and even related molecules (the *analogues*) derived by chemists from them, are safer than something totally unnatural. There is reason in this, close to being another marvelous *sequitur*. A molecule is hardly likely to be a universal cell poison if it is already made in cells in quantity and the cells thrive. They pass, in other words, at least a first step toxicity test (while there are certainly many toxic plants that reduce the value of this principle, it is also the case that toxic plants do not appear as traditional herbs, at least not without warnings and details of safe use, by the ancient equivalent of "on the label"). Nonetheless, there is often a need to tweak the chemistry of the natural compound because what is good or harmless for a plant cell may still not be optimal for humans, causing side effects.

For example, in 1944 Siegfried Gottfried, a Romanian physician, and Lily Baxendale, a British research chemist, got together to explore the benefits of licorice root (Glycorrhyzia, i.e., "sweet root"), funding research by the sales of over-the-counter creams, lotions, tinctures and so forth. The research led to the isolation of glycyrrhizic acid, a potent anti-inflammatory compound. The side effects here included anti-diuretic action and possible potential birth defects when taken in excessive quantity, but it led to the synthesis of the analogue carbenoxolone, much marketed as an effective treatment for stomach ulcers. We now know how it works, down to details at the atomic level, to the extent that modern computer techniques might have helped design the new analogue. The action of carbenoxolone was discovered to be the inhibition of the enzyme that makes the steroid cortisone from cortisol. The drug has many beneficial effects as a consequence of this inhibitory action, many perhaps yet to be discovered and some perhaps involving other enzyme or receptor targets. Recalling that obesity, diabetes, and Alzheimer's are variously comorbidities (tending to occur together), it is significant that carbenoxolone increases sensitivity to insulin, and ameliorates consequences of obesity. "Is 11-beta-hydroxysteroid dehydrogenase type 1 a therapeutic target?" recently asked pharmaceutical researchers D. E. Livingstone and B.R. Walker in their paper of that title, and subtitled "Effects of carbenoxolone in lean and obese Zucker rats" (*J. Pharmacol. Exp. Ther.* 2003;305:167–172). It may help Alzheimer's by reducing glucocortocoid levels in the brain (J. Warner, "Licorice root may keep mental skills sharp: compound derived from licorice root may fight effects of aging on brain," WebMD News, March 2004), improving memory, verbal efficiency, and cognition in tests on elderly males (Jonathan Seckl, U. Edinburgh).

In the second camp lies a much more mysterious phenomenon that step by step is only slowly becoming a little clearer. This involves those cures, herbal, ritual, or otherwise, that work only, or partly, because of the placebo effect. The word "placebo" comes from the Latin for "I will please" and is a very powerful effect that in many people appears to get switched on by, or is associated with, the feeling that one is "in good hands," and it ultimately results in recovery of health. The placebo effect may be one of a whole group of related physiological as yet poorly understood processes. It would be misleading and derogatory to say that the effectiveness of spiritual faith and much alternative medicine is some extension of these, that is, that they are placebos. It is more appropriate to say that whatever the truths of these disciplines in their own right, the placebo effect is an aspect of them which may be susceptible to scientific proof. Despite much ignorance of the mechanisms involved, mainstream medical thought leans to the view that the placebo effect is a physiological phenomenon as real as the workings of the immune system. Physicians have long known the power, and practical advantages, of the placebo. They frequently give a placebo or rather irrelevant harmless drug to a troublesome or "lost cause" patient to make them relax, go away, and feel better. It is so real and so important a phenomenon that it is recognized "by law": clinical trials are fundamentally based upon its truth, and a drug must do better than a placebo control study in order to be considered effective. Brain imaging and neurochemistry are at present the most fruitful in providing understanding. As far as relief of pain is concerned, several studies have shown that a placebo will activate brain areas to produce endorphins, the body's own natural morphine. The role of endorphins has long been implicated in acupuncture, and many have considered that they may be implicated meditation too. It is important to consider the placebo effect as larger than just pain relief. By extension of the above ideas, one might see the brain having many effects on the body's status and defense systems other than through the action of endorphins, and perhaps through neuropeptides or other molecules as yet unknown.

Science has yet to learn many details of how our beliefs and commitments map to physiological consequences, and the placebo effect is formally classified as a *psychosocial effect*. It is an effect that often carries the sense of being associated with an "energy," perhaps an energy ultimately to be interpreted scientifically as a set of specific features of metabolic and immunological vigor. It may be, or be related to, the process of spontaneous remissions of cancer, and so on, or the kind of energy that disappears if one's lifelong partner dies such that the surviving spouse "gives up" and follows within months.

Complementary psychological mechanisms may also somehow be related to the admission that one is sick, and the choice to become a patient. It may relate in turn to the sickness cast upon the unfortunate victim by a curse or "hex," and the relief of that sickness by a more kindly witchdoctor. The "in good hands" or "there is someone or something to lean on" sensation that activates it is one that also seems most naturally to embrace religion and other belief systems, as in Psalm 23:4: "Yea, though I walk through the valley of the shadow of death, I will fear no evil; For you are with me; Your rod and Your staff, they comfort me." The interest in the link of faith to physical health is no less important in Islam, and today perhaps even more so, with much attention paid to the healing power of the Koran. There is of course the view of the atheist as in *The Future of an Illusion* (*Die Zukunft einer Illusion*), a book written by Sigmund Freud in 1927 describing his interpretation of religion's origins, development, and future, from the perspective of psychoanalysis. Yet the irony for the atheistic argument is that if the placebo effect itself is more than just an illusion of well-being, faith has a hugely important role in well-being, at least for many of us. It seems that phenomona like the placebo effect can prevent physical disease and perhaps bolster the effects of chemical therapeutics.

But there's still more in this for the pharmaceutical industry! Because it seems to be a real physiological phenomenon, one can also imagine a drug that actually triggers the placebo response by a molecular mechanism. It would, of course be a curious drug to test in view of the current requirement that a drug must do better than the placebo effect. That could actually be already a problem in studying drugs that enhance production of interferon, an inhibitor of viral replication and a molecule that might also be unleashed in the placebo effect. Interferons cause antiviral resistance not directly, but by activating several cellular genes for antiviral proteins, and they thus serve as an example for the complex flow through a chain of physiological command that a placebo might initiate. "Feeling low? Take X!" But what would a "placebogenic" drug "look like"? Such a drug would seem to need to involve, at very least, a boosting of the immune system and a sense of well-being. Some traditional drugs that are said to increase "energy," notably ginseng, may provide a lead, assuming of course that this is not an illusion of energy: that would make it still very valuable as a placebo, but not be of much value in yielding a "placebogenic" molecule that will more *centrally* trigger the required effect. One recalls the claims that ginseng strengthens the heart and nervous system, builds mental and physical vitality, builds resistance to disease, and stimulates endocrine glands (http://www.dacom.co.kr/O/o7Ekkm55/moreinfo. html), and it is recommended for weakened health conditions, hangovers, fatigue, cool or hot feelings, stress, menopause, mild symptoms of diabetes, male impotency, and weakness surrounding childbirth, by increasing strength, stamina, athletic performance, stress management, and recovery from illness (http://www.tenzing.com/g.htn-d). These do seem to fit the mould. A possible molecular candidate is the molecule ginsenoside-Rg1 (G-Rg1), which acts by binding to the glucocorticoid receptor (Y.J. Lee, E. Chung, K.Y. Lee, Y.H. Lee, B. Huh, S.K. Lee, *Mol. Cell. Endocrinol.* 1997;133(2):135–140).

Oddly, however, a "placebogenic compound" would not necessarily be a blockbuster drug, in the sense that pharmacogenomics apply no less here. Only about a third of the population seems to be strongly susceptible to the placebo effect ("First 'placebo gene' discovered," *New Scientist*. online version retrieved on December 31, 2008). That might of course mean, however, that about two thirds of the population requires a drug to "switch on" the placebo effect. And the placebo effect, currently poorly understood in physiological terms, may vary both quantitatively and qualitatively from person to person and situation to situation, so various drugs might potentially "switch on" various parts at the right time.

THE SEEMING ODD MIX OF IT AND ALTERNATIVE MEDICINE

In the application of IT, there is a recent and rapidly increasing tendency by many to use "holistic" to mean simply "consideration of all factors for the patient," but nonetheless essentially meaning only those factors that are the focus of Western mainstream medicine. Presumably, this restricted use of the term is intended to give an air of establishment respectability, while the idea still confers a significant improvement on current healthcare. In contrast, everyday use of "holistic" continues to incorporate *alternative medicine* and the emotional, philosophical, metaphysical, and spiritual aspects of well-being. It would be very sad if this were lost from the definition. The goal of the traditional holistic approach is a wellness that encompasses each and every person in entirety, according their belief systems, and not just the lack of physical pain and disease (see, e.g., http://en.wikipedia.org/wiki/Holistic_health), in complete accordance with the definition of health by the WHO as mentioned above and discussed below.

An immiscible diet of IT taken with alternative and sometimes more spiritual medicine is something that we might have to swallow in entirety if we believe that IT can deliver a holistic approach. How the IT prospective is enabling, or has anything to do with what we mean by an alternative, holistic, and more spiritual approach has much to do with the extension of IT to include aspects of our physical, mental, and social selves as discussed before. To a very different atmosphere pervades out discussion be sure, of ancient and alternative medicine. Nonetheless, today, many on both sides of the cultural divide, with as many diverse ideas, are coming together to try to plot the future of human well-being.

CONCEPTS OF WELL-BEING AS A FOUNDATION
FOR ALTERNATIVE MEDICINE

The struggle ahead should not be too hard, since most of us would recognize that there is much wisdom in alternative views of the world. Very different medical doctrines often contain features that we should not be afraid to consider and even adopt. The *holistic* approach is prominent for its consideration of all factors pertaining to human well-being, including the environment, lifestyle, and psychological and spiritual aspects by which to avoid disease.

In the attention to the individual and the importance of humankind's need for a sound relationship with the natural world, the holistic approach reiterates themes of ancient disciplines, from which derive all current medicine, mainstream and off-mainstream. Personalized treatment, with an emphasis on prevention and the whole picture, form the basis also of ancient and alternative medical doctrines that may otherwise seem to thrive on the magical, mystical, and sometimes downright weird ritual, by modern Western mainstream standards of medicine. Yet it makes good sense that a practitioner should delve into the patient's life to seek the underlying cause of the medical problem, and leverage whatever IT can provide to do that. So "holistic" ultimately means, no more and no less, than bringing together *all* information that will enhance well-being as declared by the WHO definition. In the fullest IT picture that includes your beliefs and needs. It may be that medical science plus IT will be able to predict what to the patient is likely to be pleasing and uplifting, pointing the patient in the direction of mental well-being.

Today, the physician of mainstream medicine still does not even remotely have the time to take all lifestyle factors into account (and certainly not provide any broader guidance) without the resource that IT could provide. The best that can be done is referral to a specialist, which may never happen. Neglect of a holistic view is especially noticeable when a patient's illness demands urgent attention, and all effort must be focused on the episodic and reactive (instead of proactive) treatment of the patient. Most often a so-called disease is technically a symptom, of an underlying cause that is not addressed. Symptoms are cured, but by waiting until the patient reaches a state where treatment is essential, the core problem is harder to treat. If truth be told, the inevitable and fundamental nature of any episodic and illness-oriented approach allows a patient to deteriorate to a condition of stress before action is taken. It is even defined as the moment at which the patient is so stressed that he or she takes the decision to be a patient, and often the point of illness is all that the physician ever gets of a glimpse of the patient.

So what is exactly is the nature of the holistic cure for mainstream medicine right now? It is the scientific and engineering impact of the Internet on the holistic approach that will be highlighted in the second half of this chapter. According to David Collin, MPH, American Cancer Society, Oakland, CA, who clearly shares the vision of the link between aspects of holistic medicine and modern technology:

> As severe conditions become more manageable, the healthcare market will continue to move toward removing limits and enabling optimum performance. More billions will be spent on troubling, but not life-threatening, conditions. Public acceptance of genetic interventions will follow this trend. The professions

of health will become less about disease and death and more about marketing, and their education will reflect that. More interaction with patients will be conducted by high-bandwidth multi-media and supported by heavy information processing to improve precision and lower professional time spent. Although physician/patient face-to-face interaction will be reduced, physicians will get live, rich telemetric data.

The cardiologists like Joe Flower, Leonard S. Dreifus, Alfred A. Bove, and William S. Weintraub cover our other points about the link between holistic medicine and modern technology, as described in their web article *Thinking about the Future*:

> Think of every belief you have about healthcare, every assumption (e.g., "I get sick, I go to the doctor … "). Now, turn each one over, pull it inside out, imagine how it could be made false (e.g., "What if I don't wait until I am sick? What if the doctor comes to me? What if the help that comes is not a doctor? How could that be? … "). This is the future of healthcare. The combination of demographic shifts and cost pressures and a flood of new technologies—both biological and digital—promise that the new century and the coming generation will see the creative destruction and rebirth of what we know today as healthcare. In no field is this more true than in cardiovascular medicine, situated as it is at the nexus of the most advanced technologies, the most expensive techniques, the conditions most sensitive to changing lifestyles and demographics, and the deepest scientific understandings.

However, we do not want to be presumptive at where to draw the line between what is mysticism and what is science. This is for four reasons as follows:

First, the new healthcare will inevitably demand considerations new to current mainstream medicine. Some kind of regrouped philosophical considerations, including ethical philosophy considerations, will be required for healthcare planners and administrators. Among these, notions of holism and of *well-being* will be prominent.

Second, in regard to scientific matters, the off-mainstream disciplines make useful scientific or commonsense contributions that reflect classifications and concepts of ancient doctrines, but tested over thousands of years. The trial and error testing that have elapsed are an excellent gold-prospector's sieve, or clinical trial, for what is actually useful. Biopharmaceutical companies have been founded to explore ancient and alternative medicines on that very assumption. What is left may nonetheless have analogies with modern concepts if we allow for the cultural differences and the way that available knowledge was represented at the time. So it would not be unfair to say that alternative and mystical medicine are languages that can be translated into mainstream medicine of the future, only if we understand the keys and we are tolerant about using them.

Third, the wishes of the people are always to be respected in healthcare. As we will discuss, alternative medicine is a popular choice of many people, and one that goes back to traditions that have given rise to both mainstream and mystical medicine. Much of the interest in alternative forms of medicine relates to the fact that for many people it provides a broader concept of well-being than mainstream medicine.

Fourth, there is benefit to medical science in regard to brain science and a deeper appreciation of the nature of well-being. There is a strong body of popular opinion on the value in the mystical side of some alternative medicines or doctrines. To exemplify this, we will take time out on an emerging view about Zen Buddhism, to the acme of mysticism and of holism, and related disciplines such as the Western equivalence of existentialism. Importantly, these disciplines provide insight into the complex nature of well-being that a powerful holistic system of medicine must grasp. As a bonus it seems now that the phenomena and states of being described by these seemingly unscientific doctrines have a strong basis in brain science. There are aspects of brain function that relate not only to the benefits of silence, tranquility, and meditation (which is in any case not unique to Zen), but also to the essentially pragmatic nature of Zen philosophy as brain science.

Before Western conservative medical hardliners decide to skip this chapter as pandering to unscientific faddish and cultish tastes, they should note that there are real indications that many physicians and medical scientists would at least like to turn the tide. The very conservative Royal Society of Medicine in London October 2000 had a conference on the theme "Healthcare for the Whole Person: Is Holistic Medicine More Healthy?" and it received a generally favorable opinion. The First International Conference on Holistic Healthcare was held in Copenhagen, November 1 and 2, 2004 on the scientific aspects of holistic medicine and its now being perceived no longer as an occult, or naive and unscientific approach.

Nearly three million hits were obtained through an Internet search by entering "holistic" and "medicine" together without the quotes, and well over half a million on entering "holistic medicine" with the quotes. While holistic medicine or lifestyle is a hugely popular topic searched on the Internet, *holistic medicine* is not always the two-word form used for it. *Holistic healing* and *holistic health* were more often searched. Most often it was the term *alternative medicine*, as this term yielded well over six million hits. The singer "Elvis Presley" yielded over 5 million, so roughly holistic medicine is about as popular on the Internet as the "King of Rock 'n' Roll."

What we learn from hits on the Internet, is that popular interest in the holistic approach is in marked contrast to the relative lack of interest in the application of holistic principles by mainstream medicine in the United States. Yet *holistic*, when entered with *managed care*, gave a significant 154,000 hits, but most sites were pro-holistic and anti-managed care. Still some web pages with large numbers of hits did speak favorably about early efforts to combine the two approaches. On the whole, the most common observations were about the lack of holism in mainstream medicine, the need to restore the holistic approach to mainstream medicine, and the extreme difficulty in doing so.

In particular, a web page article by Ronald Parks writing for Natural Health and Longevity Resource Center, "Holistic Medicine—Becoming a Partner in the Healing Process" (http://www.all-natural.com/holistic.html), points out the recent dramatic increase of public interest in holistic medicine. Parks and his colleagues see holistic medicine as encompassing the mind, body, and emotions, which, if nurtured and empowered, can be "a partner in the healing process." In Parks's view, the holistic approach could help the US managed healthcare system make a shift from a focus on profits and cost savings to best business practices that are ethically motivated. Parks sees managed healthcare's preoccupation with cost reduction as entangling medical care and clinical decision-making with bureaucratic red tape, with the result that the sickest patients are turned away or receive less care. We agree that despite the many positive things also said about managed healthcare, patients manifestly regard it as confusing and cold-blooded business in sharp contrast to the teaching of Hippocrates and Galen. Parks notes that the trend has been toward a system lacking clinical leadership. He sees traditional natural alternatives as providing a more caring, personalized, patient-centric approach, and cites success stories where nutrition, exercise, yoga, and group support have provided an effective complement, and even alternative, to modern medical technology.

Why is Parks's opinion relevant to IT? The motivation behind the development of IT has been to reduce costs, enhance clinical decision making, make medicine safer and more effective, and return the patient to the center. It is easy to see how IT promises an essentially holistic approach that complements, not replaces, advanced medical technology. According to the Markle Foundation, a nonprofit organization formed in the United States to "address critical public needs in the information age," particularly in the areas of health and national security, it is to meet the challenges of "an aging population, a rising tide of consumerism, escalating healthcare costs, medical safety lapses, and the increased complexity that advances such as genetic discoveries will introduce into clinical data analysis and application." Importantly, although this view is centered on the technology aspect, it pretty much corresponds to Parks's concerns.

TRADITIONAL NATURAL ALTERNATIVES

Traditional natural alternatives, which may be identified more or less with *folk medicine* (or *nature medicine*), are sometimes cynically viewed as archetypal "sub-cultural" medicines. However, natural alternatives persist today as thriving traditions are passed down through families (typically maternally) in most cultures. Alternative medicines are found both as a popular approaches in the West and in the third world. Their development reaches very far back in time, probably representing the prototype healthcare, and has in large part a scientific herbal basis. The skills acquired have not, however, been put down in a scientific manner but passed verbally from one generation to the next (it seems that many tribes do not like to divulge their accumulated medical wisdom, perhaps feeling that revelation will diminish its strength). At the other extreme, many take it for granted that folk medicine is simply a collection of medical old wives' tales. Indeed, while some erroneous science seems to have crept in along the way—and many *placebo*s so has a great deal of mystical, and botanical, wisdom. Further it should be respectfully remembered that up to the first third of the twentieth century much of mainstream administrative medicine had the same mix of usefulness and uselessness. In those days there was even the term *materia medica* that often euphemistically signified substances in the latter category. Here we pause to share two such confirmational accounts: "My father, who qualified during the Second World War, learned from his father, who started doctoring in 1910 with the truncated and largely cosmetic materia medica of the day, the value of mist. aq. rub. This was water, colored red and prescribed with confidence: the placebo." (Michael Bywater; "Trust Your Doctor," *The Daily Telegraph London*, January 11, 2003). "If the whole of the materia medica as now used could be sunk in the bottom of the sea, it would be all the better for mankind and all the worse for the fishes." (Oliver Wendell Holmes Sr., 1883).

Closely related are *spiritual medicine* and *spiritual healing*, both subjects that we use as a collective term for special forms of medical doctrine. The stronger religious aspect or miraculous aspect in these practices simply focuses on mobilizing energies, human or divine, that are not recognized as energies in the sense used by the physical scientist. The earliest candidates for healers, shaman-like practitioners, must have stood out from the rest of the tribe. It must have seemed in ancient times, as it so often seems today, that some people come with a special share of inner power on which the tribe and its individual members can draw in crisis. Whether this comes from wholly within them, or is assisted by an external divine intelligence, or whether we all have the ability to mobilize such powers, it is just that the ability or will to do so differs by widely varying extents.

The belief in *special* inner power, energy, wisdom, or whatever, has clearly persisted through the rise of the great civilizations. Is there real magic involved? The apparent magic of ancient practitioners might have simply been psychological skill and force of personality to mobilize in turn the inner strengths of the patient. Nonetheless, the remarkable energy that such powerful personalities possessed, and imaginative sense in using it to restore misbalance in the patient, has permeated the thoughts of many peoples. Having seen the wonderful things that can be done by advocates of oriental martial arts and by Indian mystics, it is not hard to see that great reserves do exist within for calling upon unexpected strength and prowess, to the extent that such acts might seem magical, breaking the laws of mainstream physics. Elevating objects and flying through the air may be a fabulous exaggeration of the potential within us, and the balance of dark and light forces may be a simplification, but magical acts all reflect some deep human need to harness the supernatural. In many cases alternative traditions provided effective medical approaches that blended with essentially scientific thinking. For example, Chinese medicine goes a long way back to Ying-Yang (the negative force and positive force) that regulate the balance of what we would these days interpret as aspects of biological systems, including hormones, metabolic pathways, neural pathways, transcription, translation, posttranslation and modification.

It is perhaps important to understand that many Eastern thinkers regard the above energies as real, as opposed to being magical in some abstract sense that would imply they were improvable. Some even believe that they represent, or at least partly involve, energy precisely in the physicists' sense of the word, and hence it should be measurable. Biophysicist Dr Shin Lin at University of California at Irvine has studied herbal medicine and the placebo effect, and the effects of many mind-body practices such as acupuncture and, especially, tai chi (the controlled physical exercise system increasingly popular in the West that also seeks to involve the mind). Although the energy produced is at a low level, there does appear to be an increase in electromagnetic emissions above the levels of the obvious "basic physical exercise" and other controls. In 2008, based on his public reputation for this work as well as for his scientific reputation in "mainstream" biophysics, he was appointed by the US Secretary of Health and Human Services to a four-year term on the National Advisory Council for Complementary and Alternative Medicine at the National Institutes of Health.

THE MEDICAL CONTRIBUTION OF ANCIENT INDIA

While medical mysticism (and mystical medicine) is so ancient that much of the story is lost, many of the story threads are known. Not unexpectedly, these stories begin, or meet, in India, a traditional home of most things mystical. However, it must first be said that there is no implication that mystical methods are a hallmark of primitive or isolated civilization, and that ancient India "knew no better." Ancient India appears to have experimented with, and maintained both approaches of its own and those imported from abroad. It did not lie off the mainstream of protoscientific Greek medicine that we associate with Hippocrates and later Galen and the Arabic culture. Long before the rise of modern medicine, the Middle East and Indian subcontinent had a particular discipline of medicine that followed essentially a scientific thread that may be traced to Greek medicine as it was further developed by the Arabs.

Much more than that, it is believed that the Indian peoples themselves contributed greatly to the early development of Greek medicine. India played a very early role in producing therapies that the ancient Greeks subsequently employed (the Greeks, however, were not content with borrowing; they subjected new therapeutic measures to their own tests before they adopted them). The Muslims are said to still respect the Indian origin of a major aspect of medicine and indeed call it *Unani medicine* (or "Ionian medicine"), though European historians sometimes simply include this as part of *Arab medicine*. *Unani medicine* is now practiced in the Indo-Pakistan subcontinent. Following the decline of the Greco-Roman empire, the tradition was kept alive mainly by the Muslims; with the advent of Muslim rule, the chain of medical development came back to India and was enriched by addition of many therapeutic measures.

Of particular interest here, however, is a thread of Indian medical history of even more ancient origin, one by which India took prehistoric *folk medicine* and *nature medicine* to a fine art, comprising a blend of herbal and more mystical matters in an essentially holistic setting. Ayurveda, a Sanskrit word that literally translates as "science of life," or biology, is believed to be a system that was formed some 5,000 years ago in the Himalayan region. Though attributing pschological diseases in part to invasion by evil spirits, the overall flavor seemed to be a pursuit of a medical system into essentially physicist's terms such as scientific knowledge allowed at that time. The scientific basis conjectured three forms of energy, *vata*, *pitta*, and *kapha*, which in modern physics might respectively translate as information (of which many physicists believe everything is composed), energy, and matter (a special form of energy, as per Einstein's $E = mc^2$). Applied to the human body, they translated more specifically as mind and biological control systems, metabolism, and the physical body and physical (but also immunological) strength. Long used herbal products in Ayurvedic practice have been clinically studied for some of the diseases that they were claimed to treat. An Indian incense, the resin of *Boswellia serrata*, was considered inferior as an incense to the resins of other *Boswellia* species, but superior in treatment of diseases such as arthritis. It does indeed appear to hold promise for treatment of osteoarthritis and joint function, and although its pharmacology has been studied, to the author's knowledge there have not yet been any detailed chemical analyses and syntheses as there were for the licorice root (see above). Since the basis of Ayurveda was essentially scientific, and the divisions of medicine, surgery, obstetrics, and ear, nose, and throat were rather similar to those of Western medicine, it could be argued that the more modern Western feel to it rendered it similarly somewhat less holistic. However, that is only because there emerged related disciplines to focus rather more on the holistic and spiritual aspects, and variously we might either see these as branches or specializations of Ayurveda, or as parallel efforts. Two of such examples are the *Siddha system* of medicine (Siddha means one who has attained immortality) and another form better known to the West as *tantric science*, which became dominant in the north of India, also known as the *Siddhar-Kalpa* system (Kalpa means panacea).

The Siddha system itself had its origin to the Dravidian (pre-Vedic) culture of India, and hence presumably thereby a link to the cult of Shiva and the worship of the phallus. According to the Siddha system, the universe consists of five elements: earth, water, fire, air, and ether, which correspond to the five senses of the human body. The seven working principles included the elementary constituents of the body: the *mizaj,* the physiochemical aspects of the body; the *akhlat,* the bodily humors; the *a'da,* the anatomy of the body; the *ruh,* the life force or vital force; the *quwa',* energy; and the *af'al,* the physiological and nutritional aspects of the body. These kinds of concepts appear very ancient and, as we will see, not dissimilar kinds of thinking emerge in Chinese and Western medieval medicine. There is even impact today. It was mentioned above that many old terms do have identifiable analogues with modern concepts. For example, we might consider the humors of *akhlat* to relate to matters of hormones in the body, including a class called *neuroptides* that determines the mood states of the brain, while a deeper consideration of *af'al* certainly makes it appropriate to include the biochemical (metabolic) processes of the body. We can also have some insightful fun by attempting to pair off these systems against the system of the new emerging medicine: among these, the genome, proteome, physiome, and metabolome as are discussed elsewhere in this book.

One Indian people in particular, the Tamils, were responsible for developing the Siddha system of medicine. The ancient Tamils focused on the mission of achieving longevity by two routes: Yoga and a form of pharmaceutical medicine. Some attribute the earliest Indian writings as 3,000 years old and of Ayurvedic origin, but others feel that the earliest mention of medicinal plants is to be found in *Thirumular Thirumantiram-Ennayiram, Tholkappiam,* and the ancient Tamil works of *Sangarm* literature whose origins are believed to be thousands of years BC. Besides plant products, arsenic, mercury, iron, copper, gold, sulfur, and other substances comprise the pharmacopoeia of the Siddha tradition. The Siddhas obviously had skill in handling inorganic as well as organic materials. Probably predating Western alchemy, Siddhas also held that he who knows the secrets of the five elements could change a base metal into gold.

There is no doubt that these approaches and their derivatives are essentially holistic, but some were very specifically so. For example, there were among the physicians in the Indian Alai period (1296–1216 BC) master physician (Ustad-ul-Atibba) Maulana Badr-ul-Dindimeshiqi who emphasized a holistic doctrine known as *Tibb.* This doctrine teaches that the body as a whole is composed of matter and spirit and its interaction with the universe, so harmonious life is possible only when there is a proper balance between the bodily and spiritual functions. The doctrine of *Unani Tibb* seeks the restoration of the body as a whole to its original state.

The folk medicine origins and the therapeutic materials used in the Siddha system described above have struck a strong chord with adherents of *homeopathic medicine.* A round table conference on tribal medicine and related matters of more herbal medicine was held in Digha, West Bengal, in January 1987, and this conference extensively considered as well homeopathy. Homeopathy is popular in India, and there are now well over a hundred homeopathic medical colleges in India. Many thousands of students specialise in homeopathy studies each year, and so there are tens of thousands of qualified homeopaths, many homeopathic hospitals dispensaries, and even home-opathy research institutions.

HOMEOPATHY

Besides the several Indian connections, and the more ancient wisdom that it seems to reflect, homeopathy as we know it now is of relatively modern European origin. Its originator was the German physician Samuel Hahnemann (1755–1843). While translating lectures on the *Materia Medica* by the Scottish professor William Cullen, Hahnemann came across some expressions such as "like is cured by like." He attempted to apply this conception to cure a disease by imitating its nature, in the sense that a medicine will produce a similar but artificial disease and so stimulate the body to react appropriately to the original disease. Hahnemann got rid of the dangerous symptom-inducing effects of his molecules by serial dilution, which would actually have removed almost all the molecules, leaving nothing but the solvent. It is often said that homeopathy does not recognize Avogadro's number, which relates to the number of molecules in a given mass. One has to therefore take the position either that the discipline is essentially based on the placebo effect plus wise management of holistic considerations for the patient, or on some indefinable effect, of the molecules originally present in the solvent. It is not clear whether his successes owed more to this philosophy or more to the enthusiasm and general medical skills of his students. In any event, it is said that when cholera struck Germany, Hahnemann's disciples treated 154 victims homeopathically. Six died, but orthodox doctors treating some 1,500 cholera patients lost almost a thousand. Still, this "modernized" homeopathy has struck a common cord with India, which embraced it officially (it is recognized by the Indian government). In homeopathy as often practiced, the holistic view is clearly taken. Although the disease for which different patients are consulting the physicians may be the same, the remedy is different for each patient. In homeopathy the physician's interest is not only the alleviation of the patient's present symptoms but also his long-term well-being. Diagnosis was, and often still is, made after pursuing the totality of the symptoms of the patient. The patient's demeanor, manner of presentation, humor, grooming, complexion, hair, and nails, are all considered. Symptoms that are special to the patients, rather than the most common manifestations of the disease, are given focus. Ideally all the symptoms of the patient fit into a specific therapy.

LIFE FORCE AS A HARMONY WITH NATURE

As noted above, a frequent common concept in these relatively mystical medical disciplines, and a concept that may define them, is that there is some kind of energy or force within humans that is primarily responsible for representing and maintaining health, fighting disease, and achieving well-being and longevity. "Siddhar" is said to be a Tamil word derived from the root "chit," indicating both perfection in life or heavenly bliss. Specifically it was developed as a concept to describe eight kinds of *supernatural powers* attainable to humans. Siddhars, as applied to persons meant someone of great, even supernatural, talents achieved in their own lifetime. This kind tradition of medical energy was not lost. In 1810 homeopathy founder Hahnemann published his *Organon of the Art of Healing.* According to him, the human body functions by a "life force." But is this force wholly within?

Over the century following Hahnemann there came into existence a slightly different view of life force associated with several rather interrelated disciplines for maintaining health. The life force was seen as inherent in a harmony with nature. This kind of approach became known by various names and in various forms, such as *naturopathy, naturotherapy, nature cure, drugless medicine, natural therapeutics, and hygeiotherapy*, and most survive today. Clearly, the general emphasis on health and interaction with nature is essentially holistic. Vinconz Priessnitz (1799–1851) started a natural cure clinic in Grafenburg. Much later (1922), Henry Lindlahr published his controversial *Nature Cure: Philosophy and Practice Based on the Unity of Disease and Cure*, and founded many other clinics. These new disciplines were sympathetic to homeopathy in some respects, but leaning heavily toward healthy lifestyle and away from chemical therapeutics and often even excessive use of herbs. It is presumably no accident that the distrust of extracts and chemicals, and the focus on the need for healthy air, walking in green fields, sunlight and exercise, coincided with the rise of the industrial revolution, with its appalling hours of labor in "dark satanic mills."

Other doctrines that seem to reflect ancient wisdom too, and practiced by many cultures, derive from *geomancy* ("earth wisdom") where by the environment, both natural and constructed, is considered for its effects on the patient. In one particular form, in the Chinese discipline of Feng Sui (see later below), this practice takes the form of a fine art. Indeed the importance of staying well by maintaining a healthy lifestyle and healthy interaction with the natural environment seems to be as old as the first emergence of humankind from the wild into civilization. Of course, historically such aspirations are not novel to us: Egyptians, Greeks, Romans, and Jews had various rules or expected practices of hygiene, bathing, massage, and sports, with varying emphases. A probable new idea that is appropriate to modern pharmacology, however, is the cynical one that drugs possess very little power to cure disease but rather suppress the symptoms.

In disease the life force, as recognized by both homeopathy and these nature disciplines, is typically considered as disrupted, but almost always it retains the capacity for self-repair. The new approaches, nonetheless, specifically associate the life force with healthy life and harmony with nature. Particularly in nature medicine, there are seen two facets of the life force. These are the material and the vital forces of well-being. The material aspect of our life or vital force consists in the human organs; the vital aspect comes from a kind of spiritual source, or supreme power and intelligence, acting through any human that is the true healer. It is this energy that always endeavors to repair, to heal, and to restore the perfect state of being human. Health is seen as the normal and harmonious intermeshing of all factors comprising the human being, while disease is abnormal or inharmonious vibration of the factors. These two states are identified with constructive and destructive principles of Nature. This constructive principle can either be maintained by the good living of the healthy individual, or deployed from within the healer for the good of the patient (or awakened in the patient by the healer) when something goes awry.

PASSING DOWN WISDOM: JUNGIAN AND DARWINIAN VIEWS

Recall that we wondered above about how real are the mystical powers and life forces in the scientific sense. If we wanted a hybrid view of the type of nature medicine popular for the first two-thirds of the twentieth century, and typically respected by both the sciences and the humanities, it might be said that this resides in the kind of underlying, human collective psyche, and reservoir of energy as proposed by the great psychologist Carl Jung. Upon that view of the world, the reader might wish to embellish her or his more philosophical mystical, religious, existential, or spiritual views about the nature of the capabilities, and the extent of the influence of a higher power.

Many scientists might instead identify this ancestral subconscious with the fact that the human race grew up not only with the experience of their own bodies but with the experience of the plants and animals around them. The Jungian subconscious would be effectively the programs hardwired into the reptilian brain, the old mammalian brain, and the new mammalian brain, all of which survive as parts of the human brain today. On the long road to becoming human, the trials of countless years must have implanted (by Darwinian evolution) at least some instinctive appreciation of what to use and what to avoid, much as the sweet smell of fruit and flowers have become innately attractive to us, or the smell of the chemicals released from rotting meat has become innately naturally repulsive to us. This implies both the evolution of specific receptor molecules in the nose, and the connections in the brain giving a good or bad sensation when these are activated. In the interest of public health and comfort, there has been a lot of research into smells that we evolved to dislike instinctively because they are associated with food in a state that would harm us. They include those involving the chemicals putricine (decaying meat and fish), cadaverine (rotting corpses), skatole and methyl mercaptan (feces), and isovaleric acid (sweating feet). Tutricine is the source of the characteristic smell from swine and from grape skin waste. A very foul stench indeed results if such chemicals are produced in small amounts with other breakdown products such as hydrogen sulfide (characteristic of rotten eggs).

Having said all that, contemplation of folk medicine makes it seem obvious that much more information about therapeutic plants cannot be so hardwired into our brains by evolution. Time was too short. Such knowledge resides in a more conscious lore, passed on verbally and by example as themes and memes either collectively or by a privileged few. It must have been the basis for almost all of tribal medicine. Intuitively, in order to justify its frequently privileged status, such wisdom must *not* be freely accessible to everyone as inherited instinct. This *learned* knowledge must provide the vast bulk of folk medicine and the rise of new medical doctrines of the ancient and modern world. Such learned knowledge passed on, that in Chapter 2 we described as an example of a *meme*, not only for personal well-being but also to the collectively organized (tribal and ultimately international) development of medicine. Intellectual activity requires the capacity to learn, the capacity to discover, and, at its finest, the capacity to creatively explore.

In such respects, our species, *homo sapiens* or "wise man" may indeed be a special case because we are not just reservoirs of instinct. We can think creatively, to meet new problems rapidly. In that respective humankind may have been superior to one of their most recent, and now extinct, competitors, the Neanderthals. An important idea, simple though it may be, is that humankind has been always as *smart* as today, at least for a significant period of time. There was a wisdom of the ancients that *intellectually* improved our ancestors chances of survival for many tens of thousands of years, maybe many hundreds of thousands of years, while only recently have we begun to use machines to augment that smartness. Our predecessors experimented extensively with diet and herbs, and indeed the dietary obligations of many religions are not without some sound basis in the conditions prevailing at the time. Such time that has elapsed since the ancient world, even thousands of years before history, is a blink of an eye in evolution. While we might think of our ancestors as primitive, it makes good sense that our ancestors could not be materially different in their intellect.

Consider the case of the Ackee fruit, popular in the Caribbean and originally from West Africa. While apparently a reasonably pleasant-looking and -smelling fruit, even when not yet perfectly ripe, it contains in that state and in certain parts a substance called hypoglycin. It is processed by the human body to molecules that look like parts of very short chain fatty acids. They interact with and confuse the metabolism concerned with breaking down fats for energy, setting off a chain of effects that causes the blood glucose level to drop, even to fatal levels. Yet Africans, and later African-Caribbeans not originally familiar with the Ackee, came to learn that it is not always poisonous, and a valuable crop. Yet, in contrast, many animals have by evolution adopted the colors or appearance of a known poisonous species and almost always avoid being eaten as a result. Animals evolve instincts to eat certain plants when sick, but that is relatively very limited in comparison. In addition many herbs beneficial to humans, as reflected in many nineteenth- and twentieth-century elixirs, taste absolutely awful but are traditionally taken for their good effects. Getting pleasures and benefits takes intellectual maturity and sifting of the benefits and dangers from the more rapidly evolving messages from our culture. It is a rare thing to find a youth who would take kindly to being sat in front a stereo playing Wagnerian opera and given a cigar and a glass of cognac. And equally tellingly, it is now a rare thing to find a bar or opera house that will even let an adult smoke a cigar or cigarette on the premises.

This illustrates that a major value of being smart rather than simply having good instinct is that the intellect is rapidly adaptive: many populations of human beings and their near-relatives have been migrating and colonizing the Earth in waves for hundreds of thousands of years, such that they are constantly exposed to new challenges and opportunities in confronting different ecologies. So, over the past several millennia, much of human smartness has been spent on the maintaining health and curing disease. That intellectual activity has been secondary only to the more immediate survival issues involving the more primitive, instinctive activities: avoiding predators, finding food and water, and having babies. If those more intellectual pursuits of health are not successful, even the more pressing instinctive activities like fighting, running away, mating, and having strong children without complications will often ultimately have greatly diminished chances of success.

COULD A TWENTY-FIRST CENTURY HEALTHCARE SYSTEM ADDRESS OUR INNERMOST NEEDS?

Albert Einstein recognized that having the ability to find solutions to our problems is the most important aspect of our minds, since it is by power of intellect that humans became adaptive to new circumstances: "Imagination is more important than knowledge, because knowledge tells what was whereas imagination tells us what will be." The importance of problem solving here is that it marks a transition point in our narrative. It is not simply that it pertains to the human phenomenon of traditional and herbal medicine but that the freedom of will and imagination can be linked psychological and spiritual health. This freedom is part of our overall health, and notably so by the broad WHO definition. Moreover the evidence is that it manifestly affects our physical health.

It is true that the current reactive (rather than proactive) healthcare system and wise physician will give advice when "red flags" are seen. The mechanisms of the connection between stress and physical health are not perfectly known but are increasingly well understood. When we experience a stressful condition, the hypothalamus situated in the brain secretes adrenocorticotrophic releasing hormone that stimulates the pituitary gland to secrete adrenocorticotrophic hormone. This then stimulates the adrenal or the suprarenal glands to secrete the stress adrenaline and the cortisol. These two hormones are responsible for the physiological effects of stress through the "fight or flight response" by making functional adjustments that evolution really intended to be temporary. About 75% to 95% of all visits to physicians are due to chronic semi-acute stress-related disorders (http://www.tm.cme.edu/03.html). Such stress leads to an off-balance biochemistry with elevated cortisol and suppressed serotonin. It can affect the onset, susceptibility of disease, and progression or course of a preconditioning disease and recovery from it. Stress has been linked to cardiovascular dysfunction, cancer, diabetes, breakdown in the immune system, and alcohol and substance abuse.

It is not sufficient for the physician, in many cases, to say "you have to take it easy." We do have and will have better drugs to deal with depression, and we may yet have drugs to deal with different shades and types of depression. This, however, is only part of the story: it masks the symptoms, it does not cure the disease.

THE LACK OF A SENSE OF WELL-BEING IN THE WORLD

The mechanisms that lead to *chronic* acute stress, when associated with a profound sense of a lack of well-being in the world, are less obvious to mainstream medicine. Some of us can be dissatisfied with a moment in our lives, with good reasons. Stress in response to the death of a loved one, ill health, bullying, and divorce may persist unfortunately longer than would seem desirable, but it is not pathological. However, the origins, nature, and response to stress are highly personalized. Some of us will show a marked stress response to a situation that another person would take in their stride, or even shine and emerge as a leader. Some not only seem to thrive on stress but are also unable to cope without it, and even get stressed if they have to do without it. There are ranked tables of situations by severity of stress suggested by various authors, and marriage and even vacations often rank high. With different statements on the character, kind, or qualities of stress, and with the current minimal data on stress, who can insist that certain stresses are not a lot healthier than endless cups of coffee?

For many of us there may be bad stress with no obvious cause or reason. There may be a sense that we are out of place in our job, with our circle of friends, or in our culture as a whole. Often the bad stress we feel is combined with a set of excuses that preempt any escape (this forms an important aspect of some thinking discussed below), or there may be no excuse at all of why we just feel alienated from the world. It is a very individual thing.

IT could help in such instances of unexplainable malaise by its power to analyze data on lifestyles and psychological and genetic differences and make recommendations, the same as for any more physical medical issue. Admittedly, to provide in the near future a more personalized service, an implementation of Marvin Minsky's "caring agents," (Chapter 9) with a broader and more spiritual service than simply connecting to a wise human being will take some "thinking outside the box." But what can be done soon is for mainstream routine medicine, through its growing use of IT, to recognize the more fundamental dissatisfactions of the human spirit.

THE FUNDAMENTALS OF ZEN ARE RELATED TO THE BASIC CONCEPT OF WELL-BEING

The term "thinking outside the box" means thinking (1) out of common bounds and (2) creatively and innovatively. To call upon creative new solutions to new problems is, however, more easily said than done. To the ancients, as to many philosophers today, the trick is to achieve radically new modes of thought.

Zen Koan, used in Buddhist training of nonstandard thinking, has a great deal to do with thinking out of the box. There are several reasons medically for breaking free from the box of everyday thought. Zen, though enduring, has its origins in natural and mystical cults, and indeed many claim it to be the acme of mysticism. However, from a scientific perspective, there is a growing understanding of what Zen is about and with that understanding, a growing recognition of the relationship of Zen with psychology and brain science. We will use this to exemplify the dangers of being too quick on the trigger to shoot down the mystical side of holistic medicine.

Zen has been a major force in Asian history, but it differs from the early religions, cults, and doctrines, and from their view on well-being, by an enduring sense of modernity. Zen does not lay any claim to being a religion. Although Zen captures much of ancient thinking, it continues today to have impact globally. Zen also takes a "holistic" view of well-being, which has becomes a strong theme in the rise of the new medicine. Because its scope can include applications in psychiatric therapy, and because it runs into another related Western discipline, *existentialism* (see below), which has had a heavy influence on psychotherapy and lifestyle treatment, we will give it some attention.

The doctrine of Zen Buddhism is based on enlightenment through meditation and intuition rather than through faith. Not least, a central theme of Zen is about reaching a state of well-being associated with an enlightened state. However, true enlightenment is distinguished from practicing tranquility and meditation (though classically these help to achieve enlightenment), and this is the hardest part of Zen Buddhism to understand. That is to say, any relation between well-being and enlightenment must be tempered with the observation that the kind of well-being (associated with enlightenment) is not necessarily some kind of mindless pleasure state or some kind of sustained spiritual orgasm. According to tradition, at least one Buddhist monk who claimed that he had reached enlightenment, when asked how he felt, replied "I am as miserable as ever." Rather true enlightenment has to do with a sense of awareness of perception of underlying or infinite truth about the nature of self and about the world. For those of us that feel at least a little alienated from the world, that seems pretty relevant. Rather than dissipating our fears and problems, it provides a way to live with them, with the consequence that this provides a solid basis for ultimate fuller well-being and health. It is, at the very least, a key part of the holistic therapy.

Be that as it may, practicing tranquility and meditation, or simply practicing a healthier and more relaxed and philosophical approach to the world, is becoming an important theme of medicine because this does seem to reduce stress. Thousands of books have been written on various aspects of meditation and related Buddhist theory, but in the final analysis, it amounts to very simple advice: create a real quiet space in your home and in your heart, convince yourself or pretend that there is nothing to be done, and try to get the knack of regularly sitting back and doing nothing at all for a few minutes a day.

The seventeenth-century French philosopher Pascal said: "All man's miseries derive from not being able to sit quietly in a room alone." Sitting quietly and doing nothing, which is the key properties of the Buddhist meditation, is the essence of the oldest and most reliable therapeutic practice in the world. The various schools of Buddhism teach many different practices, but the underlying premises all point in the direction of stillness and silence. There is a Buddhist joke that says "Don't just do something, sitting there, but try to do nothing." People need the healing balm of quiet and spaciousness. It may be next to impossible to find these things externally in the big city, which makes it all the more imperative to look within.

In the highly populated cities like New York, London, Tokyo, and Seoul, everyone seems to be in a rush. On the street, we see people running to catch subway trains, buses, or cabs, even though another one will come within minutes. People behind the wheel make their own imaginary lanes to pass the cars in front of them in rush-hour traffic with no hope of arriving sooner. Some even press on the button of the elevator repeatedly to make the elevator arrive faster. Why do we add to the pressure we have, and even fill the empty spaces with more loud noise and near-manic intensity? Is it because "the eternal silence of these infinite spaces frightens me," as Pascal pointed out?

Most people will agree that impatience is counterproductive. If you watch someone who is very skilled at what they do, you will see a beautiful economy of motion. For someone like that, every action has a purpose, and there is no wasted effort as this person does his or her job with calmness and efficiency. But watch someone who is in an anxiety-causing situation, such as the one waiting for a job interview or a driver's test. See how the hands and feet fidget, wasting energy. Such a person would be far better off taking a deep breath, centering on stillness and just doing nothing. Then when the moment arrives for action, that person will perform at optimum because his or her mental resources will be calm and collected. Managing the smooth operation of the metabolic pathways and neuropathways through well-regulated hormones in our body system, by putting ourselves in a state of calmness and happiness, is believed to be even more effective practice of preventative medicine, again, with practically no cost and no adverse effects. This way we help ourselves stay well, and we greatly help other people around us as well.

There has been substantial study into the physiological basis of relaxation and meditation. The brain vibrates much the way the heart beats, but only faster. The average heart beats normally around 70 to 72 times per minute, the brain, when it is awake but resting, beats at about 20 to 22 cycles per second (cps) or hertz (Hz). To put it crudely, as with the heart, the faster the beat, the worse is the level of stress indicated. People with high-stress, fast-paced, modern lifestyle persistently have higher vibrations than 22 Hz (cycles per second) even for the resting but awake brain. Beta waves beat at 29 to 14 Hz and reflect a conscious state of contemplation, but not attentive to new information gathering. Gamma waves beat at 30 Hz or more and are associated with vigilance and use of our physical senses. Higher frequency beta waves are associated with special levels of awareness, vigilance, or excitation, and hence with stress, tension, anger, panic, anxiety, anger, and so on. Hormones such as epinephrine, norepinephrine, and cortisol are released but are detrimental to health when sustained. At the other end of the scale, delta waves beat at 3 to 0.5 Hz. Here we are in deep sleep or coma. While regular sleep is essential to health, maintaining this state indefinitely is of course a little too extreme to be a constructive contribution to society! Of more particular interest to tranquility and meditation are the waves between the sleeping and waking levels of consciousness. Alpha waves beat at 13 to 7 Hz, and theta waves beat at 16 to 4 Hz. Alpha waves are associated with a state of tranquility; we are only semiconscious of our surroundings. Lying between wakeful state and sleep state, it can be identified with some kind of trance. At this level various neuropeptides, endorphins, dynorphine, and so on, are released. With theta waves we are in deep trance state, which goes down to a light sleep state. The lower end of the waves is characterized mainly with dozing, rapid eye movement (REM), dreams, and hallucinations.

A substantial numbers of studies have addressed the benefits of other mental states that might by achieved through meditation, or by such means as deep introspection. What do we mean by "other mental states"? Are these identifiable with the brain waves discussed above? Only to a point! And when they are, there may be an unexpected association. In some instances there may be a seemingly paradoxical positive correlation with heightened awareness and vigilance. Enlightenment is not necessarily peace, at least not at its moment of arrival. It means literally "struck by light." Zen is not just about relaxing and learning to do nothing. To reach an absolute state of enlightenment we need to readdress the very way we think. But other than a vague awareness of the matter, this relevance of Zen is obvious neither to every patient, nor to every physician or medical scientist. Does enlightenment truly lead, though perhaps indirectly, to a true and greater peace, an ultimate Nirvana, as indicated by Buddhist texts? Can the great wisdom of Zen be rationalized for more modern scientific taste, and thus brought into one with emerging medicine? Is there a scientifically compatible explanation as to how we might draw on our hidden reserves? The clearest possibility of answering such questions, not surprisingly, comes from brain science and analysis of everyday tasks.

IT MODELS FOR THE HUMAN CONDITION

It is possible to invoke examples about the way the human brain works and from IT to illustrate that Zen and existentialism (see below) have an essentially scientific and biological justification. Consider this. Non–automobile drivers can substitute travel by subway train, walk routine, or other forms of transport to work. Drivers making their daily trips to work often barely remember the journey. Weren't they paying attention? Wasn't that dangerous? Consider first that these drivers must have made many intricate decisions, and performed many complicated operations, successfully. They switched lanes in a complex maneuvers and slowed down to let pedestrians stroll across roads. To perform such tasks many times a week, we take them "in our stride," or we should say "behind the wheel." Consider that if the unexpected had occurred, the driver would have quickly become alert and dealt with it soon enough. However, if the driver had been paying attention to every minute detail, that definitely would have made the trip dangerous, as this is exactly what happens the first time that we ever drive.

Performing such tasks as driving to work may seem to us instinctive, yet it cannot be instinct in the sense that biologists use the term. We cannot have *evolved* hardwired neural programs to handle these situations. To have 100% inherited instinct, humans would have to be accorded unreasonably astronomic scales of information-capturing capacity to cells, and no less astronomic information-carrying capacity to DNA for preprogramming everything about the minutiae of handling everyday living. Cars and driving did not exist in evolutionary time, so other process must be involved. But how is it that humans achieve this state of seeming instinct, and for what biological purpose, that is, with what Darwinian advantage? We will take the liberty of repeating the answers as we see them several times and probe more deeply into them.

The first part of the question is not too hard to answer in general terms. Somehow we can learn programs and can also be taught programs that can autonomously manage extremely complex tasks that would otherwise consume our attention, and would probably be associated with a degree of stress when tackled first time—the same as when we first learn to drive. From our earliest perceptions and thoughts, our earliest steps, our first friendship, our earliest musical instrument, our first car, our first job, we learn programs. And then we learn programs that run those programs, and then again in turn we learn programs that run the programs we just learned.

The Darwinian advantage surely is twofold. Many things such as gymnastics or playing piano or other musical instruments are much more speedily and smoothly performed when programmed, because the conscious mind, a very complex machine using very elaborate techniques, is rather slow. One thought per second is a frequent estimate; applied to movement that is not too good a speed for a racing car driver, a black belt in karate, or for winning a gold medal on the parallel bars. The other Darwinian advantage is this. While performing complex tasks like driving again and again, your mind ultimately becomes set free from the drudgery of details, the tedium of routine tasks, or complex operations. This freedom enhances survival by the ability to focus more often and creatively on the imminent, but as yet less tangible, challenges of the day, or on attempted resolution of the unresolved problems of yesterday. Harnessing the full creative computational power of the conscious mind to handle more routine tasks, such as driving a car, would be overkill.

What is the essential value of the relationship between the learned programs and the conscious mind? The programs exist or arise to help and serve this conscious mind. They liberate it from unnecessary labor. They set filters on when to alert higher cerebral management. Normal information encountered and routine responsibility is *not* passed up the cerebral management chain. *Our experiential core is relieved from micromanagement.* We cannot waste time thinking about everything. We cannot walk if we have to think about movement and coordination of every muscle, and the gymnast cannot perform if he or she has to think even at a significantly higher level. Music is more efficient and more beautiful when we do not have to think slowly and logically about which piano key to press, and our mind is set free to think of higher musical forms, including importantly, improvisations.

Neurologist James Austin made similar observations in the late 1970s and after, and probably the most similar points are due to the psychiatrist Arthur Deikman in late 1990s. Deikman is often quoted by Austin but critical of Austin's arguments on several points. Deikman uses the term "automization" as our propensity to learn tasks so thoroughly that we pay them no conscious thought. Such tasks include those that organize tasks, and even the learned programs of cognition itself. Here, Deikman also uses the term "deautomization," meaning *disruption of our routine ways of thinking, acting, and perceiving, as the route to awareness, creativity, and innovation.* Too little automization is bad, situations in which automization fails can be very stressful, and so it seems, too much automization can sometimes feel fundamentally wrong; in any event, it may deny an individual his or her rightful energy and contributive force to society.

As Austin and Deikman emphasize, these considerations relate directly to topics that philosophical, mystical, and religious thinkers have addressed for many years, hundreds or even thousands of years. Recent novelty has been mainly in the *interpretation* of such classical thought, reframed largely in modern neurological and psychiatric terms, such as deautomization. The problem has been, of course, that the great thinkers and schools have not addressed the topic in easy-to-understand layperson terms. In fairness, this is in part because using the best terms for the modern world does require a neurological basis and familiarity with basic computer science terms that have only in recent history become available. There has also been a tendency to use rhetoric, prose–poetry, and emotional, rather than logical, tools in order to break down barriers to thought and to promote the very kind of thinking that leads to creativity and innovation. Still another important point is that the road to creativity and innovation does demand nonconformity of thought, as compared to relying on taught and learned programs, and that instills a general sense of nonconformism in the whole discipline for considering such matters. Admittedly much of the esotery in the past has also been to cultivate an area of mystery and intellectual privilege, and to attract and motivate the initiates. The ancient root "my-" in "mysticism" means exactly silent or mute. However, further clarification on the above has come from philosophical ways of thought which, in some manifestations at least, have more obvious links to Western medicine.

HOW EXISTENTIALISM AND PSYCHOTHERAPY MAY ENABLE HOLISTIC PERSONALIZED HEALTHCARE

Now we may apply the above IT model to Western thought and psychiatry. Existentialism is a natural next step on our road and a major, essentially holistic, school of Western psychiatric medicine. The neurologist Austin who has considered similar issues was also a Zen Buddhist, and (arguably) more extensively an *existentialist*. Existentialism can perhaps be considered the Western twentieth-century counterpart of Zen.

As indicated above, the hardness of life stress is a motive for looking at the Zen way. A difference is that while the Eastern practitioner of Zen pursues enlightenment voluntarily and proactively, the Western existentialist is frequently driven there reactively by necessity, and apparently often by stress itself, and does not always like what he or she finds. What the ends have in common, for better or worse, is that they are the truth. This is not religion: the truth is not faith, but whatever truth turns out to be. It is not science because the methods are very different. An existentialist and a Zen practitioner can be religious, or not, and a scientist, or not. It is not ancient tradition for a Zen practitioner to have another religion, nor be a scientist, but in modern times this independence has allowed many races, creeds, and professions to explore its paths. You can follow both the Zen and existential paths, but there is a joke of unknown origin that which you follow at any moment depends on whether you are in a good or bad mood. This is in the sense that if you have two books entitled something like "The Joyful Road" and "Misery and Death," it is a good bet as to which is which.

The existential spin on things is a useful one because (although it is not solely a clinical discipline) via psychotherapy it makes a direct inroad into psychotherapy and theories of well-being. Many (e.g. Raymond J. Corsini and Danny Wedding, *Current Psychotherapies* (Wadsworth Press, 2004)) define existentialism as something like a philosophical movement that stresses the importance of existence, of our responsibility for and determination of our own psychological existence and authenticity in our relationships, and of our use of experience of the here and now in our search for knowledge. However, existentialism as a philosophic and literary form is in fact a pragmatic, cold-blooded (indeed depressing) philosophy, preaching to "never fool yourself" and to "see things as they *really* are." That characterization has tended to give it the status of science. Yet, by this description, existentialism eschews definition, classification, or labeling, since cold analytical thinking free of comforting pre-perceptions and preconceptions is also part of what it is to contemplate anything. If you do not so eschew, you are a phenomologist, not an existentialist. But because existentialism also preaches that we are responsible and free to choose, so we chose. We can choose to try and "nail down" the common threads in existential and Zen texts, in scientific and medical terms.

In the interest of brevity, we must classify, and classify fast, the three key terms in existentialism. Existentialism follows the notion of automization, even to the point that we become robots. *Nausea* (from Sartre's novel of that name, *La Nausee*) is about the programs we learn very early to perceive and classify things in our environment, and how we feel when those programs break down. A chair is no longer seen as a chair, but an arbitrary thing in a space of properties that we learned to partition, and *label* as 'chair'. *Vertigo* is about the programs we learn from our parents, and so on and on, for morality and our position in society, and how we feel when those programs break down. *Ennui* is about the programs about our place, purpose, and motivations in life, and how we feel when those programs break down.

How can we explain the existential 'disease' caused by the glaring truth of reality in the absence of the intervening programs? According to the existential psychotherapist Karl Jaspers (1883–1969), sustained stress by a mismatch between intent and outcome, a gap between what we want and what we can get, is in fact the very factor that causes these existential conditions. Our cybernetic autopilots were there to try to close such gaps by negative feedback. Too many alerts by failures cause our 'autopilot', our learned programs, to pass warnings and direct control to our full consciousness. Like a pilot in an airliner, those alerts oblige us to look out the windshield and see the world ourselves, and be fully responsible, at the controls, without all the natural IT support we expect.

Zen and existentialism put much focus on an idea that automization is a double-edge sword. Autopilots free us up, and enable us to think. But in a curious paradox, *the service provided by the neural service programs, the freeing of the mind, as liberation, is at the expense of a reduction of the very scope of consciousness*. It is both a symbiosis and a parasitism. When the robots within our heads take over all the complex activities of life, over many levels, what or how much is left for our own human brain to do? The philosophical disadvantage becomes clear. Automation spreads upward until there is almost nothing left. It erodes consciousness. Our core is absorbed by, and becomes, our own slave system. This is, in particular, an existential position. We become *inauthentic* (Heidegger) or *in Bad Faith*, Sartre's café waiter who leads, and chooses to lead, an almost robot-like existence as a waiter. When we become almost 100% automaton, we will not be truly aware; we will not be creative for sure. It is in *Bad Faith* that the waiter lets his programs dominate his existence, even though he is ultimately free not to do so—he has the power to override the autopilot.

CONSEQUENCE 1: APPLICATIONS TO THE MEDICAL PHILOSOPHY OF WELL-BEING

Applications of existentialism to holistic healthcare and psychiatry may be simple because of general similarities. There is, for those of us who feel that things should change but like Sartre's waiter make excuses why we cannot change, counseling to bring back our authenticity. IT could, in principle, help us explore many factors from patients' records as the best way forward, given the genetics, early history, and life experiences of different patients, the same as outcomes analysis is applied to any spectrum of medical diseases, diagnoses, and therapies. The number of parameters that describe humans make all of us unique in the world in mental health as in pharmacogenomics (see Chapter 9), but we should not be so arrogant as to believe that we are unique in our problems. We will not debate here the issue of whether some factors, held in sacred trust with the psychiatrist and counselor like confessions to a priest, should ever be recorded. But certainly general aspects can be, and are. The dilemma is that we speak of preempting and preventing physical disease, and yet psychiatric issues also usually get recorded when the condition becomes pathological. This means primarily a danger or at least an irritation to society. For the inauthentic waiter this is not much of an issue for society, but that is not the case for the second type of application, as follows.

In the general case of the frustrated person with so many mismatches between what is wanted and what is gained, there is the fundamental dissatisfaction of place in the world and the desire to change the world. In the extreme, such are the heroes and antiheroes of which legends and stories are made. There is the escalating danger of being stranger, misfit, outcast, lone wolf of the plains, rebel, anarchist, and ultimately terrorist, all strong existential themes among which we may find our final level according to our genetics and early experiences. As communism is extreme socialism, and fascism is extreme conservatism, even liberalism has it extreme in anarchy. The mission of psychiatric medicine then is to restore all the kinds of mismatched individual to a mutually acceptable role in society without annihilating those wellsprings of courage and creativity that could save the rest of us. After all, society is not always right: some rebels will take the path to become true heroes, society's held-in-reserve "joker in the pack" who can put things right. We just have to be helped to find our place, one that is acceptable to us and does the common good. The relative uniqueness of such individuals in the extreme case makes a kind of epidemiological and statistical analysis from medical records more sketchy, but there are enough exceptional leaders, as well as exceptional psychopathological cases, to do something. That is why in legal psychiatry and criminology, profiling is possible.

But this discussion begs some serious questions as to the significance for the majority of us for which a sense of dissatisfaction or misplacement is in a more specific and tangible context, and for which a growing sense of nausea, vertigo, and ennui is just the growing sense of a plain good old nervous breakdown. That is, according to Jaspers and others, what they are anyway. What forms can it take?

While the books of Camus and many others consider the hero, rebel, or anarchist, Sartre's character in *La Nausee* is a lot closer to most of us. So, here is a person who, the book slowly reveals, has a mismatch between "what he wants and what he gets" in rejected love. And yet he experiences from time to time a seemingly very specific effect, a sense of complete breakdown of his phenomenological engagement with reality: "Nothing seemed true; I felt surrounded by cardboard scenery which could quickly be removed. ..." If rejected love is the sole reason, why should one specific gap in the desired worldview results in an overriding of a seemingly specific mechanism? Well, the book is a work of fiction, and anyway, it isn't entirely true that this is the only mental state and experience of the character. But the main thing, perhaps, is that our innermost core is a sifting and planning entity surrounded by numerous hierarchal layers of increasing numbers of autopilot units, with interplaying feedback, as they are counted layer by layer toward the outside world. The innermost layers to us are a few top-of-the-hierarchy master controllers *broad in their scope*, and when thing go awry it is typically these that must be subjected to attention and "manual intervention" by our innermost core. The list of existential states, nausea, vertigo, and ennui, and maybe a few others, is not long. The modular brain with its great variety of centers, evolved in layers, suggests that there are many psychopathologies and many opportunities for finer unique benefits, but there are for many of us only one or very few types of *human condition*. Unrequited love, a kind of bereavement, the loss of a job, the crash of the financial marketplace, can each alone sometimes be enough to bring many of us closer to Sartre's single vision of the alien nature of cold, harsh reality.

The roads of healing, however, can be diverse, according to our genetic constitutions, cultures, faiths, past experiences, and lifestyle. If across the globe we share data on our life successes and failures anonymously and for the common good, IT would be available to help find the best ways for each of us to cope with being a simple human being in the common human condition.

CONSEQUENCE 2: LEVERAGE OF IT FOR HUMAN FREEDOM

The liberation of the mind from unnecessary labor by "automization" reduces the scope of consciousness. It seems that such reduction is not inevitable, but it is a consequence of *the finite capacity* of conscious thought through the neural computation of *Homo sapiens*, and the encroachment of learned cerebral programs for routine tasks upon it. It is as if for any portion of the higher mind, it can be dedicated either to automated programs, or to consciousness, or something between. If you like mathematics, it is almost as if *consciousness + learned automation = a constant*. If you like business, then consider that you have a budget, it just depends where you, or circumstance, end up spending the money.

How does one compensate for finite resource? Can we go for quality? Can we by in some way of teaching, training, spiritual guidance, or biological enhancement make better use of what we have? Can we go for quantity? At first glance, no. The issue clearly is not resolved by increasing the number of human brains per se, for the problems are as scalable as the benefits. But with the "finite resource" problem in mind, we might imagine an artificial, nonhuman "prosthesis" in our environment, an external computation to compensate for the finitude. It could be a train implat, but we will not pursue that idea here! Rather, we reallocate the type of computation that occupies our minds, by having more of the automated computation done elsewhere. The idea is that problem *is potentially resolvable by dramatically increasing the external resource to provide computational support for routine living.*

What do we mean by "provide computational support for routine living"? Remember how we started with the driving analogy? It means nothing more scary than, for example, having your car so smart that it drives itself. Then there is even more resource available in your brain for higher intellectual thought, as you are driven to work. And IT can extended that to include tools for lifestyle decision support, secretarial and everyday management support, and the automatic provision of the optimal choice, *whenever*, importantly, we don't have a concern or preference, or wherever we give clear instructions as to our wishes and preferences. Much of the above previous section hinges on the fact that stress arises when automization cannot cope, flashing red lights to consciousness and thrusting us into the pilot seat. With less automization within us, there is less to fail, it is the responsibility of IT. But what if IT *automation* fails? Well, the job of good IT is to have backup. Most of us do not have the same kind of scope of backup in our brains that a powerful IT infrastructure has. If we did have that, we would not feel alone, dropped, and fallen, nor get stressed and sick enough to seek out physicians, be given antidepressants, or be referred to counselors and therapists. And where IT falls short of this enormous responsibility, it has the means to detect the problem and alert the human experts.

FENG SUI MEDICAL INFORMATION TECHNOLOGY?

Feng Sui has not had a direct impact on medicine. Nonetheless, it is a philosophy whose main focus is an appreciation of the natural and artificial factors in the environment that have an impact on human well-being. Feng Sui is essentially a holistic ancient Chinese study of the environment that has been practiced for thousands of years. Feng Sui, literally means wind and water. Classical Feng Sui was a closely guarded discipline and was practiced to ensure the good health and wealth of the Imperial dynasties. In the twentieth-century Feng Sui principles were adopted in the West by some architects and interior decorators seeking to design ideal environments in which their clients could live and work, both in terms of orienting the architectural perspectives and interior décor. As in the time of the Chinese emperors, good Feng Sui is said to command prosperity, health benefits, and well-being. Feng Sui is based on the Yin-Yang principle. Balance, harmony, consistent change, and the interdependency of all things are a few of the deep meanings within this simple representation. Yang represents heat and light, and rising, and Yin represents cold and darkness, and descent. Neither is good or bad, they just are two principles, inherent in Eastern philosophy including the above-mentioned Zen.

The Feng Sui message on balance and appropriateness can be related to the expected impact of medical IT, which must be positioned appropriately balanced to make the patient attain well-being. For most of us healthy healthcare consumers, Feng Sui of medical IT will being more comfort than the Feng Sui of where to put our sofa. The basic idea is that there are contrasting themes in lifestyle guidance that present individually. That demands a significant sensitivity on the part of the intelligence behind the guidance and care that the IT system provides. It will have to grasp the general principles of what a good physician acquires as a good "bedside manner." Feng Sui will not be a challenge for a system if it has already mastered principles of the authentic and inauthentic (Heidegger), or Good Faith and Bad Faith (Sartre). These things are the same that reside, after all, in a few ounces of gray matter, and a smart system is able to act on the basis of general pattern in style and learn from specific examples.

MORE IMMINENT HOLISTIC PRACTICALITIES

The end of the twentieth century witnessed a growing appreciation of how our differing genetics give us different tendencies to disease, different manifestations of the same disease, and different responses to the prescriptions intended to cure them. For most of the twentieth century, drugs and other cures were developed like suits off the department store rack, with the idea that one kind of drug cures a disease in all people. As we have discussed, this is patently incorrect. Drug therapies need tailoring to the individual. In the 1990s it became apparent that Herceptin for breast cancer could be targeted at only the fraction of the population who had the appropriate gene for the drug to have an efficacious response, antidepressant drugs could be selected with a microarray chip to fit the specific patient genomics, and cancer therapies could be selected on the basis of specific genomic biomarkers. With these milestones came the first applications of molecular personalized medicine.

Today, medical research into molecular biology and new pharmaceutical drugs, however, still does not meet up with personal healthcare. Ideally supercomputers in the physician's office or accessed from the physician's office could treat patients based on their personal molecular profiles in real time, and select appropriate drugs. A supercomputer per physician would currently be too expensive, but local standard computers interacting with supercomputer centers are not only feasible but could be regulated. Recall the FDA amendment Act of 2007, which requires reports on adverse drug reactions from 100 million patients by 2012 anyway, and for all players (physicians, those in the FDA and pharmaceutical industry, healthcare administrators, epidemiologists, researchers) the real interest is in analyzing patient records for all kinds of associations and correlations. This includes, but is not confined to, outcomes from therapies. The end of the twentieth century brought us such a vision, but it is being hotly debated by the thinkers and the movers-and-shakers of healthcare.

The proponents, which include Dr. Roland Parks discussed above, hold that holistic medicine is an essentially ethical approach to medicine, perhaps *to the extent that medical ethics and holism are essentially synonymous*. As we discussed earlier, among the many practices that stand out in ancient wisdom about healthcare, the holistic view is the most pro-active, universal, and all-embracing view that at the same time can be highly personalized with regard to wellness, disease, and therapy. Well-being was not a question of waiting for a disease to happen, and hoping for the quick fix of a single herb; it is an issue of how life is lived.

The absence of a holistic view in the US Managed Healthcare is a characteristic of the entire Western world. Twentieth-century medicine neglected the personalized approach and rejected ancient holistic practices in all their forms in mainstream medicine. Medicine was presumed to be an analytic and focused science, and for the most part too few physicians were treating too many patients and were short on time. There was also no easy way to gather or assimilate all patients' lifestyle data. After IT was applied in genomics research to assist in the capture of data, to turn data into knowledge, and to turn knowledge into wisdom, it became evident that traditional notions of preventative medicine, personalized treatment, and holistic, lifestyle-cognizant treatment, could be made possible.

Recall from Chapter 1 the two medical principles thought to be of value in reorienting medical practice in the last half of twentieth century toward the personalized and holistic medicine that considers humans *collectively*: (1) *autonomy* of the patient for his or her self, including privacy, and (2) *solidarity* or *cooperation* with the patient in what we learn from the patient on the medical information that he or she is willing to share that can be pooled for the common good. Personalized medicine, with its focus on the individual, emphasizes autonomy, but its effects critically are far-reaching, extending the knowledge gained to the greater good of humanity.

Medical ethics always has to be a point of reference. In all cases it is what means being human. Whatever the culture the basic premise of ethics is to retain the right to be what you came to be while holding ready the right to be what you might want to come to be. The implication is that being at one with nature gave rise to the individual in you. While having genomics on the record is not popular with everyone, despite the imminent personal medical benefits, for those who are a descendant from Viking colony in Iceland, or Inuit, that heritage is an important part of "being in the world." Genomics, it seems, is more appreciated in the cultures with just one or two racial groups, as the company DeCode Genetics discovered in their dealings with Icelandic healthcare.

The dramatic transition point of medical advances in the late twentieth century is just beginning to reach the global population. How much can the traditions of the remote corners of the world and the wisdom of the ancients be served and serve us? Revolution in healthcare will present many dilemmas. Recognizing our common humanity and the global human experience will keep us on the right path.

HOLISTIC ASPECTS OF PERSONALIZED MOLECULAR MEDICINE

As we have shown, personalized medicine at its fullest takes consideration of individual's hereditary, environmental, and lifestyle variances, and hence is not very far removed from the notion of holistic medicine. In clinical practice, holistic medicine has rapidly become the dominant theme in oncology where the therapeutic index of the drugs is perhaps the narrowest. A further development of such personalized medicine may be medical diagnostic devices in the home. A medical diagnostic device in each home could personalize monitoring, since families differ in their genomics and lifestyles and the risk factors implied by both of hereditary traits and phenotypic variances.

Currently such technologies are largely confined to chronic care patients at home. The general idea is that with the new molecular diagnostic devices located in homes, all traditional first-check methods will no longer begin with the physician. The physician would be only involved by telemetry. The diagnostic devices would include stethoscopy, blood pressure readings, body temperature readings, plus cardiograms, and ultimately medical imagining facilities all done in the privacy of the home. These devices could also include sophisticated diagnostic detectors that can read molecules and their concentrations in blood, urine, and saliva and cheek swab samples.

In 2008 Lawrence Livermore National Laboratory took a device their scientists first developed for the detection of malicious use of pathogens by terrorists and demonstrated its capability to detect and distinguish in sputum even closely related bacteria such as tuberculosis and mycobacterium smegmatis. While detection of pathogens is important, the sensitivity and the already long existence of devices for doing bloodwork chemistry help us see how differences among individuals can be accommodated. Retinal scans with spectroscopy might eventually become a valuable tool to monitor blood health, although a tiny pin-prick, as in a diabetic's blood sugar monitoring device, is probably acceptable to most of us. Particularly conveniently when done at home will be routine cancer screenings, as in diagnostic checking for prostate and other cancer markers in the blood.

With genomic criteria established for family members, proteomics will become important in determing how the family member's genes are differentially *expressed* by the RNA and proteins they synthesized, in space over tissues, over time, and during the onset, duration, and recovery from disease. Then, after the genomics and risk factors are adequately identified for an individual or a family at home, along with each member's proteomics, there are the applications of DNA and pathogen DNA diagnostics to consider. Recall that these are *somatic mutations* that occur in our bodies, healthily as part of the development of the immune response, and unhealthily in cancers and other conditions. Particularly indicated may be monitoring the health of our mitochondria, those multiple bacteria-like structures in each of our cells that *were* bacteria billions of years ago in the primordial soup. A simple swab from the cheek inside the mouth is all that is required. The mitochondria do undergo mutations in their DNA as we age and in a few disease states, dramatically so. Will this be just too much for much of the general population to grasp, reducing the comfort level of the "end user" and making compliance difficult? For the kind of health education that epidemiologists call *primary prevention*, it may be that basic forms of cell physiology relating to these issues will have to be taught at an early stage in schools, perhaps along with hygiene and sex education. But then, the harder and more fundamental concept of DNA has been embraced already by the popular culture, and it must be a remote place far from the beaten track where that word has not been heard.

In the recent years heart disease, stroke, and cancer are regarded as the top three killer diseases to monitor in the Western countries. Also most research funds are being allocated for research in those three diseases, especially cancer. It is important to be able to restrict the prescription of potent, relatively toxic therapies to those women at highest risk and greatest chance of benefit, but to spare such therapies from women with significantly lower risk. Wherever patients are monitored, diagnosed, and treated, rapid influx of information from translational research could be critical in regard to genomics. Translational research is the research geared up to feed new findings into clinical practice at high speed. Recently there have been consortia of major pharmaceutical companies such as the (genomic) Biomarker Consortium, and efforts to get feedback about the performance of drugs from many patients. There is an increasing focus on cooperative co-morbidities, namely diseases that tend to occur together or precipitate each more than would be expected on a chance basis, like obesity and cardiovascular disease, and obesity and diabetes, and even diabetes and Alzheimer's, showing a domino effect of risk. Such research is paving the way to personalized medicine.

The general internationally coordinated research studies underway into major diseases are frequently considered translational research, although times of delivery of results may differ. Few (if any) results are at present immediately fed to the physician and home clinical and lifestyle decisions support systems in real time except by the Internet, so the issue of whether such a delivery method constitutes translational research is debatable. Often the studies are of a traditional epidemiological type, but with greater "drill down" into individual molecular (and lifestyle) differences. Remember, epidemiology is not confined to epidemics; it considers the statistics and distribution in time and space of all diseases, and is the basic science of public health. There is also greater "drill down" into the molecular biology and the genomics basis of the differences. For example, 42 countries, including the United Kingdom, Germany, Austria, Denmark, Sweden, Belgium, Italy, Australia, Japan, and Russia, have launched an international collaborative research initiative for a translational oncogenomics research with a focus on breast cancer. At the time of writing, about 600 cancer research centers participate around the world, including the Institute of Cancer Research, the Breast International Group, and the Roche Pharmaceuticals and Diagnostics. As mentioned in the previous section, in North America and much of Europe, Herceptin is approved as immunotherapy for the treatment of patients with metastatic breast cancer, for the patients whose tumors overexpress the HER2 protein and who have received one or more chemotherapy regimens for metastatic disease, as well as in combination with paclitaxel in patients whose tumors overexpress the HER2 protein and who have not received prior chemotherapy for their metastatic disease. *The main objective of the international and interdisciplinary research in breast cancer is to predict individualized outcomes for women with HER2+ early breast cancer through analysis of the RT-PCR gene set, expression array, and proteomic signature and to assess oncology therapeutic response on an individual basis, in consideration of the individual patient's genetic, environmental, and life style variances.*[1]

Another large cancer-oriented program was launched in 2001 in the United Kingdom (which provides public healthcare) as a national collaborative cancer research initiative. The National Translational Cancer Research Network (NTRAC) is working to improve the quality of cancer care. The national network of cancer research centers is embedded in the NHS, which integrates scientific and clinical expertise, and shares knowledge and resources for the benefit of cancer patients (ref: www.ntrac.org.uk) by integrating the expertise of the clinical researchers with the front-line clinicians to support translational research for the integration of research, treatment, and care for cancer patients. The principal aim of NTRAC is to build research infrastructure and workforce capacity that will support the advancement of novel anticancer therapeutics from the laboratory into the clinic and to test their promise in early clinical trials and diagnostics. *The approach taken for the cancer research is, again, to understand the fundamentals of disease mechanism, not only to find the most effective treatment (therapies, drugs) based on individual patient's responses to the treatment but also to find a way to let the immune system cure the disease without any external aid.*

---

[1] M. Piccart-Gebhart, M. Procter, B. Leyland-Jones, et al. A randomized trial of trastuzumab following adjuvant chemotherapy in women with HER2 positive breast cancer. *New England Journal of Medicine* 2005;353:1659–1672, Vol 16.

Several other *international* efforts involve consortia. In fact the leading causes of human deaths worldwide are not heart disease, stroke, or cancer, but diseases of malnutrition and infectious pathogens. The top three killers are diseases of famine (e.g., anemia), malaria, tuberculosis, and HIV (human immunodeficiency virus)/AIDS (acquired immunodeficiency syndrome). Malaria is considered as the foremost killer of children, whereas AIDS is considered as the world's foremost killer of adults. Millions of children in Africa die of malaria every year.

The pharmaceutical industry has given attention to developing antimicrobial drugs to kill bacterial, parasitic, and viral microorganisms. One problem with the traditional pharmaceutical approach is that developing a new antimicrobial drug and bringing it to market takes about 15 years, while it can sometimes take much less than 10 years for a pathogen to mutate, or resort its RNA or DNA with other strains, or for microorganism to develop resistance to an antimicrobial drug. The traditional scenario thus makes our fight against the infectious diseases an ongoing up-hill battle. For example, while there has been a growing sense that the common strains of HIV virus are getting weaker in the United States, a 2007 press release by pharmaceutical and diagnostic giant Abbott indicated that new US strains were emerging (http://www.abbott. com/global/url/pressRelease/en_US/60.5:5/Press_Release_496.htm). Another problem is that killing the pathogens with antimicrobial drugs does not necessarily help the patients get well. Medical students learn, usually in the first year, that the clinical outcome of all infections in humans depends on two important factors: (1) the pathogen that infects an individual and (2) the individual's response to the pathogen. The traditional approach has been focused on the pathogens that infect human. In some cases like leprosy or Dengue fever, it is the reaction of the human immune system that does most of the harm, and treatment often comes too late. The immune system of the human body produces inflammatory cytokines to kill the pathogens when infected with the diseases like malaria, and the people suffer from the complications caused by the inflammatory cytokines.

The need for more personal and holistic medicine is particulary evident in regard to cytokines. These represent a class of substances that are produced by cells of the immune system and can also be synthesized in the laboratory by recombinant DNA technology and given to people to affect immune responses. The problem is that many people produce excessive inflammatory cytokines and consequently suffer from complications. There are drugs to treat these complications for malaria, but the chemical entities such as antimicrobial drug molecules for malaria do not travel well to the brain (or cross the blood–brain barrier). This leaves blood vessels in the brain to swell and consequently cause convulsions, coma, and even death. More recently, the war against malaria may have had a lucky break; this quick aside is of interest in this chapter because it is partly based on a natural product. Coartem® has proven to be a relatively very safe product developed by Novartis in partnership with Kenya-based East African Botanicals to significantly increase agricultural cultivation of *Artemisia annua* and extraction of artemisinin. The latter is used to produce artemether and is one of two active ingredients in Coartem® (artemether-lumefantrine), provided by Novartis on a not-for-profit basis to the public sector in malaria-endemic developing countries. Incidentally, only distribution problems seem to be holding up a near-total eradication of malaria, and the authors speculate that distribution of tablets in cigarette packets might solve it (the prevalence of malaria is about 9% in Africa, while Africans are becoming big smokers, with the prevalence of smoking at probably well over 20% by now). Nonetheless, researchers focusing on personalized medicine are now paying attention to the individual's responses to the pathogens. Of two people who contract the same type of malaria bitten by the same mosquito, one might live and the other might die. The outcome depends on the second important fact all medical students learn in their first year: the clinical outcomes of all infectious diseases depend on the individual patient's responses to the pathogens. It may be that we would not need any antimicrobial drugs to cure some infectious diseases if we could figure out how to help the human immune system regulate the production of inflammatory cytokines to the right amount to kill the pathogens when infected with the diseases like malaria.

As to be discussed in Chapter 9, many of the variations among individuals arise from genomic differences like those in HLA genes, which are involved in the response to infection. These are genetically highly variable; seemingly it benefits evolution to find at least a tiny percentage of the population that has the right HLA protein structure to survive an epidemic. Many other factors are, however, as yet unknown to science.

An issue of provision of dugs to the less industrialized and emerging nations is not, of course, solely one of the times it takes to produce a drug or vaccine to a new strain. It is unfortunately also because of financial, distribution, and sometimes political factors. With all these unfortunate barriers, there are more traditional methods that can be pooled from the histories of many countries, and that can help. Eastern and Western medicine can complement each other wonderfully. The former has been focusing on the individual's responses to diseases and on stimulating or boosting the patient's immune system to self-heal from the disease. The latter, in our opinion, has been focusing on the pathogens and on killing the pathogens using antimicrobial drugs, although that sometimes makes patients suffer from or die of complications. For medical care generally, Eastern medicine can offer a substitute. In Eastern medicine, which has been practiced for thousands of years, diseases are diagnosed based on heartbeat pulses and patterns, color changes in facial skin, eyeballs, tongue texture, and other such analysis of the human organism as a whole, and consequently a mixture of various kinds of herbs is used to boost the patient's immune system to fight off the disease. That all said, the benefits of the latest Western and traditional Eastern methods are only at their best when merged. Although many AIDS patients have turned to Eastern and traditional folk medicine to boost their immunity and general health, very few would find any traditional medicine useful in treating global HIV and other infectious diseases, nor as an adequate substitute or acceptable excuse for the failure in responsibility of the rich industrial nations to provide vaccines and antibiotics.

HOLISTIC MEDICINE AND NUTRITION

The holistic approach, including the traditional Eastern approaches, does measure up well in regard to nutrition. We take medicine only when we become ill, while we eat everyday and usually three times a day. Studies have shown that many diseases and illness are psychological and caused by stress (e.g., high blood pressure, fatigue) in modern life, and that many illness are caused by what we eat (e.g., food poisoning, food allergy). Remember the saying "You are what you eat." Indeed we may be able to prevent illness by better managing stress in our daily life and being disciplined about what we eat in consideration of our hereditary and environmental properties. For example, people allergic to peanuts avoid any food that contains peanut, and people with high blood pressure take anger management courses. The truth is that there may be many subtle effects of food factors of which we may not be entirely aware but make us feel a little less than optimal. For genomic reasons, a large number of Caucasian males over fifty can feel "a little rougher than they should" the morning after drinking red wine. On the other hand, quite a lot of people become somewhat sensitive to the sulfites in white wine.

The foods that can cause that suboptimal feeling in many people are as diverse as their genomics and prior immunological exposures to substances, and these differences may only show up with careful records. We all have had experiences with certain foodstuffs that do not agree with us, that we like or don't like. They range from foods as diverse as duck meat and sardines, and often it is the preservatives and other food additives that turn out to be the cause, which provides an even stronger reason for keeping careful records of brand names and contents. It is also likely that low subclinical levels of harmful bacteria are constantly present in our foodstuffs, to our deleterious effect, especially in consideration of the rises of frequent "common source" epidemics recently of *E. coli* and *Salmonella*.

In a typical genomic approach to nutrition, the pharmacogenetic polymorphisms or SNPs are compared and contrasted with the long-established inborn errors of amino acid biochemistry (exemplified by phenylketonuria), suggesting ways in which the approaches of pharmacogenetics might inform the safe and effective use of amino acids as food additives and supplements (see, e.g., the *Journal of Nutrigenomics*). This way family doctors would be able to take their patients' genetic profiles, identify specific diseases for which they may be at risk and create customized dietary plans. The promise of nutritional genomics is not to overturn a century's worth of dietary advice but to understand the scientific fundamentals of dietary impact on health on the most basic level and to study how health is affected by the interplay of nutrition and genes—the same as has been studied extensively on the impact of alcohol consumption and smoking on health. The model for nutritional genomics is the work that has already been done on drug–gene interactions. But food interactions are usually far more complex. Consider that, there are at least 150 gene variants that can give rise to type 2 diabetes, and 300 or more that are associated with obesity while these two diseases, among others, have direct link with dietary patterns as well as genetic variances.

Amino acids, along with vitamins (the accessory factors needed for enzymes to work), are mostly essential to diet. Nonruminant mammals like human cannot synthesize all amino acids, which are essential ingredients of proteins, and need to intake them from external sources (actually even ruminants generally rely on bacteria in their guts for synthesis). We believe that somewhere on the road to our evolution, certain important amino acids were so abundant in our food that we lost the ability to make them in our own bodies. The food proteins will be decomposed by our digestion system into amino acids that are used as parts for synthesis of human proteins. Our DNA sequences are used as the assembly instructions for generation of human proteins used by our body systems to generate new tissues to replace old ones or damaged ones. When something upsets protein expression in our bodies, we basically feel not well or become seriously ill. We are born with DNA and therefore we do not have much control over it. But we could try to get good quality amino acids from what we eat. Of 20 amino acids required for the synthesis of proteins, isoleucine, leucine, valine, methionine, threonine lysine, phenylanine, and tryptophan have to be present in our food. A foodstuff containing all of these is called a *first-class protein source*. A diet lacking any one of these amino acids will ultimately lead to failure of protein synthesis, although death may take months. Such deficiencies are common of plant foodstuffs. Foodstuff like beans and rice are individually so-called *second-class protein sources* because these are relatively deficient in certain essential amino acids. However, like beans and rice, they are not necessarily deficient with respect to the same amino acids. Eaten together, rice and beans provide the full compliment. The message here is that vegetarians should mix and match intelligently. Soy beans are unusual in being first-class protein sources. After all the complexities described in the next paragraph or two, the ancient Eastern recommendation will probably stay the same: eat more soy!

Beyond these rudimentary dietetics, things are a little more complex. Although manufactured within us, arginine and histidine are made only slowly in human tissue, so these amino acids are also required in the diet during pregnancy, growth, and convalescence. In other cases, we may have slightly defective genes for making certain specific peptides and proteins, but this might be overcome by "mass action," by providing excesses of certain amino acids to force production. For example, it appears that excess methionine, and possibly cystine, might overcome low levels of production of the important internal antioxidant peptide called glutathione. Certain neutraceutical and vitamin companies sell these specifically for that purpose. In still other cases, amino acids need to be controlled in certain ratios so as not to interfere with each other.

Foodstuffs taken as herbs in Eastern medicine include ginseng, garlic, ginger, and gingko, all known to boost our immune system. The active ingredients are not understood in every case, and even when their actions are not known in detail, it is held that ginseng helps boost our immune system, garlic improves our liver functions, ginger boosts our digestion system, and gingko helps our brain functions according to Eastern medicine. Ginseng is certainly at very least a healthy mental stimulant with an alkaloid-like action, and garlic is known to act also as an antibiotic. We note that the names of those herbs start with "g," the first letter of good. What a coincidence! We are well aware of the old saying "An apple a day keeps the doctor away." We should probably add those g-herbs to our daily diet. In addition the more prosperous nations engaging in intensive farming need to watch that some essential minerals are not leached out. Selenium is particularly a important mineral present in a diet that includes poultry, eggs, mushrooms, and shrimp, among other good sources. A deficiency in selenium is associated with an in increase in risk for a number of cancers, such as prostate cancer. Another "cancer-preventing" food component is the plant-based chemical sulforaphane. The role of selenium in the antioxidant system is well understood. Also researchers studying human cells in the laboratory have discovered that combining the food compounds selenium and sulforaphane (found in broccoli) has an increased effect on cancer genes than as compared with each being used separately. Almost all plants that we eat have a whole spectrum of chemical factors that are classified as cancer-forming or cancer-inhibiting agents. Getting the balance right with a broad range of vegetables is important, but those that have a predominance of cancer-causing agents cannot be neglected because of their other nutritional benefits.

Although the mechanisms of action are often unknown, it is possible that many other substances have direct action in switching on or off some of our genes. Some dietary substances are known to do so. Raymond Rodriguez, who heads the Center of Excellence in Nutritional Genomics at the University of California, Davis, has identified a soy constituent called lunasin that increases, by his count, the activity of 123 different genes in prostrate cells. Among them are genes that suppress tumor growth and initiate the repair of damaged DNA. The genetic factors predisposing men to prostate cancer can, in principle, eventually be identified and calculated for each individual. In another study at Harvard Medical School the interaction of two categories of drug-metabolizing enzymes (phase 1 and phase 2) were observed to work in sequence to eliminate certain toxins from the body. It is desirable to have a balance of the two enzymes, but some people have a variant gene that speeds up the phase-1 enzymes, so they form carcinogens faster than the phase-2 enzymes can get rid of them. This gene is found in 28% of white Americans, but roughly 40% of African-Americans and Hispanics and nearly 70% of Japanese-Americans (who, as it happens, have a high rate of stomach cancer).

But there are ways to tweak the system: garlic contains nutrients that slow down the phase-1 enzymes, and a substance known as sulforaphane boosts levels of the phase-2. However, the sulforaphane molecule is also an antagonist of the nuclear receptor PXR that regulates many of the drug-metabolizing enzymes and transporters so that it can "turn down" the enzymes.

There's not much chance that nutritional genomics will ruin the pharmaceutical industry. Rather, the field has been creating opportunities for drug companies to isolate, concentrate, synthesize, and improve on the compounds in nature, as drug entrepreneurs have been doing for a hundred years.

GETTING READY: MAKING MANAGED HEALTHCARE PERSONALIZED AND HOLISTIC

Holism requires both a patient-centric view and the spread and sharing of information. Still there is a general consensus among the industry analysts: the healthcare industry is far behind other industries in adopting IT. Much of the IT required is already used in other areas of modern life (e.g., financial, insurance, retail, travel, manufacturing, education), and most of us take IT for granted. Concern over medical errors, radical changes in recommended best practice and law, and the enthusiasm of the Obama presidency for healthcare will cause great change, but it is not quite here yet at the time of writing. Some industry consultants even contend that the healthcare industry is still lagging more or less 20 years behind other industries in the adoption of IT. For example, a travel agent can make complete travel arrangement for flights, hotel, and rental car, with just a few clicks of the mouse. Compare that with healthcare, and you will see the patient's journey to be unnecessarily elaborate. For example, why should the patient have to personally see the general practitioner (GP) for a referral when the disease presented is obvious? Then, to find the appropriate specialist for the patient, the GP (or an assistant) has to call the specialists one by one, until a specialist able to see the patient is found.

Such needless delays of treatment are due to the healthcare industry's relying on manual processes for its service delivery, administration, monitoring, and management. Consequently healthcare services have been administered and managed in a fragmented and uncoordinated fashion. Since the existing system only initiates action when the patient "cries for help," current healthcare focuses on treatments of episodic illness as opposed to preventative wellness programs in a holistic, integrated way. In the United States, there is the additional challenge provided by managed care, or managed healthcare, which is an ingeniously phrased euphemism for healthcare run by business managers. It also relies on individual service providers, and as discussed above, the outcome is measured from the financial perspectives as opposed to assessing the performance of the clinical outcomes rendered from the wellness perspectives.

With US states spending so much less on patient treatment than countries with social medicine, there is a great deal more money to be spent on medical research (though some may say not always wisely). Still very sophisticated medical treatments are available, at least for those who can afford them. This medical research includes much of the aspects of molecular science and some aspects of IT, which is growing and poising itself for use by the US healthcare systems.

An important force for change is that the days of the existing US healthcare system are numbered. The baby boom of the 1940s and early 1950s is usually blamed. Demographic projections on the baby boomer problem are predicting impacts more-or-less equally badly for both the managed and relatively social systems of healthcare, and the fear is that today's healthcare systems will be unable to keep pace with the growing aging population. In order for governments to provide *sustainable programs that ensure the availability of high-quality medical services*, healthcare systems must focus on patients' wellness through preventative medical care. Such integrated healthcare services require close coordination and maximum information sharing among the healthcare professionals, which is closely related to the fact that with the significantly improved longevity and quality of elderly life due to technological advancements in medicine, healthcare costs will be increasing exponentially. Already the healthcare spending in United States has been exceeding $2 trillions a year ($2.3 trillion in 2007), and the federal government of Canada has been spending more than $150 billion a year ($160 billions in 2007) for healthcare. So these costs will be ever increasing.

Yet it may be the very nature of personalized medicine driven by new technologies that will shake up the US managed healthcare harder than other factors. Optimists would note that already rapidly proceeding in the United Kingdom is the development of digitalization of the patient record, and the genomic sampling of patients. The UK healthcare system now intends to thrive on such progressive developments, and Canada, Belgium, Singapore, and Japan are also rapidly re-engineering their national healthcare systems for an effective and universal healthcare.

Be that all as it may, the US healthcare industry is not static. The holistic healthcare industry in the United States is at an embryonic stage, but with IT there is hint of a radically new future emerging. It is imperative that as healthcare systems change in terms of business function models and technologies, the goal is kept to develop and integrate technologies that will enable the transformation from episodic care to a continuum of care and from a focus on illness to a focus on wellness. Achieving this goal will require the elimination of the data isolation that is prevalent throughout the healthcare industry. The medical information including patient data must be made available to all the constituents of the healthcare delivery system, from the home to clinicians to care managers. The healthcare solution needs to include functions such as the right management, security, and extended transactions (e.g., embedded workflows). The security aspect of the new healthcare system is critical to its successful deployment because of the privacy concerns associated with patient information. Healthcare solutions that use human–computer technologies to create more "natural" ways of capturing and retrieving medical information need to include speech recognition and mobile devices. Mobile technologies are important because they provide the ability to capture content at the point of care.

Bureaucracy will have to fundamentally change. Both government and industry initiatives for a new healthcare system have been launched recently from time to time in Canada. The key business objectives of the provincial initiative were (1) sharing relevant information about health and healthcare with all health system stakeholders and decision makers (patients, policy makers, administrators, researchers, physicians, pharmacists, nurses, and other health professionals), (2) maximizing accountability within the health system, and (3) protecting privacy of individual health information. An independent nonprofit organizational entity has been established to provide an information sharing and management infrastructure and common sets of core business functions accessible to the health system stakeholders.

FINALLY GOING HOLISTIC

For holistic medicine to be effected, an adequate, stable, and sustainable program must be in place to ensure the availability of, and access to, the high-quality medical services. Because the focus of holistic medicine is on patients' wellness through preventative medical care, the integrated healthcare services will require close coordination and maximum information sharing among the healthcare professionals. The steps toward this objective must be legislative and administrative. By "legislative" we mean strong guidelines and mandates with timelines from the central government, though it is likely to be with a "soft hand" and in a period of changes phased over time, say the next 10 years. By "administrative" we mean the ability to keep track of and to analyze the outcomes of patient care in terms of clinical efficacy as well as financial outcomes of healthcare plans and programs.

As we noted several times before, a driving force is wide recognition, at last, of the existence of critical errors in healthcare and the need for systems for correcting errors and ensuring quality control. A study by the US Institute of Medicine has outlined 10 such objectives, several of very holistic flavor, that would to "make the health system more responsive to patient needs and preferences and to encourage their participation in decision making":

1. *Care based on continuous healing relationships*
2. *Customization based on patient needs and values*
3. *Patient in control*
4. *Shared knowledge and the free flow of information*
5. *Evidence-based decision making*
6. *Safety as a property of the healthcare system*
7. *Need for transparency* (information to be provided for decision making by patients)

8. *Anticipation of needs*
9. *Continuous decrease in waste*
10. *Cooperation among clinicians*

Most of these objectives clearly correspond to matters of personalized and holistic medicine. The conclusions of the Institute of Medicine came within a month of a 54-page report issued by a group of 13 health and IT organizations to the Bush administration with recommendations for just such a roadmap for a national health information network. The group providing the report included the American Health Information Management Association, the Healthcare Information and Management Systems Society, and the Liberty Alliance Project, and was coordinated by the Markle Foundation in New York. Among the principles indicated that should guide the creation of such a network were the need for open, nonproprietary technical standards for communication across the network. Patient information must be capable of being sent across the network easily and securely to hospitals, laboratories, specialists, insurers, and researchers if the promise of improved care and reduced costs are to be achieved. "The issue we tried to address is how do we mobilize America's incredibly fragmented health system to really get this done," said David Lansky, a director of the health program at the Markle Foundation.

Interestingly the report also concluded that a national health network should not include a central database of patient records nor should it require individuals to have "health ID cards," as some have proposed; rather, patients should control their own records, deciding whether their information can be used in studies for effectiveness of certain treatments and drugs.

In Canada, a two-year study done by a multivendor team of healthcare professionals for the province of Alberta similarly characterized the current Canadian healthcare system to be provider-centric as opposed to patient-centric and to depend on episodic and illness-oriented (as opposed to wellness-oriented) fragmented services provided by the individual provider in a facility with very little coordination. As in the United States, the outcomes are consequently measured from the financial perspective rather than the clinical efficacy perspective. In Canada the multivendor team of healthcare professionals recommended that the healthcare system make the transition to a patient-centric, outcome-driven, and wellness-oriented system that provides integrated continuum of services with close coordination among the providers and institutions.

FINANCIAL ASPECTS OF THE MOVE TOWARD HOLISTIC HEALTHCARE

Holistic systems may well put the patient far above monetary considerations, but every doctrine has to have some kind of economy to fuel it. After all, whatever the philosophical, ethical, and social merits of communism, the largest block of it disappeared because it went broke. At present, there are many barriers to overcome before the concept of the holistic medicine, enabled by IT, can be realized. For example, efficient one-on-one interaction between physician and patient, spanning many aspects of ongoing life, ultimately requires telemedicine. While opportunities for telemedicine continue to be identified, some complications are a headache for US medical service organizations. For example, will reimbursement for telemedicine services be covered under a country's health insurance plans? On the whole, there are many macro- and microeconomic factors to consider, and the situation is quite complex.

Inspired by holistic and personalized medicine, or not, it remains hard for any healthcare system to switch who pays. To repeat, in 2007–2008, the United States spent $2.4 trillion on healthcare, which is about $6,900 per person. That is 4–5 times what is spent on US national defense. To estimate what it is at time of reading, note that it is rising at 7% per annum (staggering when one considers that is currently about twice the rate of US inflation). The US body known as the National Coalition on Healthcare expects healthcare spending to be $4.3 trillion by 2017. Managed healthcare means, of course, that citizens and residents take the burden: in 2008, employer health insurance premiums increased by 5.0 percent (the annual premium for an employer health plan covering a family of four averaged nearly $12,700, and the annual premium for single coverage averaged over $4,700). Some 46 million Americans are uninsured, but the United States spends more on healthcare than other industrialized nations who provide health insurance to all their citizens. Healthcare spending accounted for 10.9 percent of the GDP in Switzerland, 10.7 percent in Germany, 9.7 percent in Canada and 9.5 percent in France, according to the Organization for Economic Cooperation and Development (http://www.nchc. org/facts/cost.shtml). The $276 billion to be spent in US physician and hospital centers over *the next 10 years* for information-based medicine is indeed an exciting first step, but in comparison to the overall expenditure it is small. Total Asian healthcare spending is predicted at a comparable $1.5 trillion by 2025. In Canada, with roughly a tenth of the population of the United States, and with a healthcare system that is relatively efficient, the healthcare operation budget alone is well over $150 billion a year. Over the next 5 years US healthcare spending is estimated to rise from 17% to perhaps 19% of GDP. The authors are alarmed to note that these estimates have risen several percent since we began this book. Expenditure could well be higher because of the "promise" of $276 billion for healthcare IT during the Bush presidency, and "upped" by the enthusiasm of the Obama presidency, but this barely conceals the variation that may result if the GDP rises faster than or falls a little below the rate of growth of healthcare spending. Yet again, we note that many people die each year from errors called "adverse events" in hospitals. The numbers quoted in the preceding section are higher than for car crashes, breast cancer, and AIDS. The issue is not just justly humanitarian as hospital errors also cost the US economy $15 billion in loss of the patients' contributions to society and home life, and about the same again in direct losses on the healthcare balance sheet. An article published around the same time in the online version of the journal *Health Affairs* estimated that $78 billion a year could be saved in the United States in 10 years by moving to electronic patient records in a network with open communications standards or interoperability, in computing terms. This is interesting in comparison with the US estimated cost of $276 billion over the next 10 years because it means that a third or more of the cost would effectively be recuperated in addition to other benefits. Due to the recent financial turmoil leading to a global recession, significant changes are anticipated to the projected healthcare spending mentioned above.

Health insurance systems may be a barrier to holistic healthcare. A key reason, though it is being addressed to some degree, is exclusion of coverage of certain diseases on ground of prior illness. It requires no explanation to say that this position is *fundamentally against* the principles of personalized and holistic medicine. On the other hand, given the US system the way it operates for better or worse, there is clearly something fundamentally wrong in the picture of a prosperous person who took out no or minimal coverage all of his or her life, and contributed nothing to the healthcare system, but then develops cancer and immediately takes out coverage for cancer. It is almost like taking out hurricane insurance as the hurricane is starting to take off your roof. In the absence of a uniform distribution of fair-minded healthcare players, the cure here is obvious: do as many other countries do. That is to say, develop a socialistic welfare system, pay for it through taxes, and have it be done. The problem, of course, is having the American taxpayer swallow that bitter pill, especially with a history of relatively lower US taxes designed to promote enterprise and innovation. Moreover it rankles taxpayers that this could in practice lead to the taxpayer paying for those residing in the United States who are not supposed to be there. But that issue could be countered by the fact that the large number of immigrants not covered by healthcare come awfully close to representing a rather convenient tacit slave labor force. So we may have to take a truly holistic view of all players in society before a truly holistic healthcare without awaiting a cure for *all* the ills of a great nation.

Another argument for a tax-funded, more socialistic healthcare system is that otherwise you tend to get the medical care you can afford. Few would feel that the life of an underpaid but productive academic medical researcher, or exhausted nurse or paramedic, is worth less than that of, say, a prosperous weapons dealer. The only other "obvious" way out of that would be to award healthcare-access merit points for contributions to the common good like some countries have for residency or citizenship, but who feel able to quantitatively weigh the contribution of us all with our very different roles in society? Right now, money does count for a lot. At the current rate of technology growth, it could be argued that if you have infinite financial reserves, you could live forever (see Chapter 10) with new fangled devices that are too expensive for the average patient. In practice, increasingly sophisticated medical technologies and pressures on central government budgets compel providers to deliver treatment in a more affordable manner, yet the wide variation in levels of spending on healthcare and its technologies, and differences in the forms and quality of medical services ensure variability in each country's response to these changes.

The labor cost of providers of patient care such as physicians, nurses, hospital administrators, and radiology technicians remains high among expensive items in healthcare budgets. The payment of physicians on a capacitated basis (a flat payment to cover treatment for a fixed period of time or a fixed number of patients) and consortia among healthcare providers for the purpose of exacting discounts from suppliers of medical equipment and pharmaceuticals are becoming prevalent internationally. Since 1980 the high expense of inpatient hospital care has induced practically all Western European countries to cut the total number of hospital beds substantially and explore more cost-effective alternatives. In the wake of severe economic downturns in the East Asian economies, the movement to rationalize healthcare systems in order to reduce expenditures should gain even greater momentum.

Tensions between the path to a highly humanist and highly material medical doctrines are significant, 60th philosophically and economically. Capitalism and welfare are not the same thing, so a nation can be a capitalist state and a welfare state, and the doctrines can be bedfellows, albeit surly ones. That is a nation can be capitalist and provide sound social-style and even holistic medicine, and without conflict at least in principle. Capitalist-style competition is not necessarily bad for holistic medicine either, and it is not necessarily good to go to the other extreme, showing aspects of what some UK critics call "the nanny state." Competition within managed care markets is still narrowing price differences among health insurance plans, so in the future consumers might switch plans on the basis of quality of care rather than price differences in premiums. Nonetheless, the tendency toward more vigorous competition in the delivery of healthcare services is not without challenge or political opposition in most countries. The downside of the common valuation of healthcare, as a universal right with significant public welfare and ethical dimensions, is that the healthcare sector will remain highly regulated by the state, and as for-profit activity it thus carries the burden of proof. The other side of the coin, namely allowing extensive competition, has its drawbacks too. Fierce commercial competition in the US healthcare industry has resulted in slim or no profit margins for some hospitals, home health agencies, and managed care plans, including HMOs (health maintenance organizations) for a group insurance that entitle members to services of participating hospitals and clinics and physicians. Still most providers have done well in the marketplace.

Because of the more humanist nature of holistic medicine, this new medicine may drive a move to a more state-run system. For example, before the arrival of managed care, which we remember is healthcare management run on business principles, healthcare professionals focused mainly on providing medical care to patients. But now they have to focus on costs and management issues as well (in response, many physicians have been forming their own provider groups). Many have expressed their desire to return to the earlier form of pre–managed care medicine.

Still, in the United States a holistic system will need to first build on managed care. To be fair, managed care has effectively reduced healthcare costs thus far, and with some adjustments it could continue to contain costs well into the next century. Putting the problems of Medicaid (care for the retired) to one side for the moment, the situation is not so bad to all eyes. Managed care offers enrollees lower premium costs, better benefits, reasonable co-payments, and lower deductibles. Managed care may still be expected to dominate the industry with a market share of about 90%. Managed care will likely incorporate IT and contract with specialists to better control high-cost disease treatments. Mergers and acquisitions will continue to occur among healthcare organizations, but at a much slower rate than that observed in the early 1990s. Small and inefficient managed care centers will be taken over by larger ones. In recent years many employers have expanded the range of health plans they offer their employees to include managed care plans that have much lower average employer premiums than do traditional indemnity plans and that tend to control utilization through gatekeepers. The best-known managed care plans are HMOs and PPOs (preferred provider organizations), which offer a wide range of preventive services. HMOs continue to offer comprehensive benefits. All HMOs cover primary care visits with no limit on the number of appointments, and their co-payments are as low as $3 to $10 for primary care visits and prescription drugs. Managed care plans tend to restrict patient choice, use primary care physicians as gatekeepers for specialized services, and negotiate fees directly with healthcare providers.

It is difficult to get a sense of which way things will go, however. Somewhat anecdotally, in speaking to many medical students in 2008–2009, we find that many do wish to return to the earlier days where the physician can practice patient care. But others see a modern world as a business opportunity in which the group-practice head as primary care physician acts as not only a very basic shunting mechanism for dispensing patients to specialists, but also even more directly to junior members of the group practice or care consortium.

From a global perspective there are conflicts of philosophy about the way medical practitioners want to run their business. This is because private spending for healthcare services is increasing in the majority of countries, largely because the middle class grows and populations grow old as people get to live longer. Governments face intensified demands for better health treatments and so greater pressure on budgets. These issues have contributed to the popularity of US-style managed care schemes in the outside world even where foreign physicians are reluctant to accept the lower fees and decreased autonomy and flexibility. A look at international healthcare systems from region to region reveals differences in attitudes and approaches to those issues, not to mention strong resentment over US investment. Latin America remains the most promising region for US healthcare providers. Western Europe is a strong prospective market because of its affluence and large middle classes.

However, it has not increased its healthcare service opportunities commensurate with its potential. Restrictions on for-profit medical activity and a high state regulations of delivery systems discourage entrepreneurs.

We pause for one last warning. For those who like to extrapolate nice smooth curves over the years for economic trends, healthcare economics is complicated even in short-term projections where forecasts can be more predictable than in the long term. As in all business sectors, the economics of healthcare is not static. Neither is every aspect a gently rising curve. Premium rates usually follow a cycle. Historically a period of high profits in the industry usually is accompanied by low premium rates. At the time of writing, the industry is preparing for higher rates of premiums. As rates decreased through managed care, enrollment increased. Currently there is a debate about the changes needed in managed care, particularly in the areas of quality, accountability, access, and cost. One pivotal issue involves achieving a balance between patients' rights and reasonable profit for providers of healthcare services. In the next few years the number of home healthcare entities may shrink as a result of limited sources of funding; however, the number of nursing home patients will likely increase. Many government proposals made over the last few years, in many countries, are yet to be fully implemented at the time of writing, and could cause significant health–economic swings. They include extending Medicaid to cover more children and legal immigrants, providing more funding for biomedical research, enacting rules to protect consumers in managed care plans, and expanding health coverage to some 50 million uninsured persons. In the midst of the world economic slump, House leadership under new President Obama moved quickly to liberate additional funding over planned amounts by $4 to $5 billion for key scientific and engineering agencies as part of the latest economic stimulus package, now called the American Economic Recovery and Reinvestment Act of 2009. Similar developments are under way for medical research where that can generate economic wealth, but otherwise investment may be more in direct healthcare provision, say, in electronic health records and integrated medical systems. A healthcare part of the plan, crafted in January 2009, shows expectations to include $20 billion for health IT to jump-start investment in health IT, to curb healthcare costs, and to improve healthcare quality.

There has further been an issue in the United States allowing individuals who are approaching the age of 65 years to buy into Medicare. Recall that Medicare is one of the closer approaches the United States makes to a public welfare system. The program covers most people who are 65 and older but also some younger people with disabilities and people with end-stage kidney disease. Getting into Medicare is at the time of writing moderately complicated, however. When people sign up for Medicare, they get Part A, which covers hospital bills. Most people do not have to pay a monthly premium for Part A because they or their spouse paid Medicare taxes while they were working. Medicare Part B, which pays for doctor bills, is optional. They can sign up for Medicare Part B within eight months after they are no longer covered by group health insurance. Patients have to pay a monthly premium for Part B. They can sign up when they first go on Medicare, turn down the coverage, or wait to sign up at a later date if they are still working and already have group health insurance from the employer or spouse's employer. But, if they wait to sign up for Part B, the premium could go up by 10% for each year that they could have had Part B but did not. They will then pay that extra cost as long as they remain on Medicare. So they need to appreciate that they won't have to pay more for Part B if still working and covered by group health insurance when they sign up for Medicare Part B, but if they don't think they meet these conditions, they will have to pay more for Medicare Part B when they actually get it.

Well, it is not *too* complicated, but compare this with a fully public welfare system where Part A is "pay taxes on what you earn from age zero till you die," and Part B is "if sick, get cured." It would be nice if a holistic US health-care system could capture such all embracing simplicity. All things considered, however, the quality of what a holistic, information-based approach can deliver in any national context, ideally with an effort rendered transparently invisible by IT, is persuasive. Holistic healthcare transcends issues of capitalism and humanism, yet can serve and draw from both. Also it fundamentally extends the marketplace from a population of patients to include the currently healthy population to provide the broadest possible guidance respecting personal genomic, lifestyle, and diet preferences for those persons who want stay well, be fit, and even improve their health by utilizating all available information. As a bonus the associated IT reduces paperwork, bureaucracy, risks, errors, and litigation. It gives the physicians more time to do what they do well, and more time for patients to be well.

SOCIAL HEALTHCARE UNDER STRESS

The British newspapers such as the *Daily Mail* have been critics of the nastier aspects of otherwise worthy social medicine for decades, but clippings from 2005 to 2009 give a sorry account of how the health of the nation seems to be constantly getting hit from all sides. This, it may be recalled, was a nation that was still living stoically in the aftermath of two decades of veterinary and medical tragedy, for example, radioactive sheep pastures from the rains following the Chernobyl reactor disaster, outbreaks of Mad Cow disease (BSE, bovine spongiform encephalopathy) and foot and mouth disease, and the 2004 panic that BSE had spread back to sheep (from which it originally, as scrapie, had come). Concerning the health of our nation, and a snapshot of social health under stress may be newsworthy developments that have been brewing quietly for some time. Male infertility seems to be hitting an all time high, and infertility treatment is at an all time low. Obesity also seems to have hit a new high, and junk food is identified to be one of the main rising causes of type 2 diabetes. Heatwaves send air pollution to dangerous levels, increasing respiratory problems and straining the medical system; the heat even upsets the ecosystem, unleashing plagues of caterpillars reported to be toxic to the touch.

Clinical practice and physician competence have seemed to be in poor shape. In one news article, a physician was charged with prescribing huge doses of epilepsy drugs to some 700 children. In another article, a retired fireman with a broken hip lay neglected in a bed for more than a week; in surgery, which should have been performed within 24 hours, a blood clot that had formed in his legs traveled to his lungs and killed him. Crowded wards, lack of isolation facilities, and "high bed occupancy," where one patient arrives as the other leaves, were blamed for falling hygiene standards and overworked staff. Another article discussed how hospital managers put patients at risk through "slavish pursuit of government targets."

Far more devastating still, in terms of sheer numbers of patients hit, is the problem that hospital conditions have provided the catalyst for the rise of the so-called superbugs. "New" pathogens for which there has been little monitoring, like *Clostridium difficile*, which cause severe diarrhea, increased in 2005 nearly 44 times. Thirteen patients died of infection at a hospital in Exeter, New Hampshere. And these old enemies came back better armed. Another leading article raised concern about hygiene in hospitals and especially the presence of dangerous *methycillin-resistant Staphylococcus aureus* (MRSA) bacteria. The pathogen carries a plasmid or secondary chromosome with many defenses originally targeted against the world of weapons of fungi and heavy metals, and this plasmid can be donated directly to other Staphylococci. Since current medicine borrowed heavily from the chemical "ideas" evolved in the fungal armory, most drugs are ineffective. The problem in 2005 was 15 times worse than in 1992. One in 11 patients became infected, and 40% of hospitals were losing the battle with more than 300,000 patients infected in one year.

Will holistic medicine cure all this? Not, evidently, if we simply equate holistic healthcare with socialistic healthcare. The truth is, as stated above, that any healthcare system is amenable to an integrated, efficient, IT approach encompassing anything it takes to ensure well-being. But what, specifically, does this mean?

MORE SPECIFICALLY: THE HOLISTIC HEALTHCARE FUNCTION MODEL

The difficulty in all current medical systems is that information overload, the high human and financial costs of medical errors and adverse drug responses (ADRs), and the need for speed, mean that physicians cannot practice high-quality evidence-based medicine (see Chapter 10 for the increasingly popular formal form of this) unless they move toward having decision support systems at the point of care. Such IT will naturally render the system more holistic because it can collate all data. However, if we are to consciously and aggressively go for a holistic form of medicine, then the need to achieve a more intimate and extensive interaction with the patient clearly creates an even greater demand for information support technology.

A new breed of researcher has arisen to address the fundamental considerations about future healthcare systems based on IT. Such research requires thinking about the bits and pieces that comprise any healthcare structure, how they are linked together into a network, the workflow through that network, the nature of the information being transferred, and the guidelines and constraints on all of these. For example, the agricultural industry has toyed with automated management of complex flows for its agricultural research and development of engineered crops, including highly automated labs with robotics. Thanks to the universal character of living (and certainly eukaryotic, plant and animal) cells, some aspects of this look quite like data in medical labs, so exiting technology could easily be transposed, though sample sizes will in many cases doubtlessly differ.

One big problem the new researchers face is that the systems to be implemented will be large and complex, maybe tens of thousands of nodes and often with much more complexity going on inside. Because of the hard work and cost involved, not to mention some possible disruption of the organization it is seeking to automate, we need to design an IT system that will be robust and not have to be rebuilt from the ground up just because there is some administrative, legislative, resource, or standards change and, importantly, such that things will not fall apart just because in a practical world, rightly or wrongly, workers and workflows can deviate from set patterns and guidelines.

Thus several of these researchers have begun to think about designing "process-oriented healthcare information systems" that adjust naturally to changes in resources and organizational structures. Computer-interpretable models based on clinical workflows have already been implemented within the context of specific different fields, such as stroke and cancer therapy. A snapshot of part of an automated laboratory workflow is in Table 7.1.[2] These authors as well as others have considered special kinds of networks for healthcare workflow that issue simple reminders and serve as an organizer in a healthcare office environment in which duties are widely shared.

There, of course, remains the possibility that healthcare professionals may be noncompliant with guidelines for a variety of reasons, and that even workflows themselves may deviate. For this reason a general framework for *guideline-based* healthcare organization management has been proposed by Kumar, Smith, and Stefanelli, whereby work items are assigned to teams and to individuals. By guidelines we mean items like the National Institutes of Health hypertension guideline. By this guideline the tasks of hypertension management is divided into blood pressure measurement, classification of

---

[2] A good example for a more general workflow approach is in the paper "A General Framework for Implementation of Clinical Guidelines by Healthcare Organizations" by A. Kumar at the University of Pavia in Italy, B. Smith at the University of Leipzig in Germany, and M. Stefanelli also at the University of Pavia (this is a conference presentation, which may be downloaded at http://www.uni-leipzig.de/~akumar/aime_2003.pdf).

TABLE 7.1

WOKFLOW NODE = 86		
PROCESS = Receive approved samples for metabolic screening		
IN(1) = 55	CONTENT = stuff:lyophilized sample	CAPACITY = 0.2 gram
OUT(1) = 87	CONTENT = stuff:lyophilized sample	CAPACITY = 0.2 gram
STATE(1) INDICATES = saturated IS NOW = saturated		
IF = saturated ACTION = slowdown node 70		

WOKFLOW NODE = 87		
PROCESS = Weigh & Prepare samples (600 samples per day)		
IN(1) = 86	CONTENT = stuff:lyophilized sample	CAPACITY = 0.2 gram
OUT(1) = 88	CONTENT = stuff:lyophilized sample	CAPACITY = 0.2 gram
OUT(2) = 89	CONTENT = stuff:lyophilized sample	CAPACITY = 0.2 gram
STATE(1) INDICATES = saturated IS NOW = saturated		
IF = saturated ACTION = slowdown node 70		

WOKFLOW NODE = 88		
PROCESS = Store excess from sampling		
IN(1) = 88	CONTENT = stuff:lyophilized sample	CAPACITY = saturated
OUT(1) = 150	CONTENT = stuff:lyophilized sample	CAPACITY = saturated
STATE(1) INDICATES = saturated IS NOW = saturated		
IF = saturated ACTION = slowdown node 87		

WOKFLOW NODE = 89		
PROCESS = Extract Sample (2 ml) (2 systems)		
IN(1) = 89	CONTENT = stuff:lyophilized sample	CAPACITY = 3–4 samples/hour
OUT(1) = 90	CONTENT = stuff:extracted samples	CAPACITY = 3–4 samples/hour
STATE(1) INDICATES = saturated IS NOW = saturated		
IF = saturated ACTION = slowdown node 87		

blood pressure, and cardiovascular disease risk determination. These data are suborganized into classification of blood pressure, determination of major risk factors, and determination of target organ damage. The guidelines also include advice to the patient as to the benefits of lowering blood pressure, ambulatory blood pressure monitoring, self-measurement of blood pressure, patient evaluation, treatment, management of special situations with hypertension, improving hypertension control, and community program management.

Besides such a framework as conceived by the above-mentioned authors, the realizations of workflow processes may deviate from the norms set forth in the process definitions themselves. In line with the proposed stratified implementation, designers can define different levels at which an organization's implementation of the clinical guidelines can be described.

A hierarchical view is need to achieve the stratification. The concept of hierarchy is in fact a common feature of thinking about systems, so it is worth pursuing what Kumar, Smith, and Stefanelli were thinking as an example of what this means. The hierarchy is a tree-shaped graph that has several main components of a typical health organization or institution, namely its *physical structures*, its *human resources, the tasks capable of being performed by these human resources,* and *the tasks recommended in the guidelines themselves.*

The hierarchal systems approach is a general but useful way primarily for describing the workings of an institution such as hospital. Such an institution can be split up into tree branches for different departments such as internal medicine, surgery, and cardiology. The department of internal medicine, for example, may then be further subdivided into outpatient wards, procedure room, inpatient wards, intensive care unit, and so forth. This hierarchical structure can persist down through teams and individuals in the organization, and through them to the level of tasks. The healthcare teams in the organization might consist of internal medicine team A, internal medicine team B, general surgery team, cardiology team, and so on. Then in turn, internal medicine team A might itself consist of physician, resident C, resident D, nursing staff E, nursing staff F, nursing student G, and so on. For each team the tasks performed by human resources can be divided into diagnostic procedures, therapeutic procedures, and so on. Diagnostic procedure can be further subdivided into medical history taking, physical examination, laboratory procedures, as necessary.

For the overall healthcare system, say of an entire state or nation, we can benefit from the hierarchical approach, but this should not be excessively detailed. Imagining a more general flowchart type of network rather than a tree, seems to work better at the larger level. Of course, this can include the tree-structured organizations of institutions, with trees made into graphs by cross-linking some points in the tree. In any event, the idea of breaking things down into well-defined bits and pieces that communicate with each other works well.

For the larger healthcare picture could enable a holistic approach, the "healthcare function model" is a model used by several researchers. It enumerates system components (defined as services) as precisely as possible. Since the healthcare domain services depend on the healthcare model (e.g., open vs. closed, public vs. private) and organizational structure, among other things, it is a challenge to provide an exhaustive list of services, but we list below the components that are compatible with the most holistic view.

The "healthcare function model" of a patient-centric, wellness-oriented, and outcome-driven healthcare system for holistic management of healthcare with continuum of service can be categorized into two sets of services: (1) cross-domain horizontal services and (2) domain-specific vertical services.

> The horizontal services include (but are not limited to) demographic registries, services for dynamic construction of lifetime personal health record, electronic health record management services, global person identification services, clinical and financial data integration services, information management services, electronic collaboration services, clinical decision services, and interdisciplinary coordination services.

> The vertical domain services include (but are not limited to) clinical event management services, ADT services, diagnostic information sharing services, provider office system services, pharmacare services, telemedicine and telesurgery services, continuing or community care services, and public health and surveillance services.

- The *telemedicine and telesurgery services* are, with leverage of telecommunications and computing technologies, to provide delivery of healthcare at a distance.
- The *provider office system services* provide integrated productivity tools for healthcare service providers such as physicians and nurses. It consists of electronic visit panel, examination panel, electronic diagnostic panel, electronic procedure panel, electronic prescription panel, personal health record, electronic mail, and calendar, among other services.
- The *continuing or community care services* are to identify the requirements associated with supporting the delivery of services in a larger community setting.
- The *clinical event management services* are to identify and integrate the initial, minimum, person specific, service event data to be shared among healthcare service providers from clinical services.
- The *pharmacare services* are to optimize drug prescribing and dispensing by integrating electronic communication among physicians, pharmacists, and service recipients; providing access to online drug interaction checking and guidelines; generating electronic prescriptions and real-time claims adjudication.
- The *public health and surveillance* services are to identify the requirements for monitoring population health and surveillance to support the prevention, promotion and protection of population health.

- The *diagnostic information-sharing* services are to integrate the results generated and reported from diagnostic service events into the personal health record in order to expedite the sharing of this information among healthcare service providers, and permit access to laboratory results to healthcare service providers and other approved healthcare professionals.

- The *interdisciplinary coordination services* are to provide the capability to support coordination of service delivery among providers, program areas, and across regional boundaries for the utilization and contribution to aspects of the personal health record.

- The *clinical decision services* are *to* provide evidence-based decision-making activities by all levels of healthcare professionals within the health system at the point of care. Its tools include, among others, diagnosis, prognosis, critical paths, clinical practice guidelines and standards of care. The care providers, the recipients of care, insurers, and policy makers will all benefit from the results of informed decision making.

- The *clinical and financial data integration services* enable associating financial data (resource consumption and utilization data) with each specific clinical service event (e.g., involving beds, facilities, and equipment). Data will be used by policy makers to support financial administration and planning.

- *Longitudinal electronic health records* as the term is often used not only to the reference to the digital patient record but also to imply capture and abstraction of clinical data. It may include the ability to encode (categorize) diagnosis and procedures.

- *Dynamic construction of lifetime personal health record* is a function that manages the dynamical assembly of the digital patient record out of relevant personal health information retrieved from many (e.g., laboratory) sources. It is intended to be life long, longitudinal (i.e., all events) and cumulative over time. Access to personal health record by healthcare service providers and service recipients will be controlled for confidentiality and protection of privacy in areas and to levels conditional on the viewers' professional role.

- The *demographic registries* establish and provide secure shared access to appropriate information about stakeholders, service providers and organizations, and delivery sites. They administer common unique identifiers that can be used to uniquely identify the individual stakeholders across the health system.

The following list provides typical clinical support applications that can be integrated with the health informatics solution for decision support and outcome analysis. The applications that exist throughout the regional health authority jurisdictions can be categorized as follows:

Radiology/diagnostic imaging refers to support of the administration, image requisition, reporting (clinical interpretation), film management, and workload reporting for radiology and diagnostic imaging departments.

Pharmacy applications is that set of application modules that provides support for tracking the drug inventory, the formulary, and distribution, including manufacture and reporting.

Order entry is the generic description for a focused application set that provides generalized requisition facilities to a number of backend functions (laboratory, pharmacy, diagnostic imaging, purchasing, etc.).

Laboratory applications support the administration, specimen handling, reporting and interfacing to laboratory instruments that support the operations of a clinical laboratory.

Results reporting refers to a broad arena of reporting results from the labs, diagnostics imaging reports, transcribed clinical reports, and so on, when they do not fit more specifically into those categories.

OR scheduling includes both the automation of the operating room with attendant scheduling, physician times. It generally includes the entry of basic clinical information as well as the capture of workload statistical data for subsequent reporting.

Dietary/nutrition applications cater for bed tray management and recording of special diets. Inventory management, purchasing, and recipe management as part of the functionality may typically be included.

Nurse workstation/ward refers to any application facility that is specifically designed for the use of nursing staff, including bed management for ADT, flowcharting, nursing care plans, and nurse staffing systems.

Physician-specific system refers to any application that is specifically designed for the use of physicians such as physician ordering systems, review of patient data, and physician sign-in systems.

Homecare applications refer to any functions related to activities of homecare clinicians. Examples include intake systems, and the recording of vitals and nursing plans and reports. Under this rubric fall also clinical prescription data, and workload data. However, all these data are only in regard to the home care environment.

Long-term care refers to any functions related to the clinical or administrative duties carried out in a long-term care environment (but not generalized acute care or other administrative applications that just happen coincidentally to be used by long-term care facilities).

Community care refers primarily to those applications involved with the operations of the Health Units or Community Mental Health clinics. Issues included are intake, workload, and features capture of immunization data and mental health information.

ADT/CPI is relates to the recording of *admission, discharge, and transfer* movements of patients and the use of a personal health identifier in a way consistent of to preserve unique identification across many interactions with the patient ("encounters") within the healthcare system. This often includes bed management aspects, although they may also be treated separately.

Staff scheduling relates to those applications that support the maintenance of appropriate levels and mix of staff. It considers the patient load, the required staffing mix, and staff rotations while noting availability. It may also consider time entry for payroll purposes.

Patient scheduling relates to those applications that provide for registering and subsequent planning of events (consult schedule, X-ray room and time slots, laboratory collection times, etc.) related to the provision of health services to a patient or client.

Nursing workload measurement are those applications designed to capture nursing workload data by time (or via standardized time) measurements. These systems normally are functionally based around nursing tasks. This category also includes the *reporting functions* for nursing workload.

In addition administrative functions are required to enable the sharing of information and computational resources among all stakeholders of the health system. The key administration functions are to (1) plan and manage healthcare activities, (2) facilitate communication among stakeholders, (3) manage healthcare infrastructure, (4) manage information, (5) facilitate information management standards development, and (6) evaluate effectiveness of sharing the health information.

FUTURE SCENARIO EXAMPLES

When Howard Carter punched an eye-hole into the tomb of Tutankhamen, and was asked what he saw, he said "Wonderful things!" Sometimes a glimpse of the world of our ancestors deserves more respect than a glimpse of the present or immediate future, and this is so with holistic medicine. A glimpse into the most immediate future will not necessarily show dazzlingly "wonderful things," but we can at least hope for a system where there is better clinical decision intelligence, and more efficient hospital conditions that can prevent blood clots, superbugs, and many other woes. Over time holistic healthcare should lead to better informed and more effective handling of public health. Indeed is the scenano described below a patient's relapse might have never occurred if physicians had the whole picture. However, the scenarios help us think in the right direction, and about vast improvement over our present circumstances. If we cannot deliver the ability to envision scenarios with immediate applications for a troad holistic framework, we will not deliver such a holistic framework.

It is inevitable that in the near future holistic healthcare will have very specific implications for management of hospital treatments, and all the multiple interactions handled for each individual patient. IT systems will be basically charged with integrating all information that humans (not yet devices and robots or tiny submicroscopic machines) provide. This aspect of holism IT will most easily provide.

But say in our glimpse into the near future a young child living in a rural area begins to experience severe breathing problems. Her mother calls an emergency line (in North America, 911). The emergency operator contacts the nearest physician on call. After learning about the symptoms of the child, the physician signs on to the new healthcare system and, with the mother's consent, accesses the child's lifetime health records online from the physician office system at his office. He learns that the child has a history of asthma-related illness and also has serious reactions to certain kinds of medications. He again checks online the medications she is currently taking and rules out the possibility of drug-related problems. He then contacts a specialist at the Sick Children's Hospital over the network, and in collaboration they view her symptoms and history. Together, they decide that the child be airlifted to the Sick Children's Hospital. Within half an hour, the child is transported to the Sick Children's Hospital. While on board, her symptoms are monitored continuously and transmitted to the attending physician at the hospital. *When the child arrives, the attending physicians and nurses at the hospital emergency room are already familiar with all her previous health history and know the current symptoms.* The hospitals are clean and not crowded, and with constant antipathogen monitoring; the staff are alert, and smoothly running tests so that *there is no delay in treatment. The attending physician at the hospital emergency room, though, is uncertain about some of the symptoms. Through the new healthcare system he connects with both the original specialist who was involved and an asthma specialist at the nearby university hospital. He relays the critical information about the child's condition over the network, and quickly receives the specialist's advice. With that information, he prescribes a new medication. Treatment begins and the child quickly begins to recover. After a short stay in hospital, the child is well enough to go home.* Information about the child's new medication and recommended follow-up treatment is available through the new healthcare system to the child's family doctor, the specialists, the pharmacists, and her parents wherever they are.

Now we can consider a slightly more advanced scenario. The physician's office receives a call, and the receptionist schedules an appointment online. The patient encounter is registered by reading the patient ID embedded in the microchip in a smartcard or implanted under the skin of an arm. Patient identity and eligibility are validated. The patient goes to the examination room: the nurse records the "vitals" and adds to patient's office health record via electronic data capture along with speech recognition. The paramedic or physician reviews the patient's health record and obtains an authorized view of the patient's integrated health record to assess history. The patient is assessed, using an appropriate treatment plan. The physician accesses the references of interest online, makes initial diagnosis, and records these into an electronic visit record. An ECG (electrocardiogram) and lab work, including lab instructions, are requested by voice dictation. The receptionist provides information about the locations of the diagnostic laboratories. The patient chooses one at a convenient location, goes to the diagnostic laboratory, and gets tests performed.

Behind the scenes the family physician receives a notice that the ECG (electrocardiogram) results are in the patient's integrated health record and a notice when the results of blood test are available, and reviews results when they are complete (or optionally, while in progress if multiple steps). The physician finds that the tests reveal reduced arterial flow, completes and records diagnosis via voice dictation, establishes a treatment plan with reference information accessed, and a drug is identified. Next, allergies and drug interactions are checked, with some reference to the patient's genomic data. The appropriate drugs are authorized for dispensing online. A referral is created to a cardiovascular health condition program for follow-up, and the need and timing of next visit by patient is confirmed. The physician or an assistant identifies patient education resources and contacts patient to discuss results, diagnosis, care plan, and follow-up visits. The patient is informed of the results, diagnosis, drug, cardiovascular program, and availability of education and reference material. The time of the next visit is confirmed, and submission of the claim is authorized. The logistics and inevitable financials, including reconciling claim payment, is dealt with.

Things will sometimes go wrong. The following illustrates another hypothetical scenario of a more complex case. It describes the activities and events from different perspectives, such as from the perspective of patient, physician, acute care unit manager and regional health authority. It then briefly describes the events occurred behind scenes. The hypothetical scenario starts with a citizen experiencing some mild chest pain while at home, tries simple remedies (e.g., antacid, Tylenol), but pain persists. This scenario starts with the patient perspective.

The patient calls family physician's office and is instructed to come in that afternoon. She arrives at physician's office, activates personal health card (e.g., a smart card is activated by the patient's thumb print), hands it over to the receptionist; the RFID microchip in the health card is activated by the reader at the physician's office and the electronic patient record is open. The patient is shown to the examination room; a nurse takes vital signs captured via an electronic data capture system including voice dictation. The family physician sees her and orders an ECG (electrocardiogram) test. The patient sees the receptionist; the receptionist finds the laboratories nearest to her home; gives her the addresses of two nearest laboratories. The patient goes to the nearest diagnostic laboratory. The RFID microchip in the health card is activated by the reader at the laboratory; ECG (electrocardiogram) is performed, blood is drawn (test location records ECG results, notifies physician of ECG completion), and the specimen is sent to a second location. The patient waits at home for a call from her family physician. The blood sample arrives at the second location; tests are completed and results added to health record and sent to family physician. The family physician reviews results and makes diagnosis. The patient is called by family physician, who informs the patient that she has angina and explains the cardiovascular health program to be used for follow-up, prescribes a drug, describes its benefits and effects, and suggests a follow-up visit. A follow-up notice postdated is in the schedule for a phone call or another visit. The patient goes to a pharmacy of choice where her identifier in the RFID microchip in the health card is read (verifies identity and eligibility). The pharmacist checks drug interactions and allergies, dispenses drug, and prints label and instructions. The patient goes home and takes the drug. Things seem to go well. There is an apparent positive outcome for patient. The drug chosen was effective. The repeat ECG (electrocardiogram) and blood work showed improvement. There was adequate correction to diet and stress was modified. An exercise regime was followed, and the patient returns to work.

Unfortunately, some months later, the same patient collapses with severe chest pain while at her home in a rural location; her husband calls 911. The patient's husband is advised what to do by a nurse, who was connected through by the 911 operator, while an ambulance is on its way; her card not readily available, so secondary identification is processed. Assessment and initial treatment are performed; the patient is transported to the closest hospital with appropriate and available services. She arrives at the emergency in a rural regional hospital, moved to treatment room, and testing/procedures are performed. The patient's husband confirms registration information. The patient is stabilized in the emergency room and then admitted and moved to the cardiac care unit (CCU); a key person is assigned to facilitate liaison with the family and communicates her role to patient and family. Sadly, the condition deteriorates; consequently the rural hospital physician contacts an urban cardiologist for consultation via the *telehealth* infrastructure. The cardiologist reviews electronic record; the cardiologist collaborates with the rural physician and a liaison officer. A diagnosis reached: coronary artery occlusion. Surgery is urgently required. The family physician discusses options with the patient and her husband, recommends and receives patient consent to an innovative new procedure, which is available only at a tertiary-care hospital in another region (air ambulance is scheduled). The liaison officer discusses the surgery and transfer by air ambulance of the patient and her husband; the patient is transported by air to tertiary-care hospital and admitted. Surgery is performed (the innovative new cardiovascular bypass surgery). The patient is moved to recovery room, then to cardiac care unit for monitoring. The cardiologist, in collaboration with rural team, prepares postoperative treatment plan, drug prescriptions, transfer back to rural hospital, and so forth. Patient is transferred by ambulance back to rural hospital medical surgical unit for recovery. The liaison officer reviews the health record and treatment plan. The patient's family physician and liaison officer collaborate to establish ongoing rehabilitation/treatment/home support plan. The liaison officer communicates with patient and family, discusses patient selection of options available and the discharge plan, including an assessment for home care with consideration of insurance coverage. The patient is discharged and returns home. She receives assessment visit, and home care resources are coordinated. The patient receives home care by various providers. The patient gets reminders of routine follow-up provided by local cardiovascular rehabilitation program and checks with the physician.

The kinds of scenarios discussed above are those used by healthcare administrators with IT specialists to plan the healthcare system of the future. We will not labor the reader by putting in prose form every possible scenario, nor every possible perspective of each scenario, which is also very important to do. In fact the healthcare and IT experts help develop and look at a rather stylized presentation of each scenario, represented by a *workflow* or *protocol* that is very like a computer program, although it will (at least in the near future) have humans executing many of the steps. We won't present them as workflow diagrams, meaning primarily that we won't describe things like "do this if that happens, and do that if it doesn't." As with the prose above, we'll assume a linear sequence of steps in which we nail down what happens so that the branch points aren't an issue.

CAN SYSTEMS BIOLOGY FORM THE PHILOSOPHICAL BASIS OF A HEALTHCARE SYSTEM?

As discussed previously, *systems biology* is one of the most frequently cited terms these days in the academic medical research community, the biotechnology industry and the pharmaceutical industry, not to mention at those healthcare cocktail parties. It is well anticipated as a general consensus across academic, biotechnology, and pharmaceutical industry sectors that systems biology will "revolutionize" our understanding of specific diseases and radically improve treatment of such diseases, and subsequently prevent illness and help us realize the concept of preventative medicine for wellness-oriented healthcare. It implies a holistic view of the patient as a hierarchical collection of systems from organs through cells down to molecules, and concentrates on how all components work together. This also implies possibility of extension to a larger hierarchical system, healthcare itself, in which the hierarchical structure that we call the patient resides.

Can we really use a systems biology definition as that for *systems healthcare* as laid out in Chapter 4. Not all even agree? In the industry about a definition of systems biology. Dr. Leroy Hood, who is a co-founder of the Institute for Systems Biology (ISB) and is widely regarded as the founding pioneer of modern systems biology, has defined systems biology as "the study of all the elements in a biological system (all genes, mRNAs, proteins, etc.) and their relationships one to another in response to perturbations." This has little extensibility to embrace the entire healthcare system. But other definitions of systems biology are much more encompassing than what is defined by Dr.

Hood. Assorted definitions are captured in the following amalgam: "systems biology is the science of integrating genetic, genomic, biochemical, cellular, physiological, and clinical data to create a system network that can be used to predictively model a biological event(s)."

This definition is close to an IT-based view. But for holism we can still modify it just slightly: "systems healthcare is the science and practice of integrating genetic, genomic, biochemical, cellular, physiological, clinical, and socioeconomic data to create a system network that can be used to predictively model and take best action on medical events."

Part of the difficulty in defining systems biology lies in the fact that it is perhaps more appropriate to consider systems biology as a process rather than a new subdiscipline of modern biology. As we noted previously, it is the integration of "-omic" as well as clinical, physiological, and imaging measurements that is central to the paradigm shift of systems biology. But healthcare is very much a process, and essentially a hierarchical system that is in continuum with the hierarchy of human biology.

The systems concept as we have seen has been around for several thousands of years in Eastern medicine. The ancient view typically stratifies the patient into about five categories, in consideration of the metabolomics of the whole organism of human being in his or her environment as opposed to our Western approach, which is concerned more about individual organs.

Eastern medicine categorizes patients as water type, fire type, tree type, earth type, and iron type, and by a continuum of interdependency among them: water puts out fire, which burns tree, which grows on earth, which decomposes iron, which tames water, all in the form of a circle. Patient stratification is not based on gene expression analyses, SNP (genomic biomarker) analyses, protein analyses, or metabolome analyses, or advanced medical imaging. It is done based on the patterns of the heart beats felt by the Asian doctors on the patient's wrist or neck. Sometimes, the patient's birth year, date, and time are considered in conjunction with the heart beat. The herbal medicine is so prescribed that the individual patient's genotypic and phenotypic characteristics within the patient's stratification (e.g., water type, fire type, tree type, earth type, and iron type) are considered for high efficacy on an individual basis. It may not be overly exaggerated to claim that Eastern medicine has been providing personalized medicine based on the concept of the systems biology for several thousands of years, although the theoretical background has not been fully explained and articulated. For example, almost all herbal medicine prescribed for a patient includes some amount of ginseng (or insam) as it is proved to be the most effective booster of the human immune system, except for the "fire-type" patients who will adversely respond to ginseng.

As in Eastern medicine, Systems biology aims to understand the human organism from holistic view point, and to diagnose and treat illness with consideration of individual's genotypic and phenotypic variances and lifestyle characteristics. Asian doctors prescribe personalized (herbal) medicine for each patient. They do not prescribe one-fits-all type of medicine except for treatment of external injuries. However, systems healthcare can be achieved only with consideration of the IT. The ideal form of systems biology calls for very precise descriptions that would be, for the most part, broadly utilized by the full hierarchy of systems healthcare.

While we think that the systems biology view can be extended to include the healthcare system, we left the jargon of systems biology and systems theory in general partly intact for comparison. We do not attempt at the details of the healthcare workflow process in extrapolation because in systems biology the human, animal, and plant metabolism and physiology is even more complex than the healthcare system. Although our account is sketchy, it provides a plausible top-down healthcare architecture, and hints at what a deeper systems analysis would give. In the more ambitious picture, family, friends, pets (as domestic companions), colleagues, religious ministers, counselors, financial advisors, and other players in the patient's life and lifestyle, are not just data but dynamic components within the big system description.

A CHALLENGING HOLISTIC CONCLUSION

Holism has a vital role in pursuit of health and well-being. It is an ancient view to which we must return, and now that it is possible through IT. Holistic medicine is personalized medicine because it considers the impact of diverse factors that make us unique. A system that takes care of us all must adopt principles, however, that embrace a variety of tastes and personal beliefs about what constitutes the universe and our place and well-being in it. In the past, holism was practiced *within* cultures and ethnic groups, or within a limited number of cultures. We need now a system that can embrace all such knowledge. It will be a challenge. We are obliged to architect a system with enough power, flexibility, and respect for our individuality that will allow us to adapt to and conquer the challenges of that journey.

8

ARCHITECTING IT ALL

The difficulty lies, not in the new ideas, but in escaping the old ones.
—John Maynard Keynes, British economist

A PROBLEM SHARED, DISTRIBUTED DATA AS YET UNSHARED, AND KNOWLEDGE FROM IT

We would like to share our problem with you. Writing this book has taken us years. Of course, we have our everyday jobs to do. The interesting thing is that these jobs often consisted of *unexpectedly* helping build the very things that we were writing about as future healthcare needs. Almost every time that we sat down and started predicting what we thought would be needed in two to five years, somebody wanted it right now, and even though they would typically have no idea what we were writing. The time lag between starting a new IT theme in the book and someone actually wanting it has notably shortened over three years. Some of these tasks would be big jobs, requiring "burning the midnight oil" for many weeks or months, taking us away from the book, and giving a growing sense that we could never catch us with the rate at which not just ours but many people's dreams were crystallizing into reality. In many ways the book became a diary of the evolution of thinking and of the IT market place, though the thematic structures of the chapters hide that as a sequential flow.

The Engines of Hippocrates: From the Dawn of Medicine to Medical and Pharmaceutical Informatics, by Barry Robson and O.K. Baek
Copyright © 2009 by John Wiley & Sons, Inc.

The advantage, in principle, is that we could remove those things that turned out to be off track. In hindsight, however, there is nothing of significance that we can think of that was removed. Our errors as far as the IT part is concerned would be occasionally in overestimating when things would actually happen, and most often in underestimating that. In some cases it would be a mixture of the two. For example, while the explosion of clinical, genomic, proteomic, and particular medical imaging data is happening, and may even accelerate beyond our expectations, the means of sharing that data for global medical benefit is being slower to develop, even though there are technological means to overcome the issues of geographical distance and communication network bandwidth, and means of keeping confidential data on site but abstracting general principles for the common good.

We will describe aspects of that in this chapter in terms of data-centric models of computing, where we are sticking out our necks a little more as to what form the solution will take. The solution covers the case of *translational research* (rapidly capturing medical research data such as new genomics) for speedy incorporation into clinical, healthcare administrative, and pharmaceutical decision making. It must cover also the integration of many bodies for epidemiological purposes, as described in Chapter 9. Importantly it must also cover the case of the collection of data from physicians and patients to feed back information to pharmaceutical companies and the FDA, or equivalent national body, as to how pharmaceutical drugs are behaving (*pharmacovigilance*), for relationship to genomics (*pharmacogenomics*), for new applications of existing marketed or research pipeline drugs (the *"Viagra break"*), and for better assigning the cost of drugs (*drug pricing*). Similar feedback issues arise and are arising right now in assessing the worth of surgical procedures and new kinds of medical equipment, including stents, and more generally about the most successful means of diagnosis, prediction, and assessment of risk. These diverse applications all share the common themes of being widely dispersed heterogeneous data with issues of privacy and security. There is commonality also in that the work of physicians with their patients is a kind of translational research in a sense, a vast and continuing clinical trial because that has been the eternal nature of medicine, reflected in the Hippocratic theme of acquiring and passing on new knowledge. Since the ancient days of village medicine with high physician-to-patient ratios, however, much of that knowledge has not been captured.

The theme of knowledge itself has also emerged with increasing pace in recent IT solutions, and must be explored. Much work has also been going on to highly automate the R&D workflows of pharmaceutical and biopharmaceutical companies, which must also join with the business decision process and the data from translational research and from patients. The automatic extraction of information from millions of patents is a recent exciting example of the kind of information flowing in. The problem of concern to the life science industries is that even the smooth joining of diverse heterogeneous data does not in fact produce knowledge but just more nicely collated data.

Data federation systems with query interfaces do allow the human being to extract the knowledge using the invaluable natural computer between his or her ears, but the veritable tsunami of data that is starting to pour in exhausts the number of experts and the time that they have to do such a chore.

There is thus a growth of interests in *knowledge-centric systems* or some other term that inevitably includes the word *knowledge*. To get IT to handle that with a high degree of hands-off automation, however, begs the question of what *knowledge* is. It seems at first glance remarkable that there is no agreed simple answer. Dictionaries such as the *Oxford English Dictionary* variously define knowledge as (1) expertise, and skills acquired through experience or education and the theoretical or practical understanding of a subject, (2) what is known in a particular field or in total, or (3) awareness or familiarity gained by experience. According to the current entry in the Internet's Wikipedia, there is no single agreed definition of knowledge presently, nor any prospect of one, and there remain numerous competing theories. It preoccupied the ancient Greeks, as with Plato's description of knowledge as "justified true belief." Aristotle in his *Posterior Analytics* said: "We suppose ourselves to possess unqualified scientific knowledge of a thing, as opposed to knowing it in the accidental way in which the sophist knows, when we think that we know the cause on which the fact depends, as the cause of that fact and of no other, and, further, that the fact could not be other than it is. Now that scientific knowing is something of this sort is evident—witness both those who falsely claim it and those who actually possess it, since the former merely imagine themselves to be, while the latter are also actually, in the condition described. Consequently the proper object of unqualified scientific knowledge is something which cannot be other than it is." (E. L. Allen, *From Plato to Nietzsche* (New York: Fawcett Books, 1988), and H. Treddenick, *Notes and Appendices to Aristotle's Ethics*, J. Barnes, ed., J. A. K. Thomson, trans. (New York: Penguin, 1976)).

From the statements above it is clear that most thinkers in the field would consider that the developments to be described later fail to capture and utilize the full answer as to what knowledge is. The sense in that field is, however, that steps are being made in the right direction. There is much to be built that is pressingly needed without needing to understand the true nature of knowledge, because at least we know it when we see it. And the idea anyway is that currently emerging systems architectures as health informatics solutions and biomedical informatics solutions will provide the essential bedrock for what comes next.

Moreover, by building our structures and seeing how they weather the sunshine and hurricanes of real experience, building for healthcare will become a living and evolving experiment that will converge slowly to the answer. Clearly, thousands of years of philosophical, mathematical, and pure scientific contemplation has not. So then what chance has the computer systems engineer of succeeding when these basic disciplines on which engineering is founded have failed to academically qualify the nature of knowledge?

Computers handle it and enable it, but knowledge is still the mysterious beast that somehow they help manage, tame, and even farm, but cannot *harness* 100% without human experts.

But who said anything about engineers? A computer systems *architect* is not a computer systems engineer, who in turn is not a computer scientist. They work together and talk together, but they are not the same thing. As human thought resides in the systems architecture of the brain and its flux and flow of information, not in the details and neuronal fabric of it, so computer systems *architects* may pave the way. Architecting is a larger, broader, extended, and creative pursuit.

ARCHITECTURE IS A COMBINED DISCIPLINE OF ART, SCIENCE, AND ENGINEERING

The term "architecture" has many definitions and means different things depending on the context. Words like "art" and "style" frequently appear to cautiously hedge the definition. The *Merriam-Webster Dictionary* defines "architecture" as the art or science of building something; the formation or construction as the result of conscious act; or, specifically for IT, the manner in which the components of a computer or computer system are organized and integrated. The former of these emphasizes the process of achieving the latter. In the latter case we can speak of "an architecture." The *Oxford English Dictionary* favors that sense and defines the term as follows: (1) the art or practice of designing and constructing buildings; (2) the style in which a building is designed and constructed; (3) the complex structure of something. For IT, "an architecture" is the conceptual structure and overall logical organization of a computer or computer-based system from the point of view of its use or design. For the financial aspect of IT, an architecture is a set of investment principles with advanced mitigation of potential business and technical risks.

In simple but more tangible terms, *systems architecture, information technology architecture*, or usually just *IT architecture,* is the description of just how computers, their application software, middleware components used by the application software, operating systems, their databases, peripheral devices, and their networks fit together and work with each other. An information technology architect is the person who works that out in a broader and extended scope and perspectives. The architecture he or she conceives is less concerned with the bolts and nuts of the underlying infrastructure, but more concerned about the overall processes and functions from a holistic view point. Holism "rules supreme" in the architecting of knowledge systems, limited only by the extent of holism needed in the data being processed.

Like all architecture, there is a blueprint. A simple "systems architecture" diagram of the kind that one might show in a slide for a slideshow presentation might have about a dozen boxes, or sometimes many more, joined by lines with arrows. IT architecture defines the key components of hardware and software, their structures and behavior, and the relationships and interactions among the components, such as component functions and behavior, relationships among components, placement of components on individual computer nodes, geographical distribution of components, management domains of components, interactions among the components, interfaces between components, network connections and topologies, and communication protocols. But solutions architecture is not just all that: the solutions architect must meet the needs of the stakeholders in terms of the human interfaces for human users, machine interfaces for robotic instruments and modalities, performance behaviors and response times, availability, accessibility, security, usability, reliability, privacy, and so forth! By "stakeholders" here we mean anyone legitimately involved in interacting with the system and each other, but in the specific context of healthcare it means the same as it did earlier: patients, physicians, health insurance companies, policy makers, researchers, and so on.

Not all the people involved in helping build the edifice are architects in that sense. There are, of course, the builders or assemblers who must actually pull together parts of the computers, install the machines, wire them up, install the software, and run tests. Others are variously *strategists* who plan how to get things moving in the hope of ever having an IT-based healthcare system at all, and *algorithmists* who design new classes of computer program for specific parts of the healthcare information flow, such as data-mining patient records (see the next chapter). *Programmers* or *coders* will then build (implement) the algorithms as computer programs, and an algorithmist can often code his or her own software; although usually it is a rather rough, unstable research code that a programmer will subsequently harden to industrial strength. Computer software that is less variable and closely related to realizing the IT architecture by bridging application software with the underlying operating system and/or communication network is called *middleware*. Those more replaceable are called *applications*. Generally speaking, neither *algorithmists* nor *programmers* would ever consider describing themselves as a computer architect. Nonetheless, all of us, from time to time, have to play at being a computer architect. We have to be able to read and even write at least a simple system architecture diagram, and such diagrams crop up everywhere.

Although once implemented in an organization the IT architecture is less variable than the applications that it runs, it can vary dramatically among organizations. Typically there is no one kind of standard architecture to fit every kind of organization. The architecture varies with the philosophy and practices of the organization, which is why we do not have systems in standard packages but have system architects to design them based on the problems to be solved and the business needs to be addressed. The elements to be manipulated, and hence the tasks of the IT architect at the finer level of detail, are legion. He or she needs to define where data are stored, how data can be transformed for a unified access, what the security and privacy rules need to be adhered to for access to those data, what tools and algorithms are required to process the data, where those tools and programmed algorithms can run most efficiently, what data are required by the tools and programs as input and in what format, what data are produced by the applications and in what format, how those tools and algorithms interact with other related tools, how they interact with the external systems or external collaborators, where the firewalls are placed, what security rules the firewalls must be configured for, and many other things.

Following the above, the discipline of IT architecture can now be defined a bit more fully as the art, craft, and science of *determining the needs of the users and stakeholders*, and of planning and building the conceptual structure and overall logical organization of autonomic functional components and processes, and relationships among the components, to meet those needs as effectively as possible. It is also the approach and methodology associated with planning and realization of the functional components and processes. A typical IT architecture so crafted includes (but is not limited to) architecture principles, business process model, business function model, information model, component model, security model, operational model, system management policy, and deployment and migration strategy. It provides (1) a detailed business model, process, policies, rules and requirements for an integrated business solution; (2) a definition of functional building blocks of a business solution based on a technical translation and interpretation of business objectives and requirements; (3) a definition of relationships among the functional building blocks of a business solution and the boundary interfaces; (4) implementation guidelines for quality and integrity; and (5) architecture management and governance process for currency and vitality of the architectures.

While these engineering guidelines sound solid and pretty down-to-earth, with little room for the creative touch, the word "art" is used a lot. Despite our preference for a good mix as described above, quite often it is debated whether the discipline of being an architect, IT architect or otherwise, is a science or an art. In fact many IT problems are not pre-definable as to exact solution; there are countless ways even to write the underlying software, and the architect, designer, and programmer will leave an inevitable stamps of style and taste. While the architect needs the scientific disciplines for the quality and integrity of the architectures created, he or she also needs the innovation and novelty of art for its flexibility and adaptability to future changes. Where does creativity and innovation come in? The IT architect must go in and analyze the business or scientific needs before they craft the IT system. This role relates to the older term "systems analyst." Correct interpretation of these needs can itself be an art, but the particular way that the system is crafted to meet that interpretation may require a particular high level of creativity. It is rather like the way a painter *interprets* a subject. If there is such scope for interpretation, does it follow that there can be good and bad architectures. Sure! Some solutions may be less elegant, harder to maintain, and more difficult to update than others. For example, some IT systems are easier than others to evolve into new architectures to meet evolving needs. An old system with which an organization is stuck is the legacy or "white elephant" system.

Also in considering good and bad architectures whether they are of buildings or computer systems, there is a concept of *balance*. A good IT architecture must be balanced and optimized for maximum business values as well as technical advantages, also in consideration of the organizational dynamics of people.

The main themes for development of a "sound" IT architecture include (1) usability for intuitive and personalized interfaces as natural as possible to human behavior, (2) accessibility through various communication channels and devices, (3) performance for peak volumes, (4) scalability to future growth, (5) availability for access at any time and at any place as per the business needs, (6) reliability, (7) manageability for business continuity with minimal human intervention, (8) flexibility and adaptability to future business and technology changes, (9) adherence to security policies, (10) compliance to the statutory requirements for protection of privacy, and (11) viability for development and deployment in a reasonable time and at a reasonable cost with minimal risks, among others.

A BALANCED VIEW OF ART, SCIENCE, AND ENGINEERING FOR AN OPTIMIZED SOLUTION FOR BUSINESS, PEOPLE, AND TECHNOLOGY

If we can have good and bad architectures, this implies that we can have good and bad architects. The ideal architect was defined by Marcus Vitruvius, circa 25 BC, as "a [person] of letters, a mathematician, familiar with historical studies, a diligent student of philosophy, acquainted with music, not ignorant of medicine, learned in the responses of jurisconsults, familiar with astronomy and astronomical calculations." Vitruvius was a Roman architect and the author of the famous treatise *De architectura*. His work was used as a classic textbook in ancient Roman times and rediscovered in the Italian Renaissance. *De architectura* is divided into 10 books, dealing with city planning, architecture in general, building materials, temple construction, public buildings, private buildings, clocks, hydraulics, and civil and military engines.

By Vitruvius's definition, an architect needs to be the master of everything or jack of all trades. It might have been possible then for one person to master the multiple disciplines of art, science, and engineering such as literature, mathematics, history, philosophy, music, medicine, and astronomy, as we assume those disciplines during those days were at a rather superficial level. But with advancement of science and technology, it is not possible for one person to master the multiple disciplines of art, science and engineering. It should be noted that there are more scientists alive today that all of the scientists ever lived in the history of mankind!

An architect from the view point of information technology, meaning an IT architect, is a technology expert with insight in a business domain or a scientific discipline who plans and defines the conceptual structure and overall logical organization of autonomic functional components and relationships among the components. He or she addresses the method associated with planning and realization of the functional components and processes, translating business/ scientific needs into a solution with leverage of information technology through abstraction of problems to see a forest for trees. An IT architect must have breadth in various technologies and also business acumen in a specific industry to be able to understand the domain-specific business problems, explore solution options for the business problems, evaluate technical merits and risks and for business values, choose the most optimal solution in consideration of business values and technological merits, and build consensus among the stakeholders through communication and articulation of the decisions. An IT architect is not, and should not be, just a designer with top level authority, a project manager, a specialist or an expert in certain industry or technology area, or a lone scientist. An oath like the following (one of the authors uses this oath as part of his lectures to his colleagues and clients) would help one become a good architect:

The Oath of IT Architects

Think Big;

Look beyond the horizon;

Challenge the conventional wisdom for innovation and vitality;

Adhere to the highest ethical standards;

Be frank and honest among ourselves and to others;

Fight hard for our beliefs and high quality and integrity of our work;

Make things happen with a passion;

Take pride in keeping the professional integrity; and

Take the full responsibility for our decisions.

"Think big" does not mean "oversell," but apply all vision to obtain the most comprehensive solution!

IT ARCHITECTURE PROVIDES A THREE-WAY BRIDGE BETWEEN BUSINESS, PEOPLE, AND TECHNOLOGY

The discipline of IT architecture is often compared to building bridges. Fundamentally it should always represent a three-way bridge connecting business or science, people, and information technology, based on a technical interpretation of business/science needs and organizational goals. Of particular interest to the future of healthcare is how to mobilize as quickly as possible for the patient the new insights from clinical and biomedical research. That is, the IT architecture represents a bridge from medical research to clinical practice. This idea is relatively new, however. Without any bridge, medical discoveries had to take a very slow swim across a turbulent river before reaching the doctor. To be sure, surgeons could adapt to new or better ways to do surgery rather quickly, although many would still say not quickly enough. But so far medical research and pharmaceutical research and development only meet the patient when the new drug hits the drugstore shelves, or a new device is installed in a hospital. Now we would like the physician to be much more sensitive to the latest developments while interacting with the patient.

If we think of IT architecture as in part a bridge spanning the river from research to the physician, then it has to be recognized that there are many diverse types of research, some much closer to clinical application than others, and typically implying very different landscapes on the far bank. Above it was mentioned that IT architecture has to be very flexible to accommodate different organizations and their needs. The ability to span between diverse disciplines requires an open and accommodating type of architecture, but adhering to standards so that the architect does not have to go back to basic principles for absolutely everything.

The reference model for the *open distributed processing*, the international standard for methodologies and framework for distributed processing defined by the International Organization for Standards (ISO) stretches the bridge analogy a bit further by defining five key things to consider. One might think of these as five perspectives of each river bank or, since they extend the complexity of the three-way bridge between business, people, and information technology mentioned above, literally as kind of five-way bridge. However, in the case of these considerations, they are very general and it makes sense to drop that kind of analogy and think of it as five perspectives for building a bridge to anywhere. For the record the five perspectives are (1) the enterprise viewpoint to describe the purpose, scope, context, policies, standards, obligations, and roles of a system and the overall environment and constraints to build the system on; (2) the information viewpoint to describe the information categories and associated processing of a system; (3) the computational viewpoint to describe the functional decomposition, relationships and interfaces of a system; (4) the engineering viewpoint to describe the deployment aspect of a system; and (5) technology viewpoint to identify and describe the specific technologies for implementation. That is, the bridge built should satisfy all of these perspectives, regardless of whatever many domains it attempts to span at the same time.

THE PURPOSE: HELP HEALTHCARE PROFESSIONALS TO MAKE INFORMED DECISIONS FOR POLICIES, DIAGNOSES, TREATMENT, AND PROGNOSES

In the preceding section it was mentioned that one feature that makes future healthcare system architecture is an emphasis on the bridging function, and specifically between medical research and clinical practice. This is, of course, not the only emphasis that consideration of healthcare brings up. We have noted that generally speaking, an architectural view is somewhat less concerned with the bolts and nuts of the underlying infrastructure but more concerned about the overall processes and business functions from a holistic viewpoint. However, there are some important exceptions related to factors that may significantly impact the overall quality and integrity of the system. These include seamless end-to-end process management, integrated functionality, availability, performance, security, protection of privacy, reliability, manageability, usability, adaptability to environmental changes, flexibility to usage model changes, and scalability for growth. The list is not exhausted, and these considerations are by no means particular to healthcare, but with life and a patient's concerns at stake, these issues take on a heightened importance.

As noted earlier, there is a kind of computer software called middleware that sits in a gray area between the system infrastructure and the diverse application. Middleware is required to glue the system from the end-user perspective to the system of the underlying IT infrastructure, and it also addresses the issues above of end-to-end process management, integrated functionality, availability, performance, security, and protection of privacy. Since the middleware is software, a large computer program or rather a complex suite of programs, this brings the IT architect much closer to considering the nuts and bolts than he or she would otherwise like.

The middleware technologies, as the silent and invisible partner (a good middleware technology completely hides the complexity of the underlying IT infrastructure), provide the technology foundation and the bells and whistles that are required by the functional service components, the workflow management components, security and privacy management functions, and user interfaces (e.g., display and keyboard, voice dictation) through which the end-users interact with the computer systems. The systems architect will need to keep these in mind while designing the system.

IT architecture can be considered from many levels, fine-grained or course-grained, meaning from close up or from far above. This is certainly true of healthcare, which will likely be a system at the national and ultimately international level, and also at the level of the individual patient. Let's start with the simplification of the big picture, which we will call the "thousand-foot vision" of an integrated healthcare informatics solution (such a platform does exist as Secure Health and Medical Access Network—Integrated Medical Record in an IBM Research project); see Figure 8.1. Note that the diagram has three access categories: shown at the top, bottom, and right. The patient record is central to everything. The record can be accessed by (1) the patient at home via the Internet, (2) by the physician, hospitals, and clinical-trial wards, and (3) by a variety of organizations that can use the data to provide services of public as well as sometimes commercial benefit. Such a heterogeneous archival life of patients' records is envisaged in that project. The "Anonymous record" contributions is a replication of the electronic or personal health record but without the patient's name, and all other identifying features have

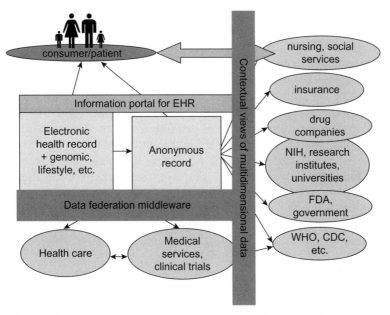

Figure 8.1   High-level view of an integrated health informatics platform

been removed as well. This category of record can only be accessed for collective viewing of all patients' records to, prevent breaching their privacy.

In accord with public concern, any integrated health informatics solution infrastructure must address the privacy issues associated with personal lifetime health records, besides provisioning the security services (e.g., authentication, authorization, confidentiality, privacy, integrity, nonrepudiation, audit trail). This is done by applying corresponding business rules based on the requester's identity, role, location, purpose, and privacy clearance (i.e., informed consent). The new healthcare system is comprised of the services and facilities to be used for dynamic assembly and presentation of the from-birth-to-present personal health information, decision support, demographic registry, electronic collaboration, and other common functions to be shared among the healthcare professionals across domains. There is more than one way to achieve privacy and one way is shown in the figure: the original patient records are effectively behind a protective firewall, and the only records that researchers and others get to access are the anonymously contributed records. Another way might be to have a single archive but with graded levels of access, in other words, through an access control based on the identity, roles, and purposes of users, and excluding types of information containing the patient's identifiers that the researcher is never permitted to see (at least, not supposed to see!). Computer accidents can happen, even though modern technology can make that unlikely; the chance of malicious access increases as the number of organizations having access gets greater and also different home accesses. All things considered, keeping the patient's identifying material physically well away from computer storage that is being accessed by researchers seems to be the safest strategy.

Malicious access is an issue that brings us back to the concept of stakeholders, meaning people with legitimate need to access the records, the most obvious being the patients and their physicians, pharmacists, nurses, and other healthcare professionals. There may come to be a time when a computer program is so smart that it functions just like a human stakeholder (imagine a robotic nurse waiting upon a patient with a chronic disease, every day of the week and all hours of the day, and not complaining at all), but we are not there yet. We must endure a system that shares information about our health and healthcare with accessible to all stakeholders. We could add to the list of stakeholders policy makers, administrators, researchers, and health insurance companies, but not all of these entities would be allowed to see data about individual patients but rather statistical summaries, and possibly archives of anonymized patient records.

For the large picture, at the most general architectural view, the main groups of stakeholders are as follows:

- *Patients* communicate with practitioners about healthcare needs, follow-up of chronic conditions, learn the results of tests, and so forth.
- *Practitioners* (nurses, physicians, physiotherapists, etc.) communicate to seek consultation, share information, educate, discuss professional matters, and plan services (e.g., call schedules).
- *Providers* of health services (laboratory information services, pharmacy information, special interest groups, patient education services, government service agencies) communicate with practitioners and patients.
- *Policy makers* (e.g., hospital administrators, regional health authorities, guideline developers, and quality-assurance staff) communicate with practitioners about practice patterns, new guidelines, and the like, and with patients about uses of services.
- *Payers* (government, third-party insurers, etc.) communicate with practitioners, patients, providers, and policy makers.

Still it should be possible to obtain, or dynamically assemble from pieces of data held at different sites, a lifetime health record on demand. The validity of the request will be based on the role of the requester and security clearance, by extracting and transforming relevant data elements from various data sources (demographic information, medication history, lab test results, diagnostic analysis details, etc.). Different parts of records may be accessed based on the professional standing and purpose of the requesting system or person. All the updates including annotations against the lifetime health record elements associated with clinical episodes will be made only through the stakeholder system.

Throughout all this, the patient's identifier will be stored in a unique space to be used by the system in identifying and locating the relevant data elements being requested in the form of information topics. So, an object identifier that is unique within the new healthcare system to be used to identify all entities— the person, the organization, the hospital beds, the operating facilities, and the ambulances. The key objective will remain to protect privacy of individual health information, in sharing relevant information about health and health-care with non–health stakeholders and thus maximizing accountability within the health system.

Figure 8.2 provides the conceptual architecture for a healthcare system where the personal lifetime health record, or personal health record, would be a longitudinal aggregation of personal health records from various sources such as physician's offices, hospitals, clinical laboratories, diagnostics laborato-ries, and radiology laboratories. This architecture is for an essentially holistic healthcare system, and it would maintain a metadata repository in a long-term data store for identification of and navigation through the relevant data sources for dynamic on-demand assembly of patient's personal lifetime health information—indeed all information that the patient wishes to contribute to ensure full holistic care. The health records retrieved from various sources for assembly of a personal health record from birth to present will not be kept in perpetual storage, but rather be placed in temporary storage for one-time viewing and analysis, although some records may be cached for subsequent analyses within the same purpose of usage. Patients should have full and direct control in managing their consent for healthcare professionals (e.g., physicians and nurses) to gain access to the personal health information. The metadata repository dynamically manages the information about the data sources so

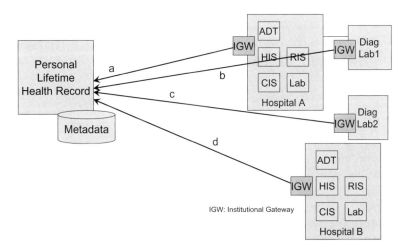

Figure 8.2 Longitudinal integration of personal lifetime health record (EHR)

that the system maintains up-to-date information about various data sources for retrieval of clinical records.

The various sources from which the system that retrieves and integrates the health records will interact through the institutional gateway systems that secure the health records for the patient with privacy clearance and ensure that a standard ontology and data formats are observed. The institutional gateway systems also determine which health information can be shared and for what purposes based on the informed consent of the patient. The basic premise is that patients own their health records, so the healthcare professionals and healthcare institutions serve only as custodians of these health records. Their providing access to a patient's health records would be governed by the statutory requirements for protection of patients' privacy.

Fragmented health records from various sources can be longitudinally integrated into a lifetime personal health record. The system for management of an electronic or personal health record (PHR) can be provided by a trusted third party for the patients, healthcare professionals, and clinical researchers. The PHR system maintains the metadata repository to keep track of data sources and privacy profiles for compliance to the privacy laws by determining which data can be made available to whom and for what purposes as well as the security profiles for validating identities of individuals or systems and for controlling access privileges. The common services and facilities refer to semantic queries, statistical analyses, and data mining.

Institutional gateway systems safeguard personal health records in accord with patients' informed consents. In cases where patients deny consent for their health records to be shared with other institutions or other healthcare professionals, the institutional gateway system has to refuse the access request from the PHR system to those patients' health records. Again, the institutional gateway systems are also responsible for transforming the health records into the standard ontology and formats for the PHR system.

CLINICAL EMAIL SYSTEM FOR SECURE EXCHANGE OF DATA AMONG HEALTHCARE PROFESSIONALS

The architecture for a holistic healthcare system will need to ensure exchanges of emails in a secure and reliable manner. With email, protection of personal privacy and also nonrepudiation (a mechanism that prevents an individual from denying involvement in an activity, whether it is a commercial or legal transaction) and security audit are still critical issues. In addition the network infrastructure will need to provide sufficient bandwidth for an exchange of large volumes of data such as medical images.

The electronic messaging system for electronic mail exchange among the healthcare professionals is referred to as a "clinical electronic mail" system. For clinical use, the management of email has to be enhanced to prevent disclosure of sensitive information. The electronic messaging or mail system, as it is used by healthcare professionals, is likely to include exchange of sensitive personal information. Disclosure of sensitive information to an accredited recipient is a matter that IT can manage in line with the statutory requirements for protection of privacy, such as HIPAA (Health Insurance Portability and Accountability Act) in the United States, PIPEDA (Personal Information Protection and Electronic Document Act) and FIPPA (Freedom of Information and Protection of Privacy Act) in Canada, and the EU Privacy Directive in the member countries of the European Union.

The selection of compatible electronic mail systems by stakeholders could require significant effort to include *gateway functions* for validation of credentials and transformation of messages among the disparate email systems. Gateway functions are literally the systems that allow the email in and out, and in theory at least let it in or out with censorship of email parts. The primary function of the gateway is to assess *message validity*.

For assurance of validity and integrity of messages, namely to ensure that the messages were sent from the legitimate sources and that the messages are delivered to the intended destination without being tempered with, the following capabilities are needed for clinical email systems:

- Confidence that a message really is coming from the purported source.
- Confidence that it has not been altered in transit.
- Ability to identify which population the message comes from (different population group may have different assumptions about security).
- Ability to identify the exact *individual* that the message comes from.
- Ability to identify each individual or institution by a unique identifier.
- Features that "point and click" a reference to an abnormal laboratory result, for example, and provide a link to the relevant laboratory reporting system and record.
- Support of digital signatures for nonrepudiation.
- Cryptography that can prevent attempts at intervention and eavesdropping.
- Ability to mark messages to indicate clinical importance or "level of emergency."
- Delivery confirmation.
- Automatic expiration of email and attachments after the date when they cease to be relevant.
- Long-term archiving for future references.

The special capabilities for provision of confidentiality and protection of privacy would need to include controlled access based on roles and identity and limited copy, print, and transfer, with an audit trail of everyone that had received and read sensitive information, as well as limited delegation and escalation. By "escalation," we mean authorization of a third party (e.g., an assistant) to review a practitioner's mail. A clinical message carry a unique identifier that assures that it gets filed correctly. Any images—video clips, audio clips, and other attachments—must allow automatic sorting by patients to see all the communications collected about them, by practitioner to see all consults from particular practitioners, by the providers (e.g., hospital) to see all communications pertaining to a particular practice environment, by priority, and by expiration date. There should be an auto-archiving feature. There should be automatic filing of messages by patients, or some other attributes, including automatic forwarding of messages to an electronic medical record system (after de-identification, of course!). There should be clipboard support, namely the ability to quickly copy materials from a message into a medical record.

In addition to the special properties of the clinical email system required for secure exchanges of health-related messages and documents with confidentiality, integrity, privacy (e.g., informed consent, de-identification of personal information), nonrepudiation (e.g., using digital signature and delivery confirmation), and auditability, the clinical email system would need to provide mechanisms for message priorities, and message expiration. The sender should be able to mark the message as urgent or high priority not only for a prompt attention from the recipient but to expedite delivery of a message by the network transport and routing protocols. On the flip side, undelivered messages must expire and be discarded after a certain period. We do not want a diagnostic report for a man to be queued in a mail server in the network for several years and then delivered to his son. Several years ago there was a newspaper article covering a story about a man who received a mail which was sent more than 70 years ago and meant to be delivered to his grandfather. The explanation for the delay of the posted letter, according to the newspaper article, was that the envelope had become stuck on the inner wall of a mailbox at a sorting station. While email messages cannot be stuck for several years in a mail server, they can be queued for delivery when there is a message routing error.*

The key properties of a clinical email system, such as message validity and integrity, are provided by encrypting the email messages and attachments and digitally signing them to protect personal privacy and to ensure data confidentiality and integrity. Maintaining email logs will provide nonrepudiation and security audit trails.

---

* A case of the domain server "omega.univ.edu" doing just that was briefly described by Michael Greenberg and colleagues in the *IEEE Communication Magazine* in July 1998. Apparently, a computer assigned to the domain name "omega.univ.edu" was decommissioned and turned off. After a few years, upon purchase of a new computer, the network domain name was reassigned to the new computer and activated to receive the emails, many of which were over three years old. The email messages had been stored "pending delivery" in mail relays on the Internet.

DIAGNOSTIC TESTS AND EVEN SURGERY CAN BE PERFORMED REMOTELY OVER THE NETWORK VIA TELEMEDICINE

A woman from Long Prairie, Minnesota, a small farming town in the central part of the state, had ulcers on her legs that were not healing. Wheelchair bound and dependent on her adult children for transportation, a referral to a dermatologist would have meant a 270-mile round trip to Abbott Northwestern Hospital in Minneapolis—a long trip for the patient and lost income for family members. Instead, her physician suggested a consultation that wouldn't require travel. Images of the ulcers were taken and electronically sent to the dermatologist in the city hospital. The dermatologist reviewed the images and emailed recommendations and a treatment plan to the patient's primary care physician, who then discussed them with the patient.

The exchange of medical information from one site to another via electronic communication is referred to as *telemedicine*, *telehealth*, or *teleconsultation*. The information can be used to diagnose and treat patients. It also can be used to educate healthcare providers and patients. Telemedicine was originated in the US space program of the 1960s, when it was used to transmit the astronauts' vital signs from space to the National Aeronautics and Space Administration (NASA).

The midterm viability of telemedicine seems uncertain because insurers have been reluctant to pay claims for it. Reimbursement and lack of acceptance by physicians and medical staff rank equally as the top operational issues telemedicine managers face, according to a survey conducted by *Telehealth Magazine*. Blue Cross & Blue Shield of Kansas uses telemedicine to reach out to rural subscribers. Being the largest health insurer in the United States with many hundreds of thousands of enrollees, Blue Cross & Blue Shield began contracting with telemedicine providers, such as Kansas Care, which also provides home health services. According to Blue Cross & Blue Shield, the thrust of the program is to monitor patients who don't need one-on-one care but need instructions or supervision to the application of medications. But the long-term goal in healthcare is to train patients to become independent in their health care by participating in their own treatment and stay out of the hospital, and consequently save money. That is basically within what we call "preventative medicine" and telemedicine will be the major enabler for patients' participation in their own healthcare management, saving money all round.

So while many insurers have been reluctant to pay claims for *teleconsulting* services, some health plans are embracing the technology as a potentially cost-effective way to reach rural subscribers who need healthcare services, especially in the countries that provide public healthcare services such as the United Kingdom and Canada. Pilot telemedicine programs at university medical centers have been expanded to nationwide networks, but this treatment protocol still represents a tiny portion of total clinical activity in the United States. Telemedicine in Canada, and similarly in other countries with dispersed populations, like Australia, is already considered as promoting better care for the population, and has led to lower incidence of disease in the population and savings on the more serious consequences of disease and illnesses. Most telemedicine sites are located at major university medical centers and were started with private and governmental funding. A telemedicine site, whether in a hospital or in a physician's office, consists of a computer and video equipment, which are used to transmit images over phone or cable lines to a similar site. Healthcare providers can interact with patients in real time or observe how patients follow instructions for rehabilitation exercises or for taking medicine. Radiologists, cardiologists, and dermatologists frequently use telemedicine, according to a recent survey by *Telehealth Magazine*, since current technology is refined enough for radiologists to diagnose using telemedicine equipment. Other uses include cardiology, psychology, emergency room procedures, ophthalmology, and dentistry. Telemedicine has also been used to improve medical care in prisons and to make medical care available on ships and submarines at sea.

Embracing the future, the US Congress has paved the way for a better telemedicine vehicle. The Next Generation Internet Research Act of 1998 authorizes entities like the National Science Foundation (NSF) and NASA to begin research on developing a new Internet that will be faster and be able to support the next level of telemedicine, in particular, "telesurgery." Telesurgery is a surgery protocol performed remotely over the telecommunication infrastructure and leveraged by the advancement of robotics and telecommunication technologies in terms of reliability, security, and bandwidth. The surgeon performs surgery on a patient in a remote location by viewing the patient through a high-resolution three-dimensional display and controlling a robot in real-time to operate on the patient.

In this scenario, a patient visits her family doctor, whose office is equipped with a workstation interlinked with biosensors, high-resolution camera, microphone, and speaker and also interconnected to the high-speed telemedicine network infrastructure. Whereas in the traditional approach, the family doctor would refer the patient to a specialist to consult with a specialist, and the patient would usually need to wait for several months to see the specialist, in this scenario, the family doctor would locate a specialist for an online consultation through the telemedicine server system. The specialist would be able to examine the patient who is still sitting in the family doctor's office. The specialist sees what the family doctor sees about the patient. The family doctor and the specialist can also collaboratively analyze the patient's medical history and also re-examine the diagnostic images at various diagnostic laboratories. Consequently the patient does not need to wait for several months to see a specialist. The family physician does not need to wait for a report from the specialist. The family physician and the specialist can collaborate online in real time through the telemedicine infrastructure.

An important extension of telemedicine is telerobotics, the remote control of a robot or robotic device to perform surgery. The first attempts were performed around the start of the new millennium at centers such as Mt. Sinai

Hospital in New York. The primary motivation originally was the thinly spread expertise around the world for certain specialized types of surgery. Another motivation is the lack of availability of any kind of special surgery in certain remote areas: ships and submarines at sea; contaminated areas due to a nuclear accident, chemical spill, epidemics, or bioterror; or in space (e.g., NASA or other remote missions providing the robots to be pre-located or delivered).

In October 2004 aquanauts aboard NASA's undersea research station *Aquarius* performed simulated medical procedures with the help of a Canadian doctor 1,300 miles away. The 11-day mission was a trial run for telemedicine techniques that could be used in emergencies on the International Space Station or on future missions to the moon and other planets. The "patient" that the crewmembers operated on is a specially designed rubber body cavity. The removal of the simulated gall bladder was done laparoscopically. Four or five small holes were made in the abdomen to allow the insertion of a small video camera and medical instruments. So far this is the extent of telemedicine. Importantly there was also a robot on board, the Zeus system, which aided in the surgery. Through the robot's arm, Dr. Mehran Anvari controlled the internal video camera. The robot had only one arm, which Dr. Anvari said was sufficient. But he typically has three robotic arms at his disposal when he performs telerobotic surgeries. Dr. Anvari has operated remotely on 22 patients in rural parts of Canada where few surgeons reside. The crew also sutured arteries together, which could be a vital operation if there was an accident on a space-faring mission. Last the crew performed ultrasound imaging of one of the living crewmembers.

But another motivation doesn't require thinly spread expertise and remoteness at all. The surgeon could be just a few yards away, and it would still be justified. Two examples of this are of interest.

The first is when the surgeon has to perform microsurgery, namely surgery on the very small microscopic scale. Effectively, the surgeon will work in a virtual reality in which the image of some delicate organ, say the brain, is amplified tens, hundreds, or even thousands of times. A movement of ten inches on the controls might actually scale down to reliable movement of a tenth of an inch on the hands of the robot, or even a thousandth. Ultimately it might even approach the nano-scale (see the last chapter), manipulating components of single cells and even clusters of atoms, although on the atomic scale one would have to perform such surgery on such clusters many times and in many places to have any effect. This all definitely sounds like science fiction. On the slightly larger cellular scale, however, there has been recent progress using atom manipulation techniques. Using microscopic lances or "microcapillaries" to do things such as remove material from fertilized eggs is now a routine technique, but the problem has been that these lances represent a crude method that almost inevitably kills the cell because the cell is badly crushed on insertion. A tiny needle can be used to aid microsurgeons and research biologists in a keyhole surgery on a single living cell. Japanese researchers turned an atomic force microscope (AFM) into a surgical tool for cells that could add or remove molecules from precise locations inside a cell without harming it. The AFM can sense the force it exerts on the cell, allowing researchers to avoid damage. The team used a beam of ions to sharpen a silicon AFM tip into a needle just 200 nanometers wide. When the needle was inserted into a human embryonic kidney cell, the cell wall was indented by only 1 micrometer. That's much more delicate than comparable microcapillary procedures, they reported. The cell membrane quickly returned to its original shape; then the insertion continued until the needle was pushed into the nucleus of the cell.

The second motivation could involve matters on the same scale, but displaced in time. This highlights the role of simulation, of building up a pseudo-reality in the computer that can be as near to or far from the real patient as suffices to help him or her. That includes simulations of predictions of what could happen, and what could happen if we did something right, or wrong. Surgery can be done in a "what if" world, and quite often in a "whoops, I didn't mean that" world. It implies, among other things, the potential for built-in systems to prevent error. It might, for example, involve performing a virtual cut on the simulation of the scene in front of the camera, such simulation using the latest data from the operation in progress to make it as much like the current situation as possible. It may then approve with an actual cut to be made seconds or minutes later. The notion is perhaps rather reminiscent of television broadcasting companies who even in "live" productions allow a few seconds before actual transmission in order to edit out any unfortunate accidents, obscenities, or libelous remarks from reaching the eyes and ears of the public. The impression created to the surgeon will be that he can backtrack from his mistakes and repeat the procedure, at least if he or she does not wait too long. However, since it may become common practice to "test run" and preplan surgery in virtual reality hours or days in advance, this will fade into the scenario above and involve hours or days of backtracking. It may become important to distinguish simulation and reality carefully, and report "real time" and "virtual time" very clearly.

There is a further potential application of simulation in telemedicine. We did not consider the detailed architectural, formatting, and standards issues involved in telemedicine, although they exist. Most privacy issues are not unlike those raised in regard to email. We note in passing, however, that it can be rather more difficult to eliminate all visual clues to a patient's identity if telemedical transmissions are intercepted or the recording is used for teaching and research. It may be that a way forward here is to use every such transmission or actual recording as a simulation that is close enough to reality to cure the patient but not reveal the patient's identity.

ACCESS RIGHTS BASED ON IDENTITY, ROLES, PURPOSES, LOGICAL LOCATIONS

So we came round to privacy again. It is odd that we sometimes feel that we are being a bit boring in dropping back from high tech to those dry sounding issues of privacy, yet the truth is that many people tend to place those issues far above high tech. Of course, there has to be a balance. There is little advantage in being a very private but dead individual. Nonetheless, healthcare security and privacy is a main concern to the public. So it is probably useful go over privacy and security again, but in more detail from the access and holistic systems architecture perspective.

Holistic medicine, which seeks to integrate so many kinds of data about the patient in order to make the best decisions, implies many doors to guard. The following abilities need to be provided for a healthcare system in regard to any kind of information, request, or instruction: to identify which population the message comes from, since each population group may have different assumptions about security; to identify the exact individual that the message comes from; to identify each individual or institution by a unique identifier; to facilitate links, indexing, and filing in other software applications; to detect and reflect any attempts at eavesdropping; to control access based on roles and identity; to limit copy, print, or transfer; and to audit the trail of everyone that has received and read sensitive information that was referred, delegated, or escalated as an authorized third party assistant (e.g., specialists and nurses).

In order to comply with the statutory requirements for protection of privacy, an individual must be notified about the purpose of collecting the personal information, as well as of the legal authority for doing so. Personal information is defined as "any recorded information about an identifiable individual." Institutions must protect that personal information by appropriate security. All the demographic and other information associated with registration must be consolidated and securely managed in one logical location for confidentiality and integrity of personal information and for accurate eligibility assessment. Access to a personal health record may be granted at the following levels: role based (access privileges will be assigned to a set of users based on the role they perform), group based (access privileges will be assigned to a set of users that are members of a defined group), and individual based (access privileges will be assigned to individual healthcare providers). Access privileges to personal health record should be constrained for delegation, referral, or escalation based on the role, purpose, and logical location, and all transactions should be logged. The transactions in this context are any activities involving the patient data such as creation, viewing, sharing with others, updating, correcting, archiving, or deleting a health record or related information.

It is interesting to think about what this means. In the future it will not be assumed a divine right, as it seems to be in many parts of the world at present, that physicians can share patient data with other physicians simply because they are physicians. The health information that contains protected (by law) personal information can be shared only after acquiring an explicit *informed consent* from the individual. The important exception to this is when the purpose of sharing the information is consistent with the purposes intended at the time of collection of the information or in the medical emergency such as the case where a person is in a critical condition but unconscious. A general consent at the time of collection, and probably built into the system as a default, might be that it may be used by appropriate medical staff if the patient has a medical emergency. The healthcare system should provide a mechanism to override the access control to a personal health record in case of emergency, such as at the emergency room, in the ambulance, or in the operating room for surgery. However, disclosure of the data must still be appropriate and consistent with the stated purpose of collecting the personal information. If a physician wants to share the personal health information with another physician for the same purpose, the first physician does not need to seek an informed consent from patient because the purpose of sharing the personal information is same as the intended purpose for collection of the personal information. In addition, if a physician wants to share the personal information about a patient with another physician for a different purpose, but that purpose is required to achieve the original purpose above, an explicit informed consent may not be necessary. Nonetheless, if it were an unrelated purpose, it is the responsibility of the first physician to seek an explicit informed consent from the patient before sharing the personal information with the other physician.

Many principles of holistic medicine strike a chord with such matters of access, since in part a broad basis for treatment does require sharing of patient data among healthcare professionals to have the broadest possible view of the patient and to provide access to the broadest possible range of medical expertise, in the patient's interest. A primary service provider typically has significant powers in a nation's healthcare system and can grant access rights on the entire health record or a part of the health record to other healthcare professionals. Typically at present, primary healthcare service providers (e.g., family doctors) have full rights to access personal health information for their patients, yet other healthcare service providers, such as specialists to which a patient is referred, have only limited access privileges for personal health information. They require an authorization based on the intended purposes for access to the personal information. At present, also, the primary service provider should advise the patient of the purposes of disclosure and to seek an informed consent in advance. This is not unreasonable but IT is required to make it slick. As such, the healthcare system needs to provide a mechanism for healthcare service providers, especially primary service providers, to acquire an explicit informed consent from their patients. We won't overlabor here the controversial matter of levels of access by health insurance companies as the key issues were discussed in regard to stakeholders to access patient data in Chapter 6.

The traditional security model can neither ensure confidentiality of sensitive healthcare information and protection of personal privacy nor conform to the governing legislation (e.g., HIPAA in United States, PIPEDA and FIPPA in Canada, EU Privacy Directive in the European countries) when healthcare services are offered through a public infrastructure such as the Internet. Obviously the security policy for an IT system will remain as only part of the traditional big picture, which includes physical security (e.g., locks for buildings, badge access to secure rooms), logical security (e.g., passwords for computers or networks, smartcards), and operational policies and procedures (e.g., oath of office, management approval). Security architecture needs to provide multiple lines and levels of defense for protection from outsiders and also policy-driven access control based on identity, roles, and purposes for protection from insiders.

THE ELECTRONIC DATA VAULT FOR SECURE MANAGEMENT OF PERSONAL HEALTH RECORDS

In this information age, knowledge and information become critical assets for business entities or individuals and need to be well protected not only for protection of intellectual properties and trade secrets but also for compliance to the statutory requirements for protection of privacy. More important, the personal information that is legally or commercially used for identification of an organization or an individual must be well protected for prevention of identity theft. The majority of information is managed (e.g., collected, analyzed, manipulated, stored, copied, disseminated, and shared) in electronic form and is readily accessible. The majority of systems managing the information are connected through a network, and the access is controlled through firewalls and validation of identity (authentication) and access privileges (authorization).

Consequently the assets, intellectual properties, and unique and sensitive personal or organizational information are vulnerable to unauthorized access or manipulation. The industry is in desperate need of a reliable means to secure and protect such information in the electronic information age. For example, the government agencies and any business entities must ensure that the personal information (e.g., legal name, date of birth, social security number, employee number, and mother's maiden name) be kept accurate, current, and in confidence at all times.

A special mechanism is required to protect the information specific to particular individuals (e.g., a person protected under the federal witness protection program), organizations (e.g., a special agency working undercover for CIA), or events (e.g., incumbent US president being admitted to a hospital for an emergency). In those cases, not only the information content but also the very existence of the information must be kept in confidence. For other information such as the information about an adopted child and his/her parents, it may be sufficient to protect the information content. The former is referred to as *sealed record* and the latter as *locked record*.

A *sealed record* requires that not only the information content but also the very existence of such information itself be completely hidden. On the other hand, a *locked record* requires that the information content be completely hidden, although the existence of such information can be known to a small group of selected people in the authorized organizational entities (e.g., the intelligence agencies of CIA, FBI, and Homeland Security).

The *secure electronic data vault* allows patients to keep their PHR (personal health record) and other personal documents in a *locked* state, whereby the content of a document is hidden from others including system/data administrators, or in a *sealed* state, whereby not only the content of the PHR but also the existence of PHR is hidden from others including system/data administrators.

The secure electronic data vault hides the content of the electronic health record and other documents from others, including system/data administrators, by storing the documents scrambled (i.e., encrypted) so that only the document owner can decipher (i.e., decrypt) the document. The *secure electronic data vault* hides the existence of a PHR as well as its content from others, including system/data administrators, by storing the metadata (i.e., the information about the document) encrypted so that only the trusted custodian may get the information about the document and by storing the document encrypted so that only the document owner can decrypt it.

People use the safety deposit box services provided by the banks to secure a tangible asset from loss or theft. The bank provides its customer with a safety deposit box with a lock and the only key for the lock. The bank keeps the safety deposit box in the vault as the custodian without knowing what is kept in the box. Only the owner of the safety deposit box knows the content of the box and has access to the content, while the bank safeguards the box itself. As a result the individual's belongings are secured in the locked box that only the owner has the key for, and the box is secured in the bank's vault that only the vault keeper at the bank has access to.

The owner of the safety deposit box may choose to share the information about the safety deposit box (e.g., name of the bank, branch number and address, safety deposit box number, secret identifier for the box) with one's spouse and children and may also choose to let one's spouse know where the key is kept. The owner may still keep secret the information about what is in the safety deposit box. The box owner may keep secret all the information about the safety deposit box for oneself and leave that information only in one's will. The former is an example of *locked record*, and the latter is an example of *sealed record*. The secret bank account with the Swiss bank is another example.

The basic idea is to apply the principles of the bank's safety deposit box to an IT solution for safeguarding electronic patient records. For the provision of services for sealed/locked records, the asymmetric cryptography technology, also known as public key cryptography, can be exploited as the base technology for implementation of a system managing the sensitive information in a "sealed" or "locked" state, for protection of privacy and for prevention of identity theft in the electronic information age.

The asymmetric cryptography technology uses one key to encrypt data and a different key to decrypt the data. Therefore the encryption key can be shared with others without compromising security as far as the corresponding decryption key is securely kept. One analogy is a lock and an associated key. There is no problem in sharing multiple copies of locks as long as the key is kept securely, and provided that no one can create a key by disassembling a lock.

In asymmetric cryptography, the locks are referred to as *public keys*, and the keys for the locks are referred to as *private keys*.

The locked record management system *completely hides the content of electronic records* from others, including system/data administrators, by storing *the electronic records encrypted with the owner's public key and again with the custodian's private key* so that only the owner of the electronic records can decrypt them in collaboration with the custodian. The sealed record management system *completely hides the existence of such electronic records*, as well as its content, from others, including system/data administrators, by storing *the metadata (i.e., the information about the electronic record) encrypted with the owner's public key* so that only the owner of the electronic records may know about and get the information about the existence of the electronic records.

A *digital signature* is used to ensure integrity of an electronic record, namely to prevent unauthorized alteration of the content of an electronic record. It is also used for nonrepudiation for an electronic transactions, namely to prevent a denial of an involvement in an electronic contract for a legally binding agreement.

Now, let us look into the fundamentals of cryptography, which is the foundation of the IT security for protection of digital data from unauthorized access.

Cryptography goes many years back into history. Julius Caesar is known to be the first person that introduced the cryptography to communicate his orders with his commanders. Army commanders used their own cryptography to keep their war strategy and battle plans from enemies (in case the liaison officer is captured by the enemy) when they are conveyed by the messengers to their captains in the battlefields. For another example, professional baseball teams use cryptic hand signals between the catcher and the pitcher.

The cryptography mentioned above is based on shared secrets between two parties, and is referred to as cryptography based on symmetric key or private key. In this private-key cryptography, the same key is used to scramble and decipher a message. To make this private-key cryptography work, the secret must be shared in advance and kept between the legitimate parties. However, conveying the shared secret to the legitimate parties in remote locations is a real challenge, especially when the shared secrets need to be revoked and replaced with new ones once in a while as a precaution that the secret may have been divulged to illegitimate parties. Imagine that one of Caesar's commanders had been captured by his enemy and tortured to divulge the secret code Caesar used to scramble his orders.

To address the challenges associated with conveying the secrets to the legitimate parties and keeping the shared secrets only between the legitimate parties, cryptography based on asymmetric keys has been developed. The cryptography based on asymmetric keys is also called *public-key cryptography* and often referred to as *public-key infrastructure (PKI)*. In this public-key cryptography, a public key is known to everyone and is used for scrambling a message (i.e., encrypting) while a private key is kept in secret by the owner of the message and is used for deciphering the message (i.e., decrypting).

As an analogy, think of the following scenario: You manufacture multiple locks and an only key for those locks; then you distribute the locks to your friends but keep the only key for yourself. When one of your friends wants to send you a secret letter, she will put the letter in a box and lock the box with your lock. Once it is locked, even your friend no longer can open the box because she does not have the key for the lock and because you have the only key for the lock. Therefore the box can be delivered safely to you even if you use some untrusted third party (e.g., courier, postman) for delivery. Only you can open the box with the only key you keep. Conversely, if you want to send a secret letter to your friend, you put your letter in a box and lock it with your friend's lock. Once locked, even you cannot unlock the box because your friend has the only key for the box. Consequently you are assured that only your friend can read your secret letter. Even if the box is misdelivered to someone else, the content of your letter is still kept secret because the box can be only opened by your friend, the friend you intended to access the secret letter. The key advantage of this asymmetric-key cryptography or public-key cryptography is that secret keys are kept with their owners and do not ever need to be shared with anyone else.

A *digital signature* is used to ensure integrity of an electronic document (e.g., PHR, electronic certificates, living will) and to prevent unauthorized alteration of the content. It is also used for nonrepudiation of an electronic transaction, meaning to prevent a denial of an involvement in an electronic contract for a legally binding agreement.

Going back to the *secure electronic data vault system*, this novel approach protects (i.e., hides or obscures) the content of the electronic record stored in the *secure electronic data vault system* even from the system/database administrators by storing the electronic record in an encrypted format. This is achieved by encrypting the electronic record with the record owner's public key and again with the public key of the custodian of electronic records. Therefore the custodian of electronic records needs to decrypt it with its secret key, and the owner of the electronic records needs to decrypt again with its secret key to access the content.

This asymmetric cryptography approach also protects the existence of the electronic record by storing the record identifier in an encrypted format. This is achieved by encrypting the electronic record identifier with the record owner's private key. Therefore only the ones who have access to the public key of the record owner can access the record identifier.

The secure electronic data vault services described in the previous section exploit the public key infrastructure (PKI) based on the RSA cryptography,[1] but in a nontraditional way using a new approach in the asymmetric cryptography. The concept of the RSA cryptography for secure exchange of an elec-

---

[1] An asymmetric cryptography developed by R. Rivest, A Shamir, and L. Adleman.

Sender encrypts a document with a personal private key code, then encrypts it again with the receiver's public key.

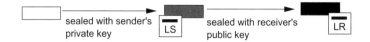

Receiver decrypts the document with a personal private key code, then decrypts it again with the sender's public key.

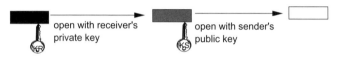

Figure 8.3   Concept of PKI cryptography

tronic document over an insecure network and of ensuring integrity of the electronic document based on a digital signature as described in Figure 8.3.

A *digital signature* for an electronic document is generated by running a mathematical hashing function against the subject electronic document to create a fixed-length fingerprint (typically 128 bits long) and then by encrypting the fingerprint with the document owner's public key. For protection of the content of an electronic document, the digital signature is attached to the subject electronic document, and then the document as well as the digital signature is encrypted with the sender's private key and again with the receiver's public key before transmission. The *digital signature* is verified by the receiver by (1) decrypting the document with the document receiver's *private key*, (2) decrypting it again with the sender's *public key*, (3) running the mathematical hashing function to the document to generate a fingerprint for the document, (4) encrypting the fingerprint with the sender's *public key*, and then (5) comparing the generated digital signature with the received *digital signature* to verify the integrity of the electronic document. The concept of ensuring integrity of an electronic document is illustrated in Figure 8.4.

"TRANSLATIONAL RESEARCH" FOR PERSONALIZED, PREVENTATIVE, WELLNESS-ORIENTED HEALTHCARE

The term "translational" means high-speed utilization of latest high-throughput research such as discovering new biomarkers; in effect it is an extension of the principles of evidence-based medicine. But it also means passing from advanced medical research to clinical applications. Some day in the near future, your doctor could screen you for known diseases, simply by

Mathematical hashing function to create a fixed-length fingerprint
Encrypt the fingerprint with signer's public key

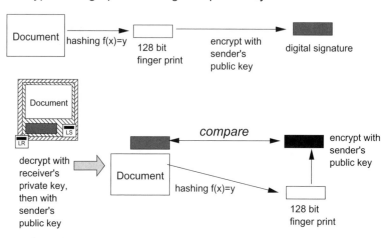

Figure 8.4 Concept of ensuring integrity of electronic document

taking a few drops of your blood, and prescribe the best medication for your condition based on your personal genotypic and phenotypic profile. This will involve physician-friendly decision support and modeling tools. Drugs may be screened in reality in microlaboratory chips, and in virtual reality in computers, and maybe even designed and synthesized in microlaboratories. In many respects all these operations are like those used by medical researchers, albeit at a much slower pace, even today. In fact one aspect of a more personalized and holistic medicine is that the research is done rapidly for a specific patient group. Contrast the fact that up to now, biomedical research, including drug research and development, has been quite separate from clinical practice, with patient diagnosis and drug development converging only at the pharmacist's counter or in hospital. The only influence of the patient on the drug choice has been that the doctor must order from a catalog of available molecular products, which are in no sense (in tailor's terms) "made to measure."

This scenario is far off right now, but in the interim the same idea, of accelerating mobilization of basic research, still stands. How then does the research get through to the healthcare system in a holistic world? The proactive, patient-centered, outcome-driven, wellness-oriented continuum of healthcare service can be enabled through IT for facilitating translational research. This bridges the patient-care domain and the clinical research domain to allow the medical researchers to leverage the clinical outcomes observed by the healthcare practitioners. It will also allow the healthcare practitioners to leverage the research outcomes derived by the medical researchers.

Translational research can be enabled with leverage of IT and other related technologies such as artificial intelligence, robotics, cybernetics (e.g., machine learning and autonomous computing) and nanoscience (e.g., nanobots). The translational research is anticipated to help us realize a personalized healthcare in consideration of an individual's genotypic, phenotypic, environmental, and lifestyle variances and to help the healthcare professionals improve the accuracy of diagnoses, the efficacy of treatments, and the patient safety (i.e., minimal adverse drug responses). The translational research is anticipated to help us realize a preventative or predictive healthcare through in-silico disease modeling and organ simulation to complement experiments based on animal models. Other industries such as automobile manufactures, aircraft manufactures, and the US National Aeronautics and Space Administration (NASA) have been exploiting IT for modeling and simulation for design of automobiles, aircraft, and space shuttles, while the healthcare industry has been instead relying on experiments based on animals and observation of only external symptoms.

The authors observed several issues in the healthcare industry that are generally agreed upon by many industry analysts. The key issues in the healthcare industry include healthcare providers heavily rely on their personal experience and opinion as the main reference of diagnosis, treatment, and prognosis; the information or knowledge gained by the healthcare providers through years of practice and experience is not shared among the healthcare professionals who can benefit from for more accurate diagnosis or for better treatment for higher efficacy (e.g., a survey conducted by the American Medical Association suggested that physicians in the United States would rather share their toothbrushes than their patient information!); the healthcare services are rather fragmented and lack of continuum of services from diagnosis and treatment through prognosis and from primary care to tertiary care; the healthcare services are provided reactively as episodic events; all the patients are treated equally for diagnosis and prognosis with little consideration of their genotypic or phenotypic variances, and consequently the patient safety is significantly compromised.

This translational research can be enabled by an integrated IT solution, depicted in Figure 8.5, that enables interdisciplinary collaboration across multiple institutions, provides transparent access to multidimensional data and tools to analyze unstructured data as well as structured data, manages vast amount of multidimensional data, provides high-performance computing, and incorporates robotic instruments as part of the workflow management. This integrated IT solution refers to a set of integrated systems that draw upon relevant information and context to enhance the activity and performance of people, robotic instruments, systems, and organizations through an online collaboration across the boundaries of various disciplines, organizations, countries, and geographical locations. The goal of the IT solution is to assist, with a leverage of IT and related technologies, a group of multidisciplinary researchers in navigating the information spaces in "real" and "virtual" environments, orienting and guiding them based on the research themes, interacting with and leveraging others to find their way in the information spaces, and sharing

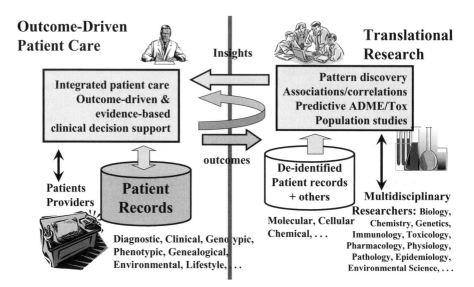

Figure 8.5 Translational research platform

discoveries and knowledge among them. The main focus is to foster trust and community in research teams, whether co-located or geographically distributed, and to support long-running, contextual interactions rather than short-term, task-focused activities, for a holistic management of collaboration among a group of multidisciplinary researchers.

The key characteristics of the IT solution to enable interdisciplinary collaboration across multiple institutions are that (1) the data to be analyzed are mainly unstructured, vast and yet scarce and noisy; (2) the users of the system, also referred to as "actors," include autonomous robotic systems as well as human users; (3) the internal users and the external collaborators need to cooperate as an integrated cohesive team, but the intellectual properties are yet to be protected; (4) the laboratory information systems for experiments and assays need to be integrated with the system; (5) the external reference systems and databanks need to be integrated with the system through a dynamic data filtering, ingesting, and transformation for transparent access to the relevant data; (6) a virtual workplace needs to be provided for knowledge sharing and online collaboration across the organizational boundaries; (7) semantic search and undirected data mining against multidimensional data are essential analysis tools; (8) very high performance computing resources, typically MPP (massively parallel processing) clusters in the range of trillions of floating point operations per second (teraflops), need to be provided as shareable services; and (9) a very high throughput content/storage management system needs to be provided for policy-driven migration and recall of vast amount of data in the range of quadrillion bytes (petabytes).

The key enabling technologies include electronic health records to be shared among the healthcare professionals and the medical researchers, electronic data capture (EDC) system to be used by the healthcare professionals at the sources of data, standard ontology and taxonomy for data representation and exchange, global patient identifier to link fragmented patient data generated and collected at various sources (e.g., general physician's office, diagnostic laboratories, private clinical offices, hospitals, clinical trial laboratories, research laboratories), cross-enterprise vocabulary services to be used among multidisciplinary professionals, integrated security services and privacy framework to ensure data confidentiality and integrity and to comply with the statutory requirements for protection of personal privacy, undirected data mining facility for discovery of associations and covariance among multidimensional heterogeneous data as well as directed data mining facilities for validation of hypothesis, and knowledge sharing and online collaboration facility among multidisciplinary professionals.

BIOMEDICAL INFORMATICS FOR ENABLEMENT OF TRANSLATIONAL RESEARCH

Key industry requirements for biomedical informatics include acquisition and integration of heterogeneous data in disparate structures from multiple sources such as integrating protocols, clinical reports, patient records, clinical trial outcomes, and adverse drug events; transparent access to multidimensional heterogeneous data on various platforms at multiple locations through either aggregation or federation; intuitive and consistent interfaces to various tools and applications running on various platforms at multiple sources; computer-assisted workflow management for intuitive usability and high productivity; common portal interface for concurrent multiple sessions with integrated security and application pipelining; policy-driven and tailored privacy framework for compliance to the statutory requirements; online collaboration and knowledge-sharing framework for interdisciplinary research; undirected data mining against multidimensional data for discovery of associations and correlations through serendipity; three-dimensional disease modeling and four-dimensional organ simulation environment; and autonomous operation of the IT system as a whole to minimize human intervention.

Autonomic computing technologies encapsulate the complexity of the underlying information technology components (hardware components and software components) and also enable automatic operation and management of the IT system with dynamic adaptation to changes without (or with minimal) human intervention so that the IT system as a whole can be used as a black box. The conceptual biomedical informatics architecture is depicted in the Figure 8.6.

The industry requirement for the acquisition and integration of heterogeneous data in disparate structures from multiple sources (e.g., integrating

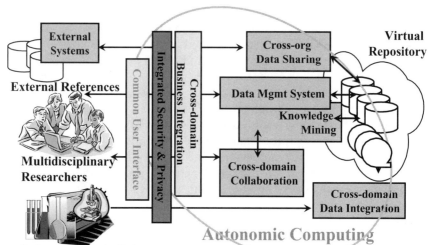

Figure 8.6   Conceptual biomedical informatics architecture

protocols, clinical reports, patient records, clinical trial outcomes, adverse drug events) can be addressed by an electronic data capture (EDC) system that is augmented with voice dictation capability and allows healthcare providers or clinical researchers to capture the data at the source through a graphical form-based user interface with pull-down menus, type-ahead features, and inline edit checks to prevent missing, duplicate, or out-of-bound data at the time of data collection.

The industry requirement for transparent access to multidimensional heterogeneous data can be addressed by a data abstraction middleware that provides composite indexing to multidimensional data and a unified virtual repository for the integration of disparate data on various platforms in multiple locations via aggregation or federation. The composite indexing will allow the researchers to access the data in various formats such as relational, XML-tagged, text, and images. The unified virtual repository will provide multiple views of the multidimensional data such as patient-centric views and disease-centric views.

The industry requirement for intuitive and consistent interfaces to various tools and applications can be addressed by a portal interface to various tools and applications from various sources via a plug-and-play interface. The portal interface also provides access to multiple tools and applications through concurrent multiple sessions and with application pipelining (e.g., automatic transfer of the output of an application to another application to be processed as the input).

Computer-assisted workflow management helps the researchers navigate through tools and data based on research scenarios, use cases, personal preferences, and usage patterns of individual researchers for usability and high productivity. Online collaboration and knowledge-sharing framework allows the researchers to interact with co-researchers through integrated email, calendaring, instant messaging, and web conferencing. The researchers will be able to insert annotations, research outcomes, and discovered knowledge and share them with co-researchers even in a different scientific discipline for interdisciplinary research.

EXTREME EPIDEMIOLOGY: INTEGRATION OF MULTIDIMENSIONAL HETEROGENEOUS DATA FOR TRANSLATIONAL LIFE SCIENCES RESEARCH

Epidemiology today is probably best defined as *the basic science of public health* or even better *the basic science of public health based on best evidence.* Certainly it is officially credited as laying the basis for evidence-based medicine, which is deeply founded in the epidemiological principle of best evidence (e.g., see Chapter 10). Older definitions of epidemiology relate to understanding the demographics, dynamics, and deduced origins of specific diseases on which health authorities and physicians can act (but not solely infectious disease, even though older definitions and public perception seem to imply study of disease epidemics). But by any definition, epidemiology was always very good in seeing its role as based on solid data in the broader well-founded scientific context, and recent definitions simply emphasize that role.

In addition, what tends to be omitted in definitions is that good epidemiologists were excellent detectives, tracking down clues as to disease source and best response from diverse sources ranging from interviews with the public through inspection of maps, to consideration of latest laboratory results. Detective work in pursuit of a killer with use of diverse data is always exciting, conjuring up for us fictional cinema characters following in the founding footsteps of a real John Snow who tracked down a cholera outbreak to a water hand-pump in 1854. Again, epidemiologists use all variety of data and add to that the challenge of including ongoing basic research data that provide the basic public health science. In other words epidemiologist are good at integrating, and inferring from, *heterogeneous data.*

It should be coming clear that we are now effectively in pursuit of "extreme epidemiology." Medical IT architects want to empower and extend the job previously done by epidemiologists and related public health analysts, but to drill down in molecular detail, not just capturing data from, ultimately at least, every patient, but also with meaning extended by research studies on animals, tissue cultures, and biomolecules. Biomedical informatics seems to be the discipline with a definition that best equates to the modern epidemiological definitions with the "basic science" and "best evidence" emphases. Biomedical informatics is an extension of bioinformatics for incorporation of medical information (clinical, diagnostic, demographic, etc.) and an extension of medical informatics for incorporation of biological information (genomic, pro-teomic, cytomic, molecular, chemical data) to enable combinatorial analyses of the multidimensional disparate data such as genotypic, phenotypic, metabo-lomic, physiological, genealogical, pathological, epidemiological, toxicological, pharmaceutical, phylogenic, environmental, and behavioral data, to name just a few.

The ultimate purpose of the classical epidemiologist was not to publish obscure scientific papers in lofty journals but to advise physicians and health-care officials. Anticipated benefits of the translational research on healthcare can be summarized as timely and accurate diagnoses; targeted treatment with high efficacy based on an individual's genotypic, phenotypic, and lifestyle variances; remote monitoring, diagnoses, and treatments/surgeries from the perspective of healthcare delivery; reduced time and cost for research and development of new drugs; novel drugs with high efficacy and safety; prevention of adverse drug responses; novel drugs targeted for genotypic and phenotypic variances; and preventative medicine from the perspective of health research and drug discovery and development; and reduced healthcare cost and wellness-oriented preventative healthcare management from the per-spective of healthcare management.

The main objective of translational research in clinical genomics is to improve patient care through highly accurate diagnosis and efficacious treat-ment based on understanding and discovery of knowledge on correlations between clinical, genetic, environmental and lifestyle variances at the molecu-lar level and disease mechanisms of the biological process at the biochemical pathways.

The typical research scenarios of clinical genomics involve two main research streams: one stream involving an identification of genes of interest, characterization of the genes, SNPs, and polymorphisms, and the other stream involving development of hypotheses based on discovered correlations between the genes of interest and diseases and validation of hypotheses based on population studies. Recall that researchers have discovered that most of human diseases are polygenetic and that even monogenic diseases are affected by other genes, and their associated phenotypes are also subject to modifica-tions by these other genes and environmental variables (see also Chapter 9).

The theme for transparent access to multidimensional heterogeneous data is the foundation for other themes for combinatorial analysis and online col-laboration. In other words, data integration for transparent access to multidi-mensional heterogeneous data is the foundation for biomedical informatics to enable undirected data mining for knowledge discovery. With undirected data mining, combinatorial analysis can be used for developing a hypothesis and statistical analysis for validation of the hypothesis.

The challenges for data integration for clinical genomics are these: the data to be accessed are multidimensional and heterogeneous, the majority of data are unstructured and exist in natural language text, the data contains personal information that is subject to statutory requirements for protection of privacy, the ownerships of data lie with multiple stakeholders in multiple organizations, new data entities are constantly added as the industry matures, the formats of existing data change constantly, the data are sparse, the volume of data are vast and growing rapidly, and so on. The main data sources include hospitals for clinical data in the clinical information system (CIS), demographic data in the hospital information system (HIS), clinical trial data in the clinical trials operational data store (ODS); pharmaceutical data in the pharmacy information system (PIS), diagnostic data in the radiology/cardiology information system; clinical laboratory test results in the laboratory information system, diagnostic images in the picture archiving and communications system (PACS), and genomics/proteomics laboratories for genomic and proteomic data in the laboratory information management system (LIMS).

We are concerned about the results of the experiments and the derived information out of the assays or tests, and not the raw or experimental data. The raw or experimental data should be managed through the LIMS or the laboratory information system (LIS), diagnostic information system managed through picture archive and communication system (PACS) and radiology information system (RIS), clinical trial operational data store (ODS) or hospital operational data store such as radiology information system (RIS) or admission, discharge, & transfer (ADT) management system.

The main theme of data integration for clinical genomics is to enable combinatorial analysis among clinical, genomic, proteomic, environmental, demographic, and lifestyle data. These data typically include patient demographic data, diagnostic test results, laboratory test results (e.g., hemoglobin, blood glucose levels, triglycerides, and biopsy), radiology results (e.g., MRI, PET, CT, US, and mammography), outcomes of treatments, therapeutic history and outcomes, genetic profiles, pathology reports, genomic assay results, proteomic assay results, environmental variances, lifestyle variances, and family illness history. A patient can be represented as an entity with the attributes of demographics, clinical history, diagnostic report, family history, pathology report, treatment outcomes, genetic profiles, biomarkers, environmental variance, life style variance, and so forth.

The data sets managed by hospitals, clinical laboratories, diagnostic imaging laboratories, laboratories for bioassays, and laboratories for clinical trials are mostly unstructured or semistructured. In addition they are relatively noisy. Therefore they are not appropriate data sets to be accessed directly via federation for analysis. As such, data ingestion through extraction, transformation, cleansing, curation, and loading is required before the data sets are analyzed or used for mining. The data sets managed through HIS, CIS, PIS, RIS, and others at hospitals; through PACS (picture archive and communication system) for diagnostic images and reports, through LIS at the clinical laboratories, and LIMS at the bioassay laboratories are not good candidates for access via data federation.

The candidate data sets appropriate for access via federation are the external reference data banks as they are not under the institutional control. Accessing the external reference data via federation ensures data currency, but at the cost of performance degradation and at the risk of security compromise. A federated access to the external data banks is generally inefficient due to the need for laborious access to various massive public reference data sources through the Internet one by one across public networks that are often overloaded during peak times because of the large number of concurrent researchers and large volume of data being transmitted on the network. This can seriously degrade the efficiency of the research process.

Data federation technology was developed at the IBM Research Division (Almaden Research Laboratory and TJ Watson Research Laboratory) to establish a virtual repository by dynamically linking multiple data sources, leaving the data at the original data sources as they are. The data federation technology allows a user to send a single query statement against multiple data sources, which can be various relational database systems (e.g., IBM DB2, Oracle, Sybase, MySQL), flat file systems (e.g., UFS, JFS), web pages, XML files, rectangular data, and so on. The data federation engine decomposes a single query from an end-user or an application into multiple queries based on the number of data sources involved in the query. It then develops a cost-based query optimization on the fly, generates separate queries for individual data sources required to perform the query, compensates the functional deficiencies of the source data management system (e.g., record sorting will be provided by the federation engine to compensate the inability of a file management system for sorting), and consolidates the results of the multiple query responses into a single reply to the end-user or the application.

The specific problems or risks associated with accessing the external reference data over the public networks based on the typical federation approach can be summarized as follows:

- Researchers' query interactions flow across the public networks (e.g., the Internet), resulting in security exposure. For example, a pharmaceutical company or a biotechnology company could figure out the research topics and approaches of its competitor by sniffing the data traffic between the competitor and the public data banks. Therefore protection of intellectual properties can be compromised and become a challenge when employing this type of traditional solution approach.
- One scientist's findings cannot be readily shared by other scientists, and annotation or updating of remote databases is difficult and impractical.
- External reference data banks contain vast amounts of extraneous data that may not be accurate, germane, or current.
- Accessing data in remote databases is often cumbersome and inefficient, not only because the site at a remote location but also because it is rarely organized and formatted optimally for the needs of a given researcher, research group, or organization.
- Data models and schema at the data sources continue to change, and consequently the "data wrappers" for the federation engine need to be modified.

Therefore, a hybrid approach may be effective for consolidating relevant reference data through online and automated retrieval of reference data from various sources, cleansing and filtering to select current and relevant data, and consolidating into a local repository based on an optimized data model that is enabled for local annotation capability. The hybrid approach essentially involves an architecture that will automatically create and maintain a buffered dedicated reference database for use by an individual or a focused group of researchers concerned with a specific domain of knowledge.

In this hybrid model the researchers can directly query against the local data repository, instead of interacting with the federated databases. In addition the researchers can add their own new entries or annotate existing entries as opposed to simply receiving the reference data published by the public data banks. The researchers can also configure the content management subsystem for their specific ongoing research needs in terms of data categories, data sets, keywords, and the like. The content management subsystem runs continuously in the background behind the scene and maintains the currency of the local reference data repository by querying the remote reference data.

Accordingly with the institutional data refreshment policies based on the needs of individual institution, the content management subsystem will access the predefined datasets at selected public data banks and retrieve additional or updated reference data sets. The reference data refreshment policy is configurable by the researchers and maintained in a human-readable as well as machine-readable format by the content management subsystem. The data in the local reference data repository is maintained in a form that is optimal for the researchers' chosen research applications.

This hybrid model solves the problems associated with federated data access across the public network, and with internally maintained local database, by combining the two approaches and automating the processes to maintain data currency and accuracy through the content management subsystem and a new software module for dynamic retrieval of additional datasets and automatic updates for revised datasets.

A number of key benefits are anticipated in the hybrid approach:

- Quicker response time since reference data are retrieved from local databases through a high-speed local area network (LAN) as opposed to remote databases through low-speed public wide area network (WAN)
- Improved security and protection of intellectual properties
- Assurance of data integrity by keeping the reference data current, cleansed, and filtered
- Improved performance by maintaining the reference data in a form optimized for local usage and query patterns
- Provision for local annotations that can be securely shared internally among the researchers

ACTIVE DATA REPOSITORY FOR MULTIDIMENSIONAL DATA MANAGEMENT FOR TRANSLATIONAL LIFE SCIENCES RESEARCH

Classical epidemiologists as disease detectives may have got there in the end, but they probably barely scratched the information that might have been potentially available somewhere, and certainly could not do so today. Understanding the properties and attributes of health informatics or life sciences informatics for translational medical research is important because scientific advancement is becoming increasingly dependent on the ability to manage massive amounts of data and solve computationally intense problems. For example, the fact that there are approximately 32,000 human genes that translate into 1.5 million proteins makes the ability to handle enormous amounts of data a clear priority.

The data that the health informatics or life sciences informatics solutions have to deal with on a daily basis are mind-boggling in terms of the volume in addition to the heterogeneity and multidimensionality. One single genome contains 300 terabytes of trace files, meaning 300 trillion bytes of data files. A typical pharmaceutical company generates over 20 terabytes a day of new data. Over 400 petabytes of new medical images are created each year. And so the list continues. Now add to these figures the fact that it takes 1.3×10^{21} floating-point operations per second (FLOPS) to fold a single protein ab initio, and we have on our hands a massive amount of data being generated continuously.

Traditional content management is based primarily on data warehousing technique and used for improvement of the decision-making process through timely presentation of relevant business information that can be used for supporting a detailed analysis of the areas the decision makers are most concerned about. Over the years these requirements have been well recognized and resulted in development of decision support system (DSS), executive information system (ESS), and management information system (MIS). These systems typically acquire data from a number of sources, run specialized tools to reconstruct the data to a canonical format, and then run queries against the data.

Content management based on a data warehouse has a very different data structure from an online transaction processing (OLTP) system for transaction management. The data in a warehouse may be (1) archived and summarized as opposed to being current, (2) organized by subjects as opposed to by applications, (3) static until refreshed as opposed to being dynamic, (4) simplified for analysis as opposed to being optimized for transactional computation, (5) accessed for read-only as opposed to being updated, and (6) unstructured for analysis as opposed to being structured for repetitive processing.

Content management via a data warehouse is based on an online analytical processing (OLAP) data structure, as opposed to the operationally tuned OLTP data structure. In terms of data access characteristics, OLAP operations access many records at a time, while OLTP operations access one record at a time. OLAP operations rarely update data and require response times ranging from minutes to days, while OLTP operations constantly update individual records and require subsecond response times for many cases, such as the online securities trading system. An OLAP environment supports analytical queries against the data at a specific point in time. OLAP data are organized into relevant data categories based on the aggregate of data from multiple sources, and structured and stored in a consistent format to execute complex queries and data mining. The main purpose of data warehousing is to separate the analytical operations from the business transactions and to prevent the OLAP operations from interfering with the OLTP operations.

The typical approach for data warehousing is to create domain-specific data marts for certain OLAP operations based on business categories, by extracting the domain-specific data from the institutional central data warehouse and restructuring the data for domain-specific use cases. The institutional central data warehouse is created by extracting, transforming, and aggregating the data from various sources for operational data store (ODS), which are typically aggregates of the online transaction processing (OLTP) data. The operational data store is a database that essentially mirrors a production data source and is used to offload query and reporting work from the production system.

An OLAP (online analytical processing) repository architecture is needed to accommodate dynamic business requirements that cannot be anticipated. Data warehousing architecture should be aligned with the organizational structure and the IT operation. Lack of fit, or rather a misalignment, between the organizational structure and the data warehousing architecture has resulted in ongoing debate on and the religious wars for which data warehousing approach is more beneficial for an organization. These debates, or religious wars, would have been avoidable had data warehousing architecture been aligned with the organizational structure.

Organizations that are highly centralized in geography and running in a centralized governance model should pursue centralized data warehouse architecture to reap the greatest operational efficiencies and business benefits. Organizations that are highly decentralized and running autonomous business units will benefit from the distributed data warehouse architecture, while the organizations that have a mixed organizational pattern and a hybrid modus operandi should take advantage of the data federation technology.

AN ACTIVE, AS OPPOSED TO PASSIVE, MULTIDIMENSIONAL DATA REPOSITORY FOR BIOMEDICAL INFORMATICS

The traditional approach for data repositories for OLAP (online analytical processing) system or DSS (decision support system) is to create a central data warehouse to aggregate a superset of data relevant to OLAP or DSS. The data from source systems are retrieved through an ETL (extract, transform, load) process in a batch mode, typically overnight. The data warehouse is a passive repository with read-only access in this case. Updated changes at the source systems will be reflected on the data warehouse as additional data with versioning. Data marts for specific domain or purposes will be created with subsets of data out of the central data warehouse.

The key characteristics of the *traditional* OLAP repository described in the previous section can be summarized as follows:

- Passive repositories exist for read-only.
- A plethora of data marts are created with subsets of data extracted out of a central data warehouse.
- Data are extracted and loaded through a batch operation.
- Data are of a static nature.

Content management based on the traditional OLAP repository will not suffice the needs of health informatics or life sciences informatics that manages multidimensional data on a real-time basis and also in an adaptive mode, especially because of the passive and static nature of the repository.

The key properties of the health informatics or life sciences informatics repository are summarized below:

- The data are multidimensional, for example, relational, nonrelational, structured, unstructured, text, and numeric, and include images.
- The data are heterogeneous, for example, XML (eXtended Markup Language) documents, BLOBs (binary large object), and CLOBs (character large object), and include images.
- The data are volatile, in that frequent changes of metadata occur in existing data sources, and new data sources are frequently added.
- The data are potentially very large; for example, trillions of bytes are stored for online access and quadrillions of bytes for near-line access.
- The data are potentially very wide; for example, a record can contain hundreds of attributes.
- The data are potentially very deep, in that they contain millions of records.
- The data are active, in that derived data need to be captured for subsequent access.

Therefore the repository to be used for content management needs to provide the following functional properties:

- Accept, transform, normalize, and populate (file based) "pushed" data in batch (traditional ETL).
- Accept, transform, normalize, and populate (message based) event-driven or time-sensitive data in near-real time.

- Dynamically transform and normalize data based on business rules as well as the business context.
- Manage versions of data to include current data as well as old data (when business rules change the old data need to migrate as a new version of the data).
- Enable insertion of derived data in separate tables or separate databases with a mechanism to correlate the derived data with the source data.
- Provide unified indexing for multidimensional data: relational, XML documents, BLOBs, CLOBs, and images.
- Provide centralized metadata management for nonrelational data such as XML documents, BLOBs, CLOBs, and images.
- Enable easy integration of new data sources.
- Scale for width, depth, and size of database.
- Adapt to accommodate business volatility.

A conceptual architecture of content management for health informatics or life sciences informatics is depicted in the Figure 8.7. There can be two types of repositories: one similar to the traditional "data warehouse" but for cross-domain general-purpose data, not necessarily a superset aggregate, and the other similar to the traditional "data marts" for domain-specific or special-purpose data. The specific data repositories can be loaded from the corresponding data sources, including file systems, while the traditional data marts are loaded from the data warehouse. The generic data repository can contain shared data sets across multiple domains while the specific data repositories contain domain-specific data sets. Back-level data can be loaded into the

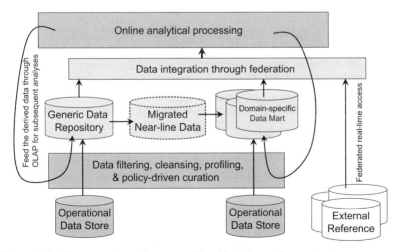

Figure 8.7 Conceptual architecture of health informatics content management

generic data repository, and the specific data repositories can be loaded through a one-time ETL batch process. Also bulky new data that are not time sensitive can be loaded via batch ETL process into the generic data repository as well as the specific data repositories.

Different data cleansing, normalization, and curation rules may be developed and enforced to the generic data repository and the specific data repositories. Derived data, such as data-mining outcomes, query results or search results that are frequently requested and can be written back into the specific data repositories. This is to enable the derived data to be used as input for processing or to be used in lieu of materialized query tables in the future, and also to enable the derived data to be shared among other systems in a specific region or in a specific domain.

For consistency and integrity of the derived data in relation to other data, the derived data are subject to the same policy-driven curation mechanism as well, although the derived data are distinct from the loaded data and likely to be subject to different policies. For actual deployment, separate tables or separate repository can be used for the derived data in order to maintain the integrity of the data.

In addition—as a hybrid solution—selected domain-specific data repository (or repositories), the generic shared data repository, the derived data repository (or repositories), and the external reference data sources can be federated for combinatorial analyses, statistical analyses, or data mining. It is envisioned that most of large installations will have a generic data repository and one or more specific data repositories although some small installations may have one data repository for both generic data and domain-specific data sets.

Based on the data retention policies of the individual institutions, some data may be migrated into auxiliary storage devices (e.g., robotic tape drives) automatically by the storage management system software for near-line access as opposed to online access. For example, BLOBs or CLOBs that have not been accessed for the last 90 days can be automatically migrated into the robotic tape drives to free up the online storage space. When the BLOBs or CLOBs are requested after migration into inexpensive near-line storage, the storage management software will automatically recall the data and load them back into the online storage (i.e., disk). This migration and recall processing will be performed automatically based on data retention policies of the specific region or domain.

FROM DATA TO INFORMATION, AND TO KNOWLEDGE, THROUGH MINING MULTIDIMENSIONAL DATA

Through the use of interviews, maps, and medical knowledge, the classical epidemiologists obtained knowledge about the disease under study. As with much human expertise, the route that was taken to that knowledge was likely misty compared to the well-defined logical chains of cause and effect in emerging and future healthcare IT systems. However, both then and today, the formal nature of the knowledge ultimately derived can be at times at least as misty, if still lying largely in the human appreciation of the information delivered. We have constantly used here the term *knowledge* in a general sense, but like thousands of years of thinkers as described briefly at the beginning of this chapter, we have as yet failed to deliver a more tangible specification of it. Knowledge encompasses so much more than mere information or data, yet falls short of reaching wisdom or innovation. The lowest rung is data, the simplest form of facts and figures. Data can evolve into information (the next rung) by validating it through imposing a structure and adding meaning to it. The next rung, knowledge, is reached by putting the information into context and adding understanding to it. From here, wisdom and innovation can be derived from knowledge in conjunction with experiences and foresight.

Because of the difficulty of obtaining a clear definition of knowledge, evidence-based medicine and other scientific disciplines have tended to take a view based on utility and flow of information that avoids the word "knowledge" altogether. For example, the following is what we consider a reasonable composite schema from many such views:

Unstructured source → [Structured data → rules] → Inference → Prediction → Decision → Action → Outcome

Note that we join together structured data and rules in brackets because rules that relate to one another can be joined up to form a network (what mathematicians call a *graph*), which is a more elaborate kind of structured data.

We need not give up so easily, however, and instead state that knowledge resides in this at about the level of structured data and rules, and maybe, or maybe not, including all or part of the inference step. Probably inference should not be included 100%, because physicians apply their knowledge from general medicine and collective patient data to make a specific inference about a patient based on input from that specific patient record. At the beginning of the chapter there are strong hints about the nature of knowledge, namely that it resides in the conglomeration and connections of facts. A first attack is that knowledge represents a kind of *mind map* or *concept map* or *semantic net*, meaning a form of structured data in which diverse items of data are crystallized as key concepts and *related to each other* in a working model with predictive capability. To this end specialist *knowledge architects and engineers* have honed new tools. There has been the important notion of *triples* (i.e., related structures), and in many cases actually being subject–verb–object or noun–preposition–noun (where we may replace subject, object, or noun with the idea of a noun-phrase in many cases). For example, triples may be read automatically from the text in millions of patents, and not least similar structures can be read from the records of millions of *patients*. But this is only a step in the right direction: we would not get very far writing this book only with sentences that are merely triples. Moreover clinical data can contain thousands of data items that may not necessarily show the same statistical behavior when fragmented only into triples. This is precisely the same as saying the data are *high dimensional*, meaning in many forms in various perspectives with many parameters. However, the triples are the most important building blocks that can be joined together by same noun to another noun to form an extensive network ("graph") which provides the big picture (albeit that this misses some cross connections—which one day will come—and hence the complete picture).

For example, a triple from automatic reading of patents is [Carbenoxolone] [binds to] [Corticosteroid 11-Beta Dehydrogenase Isozyme 1]. It is a triple because it has three parts [1][2][3]. Were it a new molecule or a known molecule with a new protein target, it is intrinsically new information. Be it old news or new news, it can become part of a network graph in which [carbenoxolone] also binds other protein targets, and the isoenzyme also binds other molecules (both are indeed the case). There will be triples for them, some containing [Carbenoxolone] and some containing [Corticosteroid 11-Beta Dehydrogenase Isozyme 1].

The triple above is a *universal categorical statement* because all carbonoxolone molecules bind to this specific isoenzyme, even though they individually bind to other things. There is no matter of degree about it unless we want to get smart and include binding strength, which is not all or nothing. If we want to assign a measure to the triple as a statement of fact, it would be assigned 100%. The only other option that arises here is that one might be able to take a triple like [Carbonoxolone] [does Not bind to] [Hemoglobin] and bring that into the same fold as [Carbonoxolone] [binds to] [Hemoglobin] but assign 0% certainty. What we can be sure of is that when in reading patents, we can come across [Carbonoxolone] [binds to] [Corticosteroid 11-Beta Dehydrogenase Isozyme 1] but never [Carbonoxolone] [does Not bind to] [Corticosteroid 11-Beta Dehydrogenase Isozyme 1]. Well we can't be sure of anything in life, including zero occurrence of errors, but that brings us to the next consideration.

The fact that doubles, triples, quadruples, and so on, are formally required can be proved, but suffice it to say here that this is because for a kind of knowledge graph of N-things, they "add up" to the total complete information that a giant N-tuple would provide. The bottom line is that the use of triples in semantic networks because they are held to be absolutely true statements that, crudely speaking, hold the network rigidly together even if data are incomplete. The need for progress in the knowledge field is reflected in the fact that few healthcare workers would claim that medicine is devoid of any uncertainty. As in other domains it is becoming clear that uncertainty is part of the aspect of knowledge.

Reading medical records we might find that for some patients the triple [Diabetes] [is associated with] [Alzheimer's] because they are both on the same record. But that is only true for some patients and their records. It is an *existential categorical statement* because the case exists at least once but not necessarily always. If we want to play the same game as for carbenoxolone, then we can write [Diabetes] [is sometimes associated with] [Alzheimer's], meaning in alternative human speech "Some diabetics have Alzheimer's," and can assign 100% certainty to that fact. Then such triples can play a robust role, and the use of universal "All" and categorical "Some" statements can have powerful roles together in inference as in the use of syllogisms. However, "sometimes" and "some" are fuzzy as to how much, and in the example above, a diabetic is definitely likely to want to know how much. In addition, to the extent that analysis of what comes first in time on the records can suggest causality (more correctly, in conjunction with other knowledge), then it is [Diabetes] [leads to] [Alzheimer's] which is of interest. [Alzheimer's] [leads to] [Diabetes] is of less interest to the diabetic.

Thus another aspect of knowledge is appreciation of *certainty* or conversely *uncertainty* of medical "facts." Future steps to follow will be able to render the kind of network above as capable of making inference, including ideally the ability to handle the almost ubiquitous uncertainty that pervades the real world. This is done first by associating the triples with probabilities or analogous measures. So an interpretation of an aspect of knowledge is that statements in joined triples such as "Obesity leads to diabetes" and "Diabetes leads to Alzheimer's" will be associated with probabilities, emphasizing that these are tendencies only and much less than 100% true and even much less than 50%.

Indeed one needs a method that expresses the fact that the risk of Alzheimer's for the diabetic is very small, it is just two to five times more risk than for the average population according to diverse sources. Moreover it might as well, according to a recent Kaiser study, have more to do with the obesity association with diabetes than diabetes directly. "A pot belly in middle age dramatically raises the risk of Alzheimer's," reported the *Daily Mail* in March 2008, "Men and women who have large stomachs in their 40s are three times more likely to suffer serious mental decline when they reached their 70s". Yet the original study also showed negligable increased risk from diabetes *directly*.[2] Not least in counselling the patient, methods should capture all this concern about obesity.

Although many of the discussions on this topic can be more appropriately placed in the next chapter, some observations relevant to architecture are worth making. Basically information in data flows from one kind of representation of *data type* or another, ultimately challenged to being knowledge, and then insight, wisdom, innovative decision, and action. Somewhere in the area of what we call knowledge involves, at present, a point in the IT architecture where a human being, likely a physician or researcher, will sit to convert it to insight. Up to a certain type of basic knowledge is as far as a machine can routinely go right now; more sophisticated forms currently require the human

---

[2] For those who may be concerned, see Whitmer RA, Gustafson DR, Barrett-Connor E, *et al.* *Neurology* 2008; Mar 26.

brain. What is that certain type of basic knowledge? A great deal of knowledge has something to do with many things that correlate or occur together, more or less than expected, or change in numerical value together more or less than expected. Robert Fano was an information theorist who defined *mutual information* between things or events as most closely related to knowledge (see also the next chapter). Some discussion about this is also important here because such measures come to the same final convergence point as mind maps/concept maps/semantic nets, suggesting that we may be coming closer to what knowledge actually is.

So information theory has something to say about knowledge too, and in quantifying things in the manner above as we did for obesity and diabetes. It says that knowledge has at least "something to do with" mutual information. As a measure it is the information in the association that you see, minus that which would be expected on some prior basis, typically a chance basis. See page 373. Actually this will be an annoying statement to information theorists in that there is an intuitively convenient but algebraically nasty switch of sign +/− in traditionally dealing with simple information and mutual information. But suffice it to say that in using the "typically a chance basis," mutual information comes out algebraically as the logarithm of the ratio of the probability of having obesity and diabetes to the products of the probabilities of having obesity and of having diabetes (together or not). Should we want to express, however, that as an existential statement, there is a way of doing that as the logarithm of the ratio of the probability of having diabetes and Alzheimer's to the probability of having Alzheimer's with or without diabetes. So, not only has qualitative progress been made over the years in terms of networks representing knowledge, but information theory gives means to quantify it too (we could just say *probability theory*, but probability ratios are not convenient and miss the opportunity to bring in some powerful tools of information theory).

Incidentally the combined use of universal and existential cases in inference could be argued as requiring two corresponding kinds of probability, a position that the author (BR) has taken elsewhere by using complex numbers (i.e., with a part proportional to the square root of minus one, to enable two kinds of probability to be quantified in a single complex value). Reasoning from quantum mechanics can then be adapted to the quantification of categorical and syllogistic reasoning. Quantum mechanics is with certain practical caveats supposed to be best practice in handling things from the smallest subatomic particle to the whole universe. That needs not concern us here except to illustrate the kind of extremes of work being done to explore definition of best practice in these areas.

There are just too many approaches to uncertainty and inference from it to fit in our brief overview, and they do not all turn out to be equivalent. They cannot all be right. Keeping in mind that medical decisions are to be made from all this stuff, it is wise to think and debate rather deeply about what best practice is, and how it can be that, if we have the right answer already, there are so many different methods.

Data mining permits the discovery of preciously unknown dependencies and relationships in the data sets as triples and indeed doubles, quadruples, and any other "uple." For example, clinical genomics research typically involves five research scenarios that start with identifying genes of interest, characterizing the identified genes and SNPs (genomic biomarkers), testing polymorphisms, correlating the identified genes with a certain disease, and validating associations and correlations through population studies. Correlating genes with diseases can be categorized into two approaches: (1) correlating one gene with monogenic traits and (2) correlating multiple genes with polygenic traits. In addition clinical genomics research involves correlating genes with susceptibility or immunity of the population to specific pathogens or allergens.

RULE TO NETWORK TO CLINICAL INSIGHT:
A WORKED EXAMPLE

For the whole network of interacting rules of varying complexity, it is actually impossible to give here a completely worked-out example. That is a job for the computer, not pencil and paper. By "interacting rules" we mean that at least two rules will touch on the same topic, say "pulmonary circulation disorder," and thus must cooperatively influence the inference process in some way. What the computer will be able to infer it can be illustrated with simple strong rules.

The value of data mining is in producing rules, and showing their use in the subsequent process of risk assessment and decision making. The example entities here called *rules* are *doubles*, one of which in a risk assessment is always congestive heart failure, since we are interested in making a prediction of risk for a patient. Actually the rules correspond to the triples introduced above such as [Congestive Heart Failure] [is associated with] [Pulmonary Association Disorder]. However, we may take the part "[is associated with]" as meaning implicit, as the default. In contrast, a connection like [binds to] in the previous pharmaceutical example would have to specifically appear in the mined data. If it did not, the part [associated with] (one might say [somehow associated with]!) would be assumed, and might be explicitly described as such in a network graph of knowledge. In Table 8.1 there should be triples, quadruples, and so forth, that can be mined have to be taken into account, and indeed in this case 6667,000 synthesized patient records were mined and analysis went up to quintuples. The doubles adequately illustrate the basic idea, and triples etc. are not included. The reason is that there are over 133,000 triples in this case, thousands of which relate to matters in the table, and some thousands of significant strength that relate to congestive heart failure. The authors and others, by the way, daily, and in this book, often refer to *pairs* or *doublets* as well as writing *doubles*, and *triplets*, *quadruplets*, quintuples, and so on, or alternatively *complexity 2*, *complexity 3*, and so on. It is just that *triples* is an

TABLE 8.1 Prediction of Risk of Congestive Heart Failure

Information	Type	Event 2 with Congestive Heart Failure (Event 1)	Patient Fit	Mutual Information ×1 for Yes x – 1 for No	Binary –1/+1 Using Strong Rules I > 1.0
1.88	association (pair)	**Pulmonary_circulation_disorder**	1	1.88	1
1.73	association (pair)	**Renal_failure**	1	1.73	1
1.60	association (pair)	**Valvular_disease**	1	1.60	1
1.49	association (pair)	**Diabetes_complicated**	1	1.49	1
1.45	association (pair)	**PCO2First(CARBON_DIOXIDE_PARTIAL_PRESSURE_mmHg:=low)**	1	1.45	1
1.44	association (pair)	**Peripheral_vascular_disorder**	-1	-1.44	-1
1.44	association (pair)	**PCO2First(CARBON_DIOXIDE_PARTIAL_PRESSURE_mmHg:=high)**	-1	-1.44	-1
1.44	association (pair)	**Coagulopathy**	-1	-1.44	-1
1.42	association (pair)	**Cardiac_arrhythmias**	1	1.42	1
1.37	association (pair)	**PO2First(OXYGEN_PRESSURE_mmHg:=low)**	1	1.37	1
1.33	association (pair)	**PHFirst(pH:=high)**	-1	-1.33	-1
1.32	association (pair)	**PHFirst(pH:=low)**	1	1.32	1
1.31	association (pair)	**BUNFirst(UREA_NITROGEN_BLOOD_mg/dL:=high)**	1	1.31	1
1.30	association (pair)	**CREATFirst(CREATININE_BLOOD_SERUM_mg/dL:=high)**	1	1.30	1
1.24	association (pair)	**Peptic_ulcer_bleeding**	0	0.00	0
1.24	association (pair)	**PTAVFirst(prothrombin_TIME_sec:=high)**	-1	-1.24	-1
1.23	association (pair)	**Fluid_and_elctrolyte_disorders**	-1	-1.23	-1
1.21	association (pair)	**PO2First(OXYGEN_PRESSURE_mmHg:=high)**	-1	-1.21	-1
1.21	association (pair)	**Blood_Loss_anemia**	0	0.00	0

1.19	association (pair)	Diabetes_uncomplicated	-1	-1.19
1.19	association (pair)	Deficiency_anemias	-1	-1.19
1.03	association (pair)	Chronic_pulmonary_disease	-1	-1.03
1.02	association (pair)	TSHFirst(THYROID_STIMULATING_HORMONE_uIU/mL:=high)	-1	-1.02
0.98	association (pair)	Other_neurological	-1	-0.98
0.96	association (pair)	Obesity	-1	-0.96
0.95	association (pair)	Hypertension	1	0.95
0.95	association (pair)	Paralysis	-1	-0.95
0.95	association (pair)	TPFirst(PROTEIN_TOTAL_g/dL:=low)	0	0.00
0.93	association (pair)	Lymphoma	-1	-0.93
0.92	association (pair)	Liver_disease	-1	-0.92
0.88	association (pair)	LDHFirst(LACTATE_DEHYDROGENASE_U/L:=low)	1	0.88
0.87	association (pair)	Hypothyroidism	1	0.87
0.83	association (pair)	LDHFirst(LACTATE_DEHYDROGENASE_U/L:=high)	-1	-0.83
0.83	association (pair)	NAFirst(SODIUM_mmol/L:=low)	1	0.83
0.79	association (pair)	Age_at_diagnosis:=>average 51.64	-1	-0.79
0.78	association (pair)	PLTFirst(PLATELETS_k/uL:=low)	0	0.00
0.77	association (pair)	CALCMFirst(CALCIUM_mg/dL:=low)	0	0.00
0.76	association (pair)	GLUCFirst(GLUCOSE_BLOOD_mg/dL:=>average)	-1	-0.76
0.74	association (pair)	Rheumatoid_arthritis_collagen_vascular_diseases	-1	-0.74
0.73	association (pair)	PTTAVFirst(PARTIAL_THROMBOPLASTIN_TIME:=high)	-1	-0.73
0.72	association (pair)	Alcohol_abuse	1	0.72

TABLE 8.1 *Continued*

Information	Type	Event 2 with Congestive Heart Failure (Event 1)	Patient Fit	Mutual Information ×1 for Yes x − 1 for No	Binary −1/+1 Using Strong Rules I > 1.0
0.67	association (pair)	**ASTFirst(ASPARTATE_AMINOTRANSFERASE_(GOT)_U/L:=high)**	1	0.67	0
0.66	association (pair)	**PTTAVFirst(PARTIAL_THROMBOPLASTIN_TIME:=low)**	1	0.66	0
0.66	association (pair)	**MGFirst(MAGNESIUM_mg/dL:=>-0.35)**	0	0.00	0
0.65	association (pair)	**Metastatic_cancer**	−1	−0.65	0
0.63	association (pair)	**Psychoses**	−1	−0.63	0
0.61	association (pair)	**PHOSFirst(PHOSPHORUS_mg/dL:=high)**	1	0.61	0
0.57	association (pair)	**TSHFirst(THYROID_STIMULATING_HORMONE_uIU/mL:=low)**	1	0.57	0
0.57	association (pair)	**PTAVFirst(prothrombin_TIME_sec:=low)**	1	0.57	0
0.57	association (pair)	**Solid_tumor_without_metastasis**	−1	−0.57	0
0.55	association (pair)	**ALKPFirst(ALKALINE_PHOSPHATASE_U/L:=>average)**	1	0.55	0
0.54	association (pair)	**WBCFirst(WHITE_BLOOD_CELL_k/uL:=>average)**	1	0.54	0
0.54	association (pair)	**KFirst(POTASSIUM mmol/L:=<average)**	1	0.54	0
0.52	association (pair)	**PHOSFirst(PHOSPHORUS_mg/dL:=low)**	−1	−0.52	0
−0.59	association (pair)	**ALTFirst(ALANINE_AMINOTRANSFERASE_(GPT)_U/L:=>average)**	−1	0.59	0
−0.59	association (pair)	**No Hypertension**	−1	0.59	0
−0.65	association (pair)	**Age_at_diagnosis:=<50***	−1	0.65	0
−0.66	association (pair)	**Pulmonary_circulation_disorder (but no congestive heart failure)**	−1	0.66	0
		CONGESTIVE HEART FAILURE		**1.60**	**−1**

industry standard in modeling semantic nets as knowledge graphs but not necessarily in data mining.

Whatever the complexity of an entity, it can be associated with a measure of certainty, and in this case a measure due to Fano, who was mentioned in the previous section. For those interested in the details, his important measure may now be described as the *Fano's mutual information* between any medical parameter A and B, such that

$$I(A;B) = \log_e P(A \& B) - \log_e P(A) - \log_e P(B)$$

P(A & B) is the probability of A and B occurring together (on the same medical record, in this case); P(A) is the probability of A occurring; and P(B) is the probability of B occurring, on any record. It is insightful to write the formula this way because it highlights that mutual information subtracts, from the joint information for A and B, the information from A and B alone, but readers out of practice with algebra may note that there is no need to take the log three times if P(A & B)/[P(A) × P(B)] is calculated first (then the log of the result is taken just once). In fact, Fano's original formula is not general enough for present purposes, needing (a) extension to I(A ; B ; C) for triplets and then further similar extension for more complex forms, and (b) treatment of finite (limited amounts) of data by replacement of the logarithmic functions by another function (actually a function called Riemann's Incomplete Zeta Funtion $\zeta(s = 1, n)$ not usually available on calculators, where in the present case n is a number of observations such as n(A & B)). Also, one needs to include such information I(~A ; B) also for "NOT A" (i.e., ~A) which is useful information (or contrary evidence) against A. Deeper discussion of all these issues would take us beyond our present scope. However, see the Bibliography and the next section, which discusses why there is a need for this more complicated approach, compared with what classical statistics and biostatistics teaches. As is standard in this kind of data mining, the natural logarithm is used whose information measure is not the binary unit or bit, but the *natural unit* or *nat*. This is in column 1, and note that the rules can be ranked in strength from highest positive to most negative value. More precisely column 1 uses the above Zeta Function estimate of Fano's measure for finite including very sparse data, but for 6667,000 patient records there are lots of data for doubles, and the estimate comes to the same thing as Fano's original measure, that is, as if we calculated classical probabilities to determine it. Column 2 shows the rule type, all here being *association rules*. Other types, which can be co-ranked in the same table, are mainly the correlations between quantitative values (as in multivariate analysis).

The idea here is that the record of the patient, including the material from the current visit, is used by the physician as if it were a kind of query. Column 4 "Patient fit" shows +1 if the patient has an entry on his or her record that matches that rule, 0 if it does not, and −1 if the rule is inconsistent with the entry. The simplicity of information theory as the numbers are simply added up to obtain the final information measure. A positive number will indicate positive risk for congestive heart failure. However, 0 in the "Patient fit" column indicates that the rule is not included because it is irrelevant or unknown for the specific patient, and −1 indicates that it is subtracted because of the contrary evidence. Of course, if the information in column 1 for the rule is already negative, the product of double negative is positive, meaning that the minus sign in column 1 is ignored when the two negatives are added. This can all be done on a spreadsheet, column 5 being column 1 times column 4, and the sum being the final answer.

In the discussion above, the diabetic patient would need to understand that just because diabetes is associated with Alzheimer's does not mean that there is a high chance of developing the disease. Degrees of certainty are important. In contrast to that, the discerning reader will perceive that the rules in the very last column are reformulated not in information units but as positive, neutral, or negative, meaning they are rendered qualitative. It behooves us to state the interesting fact that a nonquantitative approach can lead to a completely opposite conclusion: the sum of this column is −1, signifying accumulation of evidence against heart failure, while 1.6 in column 5, representing the full and proper method, shows a significant positive risk. In other words, not recognizing uncertainty, and hence degrees of certainty (expressed as probability, information, or other measures), loses information with the consequence that the finial assessment of risk, or diagnosis or clinical decision, could be radically changed.

There is more about data mining in Chapter 9, but there is an important reason for bringing it up here. When we focus on prediction such as the chance of getting Alzheimer's *and* congestive heart failure, the mind/concept maps or semantic nets expressed in similar information theoretic terms *reduce to the same inference process as described above.* This would be clearer to the statistically minded if a simple small table could show all rules, triples, and so on, especially as the technique becomes more complicated. The data could also be probabilities (in which case values are multiplied, not added), which would then bring us very close to an alternative technique called a *Bayes's net* or *Bayesian net*, after the bishop who published his ideas in *Philosophical Transactions* back in 1763.

To the mathematician, there is solace to be found in considering an *N*-dimensional mind map/concept map/semantic net with associated probabilities or information as a simplex, in which case the graph is splayed out maximally in *N* dimensions. Then our measures would relate to the corners, edges, faces, volumes, hypervolumes, hyperhypervolumes, and so forth, for that geometric object. In algebraic terms, these measures would be generated by the binomial theorem, and any incompleteness, missing edges or volumes, would correspond to what is left as an approximation. In information theoretic terms, what is missing would correspond to *entropy*. Deeper thought along these lines would bring us closer to a theory of knowledge, and preferably with a mathematical cast that can accommodate algorithms, programs, and IT.

AN ORIENTATION TO THE CLASSICAL WAY THAT HEALTHCARE LOOKS AT STATISTICS

The medical reader may find the discussion above on inference and decision support a far cry from the so-called classical statistics, which is actually much later than Bayes, and taught as "biostatistics" to medical students. It is not hard to see why. Not only does classical statistics contest the importance of combining pro- and contra-evidence (corresponding to the +1 and −1 of "Patient fit"), but it depends on a fuzzily defined contra-state of evidence called the *null hypothesis*. It then seeks to disprove this null hypothesis on the algebraically erroneous rationale that this is inevitably the more conservative way to do things, for example, that it is better to hedge one's bet by not giving a drug even if positive evidence says otherwise. To make matters worse, the result does not even relate to the probability that the null hypothesis is true given the data, but to that the probability that the data would be obtained given that the null hypothesis is true. So if that rationale is observed, the physician is not allowed to tell the patient the probability that he or she will get better given the latest data, but only the probability that the data would be obtained given that the drug will *not* work (i.e., in some fuzzily defined sense of "not get better"). The patient of course is not at all interested in seeing the mysterious probability values, but in seeing himself or herself get better.

The origin of this mess, incidentally, is that "classical" statisticians do not believe in probabilities that they cannot get by counting, an odd position when one considers their argument that the probability actually corresponds to what would be if they countered an infinite amount of data. To get to the probability of a hypothesis, they have to somehow evaluate the probability of the hypothesis in the absence of any data, as Bayes pointed out by his famous equation in his 1763 paper. There is no way to count a hypothesis. No problem, said Bayes, because you can still assign a value to it. It simply means that probabilities are not what you think and only behave like ratios of numbers (like the number of males divided by the number of males plus females) when numbers are adequately large; in general, probabilities are *degrees of belief*, with a neutral choice of value reflecting a negligible bias or pre-judgment in the absence of any data.

As circumstantial evidence that classical statistics is not really considered satisfactory even in healthcare circles, a rising new feature for evidence-based medicine (EBM) is the computer-supported counterpart information-based medicine (IBM). EBM discarded the classical approach in communication between physician and patient by introducing simple measures based on simple counting for conveying results as if they too were simple counting, such as "number needed to treat," meaning *the number of patients that would need to be treated to treat one bad outcome*. Of course, the problem is that the final measures are not real numbers of events for any one situation, and the kind of definition given above can be confusing. Other measures of EBM actually come close to being information theory without (and sometimes with) logs, however.

MORE GENERAL DATA ANALYTICS

That all said, the FDA still likes classical statistics, and so many medical systems support it, along with some other methods. The data analysis aspect of biomedical informatics involves scoring, modeling, visualization, time series analysis, bioinformatics, and data mining. All are crucial steps used to success-fully perform the analysis and of huge interest to the medical researcher, but data mining has a particular role in helping the physician make decisions. Data mining's main function is to perform predictive analyses on the data for knowl-edge extraction. This basically means that the techniques generate rules that can help the doctor make decisions. These aspects thus relate to decision support systems for diagnosis, prognosis, and therapy choice, which in turn are closely related to monitoring and surveillance systems, and are therefore dis-cussed in the next chapter. The unifying concept is that commonly used tech-niques uncover the unexpected.

The IT architect must pay attention to data types and how data intercon-vert. To get to the data mining stage, data may need to be extracted from what has been referred to as *semistructured form*. In practice, semistructured data are commonly represented by prose text, such as the notes written in legacy medical records by the physician, or as medical images from which features and descriptors must be extracted for data mining, such as the numbers describing the volume or shape of various parts of the brain. In general, by "semistructured" we mean analysis that is not as nicely tabulated as we require for direct data mining and data analysis. Any appropriate semistructured ana-lysis or data mining software that does not seem to need this intermediate step is really combining semistructured data processing and data mining in the same program, and in our opinion, this tends to reduce the quality of the data mining part, and possibly the semistructured analysis too.

Semistructured data are rather like raw data in the clinical laboratory, and both funnel together to produce or update more structured data forms such as HL7 clinical document architecture, a particular use of XML. The XML imparts a *hierarchic* data structure or *ontology*. See Fig. 8.8. It is a data type that may be called a *tree*. However, for most data minings and statistical analy-ses the XML needs to be converted to a spreadsheet form. This step is not difficult, and a spreadsheet is not the only data type that data mining can directly handle, which is fortunate because raw medical records don't look much like a spreadsheet at all, but as a *collection* or "bag," in that items have no particular order. In some ways this is rather like a paper-based medical record in which items like "broken leg" are entered and can occur more than once in the patient's record. A data type called a *list* means that the order is important. Spreadsheets, and DNA, and protein sequences, are examples of a list. There is associated metadata such as "Age" at the top of a spreadsheet column, or an implied heading, such as "column 26" or "26th item in the list." Such metadata may be considered as associated with each item under that heading, for example, Age: = 42 (see the next chapter). An intermediate data type is a *set*, in which there is no particular order but items cannot occur more than once. Lists sets and collections are all structured data, and so is the hierarchic structure of XML, which is why interconversion is relatively straightforward, as opposed to going from unstructured data such as text to any one of those data types.

Are we missing a data type? What about completely *unstructured* data? Oddly enough, if we try, we can imagine what completely unstructured data looks like: it conceptually is a simple collection or bag type of items. What semistructured data retains is some detectable relationship between items, including grammar, which might be captured in one of the more structured data forms. From this perspective the IT architect might imagine a flow from semistructured data to hierarchic data to a list to a collection, but a collection cannot go to anything else if the connecting relationships are lost. All that does remain is the description of the items such as "broken leg" and the number of times they occur. Those who like to think about such phenomena as thermodynamics, including entropy, might surmise that one can go from more structured to less structured data but never the reverse, at least not without ambiguity, because order (information about structure) is lost and not recoverable in going back in the first direction. Actually "semistructured" is a misnomer from this viewpoint. The data only look poorly structured to the human eye. The relationships are there and can be extracted. But that it is hard to do.

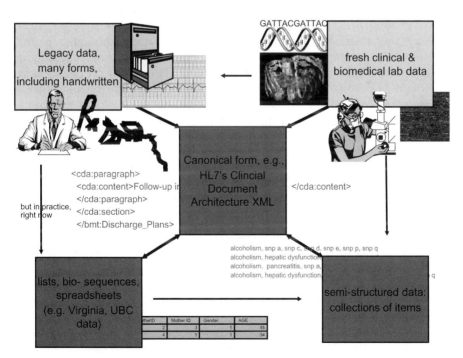

Figure 8.8 Relation of some data types in the overall architecture. Major record record collections like those at Virgin University and University of British Columbia are usually stored in spreadsheet-like form.

Similarly your DNA looks random but in fact carries a very important message about you.

Sharing of knowledge and data among scientists in real time is important. A key challenge in the IT field is the difficulties associated with knowledge sharing and collaboration among multidisciplinary researchers. To successfully implement a knowledge-sharing and collaborative system, asynchronous and synchronous options have to be available. For example, synchronous collaboration, such as conferencing, must be complemented by an asynchronous option for communication, such as email. The knowledge-sharing and online collaborative system has certain requirements to allow for efficient and effective communication among researchers and scientists. Support for both structured and unstructured data must be available to ensure that the system is capable of handling multidimensional data. Technology that will enable communities of practice, such as advanced search capabilities, an automated and rule-based workflow, the sharing of scientific annotation and data/text mining, are essential for successful collaboration and knowledge sharing.

HOW TO MOBILIZE TRANSLATIONAL LIFE SCIENCES RESEARCH FOR INFORMATION-BASED MEDICINE

Today's businesses heavily depend on information technology for their automated processes and for efficient operations with high productivity. Yet IT has become a major roadblock to businesses transformation or optimization due to the long lead time required to implement new processes/functions or changes in the business models and processes. The business processes, especially in the emerging industries, such as the life sciences industry, continuously change while pre-existing IT solutions are not flexible enough to adapt to the changes in time. Consequently there is often a mismatch between the business process and the deployed IT solution for the business.

The main source of the problem is that the current software design is based on static components. The functional behavior of a software component is statically defined, and any changes to the functional behavior of a component requires redevelopment of the component.

In the traditional approach to model a business into software engineering, a business operation is decomposed into autonomous functional units, the business functional units are mapped to software components, and the interfaces are specified for the software components to receive input data and to produce output data, and all the business rules, functional behavior, and business processes associated with the components are embedded within the functional components.

A component produces always the same output data with a same input data, regardless of other parameters, as shown in the Figure 8.9. So the component needs to be redeveloped to reflect other conditions or parameters. Any changes in the business rules, functions, control flows between functions, or data attri-

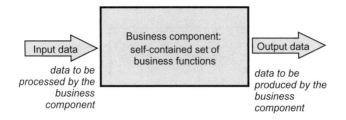

$$\text{Output} = \text{Function (Input)}$$

Figure 8.9 Traditional component model

butes or formats require the software component to be modified or redeveloped. The lead time required for the IT professionals to understand and interpret the business changes, reflect the changes into the software design, identify the affected software components, redevelop the software components, test and deploy a new system is much longer than the time for the business to change, and consequently IT has been continuously in catch-up mode.

One of way around component modeling is to implement a "control" interface for the software component in addition to the interfaces for input data and the output data, a feature already developed by one of us (OB). In this new component modeling, each business component has three external interfaces: first, an interface for receiving input data to be processed by the component, second, an interface for controlling the behavior of the component by providing the business rules associated with processing the input data and producing output data, and third, an interface for producing output data. The control interface is provided by an external human-readable and machine-readable interface. The business component can be dynamically configured or re-configured to change its internal behavior, without additional programming effort, in order to adapt it to different business rules.

This new business modeling approach is referred to as "dynamic component modeling," in contrast to the traditional component modeling where each software component has only two external interfaces: one for receiving input data and the other for producing output data. In the traditional approach the component needs to be re-designed and re-developed to adapt to changes in business rules because the program logics to handle the business rules are hard-coded within the component. The dynamic component modeling minimizes or obviates the need for re-developing a business component to address the different business rules of a specific institution.

The dynamic component modeling will be the essential foundation for realization and implementation of autonomous computing. The key functional attribute of autonomous computing is the capability of self-learning or machine learning for implementation of the main themes of the autonomous computing: self-configuring, self-optimizing, self-healing, and self-protecting.

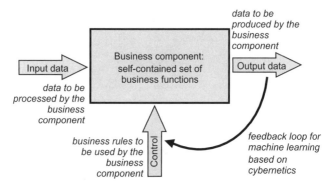

Figure 8.10   Dynamic component model for machine learning

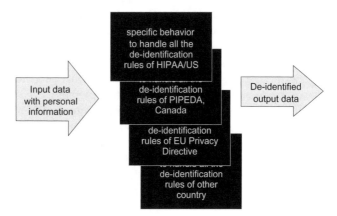

Figure 8.11   De-identification from the traditional business model perspective

The components can be extended for machine learning based on cybernetics by reflecting the output from the component on the control input so that the component can adjust the functional behavior based on the result of the previous processing. This facility enables the component to "learn from experience" and dynamically adjust its behavior and thus improve the intelligence and dynamic adaptability of the software component as shown in the Figure 8.10. For example, a software component for de-identification of protected personal information to comply with the privacy laws in one country or a specific industry may need to be re-developed, as shown in the Figure 8.11, to address the specific requirements in other countries, since de-identification rules are subject to the statutory requirements in each country and to the institutional privacy policies.

When the new approach for dynamic component modeling is applied to the software component for de-identification of protected personal information to comply with the privacy laws, the same component can be used for other

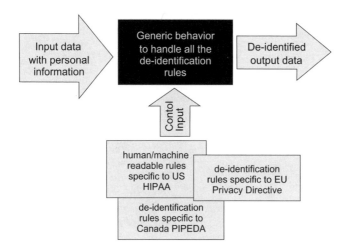

Figure 8.12 De-identification from the dynamic component model perspective

institutions, other industries and other countries by providing the control files to address the specific rules for the institution or the country, as shown in the Figure 8.12. The new approach obviates the need to develop three different components. In addition, when the control file is human-readable as well as a machine-readable document in XML notation, the business analyst or a privacy lawyer can provide the rules for de-identification.

SELF-ADAPTIVE COMPUTING BASED ON DYNAMIC SOFTWARE ENGINEERING APPROACH

Traditionally software has been engineered so that all the business rules, functional behavior, and business processes are embedded within the functional components. This way a component produces always the same output data with a same input data, regardless of any environmental parameters. Consequently the software component needs to be redeveloped to reflect other conditions or parameters. Any changes in the business rules, functions, control flows between functions, or data attributes require the redeveloped software component to be re-tested and re-deployed, causing IT to be continuously in a catching-up mode for the changes in business. This deficiency in the traditional software engineering model, among others, has been widening the gap between business and technology.

The self-adaptive software engineering model introduces a "control" interface for the software component in addition to the existing interfaces for input data and the output data. In this new component modeling, each software component has three external interfaces: (1) existing interface for receiving input data to be processed by the component, (2) additional interface for

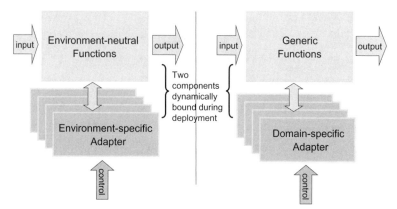

Figure 8.13   Novel software engineering approach for dynamic software components

controlling the internal behavior of the component by providing the business rules associated with processing the input data and producing output data, and (3) existing interface for producing output data. The control interface will be provided through an external human-readable as well as machine-readable interface. The software component can be dynamically configured or re-configured to change the internal behavior to adapt to different business rules or to environmental variables, without any additional development (Figure 8.13).

The software component interacts through three external interfaces: one for accessing input data ("input" interface), another for producing output data ("output" interface), and the last ("control" interface) for accepting environmental variables and characteristics to adjust the internal behavior of the software component accordingly with the runtime parameters. With this innovation, the launched software is able to discover the runtime environment and dynamically adapt to the target environment.

ONTOLOGY-BASED SEMANTIC METADATA MANAGEMENT FOR SELF-DESCRIBING DATA

In today's information age and knowledge-based economy, the main value of information technology is to engender insight and knowledge through efficient modeling, clustering, analyzing, and mining of vast amounts of data. A major challenge is an industry's inaccessibility to highly dimensional (e.g., numeric data, strings, binary data, rectangular data, graphics, audio or video images), heterogeneous (semantic and syntactic disparities, various data management systems such as flat files, binary or character objects, relational data), and dispersed data when the multidimensional data are created at an extremely high rate. The traditional method and system for data management are not able to keep up with the projected pace of the data growth.

However, data entities can be made to self-describe their properties such as semantics, ownership, version, and authorization and to provide a programmable interface for modeling, clustering, analyzing, and mining. Basically the semantic and syntactic properties of data are encapsulated for enabling data access via a set of programmatic interfaces through separation of concerns of data properties. This is similar to the *service-oriented architecture (SOA)* concept of "*information as service.*"

The semantic properties of newly generated data and the programmable interface are dynamically generated at the time of data creation whether it is machine-generated data or human-generated data. This way the problem of inaccessibility to rapidly growing, highly dimensional, and heterogeneous data is addressed by enabling the newly generated data to self-describe its semantic properties and to offer an external interface to implicitly handle the syntactical aspect of the data. So, for analytical programs to access the data without being detered by the syntactical properties of the data, the embedded functions are invoked in the data descriptor. This novel method removes dependency on data standards, which are mostly focusing on syntactical aspect of data and also lagging behind, by separating analytical programs from the concern about data syntax. In other words, the software is allowed to discover the semantic properties of the data to be processed and to access the data for manipulation independently of the syntactic properties of the data.

DATA-CENTRIC COMPUTING FRAMEWORK FOR TRANSLATIONAL RESEARCH

In the current computing model, software is "installed" on a specific machine as a stationary entity while data moves to the system where the software runs. In the exchange data across the network, issues arise, in the current computing model, about data quality, integrity, and currency, data security and intellectual property rights, privacy, performance due to network latency, software provisioning and deployment, and software maintenance. The IT industry has provisioned various solutions (but not a totally reliable solution) to mitigate the risks associated with these issues, but at the cost of end-user productivity and high cost of ownership as well as high operation and maintenance cost.

The traditional computing model where data are exchanged across the network becomes inefficient and inadequate when vast amounts of data are involved or when the data need to be protected for compliance to privacy laws. The traditional computing model where software is kept stationary on a designated system becomes not only inefficient but inadequate for pervasive computing environment.

In translational clinical research, in particular, researchers cannot access clinical information in health records that are protected by privacy laws and are required to be safeguarded within the institutional premises. Because of the limited accessibility to human data, clinical researchers instead heavily rely on animal data for developing hypotheses and for validating the hypotheses. Researchers do not have access to sufficient and reliable human data until a potential treatment option is approved by regulatory bodies (e.g., FDA in US) for human clinical trials, but only after many years of experiments based on animal data and animal trials. As a result most treatments are initially suited for animals, and the poor efficacy of treatment options for humans stems from researchers' inaccessibility to human data early in the process.

How can the healthcare professionals access the large volumes of the diagnostic images across the network in a timely manner, especially in an emergency? For example, a typical MRI scan image is in the range of terabytes (trillion bytes) and would take more than 4 hours to be transmitted over a gigabit network. All the following are within our current grasp, but the programming needs to be done with care, such that the following questions are answered in a satisfactory, safe way. How can we upgrade the software running on a medical device in an operating room that needs to be in operation for 7 days a week and 24 hours a day without any interruption? How can we upgrade the software running on a medical device on a ship or a submarine at sea? How can we upgrade the software running on a medical device on a space ship in orbit? The *data-centric computing model* where software moves to data, by way of the *self-adaptive software engineering model* and the *self-describing data based on ontology-based metadata management*, has proved to address the deficiencies of the current computing model and the current software engineering model and the data management approach.

The *data-centric computing model* allows the large volume of data or highly sensitive data to be kept at the source of collection and allows software to be launched on demand to a system of choice (see Figure 8.14). The *self-adaptive*

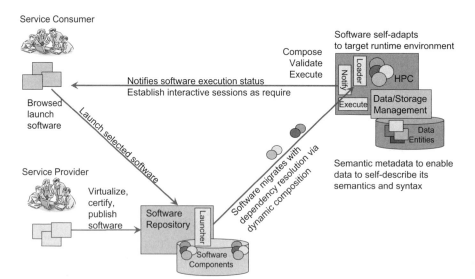

Figure 8.14   Conceptual architecture of data-centric computing framework

software engineering model allows the launched software to discover the properties of the target environment and self-adapt to its runtime environment. The *self-describing data based on ontology-based metadata management* allows the launched software to discover the properties of the data to be processed by enabling the data to self-describe their semantic and syntactical properties.

These technological innovations enable the software to (1) migrate to a remote system on demand, (2) dynamically compose its prerequisite and co-requisite software, (3) self-adapt to the target runtime environment, and (4) discover the properties of the data to be processed. With these innovations software developers can virtualize the software components, certify them with digital signature, and publish the virtualized software in a shared library, as opposed to installing the software on a designated system. This solution framework allows the end-users to search for the software of their interest in a service-oriented manner and to launch the selected software to a system of choice on demand.

By sending software to the system where data reside, as opposed to sending data to the system where software runs, this solution framework obviates the need to transfer large amount of data across the network, and consequently addresses the performance issues associated with the network latency and also improves the end-user productivity. In this solution framework data are captured once and kept at the source of collection, and consequently the system addresses issues associated with data quality, integrity, currency, security, privacy, and intellectual property rights.

This solution framework allows the software to be dynamically deployed on demand from a shared software library. Application software does not get installed on individual systems but is shared through a centralized management system responsible for maintenance, upgrade, and version control (see Figure 8.15). This way the software running on a medical device in an operating room, on a ship, in a submarine at sea, or on the space ship in orbit can be dynamically provisioned and upgraded near-real time, without disrupting operation.

When a software component is launched on demand to a remote system in a data-centric computing environment, the launched software component may not run properly on the target system because the runtime dependent software components may not be (1) available on the target system, (2) compatible (e.g., version mismatch), or (3) properly configured. The dependent runtime software components need to be dynamically composed to resolve prerequisites and co-requisites at the time of launch. During resolution of the runtime dependencies through dynamic binding of the software components, not only the required prerequisite or co-requisite software components need to be retrieved on demand from the software library but also the right version of a dependent software component needs to be selected if multiple versions of the same software components exist. This data-centric computing model addresses such requirements through

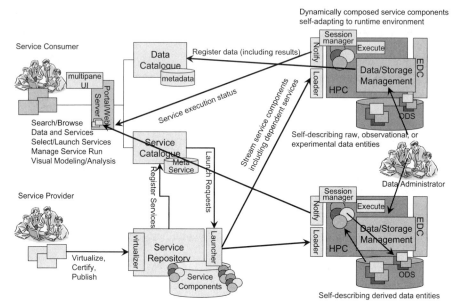

Figure 8.15   Fuller details of data-centric computing framework

the dynamic composition of application software at the time of the software launch.

SO WHAT?—A CONCLUSION

The data-centric computing solution may sound complicated, and (when we wrote this, at least) not a single line of programming code exists! That is the advantage of being the architect. Get it right, and the designers, programmers, hardware engineers, communications specialists, and all else will follow. What is the status to date? As for so many things in medical IT, 2009 is a time of transition. As yet, no such integrated, holistic system, storing, analyzing, and treating so many aspects of almost all patients, exists as an infrastructure. But many larger medical organizations like the Mayo Clinic have the elements of such a system, and many companies, and noncommercial and academic agencies, are developing bits and pieces. Clearly a single organization cannot develop a fixed system and dump it upon the world. There needs to be much debate on matters of ethics, pricing, standards, interoperability, reliability, scalability, and importantly the ability to evolve without destroying and rebuilding what we have built so far. It must be expected that solutions will grow outwards from organizations like large healthcare centers and university hospitals, the FDA, and pharmaceutical companies, incorporating pieces and evolving until the entire ecosystem of all players is fulfilled. An image comes to mind: we might see this ecosystem as a vast cave in which crystals sprout, where the strong crystals survive and the brittle die, and stalactites grow down and stalagmites grow up to meet and form staunch pillars. That is all to say that inevitable needs may be driving healthcare IT slowly in something like the direction envisaged here. At the time of reading this, subtle components may already be in position, and of the right flavor. Then some one may stand up and say that a new description is needed, and that description could be very close to what is predicted here. It will be interesting to see, and an interesting day of transition.

Of course, it is not easy to build a system that can ultimately become so knowledge based that the many facets of information to associate as knowledge act on that knowledge. Holism places a great challenge to knowledge. The whole point of evidence-based medicine, translational research, predictive and preventative medicine, and concern over healthcare wastage and medical errors, is that a few merely human brains aren't enough. Now, in Chapter 9, we may consider the broader purposes of all this.

9

GUARDIAN ANGELS: KNOWING OUR MOLECULES, DRUG AND VACCINE DESIGN, MEDICAL DECISION SUPPORT, MEDICAL VIGILANCE AND DEFENSE

1. A robot may not harm a human being, or, through inaction, allow a human being to come to harm.
2. A robot must obey the orders given to it by human beings, except where such orders would conflict with the First Law.
3. A robot must protect its own existence, as long as such protection does not conflict with the First or Second Law.

—from *I Robot* (1950) by Isacc Asimov (1920–1992)

GUARDIANSHIP

There is a far greater story to tell than one book can ever capture. Still the notion of *guardianship*, including *vigilance* over us and response to protect us, allows us now to touch upon many important topics. Our guardians, human and digital, must be able to read our state of well-being and our state of danger, and respond to save us. They need wisdom of insight into our body in molecular detail, ideally, in the far future, (and subject to fundamental theoretical limitations) near total knowledge down to almost every atom but, at least right now, knowledge of our genomics.

In the interim, IT can help provide that care, guiding, designing drugs, prescribing drugs, and nursing. IT will enhance the ability of physicians to monitor and treat patients in the different genomic strata in the population.

The Engines of Hippocrates: From the Dawn of Medicine to Medical and Pharmaceutical Informatics, by Barry Robson and O.K. Baek
Copyright © 2009 by John Wiley & Sons, Inc.

Similar monitoring will help physicians in responding and administering during disasters and epidemics. Among these and other issues the different responsibilities of medical practitioners in the patient care workflow, where IT can help with compliance and best practice in providing sophisticated molecular data.

FOUR TIMES, AND FOUR WORLDS, OF CLINICAL INTELLIGENCE TECHNOLOGY

Four people, millennia apart, have been listening to their bodies. In ancient China, lay Buddhist Su Dongpo, who actually existed, is entranced by the way he has found to speak with the atoms within his body. He is profoundly moved at the enlightenment and well-being that were dispensed from them during the night, and wonders how he can communicate it to the outside world in an essay-poem.

A millennium later, Jane O'Reilly is sitting in a room in Mount Sinai Medical Center in New York City having *her* internal status communicated to her by the skills of her physician, helped by the technology in the physician's office and medical laboratories. There is more advanced technology available to watch over the patient on an ongoing basis, but only had she been in a critical condition would she have batteries of machines vigilant around her bed, monitoring her health status. There are emerging Internet connections to help provide care at home, but only had she really needed chronic care. Sadly, healthcare providers and health systems today seem to be staggeringly inefficient at assimilating and processing information and at converting the information to knowledge. According to the Health Foundation, Health Affairs, and others, part of the problem is that the core knowledge base of healthcare—biomedical science—is expanding at a geometric rate, driven by $40 billion a year in public- and private-sector research and development (R&D) spending.

Several years later, Mgavi Smith, is somewhat less happy than these two predecessors. He thinks that he may be experiencing a technology glitch. He is staring down at a packet of frozen sausages in one hand, and a packet of cereal in the other. He is a little concerned that his bedside alarm-clock–coffee-maker didn't wake him up with his nutritional recommendations for the day. Does he need a new alarm clock? Is the server down? Is his implanted chip not reporting his blood substances status? Does the wireless connection software need upgrading? The automated help desk puts him right. Mgavi should have more faith in twenty-first century technology ... it's only 3:00 AM. He forgot to take his biorhythm adjuster pill, and he is still on European time after his business trip. He feels he must check the Internet for his Alzheimer's risk factor in his current lifestyle, now that his new affection for sausages, increased weight, and frequent trips across different time zones increase the risk factors for diabetes and Alzheimer's. But regarding the slimming pill his doctor recommended, he does remember to glance at the results of his *molecular imaging* scans, a technology already in use in research back in 2006. His suitability for a new dug has been tested by showing where the metabolically separated parts of the drug, which has previously been labeled at multiple sites in its chemistry and given in tiny dosage, ends up in his body, at the intended therapeutic targeted binding sides, as well as bad sites that may cause toxicity. The situation looks good, the associated text reports, despite prior concerns for effects on the liver and in production of excessive superoxide by the natural detoxifying cytochromes in the cells of the pancreas. It looks like he can pick up his prescription on his way to the airport for his next trip.

In 3011, a millennium later again, Charlie Schreiber-Dongpo (universal person identifier: H176Q1225A, albeit in some future script) is entranced yet again that he can speak with the atoms with his body through submicroscopic, molecular-scale devices implanted within him, and at the warmth and knowledge of well-being that were dispensed from them during the night. He knows that this is being automatically communicated with the well-being guardians on the Hypernet, and wonders only how he can communicate it to the outside world as an essay-poem.

It was no accident that the start and end of the first paragraph of this chapter brought us almost full circle. There may be millennia beyond the example of Charlie Schreiber-Dungpo with technology so advanced, so fundamental to the structure of the universe that matters spiritual and scientific become less distinguishable. "Any sufficiently advanced technology is indistinguishable from magic" stated science fiction writer Arthur C. Clarke in *Profiles of The Future, 1961* (Clarke's third law). But from now on let us concentrate on the very imminent technology and exclude for the moment nature's natural technologies and Buddhist technologies of the mind and spirit. By IT, we inevitably mean human-made computer hardware, software to run on it, and associated communication systems (though we will leave that as the "between" aspect to discuss later).

INSIGHT AND GUARDIANSHIP

To achieve depth of *insight* into our bodies and *guardianship* over them could seem like the work of God or magic. It will definitely take much greater computing power than we routinely have today and a lot of capital investment. There is no obvious insurmountable technological limit except that increasing amounts of energy will be required to get the finest details, due to considerations of quantum mechanics and entropy. One day the Earth may even run hot with guardian devices.

However, for the foreseeable future there will always be a role for the human physician, for whom IT will provide many methodologies to help get the job done better. One important reason for retaining the physician will be the need for a human ambassador between IT and the patient, a physician of wisdom and moral standing who has taken the Hippocratic Oath or modern equivalent and who will make the final choices and police what IT is recommending. There are those software engineers who look beyond even that to conceptualize software that might carry some of the caring character, wisdom, and morality of the dedicated physician. Isaac Asimov's three laws of robotics at the head of this chapter are an example of strongly built-in pro-human ethics as a kind of failsafe device, a kind of unbreakable Hippocratic Oath. But there are some "minor" practical principles of behavior too, the most basic being that the system must be capable of distinguishing between bathing the baby or boiling an egg. Marvin Minsky, regarded as the father of IT, has been extremely interested in the notion of IT systems, be they robots or boxes, as "caring agents." The Future of Health Technology Institute founded in Cambridge, Massachusetts, by Minsky's students, has concentrated on developing such "caring agents."

As in the robot stories of Isaac Asimov, some guardians of our health could literally take the form of walking-talking guardian robots, perhaps as humanlike in form as "androids." The years 2004 and 2005 were a watershed period. At St. Mary's hospital in London were introduced two such robots, named "Sister Mary" and "Dr Robbie." In Kansas City the untiring doc is named "REMi." Hackensack University Medical Center prefers to call their robot "Mr. Rounder." The robots at St. Mary's in London are in a general surgery ward, and those at the A&E Department within St Mary's and at Imperial College's Academic and Clinical Skills Unit are used for training purposes. In March 2005, UCLA Medical Center announced initial clinical tests of the RP-6 mobile robot system in its neurosurgery intensive care unit. This allows doctors to "virtually" consult with patients, family members, and healthcare staff at a moment's notice, even if miles away from the hospital. The Detroit Medical Center (DMC), also in March 2005, launched a mobile robot initiative that allows its physicians to interact with patients on demand and from remote locations. The DMC will deploy 10 mobile robots throughout six of its hospitals, the largest such deployment in the nation. The mechanical physician, Mr. Rounder, made its debut at Hackensack University Medical Center in December 2004. In a study done by Johns Hopkins University Hospital in Baltimore, Maryland, half the patients preferred a telerounding visit by their own doctor over a "real" visit by another physician. And 80% of the patients felt that the robot increased physician accessibility.

Remote Presence (RP-6) Robots, sold by InTouch Health, Inc., allow a medical expert to visually examine and communicate with a patient from anywhere in the world. The 5-foot 4-inch robot has a flat-screen computer monitor mounted on top. It is connected to the Internet via a hospital's secure wireless network. The system includes a two-way video feed, a microphone, and a speaker. The robot is guided by a physician using a joystick from a computerized control station (usually) in the physician's home or office. The doctor "controlling" the robot can view the patient, ask questions and read patient records, view X rays and test results from the console. The patient sees the doctor's image on the robots "face." Mass production of something like this may be needed soon if things get much worse. According to InTouch Health "Already today there are over 400,000 unfilled nursing positions causing hospitals across the country to close wings or risk negative outcomes. Over the coming years, the declining ratio of working age adults to elderly will further exacerbate the shortage. In 1950 there were 8 adults available to support each elder 65+, today the ratio is 5:1 and by 2020 the ratio will drop to 3 working age adults per elder person. Technology solutions that dramatically increase the effectiveness of healthcare professionals are required."

IT WITHIN US?

What is wrong with robot nurses or robot paramedics being always with us? Other devices would be like today's servers or as dispersed structures invisibly "within our walls" or even as chips implanted inside our body. Biochips are discussed in more detail in the last chapter. Already plausible for implant use are RFID chips (radiofrequency identifier chips) based on the EZ-pass toll-booth system in the United States: a radio signal provides a stimulus and the energy for a chip to transmit back information, without need for batteries powering the chip. We might call the implanted technology *invasive*, and that just outside *pervasive*. There is a rising interest in the United States and elsewhere on having implanted smart chips, say implanted in the wrist, that also contain the record and that could also perform more elaborate monitoring (and potentially action) functions. Already they are being used in several hospitals pervasively, and for cats and dogs invasively. Based on the RFID, an implant chip could do many more things for our lives. It also be read automatically in a medical emergency, or be linked to our bank account data when we walk pass a checkout at the supermarket. As discussed earlier, there is no obvious ultimate technological barrier to stop medical records and other data and software being inserted into the patient's own real DNA (both somatic and inheritable) as a sequence of base pairs ... GATTACA ... , each of G, C, A, T representing the pairs binary digits 00, 01, 10, 11. To aid that, sequencing your *entire* genome is getting cheaper, rapidly approaching the goal of the "thousand dollar genome." Tools for inserting new genetic content are known to genetic engineering and other relevant tools are being worked out by gene therapy. Also DNA sequencing or "readout" technologies that could *directly* drive a computer are becoming cheaper all the time. It may also be possible to use DNA in other information storage polymers on chips external to the body, or as components of chips implanted in the body. All such applications will require, however, significant IT support to enable queries or mining and to link the data to clinical decision intelligence systems. Of course, one might imagine a lot more computing activity to be programmable into such a chip, making it more like that in your PC.

These chips within us might at first be of the type that is merely transmitting information; even so, a degree of *local intelligence* is desirable to give us those same benefits of protection as does a physician. This is to provide a degree of *autonomy* such that a failure of an outside computer will not cost our lives. An extreme example is that smarter control could be placed over a cardiac pacemaker, but you would not wish your heart to stop beating just because the Internet is down! A caring system should be capable of still looking after the patient even when the rest of the healthcare IT structure is disconnected or destroyed.

Could the assimilation of cybernetic components, including prosthetic devices, molecule-releasing devices as metabolic controllers, mind-enhancing chips in our brains, turn us into robots? Again, we will defer such discussions (to Chapter 10) and mostly consider in this chapter computers communicating outside of us, and only such machinery within our bodies as is necessary to do that. The devices in and around us will only (at least mostly) report to the external world, not act inside our body. More spectacular and futuristic cases of artificial machinery, playing a more active role within us than simply sending the data, will be considered in the final chapter. Even so, devices that report without acting greatly concern some people. Could too much deep surveillance of ourselves by invasive or pervasive advices be abused? And as a little information begins to flow back into us, are we moving to a state in which we get so totally entwined with computers that only the basic information in our minds is retained, and our bodies and actions become simulations in a virtual reality, as in the cult movie *The Matrix*? A cynical perspective might be that these are risky routes to take, and that physicians must always be the ambassadors of the human race to speak for our humanity.

But we don't need to worry too much yet. Even those of us who feel that too much machinery inside us is undesirable might at least welcome basic internal biosensors and other monitoring devices that can only report information. Failing even that, externally worn biosensors or such devices around the home are certain to be welcomed by us all. The process has already started, and the first significant systems for home monitoring are for patients with chronic disease such as heart disease or diabetes.

AT THE SAME TIME, GENERAL COMPUTER SYSTEMS ARE BECOMING MORE LIKE US

Biological methodology in our everyday IT promises a kind of uniformity and interoperability that will encompass both medical and nonmedical computing, and mediation with implanted chips. This "biology in IT" is a methodology apart from *neural nets*, which are smart learning networks based on brain principles, represented in software. The changes of interest here are at the hardware level. It is probable that all traditional computer system architecture, medical and otherwise, will soon make the first steps to a transition to a deeper affinity with humans by adopting the concept inherent with the nervous systems of vertebrate living organisms (i.e., central nervous system and autonomous nervous system) and introducing a separate PPU (peripheral processing unit). The CNS (central nervous system) is of course the part of the vertebrate nervous system consisting of the brain and the spinal cord. The autonomous nervous system is the part of the nervous system of vertebrates that controls involuntary actions of the heart, glands, and muscles. The latter is analogous to the PPU that runs independently and autonomously from the CPU (central processing unit), especially for the health informatics and the life sciences informatics, to address the industry requirements for petaflops of computing power and exabytes (i.e., 10^{18} bytes, or one million trillion bytes) of storage management.

Already something called *autonomic computing* exists in the IT industry and is intended to exploit the same ideas as biology. One advantage for computer systems is that the system does not totally collapse for chip-augmented patients as described in the preceding section. The mainframe computers, the PPU (peripheral processing unit), will handle all the processing involving external systems and devices, such as input/output (I/O) processing through disks, communication adapters, multimedia content streaming, radiofrequency identifier and chip readers, hardware encryption and decryption, and biometric devices. In effect the CPUs are relieved from the chores of raw data processing (I/O) related activities and consequently can be dedicated for CPU-intensive activities. The CPUs and PPUs can interface through central memory (RAM). One benefit of having separate PPUs is that many CPUs now stay idle, waiting from a response from hard drives, external adapters, and diverse external biomedical data sources, and even computations on a connected highly parallel supercomputer. Processes call threading and micropartitioning do find work for the waiting, idle, processor to do, but in fact a simple preset waiting time cannot be guaranted by which data will come and go. A smarter process analyzing the statistics of how data arrives, and allocating time accordingly, would use up the CPU, but when allocated to the PPU, the CPU would be relieved for other duties.

THE PHYSICIAN AS IT INTERFACE

Monitoring our health does not necessarily imply implanted chips will signal our condition to the outside world, even in the future (though simple forms of this are technically feasible, and such a process has begun). It could simply be your physician examining you, and reporting to the computer. The physician serves as a human ambassador between IT and the patient, and it will be up to a physician of wisdom and moral standing who has taken the Hippocratic Oath to make the final choices and approve what IT is doing. The physician in the not-so-distant future will, among other duties, be charged with information gathering. That vigilance that relates to examination by physicians will be sound for years to come, and may be called *physician mediated*, but the physician or an assistant will need to enter the physician's observations, and laboratory results directly or indirectly into a computer. All that ends up in the computer, as a smart biosensor, will require that the physician stay active and "sign off" on every medical action.

Today, most physicians do, of course, have computers. Their office computer systems have been primarily for the capture and transmission of claims data to their payers, such insurance companies in the United States. The claims data are entered, batched, and electronically transmitted to claims submitter service bureaus that subsequently format and transmit the data to the payers. In the immediate future the functional requirements for the physician's office system will include electronic forums, bulletin boards, calendar of events, online newsletters, email, online lab reports for routing of lab reports to the physicians desktop, access to public domain medical information, face sheets for patient admission information as recorded by hospitals, inpatient census for listing of all inpatients showing facility, room, and diagnosis, document routing for automatic routing of clinical reports to physicians, eligibility for online verification of registry enrollment, pre-admissions for patient admission information required by hospitals, electronic forms for custom designed forms such as lab orders), and claims for online claims submission, electronic remittance advice.

At a coarser level of granularity for location grouping, physician's offices could be grouped into "rural" and "urban." Rural offices are likely to be limited to lower speed network access methods, whereas urban offices could optionally take advantage of higher speed network access methods. Over time, it is clear that the frequency, duration, and bandwidth requirements will change—particularly as more telemedicine applications and services become available. An example of physician's network infrastructure is shown in the Figure 9.1, where the physician is the mediator. The physician gathers intelligence (meaningful information) from the condition of the patient and then gets intelligence fed back from the computers to assist in his decisions about treating the patient.

MORE ON CLINICAL DECISION INTELLIGENCE

The primary IT that the physician will interface with is *clinical decision intelligence* (introduced particularly in Chapter 8). The powers of definitions are in the eye of the beholder, and in the new emerging medicine, it is particularly problematic that no one has quite the same definition. But all are agreed that there is no point in having clinical data, in any form, if intelligent decisions in the patient's interest (or collective pubic interest) cannot be made from that data. Information-based medicine can only ever be as powerful as the tools to convert that information into knowledge, insight, decision, and action. To put it succinctly, *information-based medicine must, by definition, include the capability to convert the information base to medicine*, and this already hints that

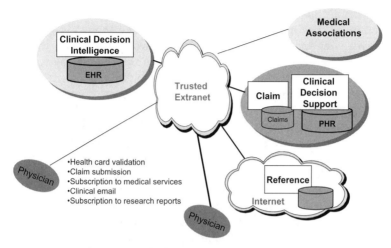

Figure 9.1   Physician's network infrastructure

any such tools related to clinical decision intelligence must play a fundamental and all-pervading role. Little or nothing in information-based medicine escapes linkage to clinical decision intelligence.

Clinical decision intelligence has been described as "the cerebral hemispheres of information-based medicine." That's not to belittle the rest of it. It works both ways, of course: digital patient records have little value if intelligence cannot be extracted from them, whereas clinical decision intelligence cannot do too much (except for medical texts, epidemiological data, etc.) without patient records. In addition we can seek to define it by what goes on with clinical *misintelligence*, in particular, all those inefficiencies and nasty medical errors. Further we might want our definition to encompass use of medical data by medical researchers, who in a way are also making decisions of importance to the health of future patients by designing new drugs. It is simply that right now those kinds decisions take years to reach the patients.

So here is an attempt at a definition. *Clinical decision intelligence is the application of IT to help gather, understand, and act on all available data in clinical practice, healthcare management and administration, and medical research, and where appropriate the automatic utilization of data to control certain clinical and research processes. Its aims are to encourage best practices; to improve the quality of patient care by enhancing speed and efficiency; to reduce safety risks and needless costs in clinical treatment, diagnosis, management, and administration; to monitor and log interactions for accountability, culpability, liability and repudiation; and to facilitate biomedical research and pharmaceutical development where based on inclusion of clinical and related data.*

The word "intelligence" bears some pondering. Intelligence in the sense used in "military intelligence" and what spies use when "obtaining intelligence" is often equated with knowledge. That kind of knowledge encompasses so much more than mere information or data, even though it arguably falls short of reaching wisdom or innovation. The lowest rung is data, the simplest form of facts and figures. Data can evolve into information by validating it through imposing a structure and adding meaning to it. The next rung, information, is reached by putting the information into context and adding understanding to it. From here, wisdom and innovation can be derived from knowledge in conjunction with experiences and foresight. Knowledge sharing is an important aspect, else it resides "frozen" in one person or group. Knowledge sharing and an online collaboration system has certain requirements to allow for efficient and effective communication among researchers and scientists. For example, support for both structured and unstructured data must be available to ensure that the system is capable of handling multidimensional data. Technology that will enable communities of practice, such as advanced search capabilities, automated and rule-based workflow, sharing of scientific annotation, and data/text mining and analysis, are essential to successful collaboration and knowledge sharing.

To really understand a definition, the extent of what it applies to is important. The scope of clinical decision intelligence comprises the following:

- *Clinical information integration.* Gathering of information from people and processes so as to support (1) telemedicine with relevant aspects of remote robotics and monitoring; (2) heterogeneous data management, including that of imaging and phenotypic, proteomic, and genomic and other relevant data and the variation of these with conditions, individuals, and populations, and aspects of architectures, grids, and workflows, and (3) formulation of standards.
- *Clinical decision support.* Understanding gained for transformation of data and prior knowledge, including use of collaboration and decision support systems and text, image, and other data analysis for profiling on such issues as management and cost containment and for bio-surveillance, simulation, and high-performance computing for prediction. This is discussed extensively below.
- *Clinical intelligence access and collaboration.* Acting on knowledge via feedback or moving humans to action by real-time on-demand access to consolidated patient, research, or other healthcare data, and including the topics of portals, shareware, identity protection, and privacy; security and consent compliance; ethical practice; and smarter solicitation and provision of services.

The claim that clinical decision intelligence is the cerebral cortex of information-based medicine is not hard to justify; at least in terms of the broad scope that it must embrace and by implication the integration of these aspects. Such broader vision is required for the following: morbidity risk assessment, diagnosis, prognosis, therapy selection, genetic counseling, lifestyle guidance, general information extraction, making sense of the flow of information, dynamically managing medical integration, medical finance and insurance amortization, medical research and teaching, pharmaceutical research, epidemiology and biothreat vigilance, auditing, validation and exception detection access monitoring and unauthorized access detection, spam and vested interest penetration into specific records and collective archives, and pharmacovigilance (i.e., detection of dangerous pharmaceutical side effects).

As we move away from a focus on reacting to disease and look toward to preventative medicine, self-improvement, and lifestyle management, it will be hard to draw any distinct boundary around medical and health improvement matters. Recall that the World Health Organization defines health as "a state of complete physical, mental, and social well-being, and does not consist only of the absence of disease or infirmity." Indeed by the WHO definition, 70% to 95% of all peoples are unhealthy right now. With extensions to cover matters as diverse as ethical, billing, mobility and handicap, public health, disaster response, fitness, sport, dietary and culinary, cosmetic, and recreational mishaps, there is much overlap with disciplines that require comparable data-exploring technologies in their own right. Just look at the relevant list to which such technologies are now being applied: emergency services, tracking hazardous activities, fire and hazards detection, disease detection (agricultural), disease monitoring (agricultural and human), real estate appraisal, taxation, and permitting, city and urban planning, financial and insurance services, retail marketing, facilities placement, facilities monitoring, peacekeeping and treaty monitoring, law enforcement, news services, environmental protection, global monitoring, resource assessment (natural and renewable), archaeological and architectural site preservation, cadastral survey and land registration, trends analysis and prediction services, navigation safety, utilities management, security reconnaissance, detection and surveillance, demographics, tourism and recreation, entertainment industry, automotive and industrial quality control, failure analysis, and maintenance contract cost control.

As indicated above, clinical decision intelligence is what happens at the smart end of all healthcare IT infrastructures, and in some views, CDI is the whole reason for existence of the infrastructure. In turning to another human being for protection and guidance, one thinks of his or her reputation for sound decisions and advice, not his or her storage capacity, format of memory records, internal bandwidths, internal information management, and so forth. These are all "under the hood." Good CDI will not at first come cheap, but what it would represent in market value really depends again on what is meant by "intelligence," and how willing healthcare employees are to embrace the upper-end, sophisticated AI-style forms of it. Generally speaking, the current inefficiencies, medical accident rate and demand for evidence-based medicine will be both a stick and a carrot (depending on who is driving the need for purchase at the time) for the most sophisticated systems possible. That is with the caveat that they are comprehensible, credible, and reliable: the physician, one recalls, will still carry the final responsibility for medical decisions.

Pharmacovigilance (monitoring drug safety) will be a driver to adoption of portals that could also serve CDI functions, as discussed later below.

For 2010, predictions of expenditure on CDI vary from about a good few millions of dollars up to $200 billion, and world predictions for CDI markets over the next ten years at $80 billion to $810 billion. The upper end estimates of these seem large, however, because there are natural ceilings of common sense: there just isn't enough money available to cover everything healthcare needs. The overall size of the world health industry for the 30 most developed countries is probably about $2,200 billion (http://mamipalgroup.com/manipal/mrbulletic_old/HVare.htm), and looking at how that cake is sliced, CDI would certainly seem be unlikely to reach anything like $300 billion worldwide in the next few years. One problem with CDI market predictions is that it is not always clear what is considered the core CDI part, and what is considered support infrastructure for it, and that could be a shifting division according to architectural philosophy. Also, the recent economic crash has disrupted forward thinking in these matters. The United States has about 45% of the world expenditure in healthcare but it may shrink to 33% by 2010, and while four fifths of US health expenditure goes on just one fifth of the population (www.globalpolicy.org/socecon/tncs/phrmas.htm); the world economic crisis and President Obama could shift that. In bad economic times, R&D into the kind of CDI system so smart that it almost thinks like a human may have to wait. Nonetheless, all things considered, worldwide by 2010, $5 billion to $25 billion is certainly possible for more basic CDI, and could be a big underestimate.

JUST HOW WELL CAN COMPUTERS KNOW YOU?

Powerful divinities are accredited not just with being all-powerful but all-knowing too. We would like our clinical decision intelligence to be of that same rank. A great power of needs great insight to see what is going wrong. But how much insight of you do computers need to have? How big can the challenge be? A wise chemical physicist once said to one of the authors "To test your equations, your models, even your ideas, look to the limits." In practice, that often mean making sure your equations give sensible results with zero and infinity as input variables. In the present context, it means looking at how our human healthcare guardians work now (zero time), and what the physical limits are to full guardianship in the far future. Not everything may be possible even in the best of all possible worlds. We do not want to extrapolate beyond what is needed, and beyond the limits of the possible!

Let us assume that we can go a lot further with IT than just, for example, monitoring our blood glucose. We are composed of far more than just glucose. To understand the upper limit to what power is needed outside (i.e., in computers), we must look first at the information that is contained within us and that is to be made known to computers.

In other words, what does a computer really need to know? How much is there in the human body that some advanced power in computers would need to monitor our eternal health and well-being? How many billion bytes of RAM (random access memory, a physical memory of a computer) would a computer need, playing the part of a health guardian?

Recall Su Dongpo (1037–1101) whom we mentioned at the beginning of the chapter. Su Dongpo was a famous Chinese essayist who lived during the Sung dynasty. Su Dongpo is said to have had "a deep understanding of the vast sea of Buddhism." In one poem, he wrote "I have heard 84,000 hymns, yet how do I tell it to people the next day?" He undoubtedly wrote this because 84,000 was said by some thinkers at that time to be said to be the number of atoms in the human body. In any event it was also used to indicate the number of emanations, or manifestations of the Buddha, within the body, with which human consciousness might resonate and potentially gain enlightenment.

Now you might say that the word "atoms" above means something far different from what it means today, and something more spiritual than material. First, we would doubt that we could or should distinguish spiritual and scientific matters as believed in those days. The ancient Chinese did have, and carefully distinguished, Confucianism and Taoism. However, one might say that the former dealt with ethics and good behavior, while the latter, Taoism, specifically mingled science, philosophy, and spiritual matters. So atoms would be a Tao matter, and in Tao, science and spirituality would be one. Second, as regard equivalence of "scientific" perspective, the word "atom" is in fact ancient Greek meaning "indivisible," and the Greeks pretty well had the description qualitatively right (even from our perspective) more than a millennium before Su Dungpo. And when it comes to the crunch, we are not so sure that the difference between Su Dungpo and us, regarding what "atoms" means, is so much greater than that between me and the person next to me on the subway train to work. Heaven knows, there is a fundamental difference of interpretation of atoms and quantum mechanics between physicists, for whom thinking about atoms is a living.

But if we accept that the Su Dungpo notion of "atoms" is at least related to the notion of atom, it remains that the number 84,000 is certainly a big underestimate as far as atoms go in the chemical sense. In 1811 Avogadro opened the way to more exact calculations of this kind, and to appreciate of how mind-bogglingly huge this number must be, he proposed the hypothesis that equal volumes of gas at the same temperature and pressure must contain equal numbers of molecules. Such a standard mass of atoms is identified by an official unit call the "mole," which avoids the need to consider masses directly and can be extended to liquids, solids, and solutions. It is not so different to using old units such as stones, meaning that the weight could be expressed in terms of a number of standard stones. In essence a mole thus represents a conversion between grams and units based on numbers of standard atoms of specified mass (mass units). By the 1970s the official deffinition of mole was based (since it had to be based on something) on material made only of a pure isotope of carbon:

1. The mole is the amount of substance of a system that contains as many elementary entities as there are atoms in 0.012 kilogram of carbon 12.
2. When the mole is used, the elementary entities must be specified and may be atoms, molecules, ions, electrons, other particles, or specified groups of such particles.

We need look no deeper than atoms, at least as long as we wish to consider the material world. All atoms of specific isotopic type, such as carbon 12, are identical, in your body, or mine, or in a lump of coal, or in the rock on a planet of a distant galaxy.

A mole consists of 6.02×10^{23} atoms. It follows that the number of atoms in the human body must be very roughly 10^{27}. To each of these ideally any guardian computer would need to know the type (or mass), position (right-left, up-down, forward-backward, or x, y, z directions), and momentum (or velocity) in every direction (again x, y, z) of every atom. We can assume that the computer will do the calculations and make predictions regarding improvements and repairs. To do this the numbers would need to be held up to very high precision, else Chaos theory would soon rear its head, meaning that any guardian computer would soon lose track. Actually calculations have to be done over very small fractions of time, say 10^{10} times to calculate effects over a second. A very extended lifetime might require a need to consider 10^{10} seconds. To do calculations spanning many years, and for a really dramatically extended life, lots of bits are required to hold the numbers to adequate precision. Overall, 10^{35} may not be an unreasonable figure.

A more fundamental approach would be to work out the maximum possible information that can be represented by the human body, using an equation called the Beckenstein bound, due to J. D. Beckenstein in a famous 1981 paper in *Physical Review Letters*. This gives something like 10^{45} bits. This, however, is the approximate upper limit due to the information that can be coded in an entity the size of a human being, this limit being the absolute maximum allowed by the structure of space and time itself. Still it might be said that the computer should really be using calculations based on quantum mechanics, so in any event it seems that a further increase above 10^{35} is required.

One thing we can be sure is that there is an awful lot of information to handle. If we have a gigabyte of RAM on our computer, then we will have to boost that at least 10^{26} times to do the job. And recalling from that millions of calculations have to be done just to emulate a second, and we want the system to be at least as fast of the real world, we will need to scale up the speed of our chip by comparably huge numbers too.

It is interesting to compare this number with the memory needs of the maximum computation which is theoretically possible. Any real computation is limited by quantum mechanics and especially Heisenberg's uncertainty principle, which places a limit on how fast energy can be processed; the velocity of light, which places a limit on how fast information can be moved from A to B; thermodynamics, which places a limit on how much information can be stored; and the age and hence size of the universe, which dictates how large a computer could be. Rolf Landauer at IBM raised essentially these issues when he pointed out that all computation is governed by the laws of physics and by the resource available. Seth Lloyd at MIT reasoned on these bases that no calculation could require more than 10 to the power 120 bits. However, if we take the worst case of information demands mentioned above, a computer of cosmic scale could take care of some 10 to the power 75, meaning 10,000 ... up to 75 zeros.

Let's take another perspective regarding how much computational power we will need. Remember the Blue Gene, a petaflop computer announced in 2000 by IBM, planned in original form as potentially powerful enough to follow the folding of a small protein, in about a year. This mission has been distracted by other pressing applications, e.g., simulating nuclear testing, drug design, and patent analysis as discussed in Chapter 10, and, as it happens, the petaflop barrier was actually broken by another IBM computer. However, these put the broader visions, at the supercomputing end of healthcare *in silico*, on schedule. To get to the size of a single cell in the patient's body, we would need to study the equivalent about 10^{12} molecules. According to Denis Noble at the University of Oxford, that would require 10^{27} Blue Gene supercomputers, each working ideally at 10^{15} floating-point operations per second, and as he notes, there is not enough matter in the solar system to use to build that number. It is worth considering that there are roughly 10^{14} cells in a human. All things considered, there would be a need for massive amounts of matter to be converted to provide perhaps 10^{40} floating point operations per second.

BIOLOGY BY COMPUTER REQUIRES APPROPRIATE LEVELS OF APPROXIMATION

In practice, of course, it is not essential to consider every atom of the body in detail. Or if we look at every atom, we need often only consider a tiny part of the body, such as the receptors, enzymes, and other proteins that are the targets for the action of pharmaceutical drugs. What one drug molecule and one protein will do, millions of them in our body will do, a principle known as *canonical assembly*. Quantum mechanics, especially techniques called ab initio quantum mechanics, are the most thorough and the most time-consuming. Actually quantum mechanics can calculate at the level of parts of atoms, meaning nuclei, electrons, and even smaller subnuclear particles. The principles of quantum mechanics are more fundamental than Newton's laws of motion, which in theory can be derived from them but in practice considered as simpler *emergent laws* arising at a higher level of complexity, meaning here on larger scales with much complex matter involved. *Molecular dynamics* is an established way to tackle *molecular simulation* that allows us to track every atom using Newton's laws of motion, but much effort can be saved if we consider structures that are collections of potentially huge numbers of atoms such as the model of an organ, namely as *anatomical simulation*, which in general use *mechanical simulation*, or as an approach called *kinetic simulation*. We'll look at those later. Molecular simulation is possible when we are only looking at very small parts of the body, such that there are relatively few, say hundreds, thousands, or hundreds of thousands, of atoms. A typical small protein might have 2,000 atoms, though our biological molecules work largely in the presence of water, and usually we should add several thousand atoms worth of water molecules too.

At that level the way to design a drug seems clear—at least to the drug design theoretician. Almost all drugs interact with protein molecules as targets (though a few target nucleic acids). Typically the drug molecules interact at some specific binding site of that protein, like a key in a kind of keyhole that nature reserved for a natural molecule of the body, say a hormone (in which case the protein is a hormone receptor), or a small molecule metabolite to be converted at that site to some other small molecule metabolite (in which case the protein was an enzyme). Hence, if the details of the protein molecule can be determined like some kind of X ray of the three-dimensional structure of a lock, it should be possible to use computer-aided design to develop a new key that will fit that lock in a desired way. For example, it could act like the natural biological key, the original natural version being deficient in some way such that body benefits from this "prosthetic molecular replacement." Conversely, it might block the action of the natural biological key if that action is excessive or otherwise undesirable (by analogy, the key would fit but not be able to turn and unlock). Of course, the theoretician would be aware of the need to consider that the flexibility of proteins and the molecules they bind should be taken into account, as well as the significant effect of the surrounding water, its salts, and any other relevant molecular players. In addition the binding of the drug molecule to other sites in the body would have to be considered; these are responsible for the side effects of the drug and so we would wish to minimize the bindings responsible for those.

Finally, there may be a need to consider interactions that can modify a molecule to the active drug form, or from the active drug form. These are challenging considerations. But all these considerations do not faze the true patriot of the rational drug design world; they justify requests for shinier new supercomputers to play with, or failing adequate corporate funding of drug R&D, stimulate ingenious shortcuts and theoretical improvements that form the basis of worthy scientific papers.

One good reason for looking at proteins or similar size biological molecules in atomic detail concerns selecting drugs for a specific patient or discovering new drugs. This is done vià *virtual screening*, also called *in silico screening*, whereby or all the atoms in the system are studied. Often a number of drugs or variants of one drug are tested against the protein target by ingenious algorithms that speed up the process. Any molecule that binds to a protein is a *ligand*; at simplest, once the ligand is in position, the computer can be instructed to make chemical changes to it, to explore whether the binding strength can be increased or decreased. There might also as noted above be considered interaction with several "further receptors," which might be an unwanted binding producing *toxicity*. The concept, much used by scientists, is that of receptor as "lock" and drug as "key," since the receptor (typically but not always at the cell surface) will trigger a certain response inside the cell. Usually the "further receptors" considered are "wrong lock," which the drug key fits at least just a bit and so initiates the undesirable side effects (still there are known cases where unlocking several different receptors is beneficial). The interactions of a molcule with a binding site in a protein can also be approximated by the 3D localization of key interaction features or "a pharmacophore." This 3D surrogate for the binding site can be used for rapid in silico screening of very large libraries of molecules in the hunt for the "needle in the haystack," namely an active molecule that could be a starting point for a new drug.

It is hard to handle hundreds of thousands of atoms: it takes a lot of computer time and memory, hence the need for a supercomputer. The need for higher levels of approximation especially arises as we move up from molecules to systems in which many molecules interact. Sometimes the way in which nature has developed control of the cell involves many interacting process driven by many locks, and simulation can be useful in finding out if and how several drugs given at the same time can interact. In addition, even without the presence of drugs, we might like to find the effect of nutrients, or sudden physiological changes like in exercise or infectious disease, or genetic defects, on our metabolism. In principle, it is possible to represent all the interacting molecules in atomic detail, but in practice, this is neither practical right now nor is it always required.

We essentially reach here the realms of *systems biology*. As with Newton's laws in comparison to quantum mechanics, we can usualy get away at the higher level of complexity with new simple emergent laws and simple new quantities to describe them. Chemical concentration replaces Newton's mass, for example. To enter first on its modest lowest steps, consider, for example, the eleven steps or so in which glucose is converted to lactic acid, a process that provides energy fast when you exercise, but the lactic acid leaves that soreness in your muscles (so you need that hot shower). The first two steps are the conversion of glucose to glucose-6-phosphate, and then of the latter to fructose-6-phosphate. The purpose of adding the phosphate bit is that ultimate cleavage and transformations of the molecule will yield energy associated with the phosphate group, and the reason for the shuffling around of atoms to make fructose is that the sugar molecule is being as symmetrical as possible, metabolically speaking, so that after a minor tweak on one of the cut products by a further enzyme, two identical "half-sugar" molecules are produced, requiring only one metabolic pathway to process them instead of two. Now, if these reactions were spontaneous without further help (which they are not really, so wait for discussion of "enzymes" below), we could replace the atomic detail by very simple equations: glucose → glucose-6-phosphate → fructose-6-phosphate. (Enzymes, recall, are *catalysts*, so without the enzyme, such a reaction would be very slow, and lost in a chaotic noise of other slow spontaneous chemical changes.) Then a study of the way these molecules all change in time can be set up using just the names (to distinguish the players), their concentrations in the cell, and so-called rate constants that show how fast the reaction will occur for a given concentration of molecules being converted. It is because of these changes in the concentrations that a fairly complicated calculation is used to sort out the net result over time. In the *kinetic simulation* case the overall model is then not an object physically represented but a set of equations showing how concentrations of molecules change given a starting set of concentrations and rate constants, with the numbers showing how much concentrations change as a function of the concentrations of reactant molecules. Note that the same molecule crossing to a different compartment of the cell or body can be treated in the same way, the change now being in *location*.

Adding the enzyme is not difficult, we just have to consider the enzyme as another molecule, the rates of binding and release of the ligand, catalytic change, and rebinding and release of the product of that change. Enzymes have evolved to have strong initial binding and poorer binding of the product, so in some simulations and conditions, these can be reduced to just two kinetic descriptors, the K_m and V_{max} of traditional enzymology. V_{max} is the maximum speed of product creation for a given standard amount of enzyme, and K_m is roughly a binding constant but actually a function of three true rate constants. The m in Km stands for molar, the physical chemist's unit of concentration, but equally well students for many years have thought it stands for Michaelis and Menten, the "discoverers" of the constant and the formula Reaction Rate = $V_{max}[S]/([S] + K_m)$, which uses K_m and V_{max}. Here $[S]$ is the concentration of molecule called substrate on which the enzyme acts. Despite the importance of these quantities and their dominance in many years of biochemical teaching, the equation is an approximation, actually, because it neglects that enzyme is temporarily used up in binding the substrate, and assumes a vast excess of substrate over enzyme. It is an aspect to be remembered in discussion of simulation of metabolism below: in cells where enzyme concentration can be high, half the enzyme concentration is analogous to, but much more important quantity than, the K_m.

Notice that these descriptions of molecular concentrations and rate constants are the new quantities of the game at the systems biology level. We could use a deeper description, and (hopefully) get the same results, by using quantum mechanics. However, that would take phenomenal computing power and processing time to address every aspect of the problem. Where it is useful at the systems biology level, it is just as the theoretical way to get the rate constants. If we can assign those empirically, from experiment, we can ignore the fact that the nuclei and electrons are the real players.

Yet, even in basic systems biology, there is one important player that must be added to kinetic simulation when it becomes a metabolic simulation. The important catch, biologically speaking, is to remember that the above-described metabolic reactions would occur only to a negligible extent, lost among other changes that could occur slowly, if the specific reactions were not selected and catalyzed by specialized proteins called *enzymes*. It is enzymes that are a foundation of a complicated road network of chemical reactions that we call *metabolism*, and since our genes code for these enzymes, our genetics carves out the road map. The mechanism of action of enzymes can also be calculated by quantum mechanics, with the nuclei and electrons all considered in the mix. But as for simple chemical reactions, their effect can be reduced to fewer numbers (see below) than we can obtain by experiment. The main action in fact is to increase the rate constant for a chemical reaction.

When the chemical transformations are governed by enzymes, as is almost always the case in metabolism, we speak of "the kinetic behavior of enzymes." The small molecules the enzymes act on (and change) the "input" are traditionally called substrates, and the resulting changed product molecule or molecules are, reasonably enough, formally called the *products*. The enzyme that has glucose as substrate and glucose-6-phosphate as a product is called *hexokinase*. The one that has glucose-6-phosphate as a substrate and fructose-6-phosphate as a product is called *glucose-6-phosphate isomerase*. The suffix "ase" indicates an enzyme, the rest usually relates to the substrate and the type of change, although "hexokinase" is a bit anachronistic because of its early discovery. All enzymes have standard numeric code names, and a published K_m and V_{max} as noted above. However, caution is required because at high concentrations of enzymes often found in the cell, a lot higher than in a test tube, the role of K_m can be replaced by a quantity that, as mentioned earlier, is half the enzyme concentration. This means that control of rates can be governed by how much enzyme the gene for it makes. When in doubt, the "whole" system with the detailed concentrations and rate constants must be used.

The rate constants are basic and allow us to represent metabolic networks as complex interlacing road systems along which matter moves with speed depending on molecular concentrations. Unlike vehicular traffic, however, there are no speed laws or road lines, even road edges, and the higher the concentration of a molecule, the faster it wants to move on to something else. The concentration (or product of concentrations of interacting molecules) times the rate constant is the speed, and this is the simple kinetic law at the basic systems biology level. Here it is almost the seeming opposite of Newton's laws underlying it, which applies greater speeds to smaller masses.

It is hard to get every rate constant experimentally, but simulation (as exemplified above for K_m and V_{max}) does not always require every rate constant to be known. The system it describes can often replace many rate constants by a single effective rate constant or another kind of quantity relating to the overall or part behavior of the kinetic system, and that single number can often be determined experimentally. A simple example of general chemical (not just biochemical) importance is that the ratio of concentrations of two molecules A and B with A converting to B and B converting back to A, when the whole tug-of-war has come to a stable balance ("settled down at equilibrium"), is most fully described by the rate constant for converting A to B and that for converting B to A. However, a number that is the ratio of these two rate constants, this ratio being the *equilibrium constant*, is sufficient to calculate the relative portions of A and B.

As noted above, a similar quantity relating to more complex systems, and important to enzymes, is the K_m, which describes the ratio of substrate A to product B in conditions *when input and output to the system is steadily maintained*. It is in fact not an equilibrium constant but a *steady state constant*. It may or may not be similar to the equilibrium constant. This applies in the test tube when substrate is present in abundance and not much product is yet formed, and often applies to metabolism too, although in the cell the enzyme is almost equally often the molecule in abundant quantity, and not the substrate. The other important number to know for an enzyme is, as was noted, V_{max} the rate constant for the chemical reaction catalyzed, as it is for a given quantity of enzyme, in the presence of excess of substrate. Like the equilibrium constants, all these are convenient summary constants that we can readily determine experimentally but that can really be determined from all the underlying rate constants.

The important point, but rarely discussed in biology and medicine courses, is that there are more complex forms of behavior of metabolic systems as they become more elaborate, and can be described also by fewer numbers. To repeat, you can imply the effect of many rate constants, not just two, for the price of one number. Such numbers relevant to individual enzymes represent equilibrium-constant-like values relating to binding (such as K_m), maximum possible speed of the catalysis (V_{max}), and possibly a few other numbers relating to inhibition (IC_{50} and K_i, the constant of inhibition) or excitation (EC_{50}) of enzyme activity by other molecules, possibly the substrate itself. Equilibrium and steady state constants are quantitative descriptors of equilibrium and steady state, and these are but points on a continuum of progressively more complex systems behavior. Physical processes can be irreversible such that all A goes to B, equilibrium, steady state, periodic (behaving in a cyclic way), quasiperiodic (coming back to the same state every time but not exactly), chaotic (seemingly random but holding to an underlying pattern called an *attractor*), and beyond into more complex behaviors. A useful word for an important type of more complex behavior was *telandic*, from the Greek teleos (goal) and so basically meaning "goal seeking." Though its twentieth-century scientific origins seem lost even to the recovery power of the Internet, it is believed to have originated as a type of behavior for goal-seeking systems coined by artificial-intelligence researchers at the University of Edinburgh.

The value of such descriptors is not confined to chemical kinetics and metabolism. They illustrate emergence of higher properties and the ability to treat lower level systems without fine detail. It is as if the fine details only rarely matter, illustrated by the fact that psychology makes only occasional reference to neurochemistry. If we knew more about these more complex behaviors, we might know an awful lot more about life and the universe. They are an essence of systems biology as a whole, and in the study of any very complex systems, yet many higher order behavior descriptor numbers may remain to be discovered. But, apart from some glimpses, we are confined at best to simulating behaviors, not fully understanding them. The branch of biology and computer science that deals with most matters above, and certainly molecular simulation of biological molecules, is more generally *computational biology*. Specifically *protein structure science*—typically a matter of studying protein structure, behavior, and interactions—in atomic detail also comes into play. Computational biology is not quite the same as *theoretical biology*, a discipline that requires integration of many types of information about living systems but interested more in the pursuit of general descriptors of behavior. Neither computational nor theoretical biology is quite the same as *mathematical biology*, a branch of mathematics that is concerned with finding mathematical solutions, not in running computer programs, to get what are essentially numerical solutions. This is much closer to the idea of finding general behavioral descriptors. Systems biology is the ideal discipline for incorporating all these pursuits and discovering new ones by simulations, but right now it remains for the most part in brute force calculation directed by constant reference to experimental input. For example, simulations can be carried out in silico with to-and-throw reference to actual tests of a drug on an experimental animal such as the pig.

As we rise to higher levels of organization through cells, tissues, and organs, the calculations we did at any simpler level become more challenging if we stick to that level of description. For example, concentrations can be much higher in the cell, interact with many other molecules, and different substrates can be compartmentalized, immobilized on specific structures within the cell, or otherwise moved around in the cell by complicated processes driven by energy consumption.

Developing the right language for modeling at the right level is sometimes a challenge, and to some the choice is a kind of special computer language. Whether in atomic detail or as a kinetic simulation, modeling the *physiome*, namely the proteins of the body and how they interact, is important. It is getting so important that there are international projects (The Physiome Project), societies to support them (notably a Physiome Committee of the prestigious International Union of Physiological Sciences), and even computer languages to help. Those who like that kind of thing might try looking up CellML on www.cellml.org. CellML is a brand of XML (recall from a discussion of the patient record that this ontology language describes relationships among things). In particular, it allows a complete specification of a model for a simulation, in terms of all the components and their interactions.

From a purely theoretical view, cells are emmergent patterns of behavior, chaotic, telandic, or more complex descriptions that arise from simpler structures assembled into complex organization. And consideration of tissues require laws of assembly by many cells, of organs by many tissues, and of the body by many organs. In moving to cells and so up in complexity, however, it still remains that we change languages of description, and even the numeric measures used in that language to obtain quantitative results. But sometimes we want to know how the quantum mechanical interactions of a tiny drug binding DNA can affect a big structure like the heart. A big issue is how the different levels of description can all talk to each other (ideally to theoretical and mathematical biologists too!), and combine to give the big picture. One of the issues (of interest to researchers in the US Department of Defense and others) is how one can represent a digital human at various hierarchical levels, of atoms, molecules, cells, organs, and anatomy, in such a way that every fine detail is not required and move smoothly between those levels. Gregory A. Voth at the Center for Biophysical Modeling and Simulation and Department of Chemistry, University of Utah, is one of several workers considering how to couple levels of representation at the more fine-grained molecular levels of that hierarchy. His approach provides an interface between atomistic molecular simulations, which he calls *mesoscale dynamics*, and a continuum of mechanics. In such studies larger structures are not considered as collections of atoms but more as complex bulk shapes for which vibrations and motions are calculated without recourse to the fine detail of individual atoms.

One of the well-studied areas in this early pioneering period of computer simulation in medicine is the heart, and this certainly addresses the issue of communication between the different levels of detail of simulation. The behavior of the healthy and sick heart can indeed be simulated at a mechanical nerve and muscle signaling level of description, and that is useful for diagnosis and therapy. In fact the heart has very few types of cell, compared with many organs in the body, which makes things a bit easier. The simulations have been used to reconstruct pacemaker behavior and to interpret the electrocardiogram in a variety of diseases states, especially the arrhythmias. In research the simulations have, for example, clarified the origins of Brugada syndrome, a genetic condition in which sudden fatal ventricular fibrillation occurs in what previously seemed a perfectly healthy individual. An important application is in assessing drug safety. About half the drugs withdrawn in recent years have been associated with undesirable effects on the heart, showing up as irregularities on the cardiogram (heart electrical activity scan) and in arrhythmias. In particular, one ion channel has been implicated in many of these problems— a potassium channel called hERG (human Ether-a-go-go Related Gene) that many drugs can bind with high affinity and disrupt the cardiac action potential.

There are at least two clear levels of simulation required in many cases, well illustrated by simulations of the heart. The cellular level includes whole cell modeling in approximate detail and, in finer detail, studies of proteins that as enzymes catalyze biochemical reactions, as transporters or gates that carry ions (charged atoms) across cell membranes, and as muscle proteins that generate contraction. The organ level involves detailed anatomical models of the heart, including the beating and the spread of electrical polarization through the heart muscle that controls that beating. Scientists have also obtained a great deal of insight by linking these two levels. For example, a mutation for the gene that expresses the sodium channel protein has been modeled, right from protein up to the motion of the heart. This mutation is responsible for a disease called long QT syndrome, which refers to a lengthening in the cardiogram of the time between excitation of the ventricles and their contraction, which can be life threatening. The simulations reveal that the mutant gene leads to production of a mutant channel in the surface membrane of heart muscle cells, responsible for a more persistent flow of sodium ions inward during the action potential, the spread of electrical charge across the cell surface that affects, and is affected by, channel behavior. This charge spread is essentially a successive depolarization and repolarization of the membrane by the opening up of channels between the inside and outside of the cells where the charge concentrations are different, representing a kind of biological battery. The defect causes an early postdepolarization phase, delaying repolarization and resulting in the extended QT interval on the cardiogram. The heart model has even been extended to a model of the whole of the upper part of the body.

Of course, simulations of these important medical phenomena mostly all use approximations except when considering a few molecules; otherwise, they are not currently done in atomic detail. If they were, it is not difficult to see how whole planets of the future human intergalactic empire could indeed be running white hot with computation in protection of our health and well-being.

COMPUTATIONAL CHEMISTRY, COMBINATORIAL CHEMISTRY, REALITY AND THE SPECTER OF ENTROPY

The major pharmaceutical company will use any tool in the armory appropriate to any level of complexity, both modeling in the mind of the computer and in real experiment, in order to get results. The interplay of reality and various levels of theoretical description is strong (in the spirit of systems biology), with emphasis on reality whenever the data are there. Input from real experiment is used to hedge R&D wisely where the pure theoretician would see such help as a Band-Aid to a defect in a perfect theory and calculation, in which only the end prediction is tested against reality. The clinical patient is not the ultimate reality: use of the drug out there in the field of healthcare is that, although presently considered somewhat after the fact for the drug company (but starting to change; see the discussion below). The more theoretical steps, however, potentially provide a powerful filter to what molecules are synthesized and tested. Moreover, in the spirit of preceding sections, we focus on computational chemistry and consider why IT alone does not *yet* take us on most of the pharmaceutical journey. Is there one recurrent theme in this? We would like to italicize this: *If there is one effect, one specter, that is free of context, that pervades all level of description in simulation and in reality, it is entropy.* Entropy is in a sense pure mathematics. It governs strongly the behavior of matter from the cosmological scale down the finest level, simulated and real. It is the problem of the needle in the haystack in massive amounts of scientific and business intelligence data to be sifted, the problem of picking the right idea and hypothesis to test, including the right drug. It is the wrong path we take, and the law that if anything can go wrong, it will. It is the information that gets lost, the information we never had, and the information we cannot get.

Computer-aided drug design, sometime called CAD but better CADD (to avoid confusion with computer-aided diagnostics CAD or computer-aided design CAD of cars, planes, buildings, bridges, and things in general) or CAMD (computer-aided molecular design), has its challenges and its tools to help overcome them. "Simulation" was certainly an appropriate term to use before, since it involved, at this level, application of Newton's laws of motion (and sometimes quantum mechanics). Challenges include getting the forces correctly modeled among atoms because the real laws underlying them are quantum mechanical. We can either go to quantum mechanical methods for docking drugs to protein targets, which are relatively slow, or refine simple Newtonian style forces based on experimental data and/or quantum mechanics. The biggest problems, however, are inherently mathematical and algorithmic and have to do with exploring huge numbers of possibilities to get the right answers. Pitfalls and lengthy calculations are related to the effects of entropy introduced in Chapter 1.

The skeptic can of course go almost totally empirical and use the older and still powerful tool of structure activity relationships (SAR) also often called quantitative structure activity relationships (QSAR). Here the molecules are represented in a very simple way and parameters are adjusted to fit facts on binding to target, stability, toxicity, and so forth. The generation and use of the basic simple equations originally handled on pencil and paper that can certainly be manipulated on the computer include predictive power about what a new molecule will do. The idea of advanced simulation, however, is to remove the difficulties and limitations inherent in such models, which is simply the lack of true molecular detail in space and also time (since many molecules can change shape). These details are essentially electronic, since the positively charged nuclei just give mass and anchor to the orbiting electrons in regions of space that the computer sees as the atoms. The masses and hence Newtonian properties of atoms are well known. Thus the difference from the older SAR methods is really mostly in the electronic details that govern the interatomic forces.

That is, with the further exception of entropy, older empirical methods can often wrap in as a single number from an experiment. We would ideally like to get entropy and so free energy right from first principles, and empirical numbers from entropy measurements are hard or meaningless to add on an atom by atom basis anyway. Briefly, the unfortunate fact is that if you want the advantages of being more detailed and hence more correct, you have to face the fact that some aspects don't break down easily into the kind of details that the computer can handle quickly. It must, as closely as possible, go through the calculation that reality does for itself, and reality is a very fast highly parallel quantum computer to beat.

How empirical can you go in this arena? Let us keep the speed of "that computer around us that we call reality" in mind in discussing a broader class of tools that are helpful in speeding the more precise calculations. All the tools described now will focus the analysis of looking at drugs interacting with their specific protein targets, called "docking" of drugs, as to activate or inhibit enzymes or receptors (both of which are, most often, proteins). This interaction, as noted above, can be a screening of a large number of drug molecules in virtual reality, testing to see which one fits the protein best in the traditional lock-and-key fashion while allowing, if done properly, for the flexibility of both the molecular lock and the molecular key.

We can be empirical and also take advantage of the fact that compared with virtual reality, "actual reality" is not only due to an incredibly efficient computer (the real world) but, by definition, is what gets the right answers and, importantly, those that better apply inside the patient. It can involve design by methodical replacement of *real* chemical groups on *real* molecules on tiny labs, meaning *combinatorial chemistry chips* and microfluidic laboratory chips (see Chapter 10). The chip does real chemistry to develop the best-fitting drug. It is a process exactly like using a locksmith's adjustable skeleton key. Since these components are on chips adapted from the computer industry, it is easy to imagine hybrid methods, as if the combinatorial chemistry chip were a kind of chemical analog processor that can talk to other digital chips in the same machine. Already computation on a separate machine is used to pick the best combinations of chemicals to use on combinatorial chemistry chips, and help process and understand the results.

In all this it should be born in mind that computational chemistry and real combinatorial chemistry are currently still not the highest scorers in the get-to-a-drug olympics. Rather, the "street talk" is that high-throughput screening in real laboratories, though admittedly now usually with robotics, is still winning most of the medals. This is, of course, more real than even combinatorial chemistry as it involves not only a target protein but its detailed interactions with the cell in the context of a tissue sample or culture, whole organ, or whole organism. But it does open an important point here. The difficulties may be not so much in the computer treatment of the drug–protein interaction, imperfect as we know they are. Computational chemistry does not seem to do much better than computational chemistry if at all, in overall, get-to-a-drug terms. There are simply more uncertainties in the downstream cytology and physiology. However, we can use computational and combinatorial chemistry as processes for selecting the molecule for the large-scale synthesis and testing. This selection is a significant in-house business decision, and implementing it is probably the biggest rate-limiting step on the long road from idea to clinical trial.

With the limitations of computational chemistry in mind, how do we best use the tools required to try to overcome the difficulties? Mostly it means that we do not yet routinely throw millions of molecular formulas at a supercomputer and keep our fingers crossed (though computers are getting faster) but take it in easy steps that have evolved in the short history of computational chemistry. As well as Newtonian simulation using molecular dynamics, they include (1) interactive docking by a research interacting with the graphics screen (typically displayed in 3D), (2) semiautomatic docking in which the computer knows some simple properties of the atoms (their sizes, and possibly their electrical charges) plus some the mathematical tricks for getting a complementary fit rapidly, (3) minimization of the energy of interaction such as to reach the bottom of a deep energy well (simply meaning a stable solution), and more accurately (4) free energy minimization in which entropy effects are included, or effective free energy minimization using Newton's laws of motion and hence *molecular dynamics*.

This last, free energy minimization, reflects the fact that the molecule is more stable, or forms a more stable binding to its target, the lower the free energy is. The computer moves atom around to minimize the free energy, which means enhancing the stability, including of drug binding.

Free energy is basically energy minus entropy, or more precisely energy minus temperature times entropy. As in the first chapter, information is negative entropy and is "good," free energy that includes both the basic energy from atomic interactions (enthalpy) *including* entropy, which is the opposite of stability. By analogy (as well as definition) of what we want for good drug binding, stability is also "good." The only caveat on this is that binding not be so strong that it sticks to the protein target "forever," or at least until the detoxification systems take the whole thing apart and flush it away.

Free energy (including entropy) calculation basically means taking account of the vibrations and other motions of parts of all the molecules involved, and the freedom of the water molecules that ultimately determines the *hydrophobic effect*, which can look like a force but is really an entropy effect. That last in turn simply means that oily parts of the molecules (i.e., mainly a *nonpolar* region on the protein and a *nonpolar* region on the drug) are drawn together for exactly the same reason that oil and water don't mix. Basically the water molecule in free water can point anywhere and sometimes find a good interaction (actually a hydrogen bond) equally in all directions, but this changes near a protein oily region, where there are no protein hydrogen bonding groups (by definition of "oily"). This restriction leads to the entropy contribution: it implies more information (and hence less entropy) about how the water molecule will orientate.

ENTROPY DEFENDED!

Entropy reflects the fact that Nature wants things random and chaotic, and more precisely so that we poor human observers have as little information as possible. To satisfy its taste for obscurity to human observers, it lets things move around overall (actually it *is* that tendency of moving around) so strongly that it can look like a force, but isn't. Putting aside some statistics that weights different arrangements of things by energy, entropy is simply proportional to the logarithm (number of possibilities after an event such as binding divided by the number before), and information, usually expressed in different units, is the logarithm (number of possibilities before an event such as binding divided the number after). Hence, by basic algebra of logs, multiplying the logarithmic result by −1 converts either one to the other. The text implies that the computer is a magic eyeglass that can penetrate that obscurity, giving information about what is actually going on—but that knowledge doesn't stop the apparent hydrophobic "force" unless we could literally grab hold of the water molecules to make them behave otherwise. It is a good job too, since otherwise proteins and all life would fall apart just by a human looking in molecular detail at it. Entropy, introduced as a bad guy, is a major player in the stability of proteins, other molecules, and molecular interactions, including drug–protein binding, the formation of the cell membrane, cells, and so indirectly tissues, organs, and humans. Nature, including biology, uses it to drive to structures that we see as complex, including life. The price to pay in having entropy around as a key player in the universe is that it will ultimately erode us all, but there is for the foreseeable future no imaginable alternative (even if we have any choice).

The calculation of entropy seems to be the key factor that impairs the performance of computer calculations on most molecular systems at this time, or put it another way, it requires extraordinary cost in supercomputer time to even approach getting the water entropy right. Good or bad (see the box) entropy is at least a mischievous guy in that (1) it can contribute the big numbers to the free energy calculation, and so dominate its value, and (2) it is terribly long to calculate in that the computer has ideally to enumerate all the possible configurations of the water for both the unbound and bound states of the drug–protein system. For folding up a protein in the computer to predict its structure, the entropy of the protein chain, which prefers to be open and freely moving (high-entropy situation), is a countering effect to the hydrophobic "forces" that try and bring the oily protein side chains together. The latter only just win, giving proteins their final stable structure. But in a drug-binding simulation, the protein is already folded, and not much is moving (actually it is moving a lot but nothing as much as the unfolded form). Also the drug may be conformationally flexible, but nothing like the open flexibility of a long protein chain. But hydrophobic binding, the burying of oily drug regions that is typically a strong feature of a drug–protein interaction, is still often the key player. Again, it lies in the entropy of the solvent and so is hard to calculate.

Solvent entropy should, if molecular dynamics is done properly and grueling long enough, fall naturally out of the calculation. The problem is that "done properly" means not only getting all the parameters for the forces assigned adequately (reflecting as much as possible the real world) but running for long enough time, and that can be computationally very expensive. Thus less exact methods remain attractive as time-saving approximations, and time is certainly money in the pharmaceutical industry. With that reason we would argue that a very fast supercomputer is an attractive and justifiable investment. The inexactness of the simpler calculations or (proactive not reactive medicine) even less perfect answers can lead to time-wasting wrong directions in drug research.

As it happens, entropy really relates to something that allows us to look at the drug design problem at another way, as a kind of puzzle like a Rubik Cube© with a (typically at least in a sense) specific solution. To solve many kinds of problem by computer simulation, there is usually some implied very complicated "function surface" that is searched. Not only does this have many hills and valleys in which one can become trapped, but it is an exploration puzzle in many dimensions, mathematically speaking (and maybe involving more complex topological objects than higher dimensional counterparts of hills and valleys).

We mean the above quite generally, since entropy really applies beyond thermodynamics to all sorts of industry optimization problems. But at level of "docking the drug," namely for modeling molecules including drug binding, the function surface is the energy surface. Some say, "ideally free energy surface," but the entropy part of free energy is theoretically a consequence of the energy surface, as the introduction to this paragraph hinted. Minimizing the energy of the drug–protein system means searching an energy surface and is analogous (albeit in more dimensions) to searching the land surface of the Earth to find the deepest valley of all (that's probably that occupied by the Dead Sea). It was tempting to say that these surfaces are like maps, but bird's-eye views are not allowed, you are only allowed local information and a record of what you have done so far, as if you are a map-less explorer. But following simple rules such as "keep going down hill" just won't cut it. So-called global minimization methods are required with a much more complex navigation recipe, involving rules such as "when you have found lots of deep valleys, draw a line from the highest valley of these to the central point between all the rest and continue on that line for an equal distance." This example assumes (hopes) that the valleys all lie on a surface with a general up or down trend, like rabbit holes in a grassy bank. Free energy minimization has the same problem, although it adds the complication that a very deep narrow valley in energy terms may not be the lowest in free energy terms (free energy gets it right; it is energy alone that is the cheap approximation). To make matters worse, and although protein scientists and drug designers have talked about hills and valleys of a free energy "surface" for years, this is a multidimensional problem in topology. Mathematical topology teaches us that we must consider multidimensional surfaces (*manifolds*) and that there there are many potential "monstrous" topological features possible, above and beyond hills and valleys. In many ways these relate to the descriptors of high-order behavior of systems, discussed above. In the end, all is math and entropy and topology.

There are some theoretically valid simplifications. Simply moving atoms around anyhow (preferably wisely) is a perfectly valid tool for solving the "hunt the lowest free energy" puzzle. One can take a thermodynamic, not kinetic, viewpoint, and one doesn't care how the right answer is reached. We don't have to get there as Nature does, but just solve it. Molecular dynamics introduces kinetics to move things as Nature does, and is a tempting tool because there might be hidden tricks that Nature uses, but that should drop out of the calculation. On the other hand, with more general minimization methods, there is the chance to use tricks that Nature cannot, such as flipping parts of the molecule through hyperspace to get to other promising situations faster. But in practice, at least so far, molecular dynamics is just another way of moving things around and hence also has the same problem. Yes, it is a satisfying tool because we know that, in the real world using analogous concepts, real molecules get there in the end. But using this idea is only at the price of enormously long runs on the computer, since a second in the real world is vastly more in simulation time. We may, however, be able to move toward that principle as much faster computers are being developed. This was exactly the kind of initial thinking behind IBM's BlueGene supercomputer, which is targeted to handle quadrillion complex calculations per second (petaFLOPS or 10^{15} floating-point operations per second), and protein folding project discussed above.

A NOT-SO-FUTURE PATENT-BASED DRUG DESIGN SCENARIO

Imagine this. You are a senior researcher in a pharmaceutical company. Your supercomputer reads millions of published patents to see what kind of new drugs and their protein targets are of current interest. It automatically detects a new area, and designs new molecules not covered by patenting. It sees if the requisite kind of chemistry is known, and tests the stability of the specifically generated new molecules by advanced quantum mechanical calculations. There could be thousands of them. It then screens them in the computer against receptor and enzyme targets to find which bind to the target protein— not too strongly, but say in the range of the natural molecule and perhaps a bit better. Many such molecules are now ranked by the results above as candidates for chemical synthesis and testing. We'll mention this again in Chapter 10. The point here is that it illustrates an important new twist. The patents are related to a rich source of molecules, protein targets, and applications, and only recently have become available for reading automatically. Their scientific and business intelligence content reduces significantly the entropy of the drug R&D problem.

DIGGING DEEPER INTO PHARMACOGENOMICS

Now we can start to pull our threads together. A major point is of Chapter 2 was that humans had a pattern of migration and recent evolution of the branches of migration. Humans differ, and so do their proteins. There is in fact no guarantee that the same lock, to which such exquisite design attention is given, is *exactly* the same lock from patient to patient. This is the basis of *stratified medicine* in which *pharmacogenomic* differences are taken account of between whole sections of the population, and ultimately *personalized medicine* in which differences between all individuals are taken into account. Stratified medicine is a first step for the pharmaceutical industry in that it is at present not commercially or technically viable to have a market for a drug that is just one patient. However, that first step is itself driven by market forces. The blockbuster drug model of a drug good for all patients has more-or-less picked most of the low-hanging fruit of common diseases. Too many drugs are recalled. It can happen early: the danger to a drug project in a clinical trial is that just one patient will get sick or die because of his or her pharmacogenomics clashing with that drug. Even the latter single failure could now throw away millions or billions of dollars that have been invested in the drugs development.

Let us review from the drug binding perspective. Two humans differ by one or two bases A, G, C, or T in every thousand base pairs in our DNA. Recall that each successive three bases in our DNA codes for one of 20 possible amino acids, and these join together and fold up to make a protein, which is a chain of about 50 to a thousand amino acids or more, each of which is one of the 20 types. Forget the biochemistry, however: statistically this means that some of the otherwise equivalent proteins in you or me will differ in at least one or two amino acids, and some by many more. That's an average over types of proteins. Some proteins like the histones, the DNA binding proteins with many important surface interactions, will hardly differ between us at all, but some like the HLA proteins of the thymus system for immunity will have many differences. In any event even one amino acid change can sometimes profoundly affect the behavior as a molecular lock for any key designed to fit it. The drug as molecular key for one patient may fit well, yet hardly fit at all for another. It may fit the lock but not turn it, potentially creating a drug with the reverse of the intended affect. The similar differences in enzymes between patients may also mean that the same drug in one patient may be processed very differently to that in another, transforming it to uselessness, or a different drug—or a poison.

The solution to meet this challenge (and sometimes market opportunity) is still not too daunting to the hardened theoretician. It merely requires that a colleague in the experimental DNA lab (or, in the not too distant future, the fully automated lab-on-a-chip) determines the DNA sequence of the appropriate gene (or genes) for the patient. Then the theoretician models the resulting correspondingly modified protein (or proteins) for that patient. In practice, it seems sufficient to hunt for key differences, maybe just a single base difference (e.g., G to C) in the DNA. Such differences are the patient genomic biomarkers.

As noted above, however, it is currently not practical and certainly not commercially viable to have a drug unique for an individual patient. In the ideal world it would imply a new molecule that is tailored perfectly to suit all the myriad interactions encountered in a patient. Yet without doubt the potential statistics of DNA variation means that we could more than distinguish every individual in a future galactic empire, let alone now on Earth. However, in a sense, the compromise of stratified medicine is possible despite of the genetic consequences of the diasporas, the ancient migrations of humans. We did not pop into existence out of the blue but have a genetic history showing that gene variations tend to travel in groups so that not every possible combination of potential difference arises and rather falls into genetic families. The potential variation is further reduced for all of non-African descent in that the last major prehistoric diaspora displaced all modern humans already outside of Africa. It seems they left no descendants (see Chapters 2 and 10).

Such stratification is only a tendency, and we each remain unique on Earth. That is, except for your twin brother or sister (or clone), and even there will be immunological and psychological differences due to different history. Nonetheless, it is a tendency that seems good enough for a whole battery of stratified drugs in the near future. We have barely begun to exploit stratification yet. The notion of a stratified market is not entirely new. The previous view of stratification, however, is that we all belong to an "ethnic group"; we are Hispanic, African-American, Inuit, Oriental, Caucasian, and so forth. As it happens, however, a lot of ethnic differences have to do with differences in demographics, tradition, religion, and culture that correlate, but sometimes poorly, with genomics. The recent popular genographic study by the National Geographic Society and IBM is based on the premise that you can still catch the original migrations and their genomics by sampling the points at which people stopped off and pitched a permanent camp during those migrations. It is clearly a correct premise, as the DNA sampling studies results show. But time is running out for such studies. The world is mixing. The Americas are, in particular, a melting pot due to immigration; in the United States the melting pot concept is almost a fundamental philosophy by intent. But mixing happens by less intent. The traditionally very Caucasian British citizen still carry genes from Africans in the Roman army and shipwrecked Moors from the ill-fated Spanish Armada invasion of the British Isles. Who is to say that one of these genes will not be crucial in some near future pharmacogenomic application?

Consider BiDil, a drug and a situation considered elsewhere, notably in the context of evidence-based medicine in Chapter 10. It is a drug combating congestive heart failure moderately well, and originally touted as a triumph for pharmacogenomics by being targeted at African-Americans. In fact, according to lawyer Jonathan Kahn writing in the August 2007 *Scientific American*, despite the beneficial effects this drug illustrates several features of poor reasoning in regards to pharmacogenomics. For the most part, as noted above, ethnic groups and "races" are not well-defined genomic groups but represent geographical and social structures. A consequence of this and other factors is that there may be well overlapping clusters, statistically speaking, such that any two individuals within a cluster have a high probability of being just as genetically diverse as any two between the two clusters. The African-American story, one might add, is somewhat different, in a way that is equally problematic—all the rest of us are just from one or two African tribes out of hundreds that may contribute to the Africans today. Pooling all remaining Africans and splitting up all descendants of those one or two African tribes into Hispanic, Inuit, and so on, is ridiculous, at least from genomics perspective. Indeed every "ethnic group" has its own special story in terms of genetic coherence or genetic diversity; what is clear is that on the whole, they are indeed a *story*, and doubtless a true one to be proud of, but not a simple genomic group at the same level of description as other genomic groups.

Although we preempt the account in Chapter 10, it needs to be emphasized that in practice, the number of African-Americans on which BiDil was tested is very small. To be fair, the difficulty is not that the drug is useless but rather there is no reason as yet to consider it as really "targeted to one genomic population": it seems it was not designed on that basis. It may even be that the non–African-American population is missing out on its benefits. However, Jonathan Kahn seems to imply that pharmacogenomics is a bandwagon in which drug companies are starting to ride to get FDA approval even when it is not pharmacogenomics at all, or at least rather primitive pharmacogenomics. Apparently Bidil is really a mix of two molecular compounds, each of which are available as pharmaceutical tablets at much lower cost. But, in a sense, it is an attempt at a "customized package."

PRELUDE TO PHARMACOGENOMIC VACCINES: THE WAR AGAINST INFECTIOUS DISEASE

While the human genome is important, very roughly half the time you go to your doctor, the genome of an invading pathogen also matters, directly or indirectly. What is considered in the next section is that your pharmacogenomics is still relevant.

Pharmacogenomic vaccines, namely vaccines tailored to the genomics of patients, provide an excellent opportunity for an interlude on infectious diseases, without which no medical story is complete. To start that interlude, let it be said that more or less 50% of the time an infectious disease depends where in the world you live. More precisely it comprises much less than 50%

of visits to physicians in North America, and much more in third world. Infectious disease (bacteria, viruses, protozoa, worms, etc.) is much more rampant in the third world. Worm infestations are also problematic in the third world but only rarely occur in industrial nations (their legacy persists to annoy us in that the part of the immune system that our ancestors evolved to deal with worms is the cause of many allergies). The only disease that is more widespread than a pathogen-based disease in the third world is anemia, due primarily to famine, although pathogens don't help. In contrast, many of the most serious diseases of the industrial nations are the longer term diseases like cardiovascular disease, Alzheimer's, and cancers. They are the diseases born within us, the diseases of longevity. Nonetheless, all of us, young or old, are always susceptible to seriously disabling attack from a pathogen, and the odds escalate in an epidemic.

Vaccines are important to every nation, however industrialized, because of pandemics (global epidemics) and biothreat. *Biothreat* can be taken as a modern term including natural epidemics because it does not have to be malicious, although it can be like the anthrax letters after the attack on the World Trade Center. Actually there has been malicious biowarfare for centuries, from hurling plague victims over the walls of besieged cities to giving American Indians blankets infected with smallpox. It may have gone on well back into prehistoric times, polluting water supplies with fecal matter and dropping dead animals into water supplies, for example, seems to be one of the oldest intertribal conflict methods in the book. Nonetheless, the maliciousness of humans is well outshone by the capriciousness of Nature. It is obvious by far the greatest number of individuals have died through natural pandemics.

Without doubt, the genomics of pathogens relating to their strains are often critical to epidemiology. For example, influenza, an RNA virus, is a well-known killer undergoing constant changes and thwarting vaccine production (which is typically based on the last epidemic). For example, the initial wave of "Spanish flu" infection in the spring of 1918 was mild, but the killer wave in the fall spread throughout the world. Healthy soldiers fell down on parade and many died within 24 to 36 hours. Some 200 million persons were affected, and 10% of them died. More than 500,000 people died in the United States, and up to 50 million people might have died worldwide. Many people died within the first few days after infection, and others died of complications later. Nearly half of those who died were young, healthy adults. *Serological epidemiology* has been used to follow the virus by analyzing adults born at earliest in the time period from 1918 to 1920. Subsequent exposure of the babies to a related flu variant induced a so-called anamnestic response to the original virus, as well as the desirable response to the new variant. This useful "ancient echo" effect is not unknown in many types of infection. Analysis of the antibodies in that anamnestic response showed that the 1918 killer was closely related to A/Swine/Iowa/30 (H1N1) stored in Iowa. Of course, with the advent of DNA analysis (by reverse transcriptase–PCR technology) like that used in modern forensic science, one might think that there is some hope to look directly at the nucleic acids of the virus from living survivors. Unfortunately, the trace is no longer likely to be detectable due to metabolic degradation of the virus, many of the viral hosts have died, and survivors who were exposed are hard to locate. However, some who died were buried in permafrost, inhibiting degradation. Also tissues from those who were infected were in a few cases archived, and now can be examined for the genetic spoor of the virus. These are formalin-fixed, paraffin-embedded tissue samples. From such sources we now have the complete sequence of the hemagglutinin gene from such samples taken from three people died of the flu in 1918.

H1N1 means immunological variant type 1 of the viral hemagglutinin protein and immunological variant type 1 of the neuraminidase protein. Immunological distinctions reflect the viral genomics. H1N1, the first known of the series, caused the highest number of known influenza deaths to date. This most serious of the influenza viruses seem to have first arisen through a mutation enabling its entry through the stomach. Subsequent very rapid generation of new strains of influenza occurred by mixing different influenza strains through a processes called *re-assortment* in the lungs of the host. That said, the original influenza type A (H1N1) viruses continue to plague us today, after being introduced again into the human population in the 1970s.

In the modern world the new flu strains change fast and move fast. Until recently, despite their names such as "Spanish", they are generally agreed to have arisen through transmission from Chinese water birds and chickens (possibly dead chickens in shops too), through the pig, to humans. In 1957 and 1958, "Asian flu" type A (H2N2) caused about 70,000 deaths in the United States. First identified in China in late February 1957, the Asian flu had already spread as far as the United States by June 1957. In 1968 and 1969, "Hong Kong flu" type A (H3N2) caused about 34,000 deaths in the United States. The virus was first detected in Hong Kong early in 1968. Again, it spread to the United States later that year. Influenza A (H3N2) viruses still circulate today. The common opinion thus seems to be that it is only a matter of time until the next influenza pandemic occurs through re-assortment, mutation, or both.

While (unlike physicians) epidemiologists generally breath a relative sigh of relief when only a few people die, a pandemic scare occurred in 1997 when a few hundred people became infected with the avian A/H5N1 flu virus in Hong Kong and 18 people were hospitalized, six of whom died. This influenza virus was different: it moved directly from chickens to people, rather than having been altered by infecting pigs as an intermediate host. Previously the receptor specificity of avian influenza viruses was unlike that of human strains; avian viruses bind preferentially to receptors characteristic of chickens, whereas human strains preferentially bind to receptors normally characteristic of humans. In addition many of the most severe illnesses occurred in young adults similar to illnesses caused by the 1918 Spanish flu virus. To prevent the spread of this virus, approximately 1.5 million chickens were slaughtered in Hong Kong. The avian flu did not easily spread from one person to another, and after the poultry slaughter, no new human infections were found. Peace did not last for long. In 1999 another novel avian flu virus (A/H9N2) caused illnesses in two children in Hong Kong. Although both of these viruses have not gone on to start pandemics, their continued presence in birds, their ability to infect humans, and the ability of influenza viruses to change and become more transmissible among people worries epidemiologists greatly.

Many epidemiologists believe it is only a matter of time until the next influenza pandemic occurs. The severity of the next pandemic cannot be predicted, but studies suggest that its effect in the United States could be very bad. In the absence of any working control measures (vaccination or drugs), it was predicted that in the United States a quite medium pandemic could cause 89,000 to 207,000 deaths, between 314,000 and 734,000 hospitalizations, 18 to 42 million outpatient visits, and another 20 to 47 million people being sick. Between 15% and 35% of the US population could be affected by an influenza pandemic, and the economic impact could range between $71.3 billion and $166.5 billion.

Nor is change of an existing pathogen the only route to a new epidemic. Animals provide a reservoir of wholly new pathogens. Despite the justifiable preoccupations with measles, mumps, rubella, tuberculosis, syphilis, and so forth, there are many very new diseases of concern: SARS, originating from animals in China like the civet, is not a flu, while AIDS is believed to originate in primates. Mad cow disease (BSE—originally a disease called scrapie in sheep and infecting humans as a form of Creutzfeldt-Jacob disease) continues to be a concern. That is not at least because, being the rare case of a pathogen that is a pure protein, a shape change of the natural precursor protein in the animal brain, can arise spontaneously in the brain, say in one in a million cattle a year.

Let us review. Escape from restriction is the commonest causes of epidemics by really new epidemics encountered so far in prehistorical and historical time. It might typically involve a mutation which, for example, overrides the immune system of a new host or permits entry into the cell of the new host. There are some 60 well-known zoonotic examples, if not exactly running from A to Z, certainly from *Acinetobacter pneumonia* to *Yersiniosis* that infect humans. The "Z disease" if it comes, may be aptly named: the analogous Greek letter omega has been used in many science fiction stories for the ultimate bacterial or viral disease; *The Omega Man* was a film in which Charlton Heston played the last uninfected man on Earth. Recent real-life examples include the recent outbreak in Toronto of bird flu (from Asian water birds), SARS (from the civet, etc.), anthrax (sheep), ebola (from rodents), and acquired CJD (sheep, mad cow).

One reason that older infectious diseases are relatively kindly is that it does not benefit most pathogens to kill their hosts or get their hosts killed by marauding carnivores in better health—at least not too quickly. The net effect over hundreds and thousands of years is that hosts and pathogens have learned to live in relative harmony. Over millions or billions of years invaders can become symbionts or symbiotes, meaning useful or almost essential organism inside the host (like bacteroids in the cockroach that make vitamins). Over several billions of years (after marriage between prokaryotic and our ancestral eukaryotic cells in the "primordial soup") they can even become an endosymbiotic part of host genome (e.g., mitochondria, which are ancient "bacteria" essential for using oxygen to burn food in our cells). In contrast, viruses may arise constantly in evolution from RNA/DNA of animals, including humans (notably most of the "Junk DNA") between genes.

Another reason that older diseases are not so harmful is because the most seriously affected humans died out. We are the descendants of the survivors, and inherited that resistance. This immediately suggests that our genomics plays a huge role and that vaccines tailored to our pharmacogenomics do make perfect sense.

PHARMACOGENOMIC VACCINES

Now to our main point. On the face of it, the popular perception of vaccines does not seem to leave much scope for personalized medicine. What is the point of a personally tailored vaccine? Is it not, after all, ultimately the DNA (or RNA) of the infecting pathogen that matters? Yes, but not only. There is interplay between the human genome and infectious disease. Moreover your history of immunological exposure to pathogens, toxins, foods, and the like, also determines part of your molecular constitution, and is potentially an important part of digital patient record. Humans differ in about one to two amino acids per protein on average over proteins. Humans also benefit from variation in proteins such that at least a few will survive an unpredictable epidemic. For example, a mutation in a hormone receptor by which HIV enters the cell makes a very few people resistant to HIV. The reason is rather like the issue of pharmacogenomics. In that case a new drug is not guaranteed to fit because of a different amino acid at the binding site, or remote from the binding site with a slight effect on the shape of the protein. It will not "bind." In the present case the protein at the molecular surface of the invading pathogen may not bind while the natural hormone may do so in some cases.

The problem is the same for those proteins specialized in the immune system to deal with invaders, as now to be described, where the molecules from a vaccine may not bind or bind less strongly. Recall that our HLA (human leukocyte antigen) genes and the proteins they make are the kings of defense and part of their secret lies precisely in their high variation. They are part of the T (thymus) immune system on cells that present on their surfaces peptides (chopped up bits of proteins) of pathogens after proteolytic cleavage. For the T-system, these are called *T-epitopes*. There are billions of possible T-epitopes because of the combinatorial mathematics of joining amino acids together, so this is a very specific recognition that excludes, if things work properly, acting against our own proteins (mistakes that happen in an autoimmune disease). Other cells now see that cell type tagged as alien, or infected, and react accordingly destroying similar alien cells.

HLA variation makes HLA genes an important part of any population genomic sampling. But that is just using HLA as a convenient population marker. The immunological importance of their variation is that there is something in at least somebody for (hopefully) almost every contingency. One person's HLA may have one amino acid or more in the HLA protein that allows a T-epitope to bind weakly or not at all. Another person will bind a new T-epitope strongly, and be "ready to go" in amassing the body's defenses. A small fraction of a human population is guaranteed to be readily primed, almost but not quite as if immunized, if a new disease strikes. Indeed a further important reason why new pathogens are dangerous is that humans without the right variation died out from plagues long ago. We are the descendants of the survivors.

HLA is thus said to be "highly polymorphic": the protein products differ between us by several more than the average one to two amino acids. The blood group factors A and B are examples of them (group O is just an absence). They reflect and determine population genomics: in Amerindians, B and almost all A blood groups have been wiped out by susceptibility to syphilis introduced by conquistadors (the detailed mechanism of this is not clear).

Vaccines need to be designed to take account of variations in human genome in regard to HLA, and also variations in our own proteins to avoid autoimmune disease. The theory of attack is to make vaccines that contain B-epitopes (bone immune system) that generate antibodies, T-epitopes (thymus immune system) that will stimulate antibody and T-cell response respectively, plus some other stimulants of immune response (e.g., "molecular adjuvant"). Briefly and crudely, the antibodies deal with the molecules, and the T response with whole cells.

Traditionally these T- and B-epitopes (detected by the bone marrow system) have been made very crudely by just injecting the existing pathogen of interest. It has been done with both killed and attenuated viruses, but the former can contain live material or infectious pathogen DNA or RNA, and the latter can revert or mutate to something worse. Either way they are a complex jungle of protein signals in which the epitopes have a small voice. The cocktail of chemical signals can cause many problems: an excessive reaction or an autoimmune response if some of the protein pieces look like those naturally in our bodies. To make matters worse, growing viruses in eggs could introduce new pathogens.

The new route is thus to avoid all contact with Nature and make vaccine synthetically, by chemically joining amino acids together to make the epitopes, and add molecular adjuvant in a very fine-tuned way. The route may be unfamiliar to many because technology in chemical and protein chemosynthesis has only relatively recently made major advances in scale and purity of these synthetic constructs, and is still in the hands of a few experts. Nonetheless, a mix of existing proteins plus synthetic constructs is not revolutionary. It has been applied in veterinary science, although the *perceived* FDA response is that it is conservative in regarding such as too new for humans.

The basic idea of manipulating T-epitopes in future medicine is well demonstrated in the related matter of transplantation. HLA diversity in humans is at the origin of the transplant problem. Our bodies learn early in life which proteins are our own, and treat new arrivals in our bodies with suspicion. So a transplanted organ or tissue looks like an invader, and gets rejected. As discussed elsewhere, in 2001 one of the authors [BR] along with research teams at the IBM TJ Watson Research Center and the IBM Haifa Research Center took a real digital patient record from an anonymous patient needing a bone marrow transplant. The patient's polymorphic HLA gene was encrypted, transmitted, automatically annotated, and used to automatically generate a model of the patient's HLA protein. The idea was to block the binding of the epitopes in the bone marrow transplant by getting a strongly binding but different-looking synthetic epitope first. The patient's HLA protein structure was then used as a starting basis for personalized drug screening and drug design, by inserting D-amino acids (mirror image amino acids) into the known binding ligands (epitopes) to which patient has been exposed in the past (and information about which can also be transmitted with the record). Sadly, it was never possible to make the synthetic molecule in time. But as an IT demonstration, at least, the importance was that this was highly automatic and could be made totally automatic.

SAVE THE LAST DANCE FOR ALL OF US: PATIENT, PHARMACEUTICAL INDUSTRY, AND FDA IN THE SAME LOOP

Computer-aided drug design may seem a digression on our current theme if we think of everything in purely clinical terms. That isn't what your physician will be involved in at least in the next few years, or is it?

The pharmaceutical industry desperately wants to access the outcomes fed back from patients about how the drugs are doing. One is for *pharmacovigilance*, that is, to see if the drugs are safe. The second is to fine-tune the drugs to the stratified population, that is, to see what is best for each genomic group of patients. The third is to find new applications for old drugs or intended drugs (called *repurposing*), as happened with Viagra. The fourth is to price the drugs correctly, according to actual use. And the fifth is to have clues for completely new drugs.

In consequence there have already been several recent initiatives to have patients, Big Pharma, and the FDA in the loop. They include the consortium placed under the management of FNIH (Foundation of the National Institutes of Health), and a separate biomarker consortium to cover the pharmacogenomic aspects. In the near future, drugs will be selected for each patient using the feedback from the accumulating knowledge in databases. In the farther future, this loop of several players could contract to drugs being selected and almost synthesized "on the spot," and then tailored for the patient.

In general, the keeping of records for patient documents is a kind of vast experiment or clinical trial. One can search patient records, genomics, therapies, and outcomes in order to gain new clues about how to focus drugs on part of the population with the appropriate profile, soon commonly to include genetics.

Medical IT and the digital medical record with patient genomics is already beginning to be used extensively in clinical trials. This really blurs research and healthcare, and the clinical trial patients receive (or should receive) an intensity of monitoring and attention to genomic and other detail that we should expect for every patient in the future healthcare system.

RIGHT NOW, PHARMACOVIGILANCE MAY BE EMERGING AS A MAJOR FORCE IN THE RISE OF HEALTHCARE IT

At present, not all impetus in the future in the above area is by the pharmaceutical companies themselves. The FDA of the United States (and similarly equivalent bodies worldwide) are concerned that adverse drug reactions in patients have been underreported, perhaps at only a 10% level. Physicians may have been nervous to declare anything that might be seen as their error, and pharmaceutical companies do not want to "fire from the hip" and recall the drug, and hit the company share price. Rightly or wrongly, they may want to balance risks and benefits and want to take some time to get the facts: it may be that the drug is behaving badly in a clearly defined pharmacogenomic group of the larger population, but saving lives in another and perhaps very much larger group. In any event, the government is not pleased, and has instructed the FDA to get the real story. By the FDA Amendment Act of 2007, the US FDA must get feedback, by IT, from 25 million patients in 2010 and 100 million in 2012. It has already awarded $2.5 billion in IT contracts. Comparable activity in the United Kingdom may now be twice that. Somewhat conceptually related, in view of the importance that data mining and analytics will increasingly have in the above kind of activity, is that the US Department of Defense in late 2008 awarded a contract, believed substantial, to the company Phase Forward to use powerful data mining software to examine the medical records of some 12 million people.

For the FDA and pharmaceutical industry, and not least patients, the real root of the problem is simple, and makes the rise of such IT systems inevitable. Clinical trials cover a small sample of a few hundred or thousand patients. This is not good in any event because adverse responses such as liver damage are often undetected when study populations are small. But importantly the trials also fail badly to capture all pharmacogenomic variations that exist outside the trial, in the larger population.

With all that has been said about our genomic and pharmacogenomic differences, it is probably no surprise that adverse drug reactions to marketed drugs are one of the 10 leading causes of death in the United States—the direct cost of harm alone is $75 to $130 billion in the United States. Under-reported they may be, but the FDA already receives 250,000 to 500,000 reports of adverse reactions to prescribed drugs from physicians and pharmaceutical companies each year (S. R. Ahmad, Adverse drug event monitoring at the Food and Drug Administration, *J. Gen. Intern. Med.* 2003;18(1):57–60; J. A. Johnson and J. L. Bootman, Drug-related morbidity and mortality: A cost-of-illness model, *Arch. Intern. Med.* 1995;155:1949–1956). While at present in the United States there will be about 164 approvals per year, there will be about 2500 drug product and batch recalls. There were about 2,072 batch recalls in 2005. It is expected to increase at an AAGR of 5.1% to reach 2,616 by 2010 (http://www.biz-lib.com/products/ZBUWP.html).

We now need a crisper definition of pharmacovigilance as the activity that seeks to attenuate the above horrors. It is the science relating to the detection, assessment, understanding and prevention of adverse effects from medicines, including both long- and short-term side effects. It also involves assessing and evaluating information from healthcare providers and patients on the adverse effects of herbal and traditional medicines. And in turn the deeper and defini-tion of an adverse drug reaction is that *it is a response to a drug that is noxious and unintended at doses normally used, either for the prophylaxis, diagnosis or therapy, or for the modification of patient physiological function.* The goals are considered twofold: identifying new information about dangers associated with medicines, and directly seeking to protect patients. In our larger health-care picture, the idea also extends naturally to vigilance over food products, which is, after all, the "F" in the FDA.

The WHO defines pharmacosurveillance and pharmacovigilance as terms used to refer to the monitoring of drug safety, for example, by means of spon-taneous adverse-effect reporting systems, case-control and cohort studies. That is, they are used interchangeably. However, this is not always the case in phar-maceutical industry speech. While pharmacovigilance is of interest as a major driver, it may be considered as part of pharmacosurveillance, which is a bigger market still. Pharmacovigilance focuses primarily on adverse reactions and on resolving issues as to whether these are general production quality, batch issues, or a fundamental property of the drug molecule. Pharmacovigilance adds in the more positive things mentioned in the previous section: fine tuning to specific genomic markets, and finding new purposes for existing drugs. It also overlaps with many regulatory aspects. In the current global market downturn, there may be less R&D and so much thought given to repurposing, and sheer panic at the thought of the recall of a blockbuster drug. We can see many of these issues in what the market analysts call the pharmaceutical *regu-latory and surveillance* industry. Given all the above it should be no surprise that the market analysts tell us that pharmaceutical companies already spend much of their budget on regulatory and surveillance issues. It is in 2009 expected to be a staggering $239 billion market, and the cost is expected to rise at an AAGR of 10% to reach $265 billion by 2010 (http://www.bccresearch.com/report/PHM047A.html).

To put this in perspective, the global pharmaceutical market in 2009 will be about $730 billion, and to access that the pharmaceutical companies spend about $67 billion on preclinical basic research (R&D) and $75 billion on clinical trials. "Regulatory and surveillance" does include submission and product quality control and distribution issues that are intimately intertwined with drug safety (e.g., drugs have a shelf life, and one which can be greatly shortened by a rise in temperature). Nonetheless, pharmacovigilance as defined earlier is believed to be a big chunk of the expenditure.

So, while pharmacosurveillance includes positive matters such as market targeting and repurposing, and so is largely internally motivated, pharmacovigilance is also facing growing external challenges by the regulatory agencies. Now the federal initiatives enforce honest reporting of adverse drug reactions, so will dramatically increasing reports, and the industry will want "first heads up," not least to prepare their defense and response in pharmacogenomic terms. A shining example of how to respond, but actually a move that long preempted these external pressures, was set by Glaxo Smith Kline, who created their own pharmacovigilance organization. Around 2002–2003, they achieved a 70% reduction in adverse event handling process complexity and a 30% boost in productivity. Their global organizational and process consistency also increased. Their system allows management to stay continually informed of the global safety operation and initiate proactive, specific improvements or corrective actions based on reliable and up-to-date data. Generally for the industry, however, post-marketing commitments have been only poorly met: 71% of post-marketing study commitments were pending in the United States in 2006. The FDA Amendments Act (2007) now gives FDA the ability to fine companies to help ensure post-marketing study completion.

In all countries, developing a nationally organized pharmacosurveillance system is not easy. There are issues such as the role of government and non-government bodies, notably the pharmaceutical and biotechnology companies. There are issues as to the nature of evidence needed to inform regulatory and reimbursement decisions. The analyses are more of epidemiological nature than in a controlled research or clinical trial setting. Cause of adverse events is usually based on observational studies rather than randomized controlled trials. It is not yet clear how to fund, oversee, conduct and disseminate the research. All seem to agree that IT is the critical tool for pharmacovigilance, which surely will rely critically on communication, data storage, security and privacy, and advanced data mining and analytics. However, though rising rapidly, worldwide pharmaceutical expenditure on IT, i.e., IT generally, is only a few billion.

So one wonders what the significant sums in the pharmacovigilance market are being spent on right now. Much at least is spent on Phase IV trials of the marketed drugs (on larger communities), to physicians, public relations, marketing studies relating to drug pricing sales and distribution aspects of safety, lawyers, lobbying government, and so forth. However, this will change. Substantial fees paid by the industry to physicians to report adverse reactions to pharmaceutical companies may decrease because the FDA Amendment Act is moving to *demanding* physician input and making analyzed data public.

Drug pricing, sales and distribution will be on rational basis of feedback from patients. The effect on marketing of drug quality based on best evidence will greatly reduce unjustified "push" marketing. There will be a massive rise in interest in data mining and data analytics to make sense of data "good and bad": whoever will best and fastest transform data to knowledge will win. There will be associated changes in the environment, some very beneficial. With standardized electronic health records, clinical trial phases will be much less time-consuming and costly to source and it will be easier to enroll participants, and clinical trials, ever far from providing the complete picture of a drug, will effectively merge with post-clinical surveillance. Physicians will be required to practice evidence-based medicine based on latest findings anyway, which will merge with that consideration. Progressively, the move will be toward a focus on pharmacogenomics and biomarkers from the very dawn of concept of a drug, to rationalize response and avoid adverse reactions.

CLINICAL DECISION SUPPORT SYSTEMS ENABLE HEALTHCARE PROVIDERS AND PHARMACEUTICAL COMPANIES TO MAKE INFORMED DECISIONS

With the above in mind, we may now return to *clinical decision support systems*. They form an important topic because it is about how we formally get knowledge out of clinical data, as well as about how we can use that knowledge to help the patient. The overall process for the clinician involves getting data from lots of patients to make decisions, through computer-augmented inference, for specific patients. This includes selection of available drugs and their mixes. For the pharmaceutical company it is at present (or soon will be) an issue of identifying target groups of patients that will or will not benefit from a particular drug (stratified medicine). Ultimately it will be for the specific patient (personalized medicine), and the role of physician and pharmacologist (and FDA) will be intimately intertwined in some way. Drugs could one day be made fast, to order.

Analysis of large amounts of data is called the *empirical* approach, as opposed to the earlier-discussed theoretical approach using a few theoretical principles. We might say that all insight and decision-making in medical practice and research that comes from Nature, whether hard-won collections of data or no less hard-won physician experience, are *experiential* or *experience driven*. For the physician that does *not* mean personal or anecdotal experience colored by old medical school learning and thus the latest "expert opinion." It means getting all the latest facts, collected and analyzed globally. This is a principle of evidence-based medicine (EBM) discussed again in the last chapter. The recent explosion of interest in EBM is that a failure to consider all the latest facts, collected and analyzed globally, injures and kills patients.

Anything much smarter than the experience-driven methods considered in this section may be experience driven but as a matter of *artificial intelligence* (AI). As noted elsewhere, that's certainly a topic of medical interest. Unfortunately, it's still largely a "not yet" topic. Except for glimpses of the HAL 2000 computer in the Stanley Kubrik's *2001 A Space Odyssey,* based on the writings of Arthur C. Clark ("HAL" being of course one letter up and two letter down in the alphabet per character from "IBM"), really good, human-like AI is still beyond the horizon. There are but a few basic examples that really get the AI name because they use some AI principles that humans have grasped, but not of course those many principles that have yet to be discovered and will be necessary for really good performance. It is possible that again we have something that relates to descriptors of higher order systems behavior, but we do not know them yet. Right now, we must be content with some basic simulations, and as described now, automatic processing of collections of rules from human experts or data, or both, to aid decisions by physicians and medical researchers. That all said, clinical decision support systems, such as things called expert systems and data mining, even as they stand right now, are still considered the smart part of clinical decision intelligence.

Much twentieth-century focus was on *expert systems.* In the 1960s and subsequently, physician and researcher decision support were studied at a number of centers, including Stanford University (Ted Shortliffe's Ph.D. Thesis) and at MIT by Artificial Intelligence Founder Marvin Minsky and students. In those days, there was a shortage of data and a plethora, relatively speaking with respect to data, of experts. Hence expert systems contained rules which specialists called *knowledge engineers* extracted from experts by interrogation.

The primary difficulty with these expert systems is that they were based on human experts, which is to say that they were based on collections of rules and rule weights (confidence in the rules) assigned by them. The limiting factor was the expert. In the view of evidence-based medicine as hinted above, the view of so-called experts is not in general now considered a good idea. Information technologists knew this from experience long before the recent acceleration of interest in evidence-based medicine. The extraction of rules from human experts and into expert systems has been notorious. It has been a very slow process constituting the famous "Feigenbaum bottleneck," after the mathematician who helped build the first expert systems (DENDRAL). Extracting knowledge from experts can be extremely difficult, since the expert may not be consciously aware of how he makes decisions. Several imitations such as distrust about sharing insider knowledge, fear of replacement by a machine, fear of being shown to have erroneous expertise, and so on, have also been identified. Regardless of the merits of the expert system shell used, there is a need (1) to get some rules by different means, notably from data mining (which we will discuss below and which can generate tens of thousands or more of rules in days) and (2) to develop better means to accelerate capture of expertise from human experts.

INFERENCE

The difficulty is illustrated by the pioneering study in medicine is the MYCIN Stanford project (1972–1982), but first let's look at the character of MYCIN and some of its more technical plusses and minuses. Incidentally, E-MYCIN (empty MYCIN) is the latter system for general rule addition for any domain. MYCIN rules were of the following types:

- "A is B." Definitional—conclusion is a restatement of the precondition in different terms
- "A causes B." Cause–effect. The conclusion follows from precondition by known or unknown mechanism.
- "B was caused by A." Effect–cause. The presence of certain effects suggest a cause.
- "A occurs with B." Associational. As in association analysis, the causal relation is not known [time order could be known if time-stamped].
- "A is greater than X grams/liter." Self-referencing. The current knowledge is used to update a value in a rule.

Whereas expert system languages for reasoning like PROLOG are universally qualified (all/all not) and nonquantitative, MYCIN allows an aspect of existential qualification (some, some not) and is quantified. The rules have both a rule form as above, and a certainty factor (CF). For those of a mathematical bent, the MYCIN certainty factor is defined by the following equation:

$$CF[h, e] = \frac{(\max[P(h|e), P(h)] - P(h))}{(\max[1, 0] - P(h))} - \frac{(\min[P(h|e), P(h)] - P(h))}{(\min[1, 0] - P(h))},$$

where P is probability, e is the evidence, and h the hypothesis.

The point here is that such equations, which are as ingenious as they look complicated, tell a story with a particular philosophy. That philosophy may have a flaw, or at least it looks that way if you hold to the competing philosophy. As we understand it, this kind of approach tries to force the positive hypothesis and the negative hypothesis, or null hypothesis, and evidence for and evidence against, into a single scalar value. This is convenient, but it is not classical. Even the worst student of classical statistics learns the difference between refuting a null or negative hypothesis versus confirming the hypothesis for something. Being from Stanford, the MYCIN gang was being far more rebellious than stupid, and as we said, the equation above is quite ingenious. However, it is not perfect in at least one sense: it results in the fact that the actual CF (certainty factor) in a hypothesis at the end of a chain of reasoning can be dependant on rule order. Such deficiencies can be overcome. For example, information theory can be considered as delivering numbers in the "right form," such that information against a hypothesis can be added to that for a hypothesis, as long as we consider the former as negative information (which simply means that you subtract the first from the second, of course). Even so, there are reasons why you might want to keep the two forms of information separate until the "last act." As a very simple example (though not a million miles from real examples), consider an instruction "Give up if the amount of information so far is not very much!" That would tend to be obeyed if the weakest sources of information were considered first. The GLOBAL language (1987–1995) that one of the authors (BR) first designed and led the development of for a pharmaceutical company before joining IBM used variables with variable parts to the variable names for the bindings and the value of the variable as a degree of truth or belief, based on an information-theoretic approach with for- and against-measures being held separate behind the scenes as a two-value variable, if required, until, for example, they hit the "IF" function when the net information value was taken and considered true if greater than zero or as a set threshold confidence value. The name GLOBAL came from the broad scope of the language as a programming, expert system, expertise capture, editing and query language, all mixable with human language that was itself defined in terms of GLOBAL, all intended to make it easy for the expert who is inexpert at IT. For example, what could have the following statement at any level of the computer system:

```
some_{{X}_proteins}}_are_not{Y} = not all_{{X}_
proteins}_are_{Y};
```

```
IF some_{{X}_proteins}}_are_not{Y} start purification_
of_{X}_proteins protocol;
```

Here, however, is the real crunch, which is by no means peculiar to MYCIN, GLOBAL, or anything else. Applied to the infectious disease diagnosis and treatment domain, work with MYCIN led to 600 rules extracted from experts, although many had say 10 parameters, and the generous upper ceiling is thus say 6,000 distinct rules. That works out to 1.6 rules per day for the duration of the project. However, on the one hand, there was a plateau reached for rules sufficient to do the job about a third of the way through the project, say 4.8/ day, while on the other hand, most rules and their weights were continually being refined throughout the project, which in some sense lifts that estimate. Unfortunately, the order of 600 rules is unlikely to serve general medicine or surveillance systems and even other systems with 100,000 rules may fall short. The domain of application, diagnosis, and treatment of infectious disease was chosen for MYCIN because of its being a focused domain with a relatively restricted, unambiguous vocabulary, with time available for several seconds of reasoning, and because of a lot of on-site quality expertise. These conditions are not true across the entire clinical domain, and typical domains required tens of thousands of rules and very fast parallel machines.[1]

---

[1] As stated in *The Age of Intelligent Machines*, Ch. 8, by Raymond Kurzweil.

Clearly, better methods of capturing human expertise are required, but we may also note that data mining can generate hundreds of thousands of rules in just a few hours or days, depending on the computer used. A character feature of these earlier periods is that there was a shortage of data and a plethora of experts. *This situation is now reversed.* There is a veritable tsunami of data, including growing number of digital patient records, and experts are in hot demand. We now have the opportunity to extract the same kind of rules from extensive archives of hard data, and update our views as the quality and quantity of data improves. (There is still nothing to stop empirically extracted rules from being mixed with those assigned by experts, and the existence of a large ranked list of empirically determined rules provides a considerable guideline to how to assign rules, where to place them on a ranked list, and what quantitative rule strengths to assign.) However, the quality and depth of the rules obtained depend on the quality and breadth of the data mined.

DATA MINING: HOW THE GUARDIANS
OF OUR HEALTH CAN KNOW US

Recall from Chapter 7, and discussions of architecting IT for knowledge, that data mining is primarily (but not necessarily solely) the means of reducing the entropy of our business or healthcare system. The unsolicited queries can amount to "find me anything interesting," and appropriately its results can ultimately be quantified as information that is the reduction in entropy. In general, the information analysis aspect of biomedical informatics involves scoring, modeling, visualization, and mining. All four are crucial steps to successfully perform the analysis. Data mining is typically now specifically seen as the input that should be used to get rules on which inference is performed rather than using rules (at least solely) from experts. This is accomplished by the discovery of previously unknown dependencies and relationships in the data sets. Data mining can be described for present purposes as the use of automatic data-analytic procedures to obtain rules (not necessarily medical) from the escalating archives of data, or some other means of providing insight from observations in such a way as to enable decisions or enhance understanding. The data archives should not be thought of as dry, fixed libraries. They may be transient, dynamically updated reservoirs of information from surveillance, and other data capture devices, the latest "hot from the press."

Data mining as the step before inference is a kind of *interrogation* of raw data or experimental data. In general, interrogation of data can be performed in two ways, either supervised/directed or unsupervised/undirected. Only the latter is true data mining. The supervised or directed method involves testing for proposed or hypothetical rules, or involves the classification of the data on grouping patterns based on prior information. The unsupervised or undirected method takes the opposite approach. It is as if the user says: "I have no ideas. I do not know where to look. Just tell me everything interesting." It "simply" clusters the material by grouping the data without any prior information. It results in many *unsolicited* associative models, such as high blood glucose is associated with a diagnosis of diabetes. Compare the directed query method, where the researcher (or in this example young student!) might ask "Is high blood glucoses associated with diabetes?" and there is just one answer. The associations formed consist of a co-occurrence of data items. Since there is no prior assumption, there are a large number of possibilities to examine (see below). It is strictly speaking the last, unsupervised, approach that constitutes real data mining, whereas the former or supervised approach is analogous to classical statistics. It would not be entirely misleading to say that data mining involves generating multiple hypotheses, each of which could be considered as being tested by statistics.

That all said, there are *several* methods that we might lump together as data mining. In all these we might argue that we are ultimately interested in probabilities, for example, the probability that a laboratory result of high glucose (A) is associated over many patients with a diagnosis of diabetes (B) and a prescription of insulin (C), with probability $P(A, B, C)$. In general, the number of things or "complexity" (here A, B, C, i.e., three things) is at least two and maybe many more.

Comparison of these data-mining methods requires a little knowledge of probabilities, but for those readers willing and able, here it goes. All such methods try to make some statement about the probability say $P(A, B, C)$ of A, B, and C occurring together, compared with prior expectation. $P(A, B, C)$ means that "the probability of A, B, and C is occurring together" or "the probability of A, B, and C is associated" and indeed this can be written $P(A \& B \& C)$. The methods may differ, not by some legislation but by tendency in what that expectation is. To some extent methods differ in the matter of *normalization*, meaning in a more general sense what probabilities it should be compared with. For example:

- *Pattern discovery.* The pattern such as $(A, B, C, ...)$ exists more than a specified number of times but does not of itself, in rawest form, state whether this is more, less, or as much as expected on the chance basis of A, B, C, and so on, coming together. It can discover very complex associations but not associations that ought to occur but don't.

- *Associative analysis.* (considered by some as synonymous with data mining). Ratios such as $P(A, B, C, ...)/[P(A) \cdot P(B) \cdot P(C) ...]$, their logarithms, or other functional forms are constructed to take account of the probability of C occurring in any event. This method can be extended to numerical data and trends by using, for example, a fuzzy logic argument relating to A, B, C, and so on.

- *Predictive analysis and knowledge discovery.* It may well be argued that *predictive analysis* is a modern trendy term for of the same thing, a euphemism for data mining after that got a bad public image from too many unfounded hopes and claims in the business sector. Nonetheless, one difference is that it has often (though not always) focused on the intuitive rule forms such as A & B … imply Z, which is quantified by the probability $P(Z|A, B) = P(A, B, Z)/P(A, B)$ and thus takes account of the probability of A & B occurring in any event. This rule basis is intuitive and widely accepted in industry, but the chance of Z occurring anyway is not considered in that formalism, while it is considered in associative analysis.

The same arguments can be applied to expert systems, except that the selection of the rules, and the notion of probability, is obtained more subjectively, from expert opinion, rather than from detailed statistical analysis. That doesn't (always) mean that they are just pulled out of the air, however. To put this all on a semi-rational footing, there are techniques by which the expert can be invited to lay bets on particular values the probabilities (or similar weight or confidence measures) might take. In any event, the fact that rules derived from expert opinion and from statistical analysis can look much the same means that both types of rule can be mixed together to generate the decision support system. It is worth noting that once you have a set of rules ranked by some kind of strength like the probability, it becomes much easier for the expert to assign corresponding weight to his more subjective rules, by sliding them in what seems to be the appropriate point in the ranked list.

The functions of data mining have the potential to greatly improve the quality and efficiency of healthcare. Technology has focused on three general trends in data mining, to best meet these purposes. There has been development in the area of mining for combined numeric or structured data and text in its natural language, mining for predictive modeling, and mining for optimization. Undirected multivariate analysis enables association studies against multidimensional data for a combinatorial analysis among genomic, proteomic, cytomic, clinical, demographic, genealogical, environmental, lifestyle, and socioeconomic factors, for example, as a means to correlate genes with diseases and to study the susceptibility or immunity of the population to specific pathogens or allergens.

Multidimensional data sets can be categorized into such things as demographic and insurance data (IDx); diagnosis (Dx); laboratory test results (Lx, e.g., hemoglobin, blood glucose levels, triglycerides); biopsies (Bx); radiology (MIx, e.g., MRI, PET, CT, US, mammography); procedures, protocols, surgical operations (Px); prescriptions, therapies (Rx); outcomes (Ox); genetic, genomic (Gx); proteomic (PRx); psychological (PSx); ecology (ECx, e.g., environmental, lifestyle, family life); and ethical, privacy (ETx). This all takes account of matters such as patient demographics, clinical events, discharge summaries, patient history, radiology, pharma/medications, clinical observations, laboratory/diagnostic procedures and test results, drugs given and procedures given outcomes, vaccinations, lifestyle, environmental, pathology, hematology, epidemiology, genotypic data (gene expression, transcriptome, etc.), phenotypic data (SNP or genomic biomarker, etc.), genealogical data, and so on. The overall data can be also classified into (1) public data and private data in consideration of the data ownerships and custodianships, (2) structured data and unstructured data (e.g., text) in consideration of the data structures, (3) relational and nonrelational data in consideration of the data management systems, and (4) protected personal data or de-identified data in consideration of the privacy implications. In the healthcare domain it is safe to assume that most of the data are private, unstructured, nonrelational, and protected data.

The clinical data such as the discharge summaries and the radiology reports are in free text format or as analog images. In order to include the unstructured text data and image data for analytical processing such as combinatorial analyses and data mining, those text data and image data need to be transformed first of all into a machine-readable format, and then need to be further analyzed to extract relevant and relatively structured data (e.g., key words and phrases from the text data, features from image data) from the unstructured data sources.

Clinical genomics research typically involves five research scenarios that start with identifying genes of interest, characterizing the identified genes and genomic biomarkers, testing polymorphisms, correlating the identified genes with a certain disease, and validating associations and correlations through population studies. Correlating genes with diseases can be categorized into two approaches: correlating one gene with monogenic traits and correlating multiple genes with polygenic traits. In addition clinical genomics research involves correlating genes with susceptibility or immunity of the population to specific pathogens or allergens.

As shown in the Figure 9.2, the system should provide a facility to extract the patient information such as gender, race, age, and clinical events from the

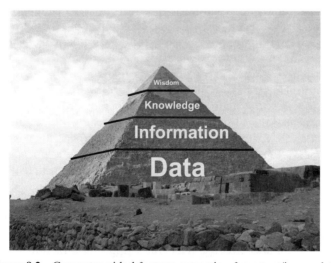

Figure 9.2   Computer-aided feature extraction from text/image data

hospital discharge summary and to extract the key features from the MRI scans and also from the microarray assays to be incorporated into a combinatorial analysis.

WHY DATA MINING IS HARD

Now we come to the major point regarding the *difficulty* in how well the guardians of our health can know us, right now. Data mining is hard when there is much diverse, heterogeneous, and multidimensional data to pull together, and that also means the patients are described by many parameters, especially with genomics, proteomics, and advanced medical imaging modalities. The number of patients is less of a problem. Data mining can tackle many millions of records of any kind quickly, as far as they are not too complex. The main problem, however, is essentially a combinatorial and ultimately entropic one, and we need to take some time to introduce this, as follows.

Medical records imply many patterns, associations, correlations, or rules such as Height:=6ft, Weight:=210lbs> or more obviously Gender:=male, Pregnant:=no>. Call these *a*, *b*, *c*, etc. The difficulty can be glimpsed by considering that if you have data with parameters *a*, *b*, *c*, *d*, ... , *z*, then there may be rules about *a* with *b*, about *b* with *c*, about *a* with *b* and *d*, about *c* with *d* and *e* and *h*, about *a* with *h* and *i* and *k* and *m*, and *x*, and about *b* with *d* with *f*, *g*, *k*, *m*, *n*, *q*, *t*, *u*, *w*, and *z*, and so on, not exactly at infinitum. But after the 26 letters of the alphabet are used up as example parameters, there are 67,108,864 combinations and possible rules. For 100 parameters (nothing compared with a real medical record of maybe 500–2,000) there are 10^{30}. In fact, as the number of parameters grows, the number of possible rules grows much faster. Mathematicians say it is an example of a *combinatorial explosion*. This difficulty, as we will quantify below, is that while a directed query or statistical test of a hypothesis is just a one off, effectively repeating these to consider all possible aspects, and hence make a discovery, can be equivalent to many billions of such queries in the worst case.

Associative data mining looks for things that occur more than would be expected on a chance basis (called *positive association*) but also for things that occur together *less* than we would expect on a chance basis (called *negative association*). Such negative associations can be so strong that some are not seen at all, for example, as in the case of pregnant males. The cases with no observation pose a problem for some traditional data methods because they have to be seen before anyone bothers doing statistics on them. As discussed below, there is even a sense in which *zero association* is important.

Correlational data mining can also (depending on the software in question) look for trends among quantitative data to find those that come together (called *positive variance between data*) or in opposite directions (called *negative variance between data*). The words "association" and "variance between data" can be replaced by "correlation" for convenience, giving positive correlation and negative correlation, for example, provided that it is remembered that correlation doesn't just mean trend in numbers (a spin on meaning that it sometimes has). Pattern discovery is similar in some respects but doesn't allow discovery of negative associations, and a pattern certainly has to occur before it can be seen. Generally speaking, it can't be said that a pattern didn't occur but should have. The researcher might also want to know that there is zero association between this drug and indigestion or some other side effect in the patient population once a drug is marketed (an aspect of pharmacovigilance). Indeed, even if zero associations are not the object of interest per se, the researcher may well need to look just to prove that there are, or aren't, zero associations.

In many cases assumptions are made such that A, B, and C can or can't come together significantly, these are made on the ground that A and B, B and C, and A and C do or don't. The second important thing to grasp is that this is only true sometimes, not in general. We cannot always ignore examining complicated rules on the assumption that they are implied by simpler rules. The false assumptions implied in the simple rules seem to show up more in regard to unexpected negative associations. For example, whereas it is often true that if A tends to be associated with B, and B with C, and A with C, then A, B, and C will tend to occur together. Medical data-mining programs deem to inform us that in some countries anemic males are quite common, and anemic pregnant patients are very common, and these are pairwise, "order 2," relationships (e.g., male with anemic—or more correctly male with anemia). But unless it has the benefit of a full artificial intelligence, and it specifically looks and counts, it could not deduce from such pairwise things that three-way things such as anemic pregnant males are a different story. It has to look at the "order 3" things specifically. Now that example is to some extent a misrepresentation because you could have found by data mining that the qualities of being pregnant and male do not occur together in the same patients. However, another example shows that in some cases no combination of pairs of things will reveal the true situation. You cannot deduce the probability of Alice, Bob, and Carol being seen on a (no sidecar) motorbike from the probability of Alice and Bob, or Alice and Carol, or Bob and Carol being seen on one. Apart from being a heated "love triangle," it is illegal in most places, for one thing. And of course it isn't the case that the most complex rules need be just of order 3. In fact complex diseases, like cardiovascular disease or cancer, may be analysis problems of order 100 or worse.

Let's first suppose we knew that we *can* consider things on a pairwise basis. The attraction of metric distance, principal component analysis, multidimensional scaling, clustering, and dendrograms is that they consider the mere $N(N - 2)/2$ parameters for an N parameter problem. The approaches are powerful and persuasive. But we just illustrated above that this is not justified in general. You just never get to miss the more complicated relationships because you never get to see them.

If, however, we also have to consider three, four, five, and more things together, right up to all N parameters (height, blood glucose level, etc.), the analysis gets really complex. This comes from the mathematical formula for taking every possible combination: $\Sigma_{n=1,2,\ldots,N} N!/(n!(N-n)!)$, where N is the number of parameters, and we are considering N coming together as rules $n = 1, 2, 3, \ldots, N$ times. The worst case (but see below) is x^N rules, where x is equal to or greater than 2. Recall that x^N means x multiplied by itself N times. This is also the number of distinct directed queries or distinct statistical hypothesis tests that would have to be performed. For a spreadsheet of N rows, $x = 2$ (and not taking out self-rules and an existence rule implied by the combinatorial math), there is exactly a worst case of 2^N potential rules. That's a staggering 10^{30} for a mere $N = 100$ items. In the spreadsheet simplest cases this includes a small number $N + 1$ of trivial rules, namely N rules that a exists, b exists, and so on, and a general or empty rule that something exists. If we wish to ignore these rules from the outset, we simply use $\Sigma_{n=1,2,\ldots,N} N!/(n!(N-n)!) = 2^N - N - 1$. For items that can repeat, say like "broken leg" several times in your record without further qualification, things are more complicated and the numbers bigger still: x is the number of possible states for each item. For multivariate analysis and whenever data are fitted by minimization, simulation, or matrix operations, there are worst cases of quantitative data, $x = 1/e$ (where $0 > e < 1$ is the error) giving $(1/e)^N$ distinct basic operations, eigenvalues, or quantitative rules. Mathematical readers who understand what we just said will also know that the easiest case is one single global minimum in the fitting surface into which the computational fitting procedure plummets to reach a single solution, and reach it rapidly, but that is rarely the case with medical data.

We say above that these numbers x^N are "worst case," but remember that in a sense, there really is always exactly that number of rules. It is just that we think of rules of arbitrarily close to zero strength, confidence, support, information, or weight as not being rules. In principle, remember, we still have to look at all the rules in order to know that we can eliminate them. From one perspective, the x^N numbers represent *exactly* the number of rules in any system of N parameters. Again, it is merely that some will have values arbitrarily close to zero for information content, rule strength, confidence, statistical support, P-value, credibility, reliability, and so on, use or call them what you will according to your expertise; hence you will typically choose to consider rules as "not rules." The difficulty is that we have to examine ideally all the rules in order to identify those values that come close to zero, and those that do not.

This x^N kind of problem arises more generally as data are analyzed or generated. The problem of local entrapment in a complex function surface is also evidenced in applications of neural networks. The reader with an interest in chemistry or molecular biology might note that the entrapment problem is directly analogous to the protein folding problem, namely that with so many combinations of shape to fold into, how can the protein find the right one in reasonable time. Indeed a direct relation between the notorious "protein-folding problem" and the generation of rules can be seen by recognizing that a polymer of N units with each unit in k possible conformational (rotameric) minimum states implies the order of maximum of k^N minima in the potential energy surface in Cartesian space. Strong evolutionary pressure in this case does typically (for thermodynamic or kinetic reasons) yield a limited set of highly statistically weighted solutions (the folded state or states), but it must still be appreciated that all other minima correspond to co-existing free energy solutions, albeit that they may be of much lower statistical weight.

Analysis of medical data for both clinical and research application reveals the need to consider the most complicated and challenging possibilities discussed above, especially irreducible complex relations involving many factors, and a significant number of interesting events that should but don't occur. For example, complex diseases such as cardiovascular diseases may perhaps involve 70 SNPs and some 30 lifestyle factors that may not be possible to break down extensively into simpler terms. To add to that burden, it becomes important for preventative medicine to recognize events that concur much less frequently than expected, including to the extent of never being seen at all (e.g., pregnant male patients). This is not something that traditional data analysis is good at: it makes no sense, in text analysis, for example, to assess all the crazy combinations of words that should occur but don't. But we want very much to find what gives negative relationships between therapy and disease, or lifestyle and disease.

Because the number of potential rules can be so huge, powerful computers and improved methods are required to help navigate through the large number of combinations of items that may need to be considered, and to develop heuristics. Here in review are the reasons why this arises when you think that it might not be the case.

1. The term *discovery* was used above. Traditional statistics is typically concerned with testing hypotheses or playing hunches; or using directed queries, traditional statistics go immediately, for example, to specific columns of data to test hypotheses about correlations between them. This is different from discovery, when we take the position that we have no prior understanding or guesses and wish to find everything that is interesting. Then we have to examine all combinations of columns (or other data structures), which gives rise to the combinatorial explosion.

2. The discussion is about potential as opposed to *actual* rules. Nonetheless, the we could think of potential rules as *actual* rules; it is simply that some rules will be weak or be zero strength rules, having an associated value expressing strength (information content, probability, likelihood, degree of belief, weight, confidence, or statistical support) within some arbitrary agreed proximity of zero. The traditional perspective is that the rules with this property are, by definition, not rules. The argument against that perspective is that, a priori, we

still ideally have to look at all 2^N of rules to determine which do, and which do not, have such values in them. Fortunately, this still allows the possibility that we may be able to think of algorithms to prune out, early in the calculation, those rules that are very weak.

3. A common assumption is that the operational number of rules is fewer because generally we do not need to state all the rules, since other rules are implied by them. This is evidently true for rules forming the matter of syllogisms. In particular, there is the common assumption that complex rules apply to patients. Empirical observation of the zero weight for pregnant male would give that away, but there are other more symmetrical examples.

ACCEPTANCE ISSUES: WE NEED TO START SOMEWHERE

Bearing in mind that there are the difficulties to overcome, will computer-based clinical decision intelligence be accepted soon by physicians and hospitals? It turns out that difficulties in acceptance are not due to the issues discussed above, of which there is relatively little awareness. Nor should there be consternation where there is awareness, since anything that can be done to make decisions on the basis of all information that can be tapped is a lot better than what was previously been done in the heads of physicians and medical practitioners, as the rising doctrine of evidence-based medicine points out (see Chapter 10). Rather the difficulty is cultural, in lack of trust, and in the pain of transition.

> The lack of trust is even more a problem with physicians than with consumers. All too often, information technology has been imposed on physicians "from above by alien, imperial powers (hospitals, health systems, or health plans)." Vendors and information managers frequently encounter physicians' fear that information systems will be used to profile them, gather information about their practices, and discipline them or deprive them of income. It is difficult to imagine a situation less conducive to the enthusiastic uptake of a new technology than one that consumes tremendous time and energy in its adoption, while simultaneously threatening the autonomy or livelihood of the user. However, there are persuasive reasons for physicians to adopt network computing, including the ability to increase the ease of consultation on complex cases, to reduce wasted time and effort in connecting with colleagues and patients, and to improve patient safety. Already, enterprise IT systems have demonstrated their ability to help physicians reduce adverse drug reactions. Combining enterprise systems with Internet connectivity to physicians' offices, pharmacies, and pharmacy benefit management (PBM) firms could alert physicians to potential drug interactions and increase patients' compliance with drug therapy. (Jeff Goldsmith, 2000, *Health Affairs, How Will the Internet Change Our Health System?* Project HOPE–People-to-People Health Foundation, Inc.)

The above was written in 2000, and elsewhere in this book we have been more optimistic. In some cases it is a case of "change or be changed," due to new pressures from bodies like the FDA for pharmacovigilance, a new US presidency, increasing alarm over medical accidents, and fear of litigation if best practice, often interpreted as evidence-based medicine, is not followed. The fact remains however that many US physicians are in single or small group practices, or even in larger institutions, where the daily thoughts are pretty much as they were 30 years ago. Concern over these coming changes has as yet had no obvious impact.

The medical industry is peculiarly reluctant to adopt some technologies, and yet very willing to embrace other technologies. Some of that has to do with medical culture. Technologies that are adapted have to fit within the cultural framework they are used to dealing with and to make life easier and save money. Another major factor involving cultural penetration has to do with the ability to limit liability. It has often been said that doctors are notoriously old fashioned about using computers, meaning that they do not want to. It should be noted, however, that the current emerging generation of physicians is entirely computer literate. Rather, the difficulty is that once a physician begins real medical practice, he or she is always rushing from patient to patient with little time to sit at the keyboard. Voice interaction with the computer may be a way to resolve that problem. But even if physicians interact with the computer system, they may not comply with the recommendations. In a sense that is good because, while clinical decision systems are less than perfect, the physician is a powerful check. Yet in some cases it may be a cultural matter. For example, physicians may resist the application of diagnostic rules that require blood test results as a primary input to their diagnostic procedure; it is backward to their training and experience.

Researchers are most likely to find clinical decision support tools easy to adopt. However, they face problems with HIPAA, database costs associated with regularizing the data so that it is possible to data mine it, reluctance of institutions to release data for proprietary reasons, and conflicts in releasing data (pharmaceuticals may be reluctant to release data if it leads to class-action civil lawsuits from severe unanticipated side effects). The data that are available for mining may have surprising difficulties associated with how the diagnostic process biases the sampling structure, how nomenclature variations may arbitrarily split categories, and how time-stamps on the results, procedures ordered, and diagnoses have been structured for mining.

IF NOT TOMORROW, WHEN? THE TIME IS RUNNING OUT AS THE POPULATION GROWS OLDER AND DISEASES ARE BECOMING, OR SEEN TO BE, MORE COMPLEX

In 2009, the new Obama presidency moved fast. As noted earlier, the American Recovery and Reinvestment Plan of 2009 is expected to include $20 billion for health IT to jumpstart investment in health IT, curb healthcare costs, and improve healthcare quality. Note that the healthcare IT plan is wrapped skill-fully in a larger plan for economic recovery in the mist of a worldwide depression, clearly therefore supporting the idea that IT enhances efficiency, reduces errors, and saves money (with the added bonus, important in the recession, that it will create jobs). Indeed, the $20 billion, to be included in multiple pieces of legislation, explicitly planned to cut red tape, prevent medical mistakes, provide better patient care, and introduce cost-saving efficiencies. In addition, a stimulus package is expected to total $275 billion in tax cuts and $550 billion in investments (according to the White House, these are thought-fully and carefully targeted priority investments with unprecedented account-ability measures built in). The health IT components in the various pieces of economic stimulus legislation are intended to focus on saving jobs, money, and lives, but most importantly call for updating and computerization of the US healthcare system.

This is fantastic news and probably only a part of things to come. Unfortunately, the healthcare system, entrenched in America much longer than President Obama, may not be able to respond so quickly. The time scale depends on a number of issues. We have some tools that fill gaps in the current technology now. Some of the problem involves cultural penetration. The particular time scale for adaptation depends on context.

In the domain where physician and patient meet, the question is whether a physician will adopt the tools. To some extent this depends on the type of information that the rules refer to (blood tests come later; physicians like their ancient predecessors start with noticing skin, hair, eyes, locution, etc.— so the rules we present should be built from databases that include that data). If the rules start with blood test results, the rules are less likely to be adopted. If the technology is effective and could be easily used, failure to use the tools may start to pose liability issues. At that point physicians are more likely to adopt the technology.

If the physician diagnostic aid started with questions that physicians were accustomed to start with, the tool would likely be adapted immediately. If the diagnostic aid started with blood test results or other items physicians considered downstream, the time delay for adaptation would be much longer.

Database management is a multi-tiered issue that includes the general protective, proprietary attitude that hospitals and medical institutions hold for their data, liability associated with confidentiality, and liability associated with failure to use information that could have saved patients' lives. Hospitals are immediately interested in getting help to manage their databases, extending the records management to include disclosure release information, and so forth. They are generally totally unprepared to handle tasks like cleansing records of identifying information to release the data for research purposes. There is immediate demand for tools to regularize database records. Yet the environment may be sensitive to outside handling, and translated records would likely each require hand-verification and signoff.

OTHER IT REQUIREMENTS TO CONSIDER

There are further challenges to solidarity, i.e. in sharing medical information for the common and individual benefit so that the guardians of our health may know us better. Medical IT isn't just software. There must be hardware, meaning storage and processing units, and bandwidths in communication links, equal to the task.

Recall Chapter 1. The base estimate assumes clinical and biomedical use will be at least 30% of 2010 total world storage, which was earlier conservatively predicted at 100 petabytes but already 400 petabytes of new medical images are generated daily. That scenario downplays advanced imaging capabilities. Advanced medical imaging will be one of the biggest consumers of computer memory: optimistic projections assuming 50,000,000 accessible population with each person requiring 82 billion (US billion, so 82,000,000,000) bytes by years 2010 to 2012. This is primarily based on an assumption that advanced three-dimensional and moving images will represent about 80% of medical storage. Projections from NASA, high energy physics, and data mining suggest that for calculations of comparable order, a petaflop processor must run for a day to clear or process each and every petabyte (give or take an order of magnitude). This depends on the order of the calculation, however. Simply storing, copying, or displaying is of order one, while image processing is somewhere between 1 and about 2.5, depending on how sophisticated it is such as in using models of the body to interpolate between NMR images to detect where a nerve is snagging.

Another supporting technologies technology will be the portals (Fig 9.3) and their graphical interfaces by which a physician or researcher communicates with the rule base. A physician's view of a portal is given in Figure 9.4. A primary consideration is how the extracted rules appear at the screen. Clearly, some smartness in the software, to make rules comprehensible to the physician and the patient at home, is required. Unfortunately, there has been evidence that some early efforts at providing such interfaces actually enhance the chance of medical error. So still much thought must be put into designing the system. In addition the display must be comprehensible to people of very different backgrounds, and to make that workable, the presentation must dynamically switch-able to accommodate the differing expertise of the user—patient, physician, clinical biochemist, clinical genomicist, biomedical researcher, and so on.

Something akin to publishing tools as are beginning to be applied on the Internet will be required to ensure that only certain data with patient consent are copied, and used only a specified number of times or on reaching a certain date, but at the same time entitling the patient to change the rules of access to that personal data at any time. One possibility is that research should limit access to an actual or effective distinct archive of anonymized records, mirroring in other respects the archive of named patient records and regularly updating from it. The gateway to ensure anonymity between two such actual or

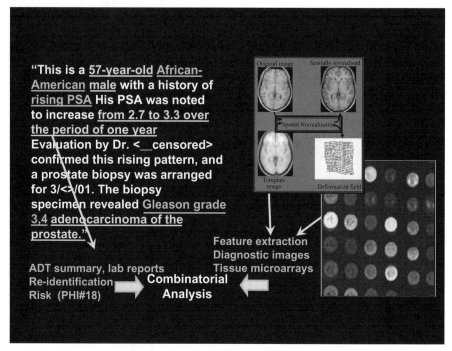

Figure 9.3 A physician information portal

effective archives is, of course, nontrivial. However, this simply means that the process of implementing the patients' wishes via e-publishing occurs at the gateway and at times of regular updates.

Going beyond data mining and basic inference, how much artificial intelligence is needed? This addresses how far the computer system should go in drawing conclusions from the basic rules. In many ways the outputted rules normally derived by data mining and related disciplines are potentially statements input to systems that derive further logical consequences. Consider the syllogisms, of which the simplest type is "All A are B. All B are C. Therefore all A are C. Here a third rule is generated by (i.e., follows logically from) two other rules. This potential 50% increase in rules can be made even larger if the new emerging rules also interact to produce further rules. The increase is, however, miniscule to the explosion in output that can occur if other types of logic are applied. We have shown that the input statements for popular types of logical puzzle can be shown to correspond to the output of typical data mining programs. For example, such puzzles ask the player to deduce from apparently incomplete information "which householder has the pet fish?" Without a focus on a specific aspect such as the fish, however, this will increase the number of rules. That is, the pets of all the householders and all other relations of little interest, such that the householder with the dog has a house

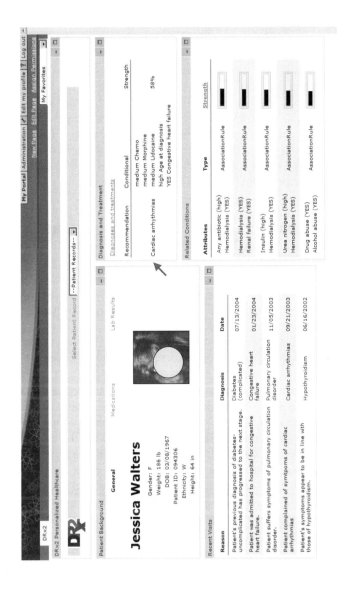

Figure 9.4 Sample clinical decision portal

447

with a green door, would be generated. Therefore this transformation is best performed at time of interacting with the user so that focusing of the rules can be applied, answering more specific questions.

The ethical views and wishes of the patient, what the authors call "ethome," are an important part of the data. Unless this information is carried in a fairly fundamental way, it is hard to see how it could be failsafe. Architectures could become unwieldy or even redundant white elephant legacy systems if such matters are not considered at the outset. An alternative approach might be to agree on an absolutely standard means of exchange of clinical data packets that can only be read and utilized if the correct information is present and satisfies internal encrypted checks reflecting the patient's wishes. But a universal standard will not be easily achieved, and a simpler core standard that can represent data within all existing media, formats, and ontologies seems to be a more practical route. Such data should, of course, be reliably encrypted both by standard and by internal encryption methods (internal that is to the simple core standard) so that it cannot be inappropriately utilized.

CONTINUOUS INPUT: LEVERAGE OF IT FOR DISEASE AND HEALTH MONITORING VIA TELEHEALTH

For our health-guardians to know us better and in a timely manner, remote monitoring of patients is usually considered part of telemedicine. If recorded, or at least temporarilly noted and sifted by computer, it is another entry in the vast heterogeneous sources to be analyzed, and possibly a continuous real-time stream of data.

This concept is not new: it predates email. In 1912 Willem Einthoven transmitted the first electrocardiogram (ECG) over a telephone line from the hospital to his laboratory. Cardiologists have been able to evaluate pacemaker function remotely over a telephone line for 40 years. Telemedicine in its most sophisticated form was originated from the US space program in the 1960s and used to transmit the astronauts' vital signs from space to the National Aeronautics and Space Administration (NASA). Radiologists, cardiologists, and dermatologists already frequently use telemedicine, according to a recent survey by *Telehealth Magazine*, since current technology is refined enough for radiologists to diagnose using telemedicine equipment. Other uses include psychology, emergency room procedures, ophthalmology, and dentistry. It is also used to improve medical care in prisons and to make medical care available on ships and airplanes.

Recent advances in sensor technologies have enabled long-term recordings of numerous physiologic parameters in patients, generating very large data sets. This development extends to implantable sensors, noninvasively applied external sensors, and the kind of diagnostic biosensor mentioned above. Examples are also electroencephalographic (EEG) recordings, hyperspectral imaging of skin and cardiovascular systems, and mass spectrometry.

Biomonitoring of patients includes, for example, cardiogram, blood pressure, and blood sugar, and urea measurements. Such patients might be critical care patients in a hospital, chronic disease patients at home (diabetes, cancer, liver, kidney, and heart disease, etc.), and in the future all patients at home, including the healthy ones, so that disease might be prevented. Monitoring occurs now in almost all critical condition wards, and it is beginning to be used for chronic disease patients at home. A classic study, in hindsight, and one that illuminates the complexities of analysis, was "Noninvasive Home Telemonitoring for Patients With Heart Failure at High Risk of Recurrent Admission and Death. The Trans-European Network–Home-Care Management System (TEN-HMS) Study," by John G. F. Cleland, Amala A. Louis, Alan S. Rigby, Uwe Janssens, and Aggie H. M. M. Balk. This study of a fairly large population of home-based patients showed the significant patient benefits of having monitoring in the home. However, the findings were complicated, causing the authors to propose a larger study. Of 426 patients randomly assigned to home telemonitoring and controls, 48% were aged more than 70 years. Days lost as the result of death or hospitalization showed no significant difference from controls, and the number of admissions and mortality were not obviously different, but the mean duration of admissions was reduced by 6 days with home telemonitoring. This perhaps suggests that at least the healthcare system is "better primed" to respond with telemonitoring. In addition, Rick Nauert of MyDNA.com, a personalized medicine web company, wrote his PhD Thesis on how home telehealth monitoring helped a poorly served Hispanic group of diabetics in Texas.[2]

Favorable reports based on objective statistics are likely to accelerate adoption of health monitoring for the chronically ill in the home, and extend it to monitoring of perfectly health patients in order to preempt disease. More widely used communications today between physicians and patients include the telephone, occasionally fax machine, and email, but things are getting more sophisticated. As discussed in Chapter 8, email will still play a role in the world of the new medicine, but some day it will include pictures and voice, and blend with telemedicine. Some time beyond that, perhaps, brain-to-brain information will transfer. More constructively, it may not be a bad idea if doctors could in some sense feel the quality and quantity and location of their pain of their patients. But how far can email go in medicine before it ceases to be email as we know it? In the previous chapter we described how a woman from Long Prairie, Minnesota, a small farming town in the central part of the State, had ulcers on her legs that were not healing. Wheelchair bound and dependent on her adult children for transportation, a referral to a dermatologist would have meant a 270-mile round trip to Abbott Northwestern Hospital in Minneapolis—a long trip for the patient and lost income for family members. In principle, such difficulties could be overcome by sending images for diagnosis as files attached

---

[2] *"Virtual healthcare as a surrogate to traditional, face-to-face medical encounters continues to be a relatively new but potentially ground-breaking area of research"*, he wrote in 2002.

to emails. However, that would be a very clumsy way to do it, and terribly slow for complex moving images.

The more sophisticated exchange of medical information from one site to another via electronic communication is referred to as *teleconsultation*. The information transmitted by real-time channels can be used to diagnose and treat patients, but it also can be used to educate healthcare providers as well as patients. While many insurers have been reluctant to pay claims for tele-consulting services, some health plans are embracing the technology as a potentially cost-effective way to reach rural subscribers who need healthcare services. The long-term goal in healthcare is to train patients to become independent in their healthcare by participating in their own treatment so they will stay out of the hospital and save money. That is clearly an early example of use of IT for preventative medicine.

Unfortunately, while many participants have email, telemedicine is expensive. A true telemedicine site consists not only of a computer and a simple video camera but also fairly sophisticated high-resolution video equipment used to transmit images over phone or cable lines to a similar site. Thus most telemedicine sites right now are located at major university medical centers and were started with private and governmental funding. An example system at UC Davis was discussed in the previous chapter. The US Congress has already paved the way for a better and more widely available telemedicine vehicle. The Next Generation Internet Research Act of 1998 authorizes entities like the National Science Foundation (NSF) and NASA to begin research on developing a new Internet that will be faster and be able to support the next level of telemedicine, for example, telesurgery. Pilot telemedicine programs at university medical centers have been expanded to nationwide networks, but this treatment protocol still represents a tiny portion of total clinical activity in the United States.

What exactly is the form in which such data are transmitted? Well, right now it is often in standard formats like those of normal TV transmissions, or general formats used in transmitting telephone analog or digital information and, of course, computer information. When there is a special format, like the PACS (Picture Archiving and Communication System) image format, that relates to the image part and not the message as a whole. However, complex, smarter, self-correcting, and importantly much more secure formats are possible for overall transmissions regarding a patient. *Messaging system*s are streams of data in a condensed format that allows recognition that a message is arriving and from a specific source, security, and error-checking. These systems could stand alone in a wired or wireless transmission, or could contain email and telemedicine information. The medical standards organization Health Level Seven had a messaging system called HL7 that has now been replaced by XML (discussed earlier), a fact that indicates that XML is itself a kind of messaging system, but one that concentrates giving meaningful structure to the data by organizing it in a classification-based way. One of the authors (BR) is responsible for a Clinical Laboratory Messaging System

(CLaMS) originally called the Genomic Messaging System because clinical genomics was the emphasis. Rightly or wrongly, this has had a good reception in the medical informatics press and a special mention from a major learned society, but the main reason for referring to the details page 426 is that it gives some idea of what a messaging system looks like, and what it can do.

STORING AND MANAGING MEDICAL DATA FROM MONITORING

Monitored data may be analyzed in more-or-less real time and not necessarily discarded after that. Generally speaking, most data that arise from monitoring should be retained in long-term storage. This is not only for back-reference to confirm a physician's recollection of something, and not only as a valid part of the patient record for the patient's future benefit, but also to maintain quality of care and even to avoid (or quickly resolve) litigation disputes.

As described in Chapter 8, the traditional content management of large amounts of data is primarily based on a technique called *data warehousing*, which moves data much the way goods are moved in a real warehouse. The system runs a specialized application to reconstruct the monitoring data in a standard or "canonical" format and then runs queries against the data. The traditional repository of large data consists not only of a data warehouse but also one or more data marts, or market-like means of interacting with the warehouse.

Such systems were discussed in the preceding chapter. The issue addressed here is that data from diverse monitoring can be considered as particularly *heterogeneous* (diverse in nature). Warehousing can divide and conquer the data by some degree of classification, but it does not alone solve the problem of *very* diverse types of data coming into it. Any file system needs to manage and process multidimensional data such as hypertext, alphanumeric data, audio streams, video streams, still images (e.g., MRI, EPR, CAT, ultrasound, X ray), large character strings or character large object, binary large objects (BLOB), arrays and large numbers, and data such as relational, structured (e.g., XML tagged, rectangular), object-oriented, semi-structured (e.g., comma separated, tabular), and unstructured data (e.g., natural language text). The technique used to put all these data together—so that they can be queried and mined as if they were all one—was described as *federalization* previously.

If the doctor wants a single patient record or two, these issues are not too much of a problem, and available techniques of warehousing and federalization can pretty much solve the major difficulties. The doctor would simply send a basic query to a remote computer asking the patient's record to be sent back to him. However, even federalized systems could imply considerable difficulty in obtaining population data to aid diagnosis and prognosis, for biomedical research, or when a public health or medical surveillance analyst seeks to protect the population by examining unusual trends in many patient records by data mining, pattern extraction or any kind of logical or statistical analysis.

Such analyses are applied to not just one but many patient records, and the more the better. So normally the demands for good overall statistics require the analyst or researcher to download the whole archive.

But why do *all* these data have to be shipped to the analyst? Recall the data-centric computing approach described in Chapter 8. It seems at first glance that one could reduce the problem where a researcher is interested in fewer representative aspects. For medical images these aspects might not be numbers for each and every pixel, but numbers relating to the "pathological-ness" of the content of the image, or the size and shape of a tumor or components of the brain, or the granularity of an image, or the volume or the fractal (branching) nature ("branchy-ness") of the bronchioles of the lung. Let us distinguish this difficulty from the problems of data mining, and the like, discussed above, which are also compounded by many parameters; here the problem is the large amount of data we wish to download. Unfortunately, we do not always know what kind of image aspect to represent in advance, namely which numbers to generate. In medical surveillance for public health we are looking for the unusual, which may not fall into the class of typical image aspects. Also lots of medical researchers want to know different things about an image, and many of them want to know different things on different days; there is not always a handful of numbers to cater for all. Similar arguments hold for other types of rich data. Indeed, not knowing in advance what kind of analysis and what kind of programs will be used to analyze data is a problem for every kind of data in large archives, not just image data. Not only we cannot but we are unable to predict what programs might ever be used for the analysis; we cannot foresee whatever programs might ever be written for new types of analyses and new research needs.

We may also recall that there is a further problem in that the data are, in general, highly sensitive and thus fully protected. To address the security requirements and to comply with the legislation for protection of personal privacy, certain personal information must be kept at the initial collection point in the original medium and is prohibited from being copied to or stored in another medium at another location. This was the reason why many workers in medical IT believed that the personal lifetime health record needs to be dynamically assembled out of the information retrieved on demand from various sources.

The model used today does not really provide well for these matters. It certainly did not provide for it when researchers had, if anything, access to a single isolated computer in the laboratory, when any new data might come by FedEx. The addition of the Internet is many times better, basically because it provides a *distributed processing* approach. Distributed processing is a good thing, and the concept has been extended beyond the Internet to use of tightly coupled computers usually called a *Grid*. It is in connection with a Grid that the term *distributed computing* is usually used (and we note in passing that an extreme case of having all the processors together in a single large box with very short wires between, not just in a single intranet, creates a *parallel super-*

computer). But whether the component machines of a Grid are brought together in the same room or building over some kind of intranet, or talk via the Internet, this allows calculations to be shared more directly across a whole bundle of computers, when it would be inefficient for one alone to handle the data.

Nonetheless, the software tends to be put on each machine more-or-less once and for all. The normal Internet and distributed computing approach for the main part assumes stationary software and mobile data. If programs are moved, they are typically for downloading only, namely as an application or small program like an applet being sent, for example to create a moving cartoon on a web page. In other words, in the current computing paradigm for distributed processing, software components stay on specific systems as stationary executable programs and move the relevant data to be processed by the software components. The main reason to keep the executable code on a specific computer and move the data to be processed stems from the fact that the executable programs are unfortunately specific to the hardware and operating systems, and dependent on the specific platform for processing. This model of stationary programs exchanging data across the network has been the design point for the distributed computing, and it was one of the givens for a distributed environment that consists of heterogeneous systems of disparate hardware architecture, operating system, or middleware technologies.

But the otherwise excellent distributed computing model does not resolve the problem of the huge data size to be imported for analysis, and the preference, even sometimes legal requirement, that the data be retained at the original site. It works tolerably well when privacy and security are less of an issue (e.g., when the data are consented and anonymous), *and* when programs are big and the data to be exchanged between the programs are relatively small. Then it would be more effective to transmit small data amounts across the network, especially a low speed network, instead of are large executable code. However, as noted above, this model causes performance problems when the data are of considerable width and depth, and when large amount of content-rich data (e.g., images, audio or video clips) need to be exchanged across the network for a time-critical transactions.

So what is the solution? If the mountain cannot go to Mohamed, Mohamed should go to the mountain. That is the data-centric computing approach. We leave the data where it is. Instead, we send the programs to go out and work on the data at their home site, where data are more secure, and to send back only the findings from the analysis, which are usually vastly smaller than the data.

But surely, even today, isn't it possible to submit queries to remote sites and get back short answers? Of course, but unfortunately, we need to remember that the queries are limited in form and cannot cover every type of complex analysis we might want to perform in the future. It is impossible to pre-conceive every type of computer program that the researcher might want to develop and use. So new programs should be in a software vehicle that makes them capable of roaming the Internet, going out, doing their work, and getting the results off-site. This is likely the way things will be done when a large number of records are analyzed collectively. In the end the solution to our problem was pretty simple, leave the data where they are.

FOOD AND DRUG AUTHORITIES AS GUARDIAN ANGELS

As mentioned above, the FDA of the United States and other regulatory bodies for food and drugs across the world are naturally increasingly interested in monitoring efficiently how marketed drugs are doing, and in collaborating not only with physicians to do that but also with the pharmaceutical companies and even academic researchers. In the limit, this all falls into the discussions above on data mining of digital patient records (or a similar but incomplete role played by billing records; see Chapter 5) and data analytics generally, and the architectural infrastructures, described in this and the previous chapter. The challenge, however, for the FDA is perhaps their historical focus on classical statistics with "the curse of the null hypothesis" discussed in Chapter 8, and a need to explore many more contemporary and emerging data analytic technologies.

But there are many kinds of vigilance issues for the FDA. They include monitoring proposals for clinical trials, and how clinical trials are going, including the need to detect a "site visit." At present, prioritization of site visits seems to be a hit and miss process, to a certain degree, where the alerts are such things as unusual numbers of patients involved, or a novel kind of therapy to which a company has usually put through clinical trials. This is all impacted by the rise of genomic biomarkers and pharmacogenomics, namely stratified medicine. What is needed is a means of defining an ideal protocol for each kind of study and, in detecting whether a proposed protocol departs from that, as well the issue of detecting that a protocol and expectations of its consequences are departing from original intent. In many respects this is like the role of institutional review boards, as discussed in Chapter 6, but on a grand scale. Moreover vigilance could be wrapped into a grand architecture, including feedback from clinical trials and from every physician–patient interaction. Above and throughout we have occasionally used FDA somewhat "generically" as standing for any nation's food and drug regulatory authority, and certainly very frequently as an important example case. However, there are many watchdogs of the pharmaceutical industry though the United States and the world. They are our ultimate top layer of guarding angels right now, at least in regard to pharmaceutical drugs (epidemics, etc., are discussed below). They include:

- United States: FDA (Food and Drug Administration), DEA (Drug Enforcement Administration), OSHA (Occupational Safety and Health Administration), and AHRQ (Agency for Healthcare Research and Quality)

- Europe: EMEA (European Medicines Agency)
- Belgium: DGMP (Directorate-General Medicinal Products)
- Czech Republic: State Institute for Drug Control
- Denmark: Danish Medicines Agency
- Estonia: State Agency of Medicines
- Finland: NAM (National Agency for Medicines)
- France: Agence du Medicament
- Germany: BFARM (Bundesinstitut für Arzneimittel und Medizinprodukte) and the Paul-Ehrlich Institut
- Netherlands: (MED) Medicines Evaluation Board and the MEB Agency
- Norway: NOMA (Norwegian Medicines Agency)
- Portugal: INFARMED (National Institute of Pharmacy and Medicines)
- Sweden: MPA (Medical Products Agency)
- Switzerland: Swissmedic
- UK: MHRA (Medicines and Healthcare Products Regulatory Agency)
- Australia: TGA (Therapeutic Goods Administration)
- New Zealand: MEDSAFE and PHARMAC (Pharmaceutical Management Agency)
- Japan: Pharmaceutical and Medical Safety Bureau

These do not of course mean they are the only players in each country. Apart from the pharmaceutical companies, the FDA in the United States has interacted in various ways with HMOs and academia. For example, Vanderbilt University, the University of Alabama, Duke University, Brigham and Womens Hospital, the University of North Carolina, and many HMOs, all in all representing 13 centers, were recently funded by a 1–2 year project on a task order by the AHRQ.

IS THERE A GUARDIAN ARCHANGEL?

Are there higher international authorities watching national food and drug administrations? A natural contender would be of course the World Health Organization (WHO), and particularly relevant are its three sections: the WHO International Working Group for Drug Statistics Methodology, the WHO Collaborating Centre for Drug Statistics Methodology, and the WHO Collaborating Centre for Drug Utilization Research and Clinical Pharmacological Services. Their mission is description of drug use pattern, early signals of irrational use of drugs, interventions to improve drug use, quality control cycle, and continuous quality improvement. These bodies seem largely responsible for introducing a third term to the already weighty dictionary of new healthcare terms: *pharmacoepidemiology*, that is, the application of epidemiologists' methods to drug responses. There are also other influential international bodies outside the WHO, notably the International Conference for Harmonization (ICH), which regularly brings together the regulatory authorities of Europe, Japan, and the United States as well as pharmaceutical industry experts. The WHO and the ICH have an integrating effect, and considerable influential powers. However these are not formally higher authorities: drug product registration controls remain under the jurisdiction of the multiple regulatory bodies in the nations where the drugs are made or marketed.

That limit to national jurisdiction must change one day. Organizations should work together internationally through IT. It makes no sense to consider wisdom and warnings in feedback just from the patients of one's own nation, when the bulk of such information lies outside national walls. So the archangel will probably be created by consideration of interoperability not only between players of the ecosystem within nations, but also between the pharmacosurveillance IT systems of nations. Planning for such international integration is actually in progress, much at time of writing in the hands of freelance thinkers and groups possibly inspired by "global healthcare system" that it perhaps portends. One visionary is Dr. Mary Wiktorowicz (Health Administration, University of Toronto), who has researched models of governance for pharmacosurveillance in seven nations, and integrated global approaches. That planning also has to consider that the players and networks are somewhat different in each nation. Space does not therefore permit deeper analysis here, and in any event the network diagrams of current plans tend to reflect institutional structure and traditions more than science and IT principles. However, good summaries of the situations and plans in many countries is given in the report "Research networks involved in post-market pharmacosurveillance in the United States, United Kingdom, France, New Zealand, Australia, Norway and European Union: Lessons for Canada" (M. E. Wiktorowicz, J. Lexchin, M. Paterson, B. Mintzes, C. Metge, D. Light, S. Morgan, A. Holbrook, R. Tamblyn, E. Zaki, and K. Moscou, at http://www.patientsafetyinstitute.ca/uploadedFiles/Research/Post-Marketing%20Pharmacosurveillance%20Final%20Report.pdf)

Some sense of the current status of organisation of phrmacosurveillance by governments can be glimpsed in the following document recently released by the European Commission (Brussels, 10.12.2008 SEC(2008) 2671):

COMMISSION STAFF WORKING DOCUMENT

Accompanying document to the

Proposal for a

REGULATION OF THE EUROPEAN PARLIAMENT AND OF THE COUNCIL

amending, as regards pharmacovigilance of medicinal products for human use, Regulation (EC) No 726/2004 laying down Community procedures for the authorisation and supervision of medicinal products for human and veterinary use and establishing a European Medicines Agency

and the

Proposal for a

DIRECTIVE OF THE EUROPEAN PARLIAMENT AND OF THE COUNCIL

amending, as regards pharmacovigilance, Directive 2001/83/EC on the Community code relating to medicinal products for human use

As evidence for the "state of the art," the specific motivations for this particular document are interesting. Titles of EC documents do not always give everything away at a glance, even to the relatively well informed. It could be more clearly entitled "how to get everyone working together and pulling their weight." The motivation is that significant weaknesses of the current EU system of pharmacovigilance were noted in an independent Commission-sponsored study, with extensive public consultation (in 2006 and again in 2007). These weaknesses included:

- A lack of clear roles and responsibilities for the key parties.
- Lack of clear obligations against which they perform their roles (and hence poor compliance).
- Slow EU decision-making on drug safety issues.
- Frequent disharmony in action taken by the Member States.
- Low levels of transparency relating to pharmacovigilance.
- Rather limited EU coordination of communication about the safety of medicines, plus complex product information with poor penetration of key warnings.
- Cumbersome oversight of companies' pharmacovigilance systems by the authorities.
- A lack of proactive and proportionate monitoring including a lack of risk management and structured data collection in the form of post authorisation safety studies.
- High degree of neglect of the patient's own feedback and hence its virtual absence from decision-making.

Clearly there are difficulties and gaps to be made up, apparently a dragging of the feet by many players and lack of sharing, even in the forward-looking European Union!

VIGILANCE AGAINST BIOTHREAT

Biothreat, natural as well as malign, is a particular challenge for guardians of our health. Vigilance can involve many players and monitoring in continuous time. The role of many players is certainly the case when vigilance generates an alert event. IT is required to integrate their efforts. In the event of an epidemic, today's physician would sooner or later be the best-informed person attending a patient and judging whether the disease poses a real epidemic risk. The attending doctor must notify the proper officers, who are usually consultants in communicable disease control. In most nations, medical consultants are required to inform a body analogous to the Center for Disease Control and Prevention in the United States, directly or indirectly. In the United Kingdom, this is typically direct (to the Communicable Disease Surveillance Center (CDSC)) and must be followed up by reports on a regular basis of each case of a disease that has been notified. In the United States, suspected cases of most serious pathogens should be reported to the state health departments, which in turn notify the Center for Disease Control and Prevention (CDC). All cases subsequently confirmed by laboratory analysis are reported by CDC to WHO.

A clinical decision support system should report at the foot of the screen all possible notifiable diseases, or diseases of current epidemic concern, for which the patient's current symptoms form a suggestive subset. For example, in the case of anthrax these are *fever, general discomfort, uneasiness, or ill feeling (malaise), headache, shortness of breath, cough, congestion of the nose and throat, pneumonia, joint stiffness, and joint pain. But such symptoms are not confined to anthrax infection, and the physician will need to take samples for tests, and pause for results if there is no reason to suspect anthrax because of exposure to infected humans, animals, or other sources. The tests will include blood cultures positive for anthrax, chest X ray, serologic test for anthrax, and spinal tap for CSF culture and analysis.*

The *communicable disease* list, which classifies over 30 different pathogens, includes the infective agents forming the four-part biohazard levels described later in this chapter. Historically, the first sophisticated statutory requirements for the notification of certain infectious diseases came into being in London in 1891. Cholera, diphtheria, smallpox, and typhoid had to be reported by the head of the family or the landlord to the local authority. The system spread to the rest of England and Wales in 1899. Originally the disease statistics were collected from the local authorities by the Registrar General's Office, where national statistics were already collected on births, marriages, and deaths (in the United Kingdom, this office became later known as the Office of Population Censuses and Surveys and is now called the Office for National Statistics). In 1997 the responsibility for administering the system was transferred to the CDSC, the equivalent of the CDC in the United States).

There are compliance guidelines even for the "do-it-yourselfer," such as might be presented on a home health guidance system. A well-informed patient suspicious about the implications of his or her symptoms or those of a family member, meaning a serious communicable disease, has certain procedural obligations in the public spirit, even before encountering a physician. In the case of suspected infection by anthrax, for example, the patient should certainly directly contact his or her healthcare provider. The patient should then go to the emergency room or call the local emergency number (e.g., 911) if symptoms develop following suspicion of exposure to anthrax powder or from being around farm animals. There is obviously need for public awareness of symptoms and prompt action such as access to medical advice via the Internet can provide help. Notably, the death rate from anthrax exposure rate is high despite proper treatment unless immediate action is taken, especially to prevent the pulmonary complications of this disease.

Still we want to emphasize the value of workflow enforced or supported by IT to help users comply with best practice. Doctors need to initiate prompt action as is appropriate and reasonable. It is not always practical to provide total isolation of the infected person from the world nor, more important, to assume that everyone who was proximate to that person is infected even if the disease is the pneumonic plague. Best practice depends on the pathogen and it's means of propagation, and on timely information about that pathogen. Gage et al. (2001) state that persons suspected of having a pneumonic plague should be maintained under respiratory droplet precautions for 48 hours after antibiotic treatment begins. Persons who have confirmed cases of pneumonic plague should be kept under droplet precautions until sputum cultures are negative. Prophylactic antibiotics should be administered to persons who have come within 2 meters (6.5 feet) of the person suspected of having pneumonic plague.

When diagnosis is not certain or a precise clinical follow-up is not well described, the most general and cautious (play-safe) practices for a variety of epidemic diseases should be adopted. In most countries mere *clinical suspicion* of a notifiable infection is all that is required to report a case of a disease. There is, of course, less regulation regarding immediate response to what the doctor suspects may be a *novel* infectious agent capable of reaching epidemic proportions. Only during the 2002 to 2003 outbreak, SARS was added to the 30+ list of notifiable diseases, and more recently avian influenza ("Bird Flu") has been added. The state of California implemented HIV reporting regulations July 1, 2002 (California Code of Regulations, title 17, section 2641.5–2653.2), and then amended by legislation at least twice around 2006. For many communicable diseases in the United States, notification is a dual reporting process that healthcare providers as well as laboratories must follow. Additional regulations may be in force for a specific disease during an epidemic.

Guidance by IT can help the physician to be aware of special exceptions in normal compliance matters. For example, the larger public interest may even override the spirit of the HIPAA regulations. The original HIV reporting regulations required healthcare providers and laboratories to report HIV cases using a non-name code. The more recent legislation, in effect immediately, requires HIV cases, like AIDS cases, to be reported by name.

Vigilance against a new epidemic or breakthrough to a new geographic area can take many other forms than just notification or the physician. Also included is monitoring of surprises in patient records or biosensors placed in towns and cities and connected to monitoring centers, analyses of filters from aircraft air systems, streamlining of video at airports, and so on. General monitoring has in the past included careful examination of the significance of unexpected increases in the sale of prescribed or over-the-counter agents. Following the maintenance of a surface water treatment plant in Battleford, Saskatchewan, in 2001, sales of antidiarrheals leapt five times in about a month, followed by a drinking water advisory two weeks later. In total, 1,039 persons were found to be infected with the parasite *Cryptosporidium*.

Vigilance and surveillance in the present context also includes biostatistical analysis and data mining of clinical and public health data to encounter unexpected events that signal or threaten a decline in human health. Over longer time scales, a careful use of biostatistics and epidemiological statistical measures over large populations has revealed other health issues. The use of real-time data capture from a variety of sources (including digital patient records), followed by data mining to spot events or numerical trends that correlate more or less than would be expected on a chance basis, promises a more rapid and methodical approach.

RESPONDING TO EPIDEMICS AND DISASTERS

Vigilance and monitoring are pointless if we cannot respond, and response certainly requires integrations of many players. There are degrees of limitations to readiness that can be completely preplanned. In home and hospital monitoring chronic care, a change in the status of a patient will result in response involving a well-defined protocol. Alerts from constant analysis of many continuously updated medical records may suggest a scenario of shift in public health for which there are well-established procedures, but it could be something entirely new. Then there are disasters that come upon us with some warning, such as hurricanes, and those with little warning at all, such as earthquakes, tsunami, toxic and radioactive spillage, the attack on the World Trade Center, and a spate of anthrax letters in the mail.

All require response, with or without prior vigilance and monitoring, and IT is an important coordinator. Responses to epidemics, in particular, but many disasters, in general, can be divided into *primary prevention* if warned in time (matters to prevent or limit the damage, e.g., vaccination), *secondary prevention* (matters to rectify the damage, e.g., as antibiotics), and *tertiary prevention* (cleaning and repairing afterward, e.g., palliative care and rehabilitation).

For a biological threat it is the response of making the right drugs or vaccines available, or even in the future developing them very rapidly, on the fly, tailored to each scenario. To put things in perspective, imagine how awful it must be to suffer a serious infection in a land with few or poorly distributed remedies, and with little hope of obtaining the appropriate antibiotic agent in time. Sadly, it is so easy for the prosperous nations to distance themselves from such situations emotionally, almost as if they were some fictional tragedy in a far-off mythical land. Somehow we rest content that we do have rapid access to widely available sources of treatment. But any advantage of the industrialized nation in regard to infectious disease *vanishes*, in the face of biothreat, when an industrial nation's population is exposed to new or unusual diseases arising naturally or by accidental biohazard, or through malicious, likely terrorist activity. Therapies, if available, may be just as poorly accessible in the developed world as in any third world situation. To date, perhaps the closest that the industrial nations normally come to unexpected exposure to diverse pathogens on a massive scale is when population groups are reduced to living in third world conditions or worse as the result of a natural disaster such as from earthquake or devastating hurricane. There is risk of typhoid, cholera, and many other dehydrating diseases, much like the situation in the third world. As in such cases communications internally and with the external world are badly hit. Mobile telephone towers tend to be the first to go, although not necessarily the Internet. For example, when Grand Cayman island in the Caribbean was severely hit by hurricane Ivan on September 12, 2004, and was almost totally submerged by 10 to 20 feet swells, the Internet server of one of the local newspapers was only briefly down whilst telephone connections were out or unreliable for days. The server was a significant source of island communication (through blogging exchanges, basically, published emails).

Currently disaster team notification systems support at least one, sometimes all, of the following communications media: telephone, cell phone, VoIP, pager (SMS, SNPP), instant messaging, email, or fax. Communications are important for many reasons, but an important concept is that they must be working so that in any emergency situation that requires human intervention, notification systems can provide a way of accepting feedback. Feedback is used to determine what tasks the system should perform. For example, a biothreat team, when notified of an event, must acknowledge that they are en route, thus eliminating the need for time spent in further notifications and panic actions in the absence of communication.

Communication difficulties appeared when hurricane Katrina hit the New Orleans area in 2005, and quickly escalated it to one of the largest natural disasters ever to have hit the United States. What is of interest from the point of view of communications in minimizing damage in future similar disasters, including a massive terrorist offensive, is the need for logistics of mobilizing large numbers of people to safety and healthcare. According to the *New York Times*, as of September 1, 2005, some 50,000 to 100,000 people remained trapped in the city, and only 15,000 could be evacuated in one day. Some 25,000 were huddled in the superdome, awaiting 500 buses while the officials issued an SOS to the federal government. Some 11,000 guardsmen were deployed, with further 10,000 mobilized; 18 research teams and 1,700 supply trucks came from as far away as Massachusetts. Another 40,000 people were housed then in 223 Red Cross shelters, in 40 of which 10,000 beds had been set up. Among many noteworthy items in these numbers, if correct, was the remarkably high ratio of incoming emergency and policing personnel to public persons trapped in the city, from 5:1 to almost 2:1 as the reserves arrived. Now we wonder in the hindsight how much the benefits of such an influx could have been reduced by more strain on the limited food, water, and medical resources.

In Katrina, and earlier in the California earthquakes of the early 1990s and the terrorist attack on the World Trade Center, communications suffered. In disasters, in general, emergency medical assistance is key to restoring communications, with supplying water, food, and medical aid quickly behind. This means that the IT infrastructure for medicine must always be built so as to minimize as much as possible the effects of a natural or malicious disaster. Communication systems should be designed such that the mobile phone transmission stations, traditionally "towers," don't fail so easily in these days of satellites and robust military communications. It is noteworthy that the poorest nations are no better off than hurricane victims in regard to IT and communications, at the time of the disaster and at least a few days following. Clearly, communications and IT should be made globally more resilient to major natural disaster health effects.

Escalation is the disaster-response term used when the criticality of an event increases before the event is finally resolved, for any reason. But escalation also applies when a small failure in a communication procedure triggers a chain of failures that can lead to events that require immediate attention. When deciding the list of recipients, a notification system might take into consideration the hours in which a recipient can be notified. Someone working a midnight shift may be available for handling emergencies between 11:00 pm and 7:00 am. The system should make no attempt to notify this person outside of those hours. A notification system could take into consideration vacation times, weekends, holidays, and the like, to prevent notifying people when they are not available. If a notification system cannot contact the intended party, it is not sufficient to let the matter drop. The system must find another person to notify, typically by scanning a predefined roster.

"Fail-over" scenarios are important in disaster response. High availability (HA) means that an IT support system must be up and running whenever the service is required, namely almost all the time. The only acceptable downtime is the scheduled time period for upgrades, which must be kept to an absolute minimum. To achieve the HA goal, software-based notification systems must be programmed to take into consideration the failure of hardware and software that provide the required services. The hardware failure could be as simple as someone accidentally unplugging a network connection or as messy as a hard drive crash. The software failure could be attributed to flaws in software design or defects in implementation. The "brains" of the notification systems are often distributed across separate physical machines to ensure that if one machine is no longer available, another system can handle sending and resolving additionally arising events.

In the United States the main responsibility for coordinating response to epidemics will in future most certainly lie primarily with the Center for Disease Control. But there are more players to coordinate than patient, physician, and CDC. The more general definition of epidemiology is "the basic science of public health," and so this also brings into play the Department of Health and Human Services and, of course, the National Institutes of Health. Overall, public health management and response procedures epidemiologically comprise primary prevention, such as vaccination or education; secondary prevention comes at the stage of diagnosis and involves appropriate consequent medical intervention, and tertiary prevention is concerned with restoring health, well-being, and normality after an epidemic event. Additional organizational entities that would be involved in cases of biothreat are the Department of Homeland Security and potentially the Department of Defense. The local police and the US military would be involved to enforce responses to such an epidemic.

Of course, a serious pandemic, whether of natural or malicious origin, cannot be the concern or responsibility of just one nation; a global integrated response is required. Critics have been asking for new international rules for many years. In 2005 the World Health Organization (WHO) approved tough new regulations that give the international agency broadened powers to fight global health threats. Under the new rules the WHO has strengthened authority to restrict travel and commerce from affected areas. In theory, WHO officials will also have access to information on the ground in the areas with outbreaks of diseases. In the past many countries have withheld such information. Governments will be required to report new disease outbreaks and provide international officials with access to data.

An epidemic can initiate a panic, which is when humans do not always act in best interests. Best practice and compliance with workflow is essential for guiding the clinical support system. The workflow may involve several organizations and accountable individuals (performing a series of significant actions as one-person and multiple-person units), and workflows may differ in each unit. Compliance can be enforced when an IT system is there to coordinate the medical workflows. It can be used also to fine-tune the workflow protocol to the *scenario type*, depending on whether there is toxic or radioactive spillage, or infectious disease, and over a time course and geographical area in accord with an actual or a potential severity.

Because an overzealous response to a minor disease can tie up expensive resources and impair a response to a more severe threat, classification systems related to epidemiology are available that dictate workflow in relation to severity. The most important of these are the Biohazard UN Codes. A biological hazard or biohazard is a biological substance that poses a threat to (primarily) human health. Examples include medical waste and leakages of microorganisms, viruses, or toxins from biological labs, all of which can impact human health. The substances could even merely be harmful to animals. The term "biohazard" and its associated symbol is generally used as a warning so that anyone potentially exposed to the substance would understand what precautionary actions to take. There is further a biohazard HCS/WHMIS logo that utilizes the same symbol. In Unicode, the biohazard sign is U + 2623 (☣). Biohazardous agents are classified by UN numbers UN 2814 (infectious substance to humans), UN 2900 (infectious substance to animals), and UN 3291 (medical waste).

An important dimension relates to the level of danger that determines the appropriate best practice. For convenience the CDC categorizes a number of diseases among the levels of biohazard, as these infectious diseases combine infectivity and pathogenicity (disease severity, fatality risk). The classification relates to the *handling* of the patient upon encounter and the patient's isolation, and the handling of samples or experimental materials. Level 1 is minimum risk and level 4 is extreme risk. However, a combination with biohazard classification (and ideally a finer-grained classification) is preferable because infective agents such as *Salmonella* may have negligible risk of infectivity among humans, and toxins such as *Staphyloccus* or *Botulinus* have none at all, but nonetheless are extremely pathogenic.

> *Biohazard level 1. Bacillus subtilis*, canine hepatitis, *E. coli*, varicella (chicken pox). At this level precautions against the biohazardous materials in question are minimal, most likely wearing gloves and some facial protection. Decontamination procedures at this level are similar in most respects to modern precautions against everyday viruses (washing hands with antibacterial soap, washing all exposed surfaces of the lab with disinfectants, etc.).
>
> *Biohazard level 2.* Hepatitis B, hepatitis C, influenza, Lyme disease, *Salmonella*, scrapie.
>
> *Biohazard level 3.* Anthrax, BSE, HIV, mumps, West Nile virus, SARS, smallpox, tuberculosis, typhus, Yellow fever.
>
> *Biohazard level 4.* Bolivian fever, Dengue fever, ebola, Hanta virus, Lassa virus, and other various hemorrhagic diseases (mostly of African origin). When dealing with biological hazards at this level the use of a Hazmat suit and a self-contained oxygen supply is mandatory, and the disease is studied and patient isolated in very rigorously self-contained environments.

At the finer-grained level, good practices in the medical responses will differ by the type of epidemic. An epidemic suggests officially a higher incidence of disease than would be usual and often a distribution of the disease in space and time. Point source epidemics are due to e.g. ingestion of chicken left too long out in the sun at a picnic. Common source epidemics are more commonly from, say, poorly washed spinach or peanut products, and proceed from a single source to many supermarkets and restaurants. But such epidemics are characterized by single spikes in the collected statistics of illness, and the toxins involved cannot be spread by the affected persons, nor are the pathogens likely to spread on their own. Flu, AIDS, etc are progressive epidemics. The appropriate responses to such food-borne epidemics are different from those geared to progressive epidemics variously mediated by contact, air droplets, or vectors typically in the form of insects. The mosquito has been mainly responsible in long-term *endemics* arising locally, and often pertaining to the West Nile virus carried and the tick is well-known as a carrier of Lyme disease. Such diseases classically appear as a series of humps in the graphs of infected persons over time, with eventual decay over a substantial later period of time. Epidemiological maps are used to show their progress across geographic areas. If an infectious state persists as in patients with HIV, or the disease cycles back into the population, the disease can be infective twice by adopting a new form. Then an accumulative or S-shaped graph results, as opposed to one or more peaks that show a rapid decline. Pandemics are the most serious because they refer to a worldwide spread of disease.

For cases suspected to be of epidemic risk, the infected persons must be isolated. At this stage the techniques used to sequence or identify the infectious pathogens and/or variants involve more sophisticated analysis of their genomes, which can be fed rapidly into the IT system. An important occasion for isolation as well is when current diagnostics do not detect a new pathogen species or distinguish a new strain, at which time a new diagnostic may need to be developed (see below). The typical objective of treatment for the individual patient is to eliminate the infection with antibiotic therapy. However, the specific means of verification and immediate follow-up depend on the symptoms produced by the pathogen. Penicillin traditionally, and currently the broad spectrum antibiotic Ciprofloxacillin, are the usual medications, but potential complications need to be addressed because treatment can vary depending on symptoms of the pathogen. Again, for the example of anthrax, these include hemorrhagic meningitis, mediastinitis, shock, and ARDS (adult respiratory distress syndrome).

NEW VACCINES AS RAPID RESPONSE TO BIOTHREAT

New pathogens require new diagnostic and therapeutic agents. Treatment of any emergent pathogen potentially opens an opportunity for rapid computer-aided design of the countering agent. Most nations and particularly the United States are exploring highly automated systems based on sound principles of biology and molecular science as a *Star Wars* style response to natural and malicious biothreats.

Currently diagnostics fall into two types: those based on nucleic acid technology and those based on antibodies. Both types could make good use of IT and microminiaturization technology to be placed on a chip or on some other surface and so represent a biosensor. To develop a new antibody by the traditional route, the infective material is injected into an animal, and the antibodies raised against it are isolated. Originally the antibodies were used in wells on a glass plate, or more often in gel media, the recognition of target material being indicated by precipitation and staining. Antibody biosensors are more sophisticated forms in which the antibody of a part of it is bound to a chip. These antibodies will recognize the pathogen when they see it again, emitting a signal from the chip by various possible physiochemical and electrical processes.

Immunization is either passive or active. In passive immunization, biotechnologically constructed antibodies are raised as in animals the same as for antibody-based diagnostics, and then injected into human beings. This procedure is expensive and so is limited to life-threatening situations when the infected patient has not enough time to produce his or her own antibodies naturally. Ideally the antibodies must be humanized by protein engineering, namely made to look human, or else they are likely to be attacked by the body as alien animal products.

Active immunization is attained through vaccination, which is based on the fact that we typically cannot catch the same infectious disease (or more precisely the same strain of infectious disease) twice. The vaccination is done in advance to prevent us from catching the disease. Bioengineered vaccines may be based on designed DNA sequences that are cloned typically in bacteria. In effect the bacteria serve as a synthetic factory for the production of vaccines. For a guaranteed fast response by vaccine design, there are several difficulties relating to achieving the correct folding of the protein, posttranslational modification (modification of the protein in a way that can only occur in much more advanced organisms), and removal of contamination by bacterial material. Moreover, because whole proteins can be relatively complex material, in vaccines they can cause autoimmune effects in certain individuals.

The peptide vaccines discussed earlier in the chapter promise an improvement, but more effective constructs for defense against epidemics in the future are *peptide cartridge vaccines*. These are peptide vaccines built in such a way that epitopes can be replaced and "upgraded" to counter new strains of pathogen, without starting the whole vaccine from scratch. Adjuvant analogues can be included, and sections can be added or removed to avoid complications such as autoimmunization.

A POSTSCRIPT ON MALICIOUS BIOTHREAT

Lack of technical capabilities is not known to deter terrorists. Existing organisms can, in contrived circumstances, spread infection. Pathogens that are relatively local in effect, like anthrax, can be broadly more deadly when dispersed by terrorists. Indeed recall our point that germ warfare is far from new. Ancient archers used to dip their arrowheads in feces and rotting corpses to infect the wounds of their targets, and armies invading cites catapulted bodies of plague victims over the walls. The first attack on the United States was not the anthrax letter attacks of September to October 2001, but in 1984 when an extreme and rich Buddhist sect in Iowa, angered by increasing friction with the local townspeople, infected the salad bars of local restaurants with *Salmonella*. Almost 800 people were infected for sure, and another hundred believed that they were, burgeoning the local medical resources. Happily no one died; the worst case was that a baby was born prematurely with the infection. The anthrax attacks, however, hitting the United States so soon after the 9/11 attacks had a more nationally devastating psychological effect. Although there were fatalities, the ill effect was somewhat compensated by the growing realization that anthrax infection could be more successfully treated than had been previously thought. Vigilance and ready defense are important factors, and one of the more serious concerns is terrorist use of smallpox.

Two letters associated with the anthrax attacks contained a short note. The first bade "take penicillin." If the contents of the letters had leaked and dispersed more readily in the mail sorting and delivery process, and if there had been widespread panic, it is unlikely that in time sufficient antibiotics and medical response would have been forthcoming for everyone exposed because the infrastructure of the US healthcare system had been allowed to decline and was woefully poorly equipped to deal with biothreat. The profound effect on the US health system was recognition of a full list of bacteria, virus, and toxins against hence the power of IT might be directed. The list includes anthrax, arenaviruses, Burkholderia, botulism, brucellosis, ricin, Yellow fever, SARS, hantaviruses and Rift Valley fever, Staphylococcus enterotoxin B, plague, dengue, ebola and marburg, tularemia, Q fever (*C. burnetii*), viral encephalitides, typhus fever (*R. proswzekii*), smallpox, Crimean Congo hemorrhagic fever, and food and waterborne bacteria, viruses, and protozoa.

In vaccine design molecular details and patterns of sugar and protein atoms in space make the difference between less harmful and lethal strains of the same virus. So understanding the scientific basis and having the technology to make use of it could put enhanced dangerous powers in the hands of terrorists, and countering power in the hands of the defenders of nations against terrorist attacks. What is the disturbing thing is that already the technology exists to make any new viral strains we want, but there is a lack of human insight and smart computer software to enable the design on a total from-first-principles basis. There is no single simple answer as to what makes a particular virus variant so deadly. It is a complex interaction that involves both viral and host gene products. The viral genes associated with pathogenicity vary from virus to virus. Design of a guaranteed killer effect and the defense against it will require a very high level of computer technology that may not be available for some time, although it behooves us to ensure that we always maintain the technological upper hand.

10

WHAT NEXT? AT ONE WITH THE ENGINES OF HIPPOCRATES

Col. Austin's legs, right arm, and left eye are replaced with cybernetic limbs which give him, the world's first Bionic man, extraordinary strength and abilities.

—The Six Million Dollar Man, ABC-TV

I don't want to achieve immortality through my work. I want to achieve immortality through not dying

—Woody Allen, American comedian.

A CAUTION

This chapter brings us back to the grand cosmological themes hinted at in Chapter 1. That the path will require our discussing more physics and chemistry as well as biology. Healthcare providers and administrators might think that they have enough to worry about without drawing in an entire universe of disciplines and the next few billion years. But future technologies may yet have a more immediate impact and hit us harder and faster than we expect, and some of the issues will be broad ethical issues that we have already grappled with on occasion and they provide a taste of what is to come. Anticipating future needs can help us set our ethical standards today. Some of the fairly new strategies and philosophies of medicine that are now being

The Engines of Hippocrates: From the Dawn of Medicine to Medical and Pharmaceutical Informatics, by Barry Robson and O.K. Baek
Copyright © 2009 by John Wiley & Sons, Inc.

implemented rapidly are due to the rise of evidence-based medicine, for example. Some have even speculated that people alive today could theoretically, given certain conditions, keep up with ongoing technological developments and live forever.

A REVIEW OF THE HUMAN STORY SO FAR, AND NEWS UPDATES ON IT

The beginnings of the human race diverged in Africa, and then spread out of it, set the genomic differences among us that make us essentially the same but individualized nonetheless. In particular, the risk factors for different diseases differ among us, and so do the responses, for better or worse, to different medicines. This consequence of not so ancient history, going back a mere 50 or 60,000 years or so, thus established the domain and game rules for *stratified medicine*, by which pharmaceutical companies and physicians distinguish treatment according to genomics. The term *stratified* is very recent. The best philosophical idea, as we stated many times, is for *personalized* medicine where all medical treatment and ideally drug molecules are tailored for the individual. On the one hand, reasonably enough, the drug companies find it hard to imagine and accept a market sector so small that it comprises just one patient. On the other, recognizing that patients do respond differently, and that there are at least multiple groups of patient types, is not just an inconvenient truth for them. On the bright side, it is a new market opportunity to break the failing revenue from the "blockbuster" superdrug-for-all idea, a way for new companies and projects to find a worthy niche and powerful knowledge to prevent failures in clinical trials and withdrawals of marketed drugs.

The latest figures on the differences among us at the level of our DNA seem to be changing significantly even as this book is being written. At first, the findings of the human genome projects around the year 2000 were that we differed by about one genetic symbol G, C, A, or T out of every thousand in our ... GATTACAGATTACAGATTACA ... DNA code. Statistically this means that many proteins in our bodies targeted by drugs will be different for each of us. This is called *protein polymorphism*. It explains the recent development of diagnostics or detectors for *genomic biomarkers* so that the right drug is given, and the science of *pharmacogenomics* to provide the right drug on that basis. If we could address the cost issues, biomarker detection "chips" would be on our doctor's desk right now. A few, like the chip for predicting the best antidepressant based on the patients genomics, could have been there several years ago. But recent estimates of the degrees of difference between us at the DNA level numbers seem to reflect surprising diversity, and recently the estimates have doubled the initially perceived diversity. If it were to keep up at the same rate, we would soon be seen to be as similar to the chimpanzee as we are to each other. That will not happen, but even if it did, another development that has recently reached popular scientific understanding is that the changes in a very few master genes matter most often in evolution. These genes control the timing and intensity of expression of the remaining genes in embryological development, and thus are responsible for many major evolutionary steps and the differences among species. The rest of the genes and the proteins from them do nonetheless remain remarkably similar between humans and other mammals, which is why there is such a thing as the laboratory animal as a substitute for humans.

At the same time there has recently been appreciation that the human race is far less genetically diverse than it ought to be. One reason discussed already is that a very few humans, maybe just a tribe or two, spread out of Africa to conquer the world. While there were modern humans (and Neanderthals) already out there, for some reason they seem to have left no descendants. They were out-battled, out-smarted, or even out-traded by some genes underlying the spirit of capitalism. While similar evolution, migration, and progress went on within Africa, the simple fact that very few tribes survived and populated on the rest of the planet is consistent with greater diversity among persons of more recent African descent, an important issue for pharmacogenomics if there is to be fair play for all.

Remarkably, however, it has very recently been appreciated that the human race is actually *very* much less diverse than it ought to be, even within Africa. Notably there is much greater similarity among human groups than among groups of chimpanzees. It is as if there was a bottleneck in human prehistory, a fairly recent moment in time in which the human race was greatly reduced. Was this an epidemic, or an asteroid collision? It would be too early for the epidemics surviving today of zoonotic origin, coming from the animals that humans lived with thousands of years ago, and there is no great geological evidence of the layers rich in certain elements characteristic of the asteroid impact that is supposed to have wiped out the dinosaurs.

According to the recently much promoted Toba catastrophe theory, it is the consequences of a massive *volcanic eruption* that severely reduced the human population. This may have occurred around 70,000 to 75,000 years ago when a supervolcano in Indonesia underwent an eruption of category 8 (i.e., "megacolossal") on a measure called the Volcanic Explosivity Index. That is equivalent to about 1 billion tons of TNT and about three thousand times of the 1980 Mount St. Helens eruption. It was not exactly a moment in time: the spread in the atmosphere ash and sulphuric acid obscured the sun and caused plants to die on a time scale of maybe 5 to 15 years. It was long enough to hit the whole food chain. Some estimate that the average global temperature dropped by about 5 degrees celsius. A volcanic eruption might have triggered the subsequent ice age, but likely it just made things worse by hastening the time when a global cooling was due anyway.

The thin spread of humans with even thinner resources probably had already encouraged the banding together into large villages, although in recent estimates for later millennia something on the order of 10 to 20 people per village seems to have been the norm. In any event, the evidence still stands that there was a much greater physician–patient ratio than in recent centuries. It naturally resulted in a personalized and holistic medicine where the physician was likely the shaman, and medicine was bound tightly with the pertaining worldview of religion, magic, and mythology. Medicine then would have observational roots in trial and error, but it was much less scientific and certainly not in the sense that we understand scientific observation today. Hippocrates was really the first physician that we know of to really make a well-defined split. It was more correctly a specialization because he remained respectful of the gods, and in the Greek spirit he for the most part distinguished ethics from religious obligation. If there have been any recent changes to our perception of those times, it is an increased sense (based on analysis of traces of written text) that even more ancient civilizations like that of Sumer may have laid the seeds for scientific and mathematical thinking that survived as a stream of thought through the pre-Hippocrates period of medicine dominated by magic and religion. In this book we have rather neglected the ancient Egyptians, with their incredibly long civilization, and so plenty of time for refinements on the earlier semiscientific methods (but still bound up with magic and the gods). Recently there has been much use of advanced medical imaging and examination of the DNA of Egyptian mummies, throwing new insight as to what diseases they had and were prone too, and what they could, and could not, treat.

Such was the impact and influence of Hippocrates (and subsequently Galen) that, in spirit, much of medicine has remained unchanged except for the recent advances in scientific research. In the course of writing this book, there has been some increase in historians' awareness of the contributions of the ancient Greeks, and perhaps the biggest growth in awareness at popular level has been about the great extent to which the fires in the great library in Alexandria destroyed so much written wisdom, even about feats of mechanical engineering. Consider that there has been no previous hint from history about the *antikythera mechanism*, a clockwork computer probably for astronomical predictions and setting dates of important events, discovered more than 100 years ago in a Roman shipwreck but only very recently analyzed and interpreted. Doubtless those fires helped precipitate, or intensify, the so-called Dark Ages; at least they were dark in Europe. Also increasingly there is better appreciation of Arabic contributions to medicine during that period.

One very recent newsworthy item, that of an important "petaflop barrier" in computing important for solving biomolecular problems and designing drugs, has been breached. General improvements in computer engineering recently promoted IBM to build its BlueGene supercomputer, specifically aimed at solving complex biological problems such as how proteins fold. A million processors are to be brought together and run at a petaflop speed (i.e., 10^{15} mathematical calculations per second), and smaller versions are already in use for helping design drugs, simulate the brain activities, and analyze millions of pharmaceutical patents. However, the goal for the processing speed of a petaflop was actually reached at the time of writing by other IBM hardware, including the Cell processor, in a device installed at Los Alamos to simulate atomic fusion. Originally designed for the games and movie industry, the Cell processor nonetheless found early application in chemistry applications, notably simulating the interaction between a drug and a protein receptor that underlies pharmacological action.

The benefits are yet to be reaped and overall picture of medical history still remains much the same, as the fundamental principles attributed to Hippocrates seem remarkably unaffected by scientific advances. So, as we leapfrog ahead in history, we can take much of what is in previous chapters as more or less unchanged: that is, with the exception of pausing for two recent developments that give some perspective of the medicine and pharmaceutical science to come.

EVIDENCE-BASED MEDICINE IS RISING AS A NEW MEDICAL PHILOSOPHY

If there is one *philosophical* shift of importance, it is the quite recent advent of *evidence-based medicine* (EBM). We have alluded to this before, and now review in a more historical and also contemporary perspective. The tangible origins of EBM date back to 1972, to a book called *Effectiveness and Efficiency: Random Reflections on Health Services*, by Archie Cochrane, a Scottish epidemiologist. Cochrane's subsequent advocacy led to an increasing acceptance of the concepts behind the idea of bringing science, latest data, and hard statistical facts in medical practice. Naturally, as an epidemiologist, he based his ideas on the established principles of epidemiology, good statistics and tracking the causes of disease, and not just infectious diseases. A major argument was that doctors were actually doing some harm. They were making bad decisions and causing medical accidents by relying on old medical school training, personal experience, anecdotal evidence, too much subjective patient perception, and so-called expert opinion. Importantly they were failing to "keep up" with the latest medical findings. Cochrane thus formulated the idea of "best evidence." The explicit methodologies used to determine best evidence were largely established by the McMaster University research group led by David Sackett and Gordon Guyatt. The term "evidence-based medicine" first appeared in the medical literature in 1992 in a paper by Guyatt and colleagues at Oxford, UK; David Sackett and Muir Gray recently ran the National Health Service R&D Centre; and Sackett founded the Centre for Evidence-Based Medicine (http://www.cebm.net) at Oxford, UK.

So why is EBM regarded as a recent update? The fact is that it did not gain immediate acceptance. It was as if a new Hippocrates and Galen had come along, but physicians had become set in their ways for hundreds of years. In addition it is hard for them to see the latest big picture when new medical information is flooding in daily from research, including now rapid translational research involving newly discovered biomarkers from genomics, proteomics, and new medical imaging modalities. It would have been an impossible task for a physician to access all the burgeoning new medical knowledge in the 1970s, and even if they could, their grasp of mathematical and statistical thinking, quantitative inference, risk analysis, and probability-based decision making was notoriously poor. The big factor that has caused acceleration has been the ability to delegate this to computers including the rise of the digital patient medical record, in other words, evidence-based medicine essentially becomes what we call information-based medicine. Still the technology has been around since the rise of the Internet (which does itself provide many web pages specifically described as representing evidence-based medicine, helping physicians and patients make decisions). What really started tipping the scale was the Human Rights Report in the United States in 2004, showing that medical accidents are now the third leading cause of death following cardiovascular disease (heart attacks, stroke, etc.) and cancer.

Again, we spill out the horrendous numbers: one out of every 25 in-patients becomes a victim of a medical accident. Some 195,000 people die of medical accidents every year. The actual figure might be twice of that, and medicine has the worst accident rate of any US industry. Substandard care in America kills over 57,000 people and wastes over $9 billion annually. Physicians drive 80% of the cost. So the Bush administration quickly committed $100 million, and congressional bi-partisan effort has been behind the introduction of legislation to stimulate electronic patient record keeping, or electronic health records (EHR).

Evidence-based medicine has recently started to be a term quoted at the US federal level, as potential litigation looms for physicians if harm is done when it could have been avoided by access to EBM resources. Certain health insurance companies have already denied coverage where EBM is not practiced, and the FDA and pharmaceutical companies are being pushed to adopt EBM. A challenge for the IT industry is that their traditional customer divisions among federal, healthcare, and industry are disappearing. The IT industry is being compelled to adjust. A major example of this fusion is that pharmaceutical companies are banding together with the FDA to check on the safety and performance of already marketed drugs, putting constant pressure on physicians and patients. There has been the formation of a Biomarker Consortium, and also a marriage organized by the Foundation of the National Health Services to collect massive amount of patient data for FDA and the pharmaceutical industries. The FDA, perceived as entrenched in the methods of classical statistics and what its critics call "the curse of the null hypothesis," is as we write making public requests for information on new and more powerful types of data analysis.

Using the correct metrics, healthcare philosophy, and underlying calculation is important in setting the price of a drug, and these are issues in both pharmacosurveillance and EBM. Drug pricing also includes the case of the drug price being fixed by a manufacturer and so the issue of whether the price of the drug makes it worthwhile. It may not be economically viable for a country with a state-funded, socialistic, welfare medical system to supply medication for a common disease if it costs $20,000 to $30,000 per patient per year. High prices can become a problem when a drug is available only as a brand-name product from a single manufacturer. A patent guarantees the holder an exclusive right to market the protected product without competition for a period of at least 20 years, but after that, other manufacturers can produce a non-branded, that is, *generic* version of the drug, and sell it usually much more cheaply. For example, fluoxetine (Prozac) sold for $2.50 per pill until its patent ended in 2001. Then a generic manufacturer brought its version to market for only $0.25 apiece. However, whatever the price, drug pricing is a complex issue requiring feedback from patients by pharmacovigilance about at what stages of the disease the drug works best, whether it works enough in achieving quality of life, what quality of life means in that case, ease of compliance, and so on. To some extent in the United Kingdom such feedback has been pre-empted by bodies such as the National Institute of Clinical Excellence (NICE) but this exemplifies and foreshadows some turmoil over what EBM actually is and how it should be practiced. Notably the recent conclusion by NICE that Aricept, the Alzheimer's drug developed by Japanese pharmaceutical company Eisai, is not worth the cost, is controversial. Was it that NICE was using a brand of EBM of its own in relation to benefit–cost model and sampling and using feedback from patients? If so, is that brand a shining model to become the standard, or does that model lie elsewhere? Part of the problem is that while few doubt the fine motives of EBM, it has developed its own brand of statistics and measures intended to help the physician who, as was noted above, is not adept at mathematics and statistics. A simple example, far simpler than esoteric pharmaco-economic pricing algorithms of at least partly EBM flavor, is EBM's best known measure, which is now considered important in pharmacogenomics. The NNT or "number needed to treat" is the number of patients who need to be treated in order to prevent one additional bad outcome (i.e., to reduce the expected number of cases of a defined endpoint by one). Particularly keeping in mind that the lower the number the better, do you find this immediately comprehensible? The new methods do not all seem to be well founded, and to be rather esoteric, and there is considerable variation and make-do in techniques adopted outside the clinic, as in economic and drug-pricing models. So physicians continue right now in much the same way as before, while many organizations like the NICE have to supplement both classical and EBM statistical thinking with new methods from diverse sources.

With the growing importance of keeping costs down, the impact of EBM on personalized medicine is at present largely in judging whether drugs or drug combinations targeted to a particular group in the population do anything much. Although about half the pediatricians in Washington, DC, around 2006 recommend that children under age 2 can be given diphenhydramine to help them sleep, the first study to look at effectiveness of the agent in children who are that young found no benefit. More recently BiDil, a drug combating congestive heart failure moderately well, has come under some attack, although it was originally touted as a triumph for pharmacogenomics by being targeted at African-Americans. In fact, according to lawyer Jonathan Kahn writing in the August 2007 *Scientific American*, this drug, although beneficial, illustrates several features of poor reasoning in regard to pharmacogenomics. For the most part ethnic groups and "races" are not well-defined genomic groups but represent geographical and social structures. In some instances there may be overlapping clusters, statistically speaking, such that any two individuals within a cluster have a high probability of being just as genetically diverse as any two between the two clusters. The African-American story, one might recall, is somewhat different, in a way that is equally problematic—all the rest of us are just from one or two African tribes out of dozens that may contribute to the Africans today. Pooling all remaining Africans and splitting up all descendants of those one or two African tribes into Hispanic, Inuit, and so forth, does not always make a lot of genomic sense. Indeed every "ethnic group" has its own special story in terms of genetic coherence or diversity. What is clear is that on the whole, they are indeed a *story*, and doubtless a true one to be proud of, but not a simple genomic group at the same level of description as other genomic groups are. In practice, the number of African-Americans on which BiDil was tested is very small. The difficulty is not that the drug is useless but rather that there is no reason as yet to consider it as "targeted to one genomic population"—apparently it was not originally designed on that basis. It may even be that part of the non–African-American population is missing out on its benefits. However, Jonathan Kahn seems to be effectively suggesting that pharmacogenomics is a bandwagon in which drug companies are starting to ride to get FDA approval even when it is not true pharmacogenomics at all, and it does not inspire confidence in that Bidil is really a mix of two molecular compounds each of which are available as pharmaceutical tablets at much lower cost.

In addition there are ethical issues now arising. It is a simplistic statement but some models put the cost of human health as worth about US $30,000 a year, anything higher being to an increasing extent "not worth it" at least for the larger common good. Also, what does it mean to say a drug is "good" or that it "works"? EBM is rich in themes of outcomes analysis, but what *is* a desirable "healthcare outcome"? Does a drug or procedure that promises a happier life but with high mortality risk outweigh one that offers a longer life with disability or pain? Are essentially sedative drugs for psychotic patients, which makes them more manageable, meaningfully subject to the same measures? Can a drug that is said to be "working" be one that helps a patient with a disease like Alzheimer's to be happy, content, and more manageable? And how does one assess some drugs that have multiple and diverse pharmacological effects? Here marijuana actually has not only the obvious but also apparently other Alzheimer's benefits. Or is it better to help the patient to be more aware and restored to normal role in society even if they are less happy in that state?

USE OF PATENTS?

A very recent unexpected development and still accelerating, relates to making better use of medical information sources while we await better "master archives" of universal medical knowledge. It is now possible for computers to read millions of patents from the pharmaceutical (and other) industries, making quickly and expressly available the molecules and applications, and making proposed improvements. Although a patent is a bargain with the state to have first commercial options while making inventions and discoveries available for the future common good, there are undoubted commercial advantages in keeping a novelty as quiet as possible for a while. Widely and vigorously advertising your patent is a strategy for start-up companies, but not for "Big Pharma." Not least, the patents reveal the research and strategies of competing companies. With the "bargain with the state" principle above in mind, there is much to be said uncovering that data, and it is a very convenient and readily accessible source of large amounts of such data compared with other text sources. US patents can be accessed over the Internet. The trick is to access millions of them, and understand their content, quickly. Others shifts involve analyzing "anonymized" data from digital insurance claims, a good source of medical information where full-blown digital patient records are not yet available.

OUR MAIN THEME AND CONCLUSION, UP FRONT

Above all things, our theme has been that IT can restore something good in medicine. Personalized and holistic medicine on a family and tribe basis, with a small patient-to-physician ratio, was a good feature of early human history. To repeat: this relationship was lost with the advent of the Industrial Revolution in the nineteenth century, and even with the advanced medical technologies to come, patient–physician contact diminished. Today, the doctor is not only overwhelmed by the number of his patients but by the escalation of medical knowledge that he or she should apply to them, especially of a molecular nature. However, IT creates a global village that restores that access to knowledge of the patient and the latest developments by gathering, ordering, and appropriately presenting the necessary data. It is still to be proved on a large scale, but forces are driving IT to an inevitable destiny with medicine, ultimately across the globe. Patients would become an important part of a global IT infrastructure, and physicians would delegate more and more to the information processing by that global infrastructure.

Those readers who must be concerned about the next patient or next healthcare budget can close the book now. But a further reason for underlining such conclusions early in the last chapter of this book is because advanced medicine and involvement of IT also raises several deeper issues for the distant future. These questions are in particular:

- How far can it go?
- How far should it go?
- Exactly *how* might it go?

PREVIEW: THE COMING MEDICAL SCOPE OF IT

It is Saturday, and Jane is reading the weekend paper. She feels a mild pain in her left chest and persists. She opens her computer and asks the calendaring agent software to book an appointment with her family doctor for chest pain. She continues to read the newspaper. (The calendaring agent software makes a copy of Jane's calendar and travels through the Internet to visit the family doctor's office system and finds the doctor is away on vacation for the next two weeks. The agent software travels to the nearest hospital system and finds an on-call doctor who is available for 1:00 pm in the afternoon. The calendaring agent software makes an appointment for 1:00 pm with the on-call doctor and returns.)

In about 15 seconds or so, Jane's home computer tells Jane that an appointment has been made for 1:00 pm with Dr. Smith.

At 12:55 Jane arrives at Dr. Smith's office, and Dr. Smith's assistant greets Jane and activates the RFID reader to read Jane's global person identifier. The clinical encounter is recorded in the physician's office system. The physician's office system retrieves Jane's health records from various places based on Jane's global person identifier.

Jane is shown to an examination room, and nurse draws blood from Jane and takes vital signs, which are captured into the clinical encounter record for Jane. Dr. Smith comes into the examination room and sees Jane and performs an ECG (electrocardiogram) test as well as a functional MRI (magnetic resonance imaging) scan for Jane's heart.

Dr. Smith analyzes the results and explains that Jane's irregular work schedules and frequent overseas trips as well as the stress associated with the aggressive plans might have weakened her heart. Dr. Smith inserts (via voice dictation to the system) a prescription for Jane and the system comes back with a list of brand names of drugs. Dr. Smith selects a set of drugs and enters an electronic prescription.

Dr. Smith, after getting Jane's consent, implants a microbot in her chest to monitor her heart function. The implantable microbot, also referred to as micro-electromechanical system (MEMS), operates on chemical energy transformed into electric energy.

Jane leaves Dr. Smith's office and goes to the nearest pharmacy. The RFID reader at the pharmacy reads Jane's global person identifier as she enters into the pharmacy and retrieves the prescription ordered by Dr. Smith. The pharmacist checks for drug interactions and allergies. The pharmacist dispenses the medicine for Jane and describes dosage and frequency of medicine, and its benefits and effects.

In a week, Jane completes the medication, and she feels fine.

Three months later, Jane is taking a walk in the Central Park on a Sunday afternoon. A sudden large noise startles her. The microbot implanted in Jane's chest detects irregular heartbeats and activates the automatic implantable cardioverter defibrillator, and makes an emergency call (911) via the Medical Implant Communication Service (MICS) interface and cellular communication.

The Health Emergency Response System (HERS) at the Mt. Sinai Hospital receives the call, locates Jane based on the microbot signal through the Global Positioning System, and dispatches an air ambulance to pick her up.

A physician on duty is alerted by HERS (Health Emergency Response System), and Jane's microbot is now linked with the surgeon's workstation. The physician analyzes the heart condition online based on the data being transmitted by the microbot.

The national e-Health Informatics System dynamically retrieves Jane's health records from various places where Jane has ever visited (e.g., physician's office system, hospitals, diagnostic labs) based on Jane's global person identifier and dynamically constructs an integrated health record up to date from birth, which includes Jane's genetic profiles and lifestyle data. The physician then analyzes Jane's personal health record for analysis of clinical and treatment history.

The physician notes that the appropriate drugs target a limited number of proteins both as the therapeutic target and as side effect decoys. He then activates his link to the supercomputers at the pharmaceutical companies and at the FDA to model some of the patient's proteins (those that carry some fairly unusual amino acid replacements) and screen the likely drug candidates in virtual reality. The results are confirmed experimentally by a rapid assay using a smear of Jane's cheek cells on a microchip.

The physician then uploads itinerant agent software modules into the microbot to monitor other conditions. The mobile intelligent agent technology allows physicians to launch or upload software programs with specific itinerary or mission to a remote system such as the implanted microbot. The newly uploaded itinerant software module then activates the implantable drug delivery device (IDDD) to release the drug compounds into Jane's blood stream.

The IDDD releases the drug compounds into the blood stream and starts sending the drug metabolism data to the microbot, which then relays the data to the physician's workstation for monitoring and analysis while Jane is being transported to the hospital.

Jane is bored in hospital. She laments that the future will see her as living in a dark age of medicine. She looks forward to a much heralded time when myriads of much smaller and more sophisticated devices will repair her on the spot.

Clearly, the future of IT had for Jane already manifested itself in many more ways than the PC on your desk. Via the increasingly powerful Internet you will be able to interact with very powerful supercomputers as if they were your own. Remember that, at the time of tidying up this book, IBM hardware broke the petaflop barrier, at 10^{15} floating point (arithmetic) operations per second. Many distinctions between local and remote computing will vanish. The PC is already vanishing, being replaced by hand-held devices. There are and will be a broadly distributed set of pervasive devices in the walls, in your car, in your clothes, inside your body, and even perhaps in your brain.

That does not exhaust it. On the side of mechanics, the future of IT in everyday life potentially also includes *biorobotics* (recall that robotics is a current industry term that first appeared in the science fiction novels of Isaac Asimov), and hence more subtle forms of half robotics that mean enhancive replacements of ailing human parts. For many years patients have already been able to have artificial replacement materials, pins, joints, various prosthetics, pacemakers, and artificial hearts. They have also received transplantations and insertions made of natural materials. This trend will doubtless continue to chips and robotic components to restore lost and damaged physiological, neurological and biochemical functions.

On the side of biology there will be no less sophisticated developments. Genetic engineering could, of course, potentially enhance human beings, for example, making them stronger. We know that is possible because the June 24, 2004, *New England Journal of Medicine* reported a baby boy with a natural mutation that enhances muscle growth. Well before the boy was five, he could hold seven-pound weights with his arms extended, which is something that many adults cannot do, and he had muscles twice the size, and half the fat, of other children his age. One might imagine that potentially enhanced soldiers, police, and security guards could be bred by introducing the same genetic change artificially. Genetic engineering can be leveraged for fixing genetic defects by turning off the genes that are responsible for susceptibility of certain diseases or turning on the genes that provide immunity to certain diseases.

Biological and nonbiological technologies may ultimately converge, and the distinction may disappear. In line with Jane's dream, progress will also include *nanotechnology*, a discipline that some say could transform us not at the deepest molecular level to something better than human. Instead of simply adding mechanical extensions to our body, there will be, according to the visionaries of the field, myriads of minute molecular-scale machines that will ultimately transform us atom by atom. This time it will not be to something that will be a blend of human and machine, but a new concept built from the first principles.

Let us address some controversial issues on what is emerging now.

CLONING

Dolly, a sheep (a ewe, actually), was the first animal to be cloned from an adult somatic cell by Ian Wilmut and colleagues at the Rosalind Institute in Scotland. Because cloning was done successfully in a mammal, it has raised interest in the possible use of cloning for humans. But real-world cloning must be distinguished from the instantaneous replication of an adult human being (often complete with the same memories and even with identical clothing!) seen in science fiction movies. Instantaneous replication like matter transportation, if ever possible, lies in the realm of physics of *Star Trek*, not biomedicine. Cloning in that sense is more as if one of the embryo from an identical twin were put in suspended hibernation and brought to life at some arbitrary time.

While cloning is not exactly an IT issue, IT does provide continuing support to biomedical research up to analysis and simulation of molecular details. So beyond that there is little more to be said except for two things that will shortly become reminiscent of some other issues that are more IT related.

First are obviously the strong ethical, even deep-rooted archetypal concerns, affecting as well other future medical issues discussed below. As we have done before and will continue to do even more vigorously below, we will make reference to mythology and contemporary fiction that say much about social attitudes regarding these matters. The more ancient roots of concern in cloning might be expressed in the idea of the *fetch* or *doppelgänger* as the ghostly double of a living person. The implication is usually evil: indeed how can a soul be duplicated along with the body? At least, for atheists, how can there be two distinct consciounesses? The ethical considerations and potentials for misuse have been addressed several times in recent fiction. Notably there was Ira Levin's 1976 novel *The Boys from Brazil* about the multiple cloning of Hitler that was significantly followed very quickly by the 1978 movie with a prestigious cast of Gregory Peck, Lawrence Olivier, and James Mason, and also by a succession of novels by other authors of almost indistinguishable plots. Notably, in the circumstances, Levin's even more famous novel is *Rosemary's Baby*, where the baby is literally the devil.

Second, there are still serious practical issues. While to be biologically practical about it there seems no more harm in cloning than in having an identical twin, cloning per se may "inherit" some of the age of the source human, notably the shortened telomeres of the chromosomes that, like a candle burning at both ends, shrink as we age. Dolly lived about 7 years, but very like dogs, sheep typically normally live 10 to 12 years (and not unusually 20). Dolly's mother was a six-year-old, so in that sense Dolly died at about age 11, which is suggestive not least because most of us, cloned or not, might like to alter the clock that fixes our life on Earth. Although cloning might some day be biotechnologically fixable, we are left again the primary barriers as those of human taste.

STEM CELLS

Among the other growing issues of "how far can it go and how far should it go?" one no less red hot controversy is the issue of *stem cells*. After all, one long standing vision of future biomedicine is to be able to re-grow whole organs, and perhaps limbs. That is after all what we all did once before in our mother's wombs. Moreover amphibians can re-grow lost limbs. Their ability to do so is because unspecialized cells retain the ability to redo the same tasks that were performed in their embryological development. The catch is that cells that can do this, and that were responsible for our development in the first place, are those notorious stem cells derived from human embryos. The stem cell issue is worth its own book, and there is plenty of Internet source material for authors and casual researchers alike. In mid-2008 there were 19,200,00 Google hits on "stem cell," but this fell to 13,500,000 in late January 2009, presumably reflecting some decline in concern combined with Google's "tidying" of secondary references. So the issues will not be debated here, except to say that the use of stem cells from human fetuses, and so distasteful to many, may soon disappear with the use of modified animal cells, tissue cultures, and so forth. They may even come from our own adult bodies, since medical science has long distinguished embryo and adult stem cells, the latter currently with a limited potential for replacement and repair but could, in principle, be extended. Again, we cannot resist mentioning two things.

First, stem cells may not be the only solution, but at best (or worst!) just part of it. Even if use of stem cells for organ replacement is well accepted, it might (or might not) turn out that the real challenge is the more complex organs that function as an internal biochemistry laboratory, the liver, kidneys, exocrine pancreas set to deliver digestive enzymes, and endocrine pancreas and other glands set to deliver hormones. A purely stem cell solution might (or might not) be extremely difficult for complex systems, at least in the near future, and the others parts of the solution may be more closely related to the IT industry as described in the next section.

Second, the science of organ and limb development is, alongside brain science, one of the last and toughest frontiers of medical science. The current state of stem cell science is for the most part that we know scientists can do it somehow. We do not have total understanding and hence control. We might yet build a heart starting only from such seemingly simple cells, but the stem cells will do all the work. How do they do it? Less grandiosely, how does the body dictate that your arms are of the same form and length, but of considerable different form and length from those of other animals?

That all said, progress in the understanding of a handful of *homeobox genes*, similar across much of the animal kingdom and controlling crucial clocks and switches for growth and form, may accelerate medical capabilities much faster than human taste can evolve. So, if we wish it, IT may play a very strong role in analyzing and simulating the control systems of embryonic development, and that may be a game worth playing even just from the perspective of enhancing repair and helping prevent errors in fetal development.

So, if stem cells will be at best part of the solution, what is the rest?

BIOCHIPS

In the current absence of a total understanding of embryonic development and limb growth, hybrid or even stand-alone biomachine devices inside the body, could replace a 100% stem cell solution for some applications for glands and some organs, with the potential in future to dramatically extend our slowly evolved biological capabilities. An example here is the liver, which is primarily a biochemical laboratory, so why not replace it with an actual, albeit very small, state-of-the art biochemical laboratory?

Devices often called *biochips* are not the whole story, but they represent at least part of what is within our grasp. The term applies most generally to any kind of chip-like entity used in the body (and occasionally more broadly for any biological application). The keyword "chip" reflects the fact that historically the solution path has involved the computer chip industry, albeit usually somewhat indirectly, by smaller companies using IT industry technology. In any event the relevant advances have come from the challenge of making smaller computer chips. However, of particular interest here is not (just) the movement of electrons and digital information on the chip but liquids.

Anatomy and biorobotics alike in their most general definition include not just movement of human limbs but movement of human liquids (among other things). The new science and engineering required is that of *microfludics*. Why need it be new? On the nearly microscopic scale, movement of liquids is not trivial engineering because of issues of surface tension, viscosity, and particularly mixing. Engineering principles are emerging rapidly, however, and devices based on such principles could play medical roles both outside and inside the body. This serves nicely to bring up also the notion of MicroLabs, effectively biochips destined for the physician's desk and yielding quick results form patient blood, urea, or tissue samples. They are basically portable (and pocketable) labs whose mechanisms are based on microfludics. Similar solutions for on-the-spot patient DNA analysis are already being deployed. The benefits of microfludics for such currently more credible applications are that the primary driver of the perhaps more incredible technology will provide biochips within us.

In most people's jargon, "biochips" are not confined to microfluidics. Among many other roles, microfludics adapted from MicroLab technology can be extended for implants to deliver neurotransmitters or inhibitors in Parkinsonism, depression, schizophrenia, and so on, in a targeted and still microfluidic way without need for clumsy and not-so-effective oral administration. Nonetheless, when it comes to the brain, the original electronic and digital capabilities of the products of the computer chip industry are as much in the forefront of the news as their microfluidic potential, to say the least.

There has been for a long time an interest in controlling epilepsy, and computer chips have already been explored as brain implants and used to repair deafness. The ability of the brain to learn the language of the chip and so soon hear distinct sounds is a remarkable demonstration of how the human will accommodate when something is there to help. While the difference is, of course, that the microfluidic chips most discussed involve moving fluids and process molecules, not electrons, the computational ability of chips is important to interface with the brain. Moreover hybrid and microfluidic chips at some stage, because the more sophisticated microfluidic systems, like any modern factory, necessarily involve computer control. Microfluidic implant technology may thus not move too far for too long from its IT industry origins.

FOR THE BUDDING BIOCHIP ENGINEER

The future of medical technology is such a plethora of converging technologies that a single book cannot follow every technology in detail, but for the reader of an engineering inclination it may be useful to drill a little deeper into biochips. Others too may want to read on. For one thing, it is a hint about how those IT engineers who are building the engines of Hippocrates can contribute to medicine in other ways than through powerful computers. For another, it gives pause to wonder at how biological evolution has addressed the challenges in what are currently, admittedly, much more elegant ways.

The manufacture of digital chips as *digital* implants is basically straightforward to grasp, but how is this extended to move and process liquids? Currently almost classical computer chip techniques are still used in the first step. A *negative photoresist*, the mask, is laid on a silicon wafer. The bits we do not want (the unmasked regions comprising the material around the planned channels) are etched away. A polymer called polydimethylsiloxane (PDMS) is then cured on to the remaining raised bits. Curing involves the application of heat to set the polymer on the raised regions. The cured layer is peeled away from the underlying base, and laid against a new silicon-based material such as silicon, glass, or even PDMS again. The new structure is exposed to a beam of plasma gas charged particles that oxidizes the surfaces molecules of PDMS structure to silicon hydroxides Si–OH. This is essentially a priming step: where the primed surface is laid against a further silicon wafer, the process forms a –O–Si–O– chemical bond. We now have a two-wafer sandwich. Holes to inject liquids, wells hold them, and pit areas for analyzing constituents are now added. In a related process called *multilayer soft lithography*, the middle layer of the sandwich is deliberately left incompletely converted to silicon hydroxides. This means it is free to move quite a bit, allowing the engineers-of-the-very-small to design pumps and valves like those in the heart, and other complex systems.

This seems quite straightforward, so what are precisely are the challenges being addressed? It was hinted at above. When we watch analysts in a clinical lab, they are moving and mixing liquids all the time without much problem. However, the very small scale of these devices emphasizes properties of liquids that aren't the same as in classical labs. Fluids on the micro/nano scale tend to stream ("laminar flow") rather than mix ("turbulent flow"). For certain purposes the speed aspect of streaming is good news, but it is bad news for mixing things. Methods of tackling this difficulty are introducing bumps into channels where mixing is to occur, or to inject a thin stream into a larger volume. It is of value that simulation can treat both laminar flow and turbulence, but the latter is much more complex. We can also exploit the fact that molecules being moved in liquids can come naturally electrically charged, selecting out molecules by electrophoresis in an applied charged field, or by electrosomosis across semiporous membranes in an applied electric field. Other ways of moving fluids could include systolic pumping motions of channels, using contractile molecules functioning like the smooth muscle fibers of our intestines, that is, by insertion of bodies in the channels that move forward on whip-like outboard motors like the flagella that move bacteria.

It would be too much right now to give such chips their own brains, eyes, and ears, but a nose of sorts is definitely needed. Having moved and mixed our liquids, they may need to do analysis and to check the existing level of something, say before doing synthesis to replace it. As discussed below, antibodies can be created in the biotech lab to bind to and signal the presence of a variety of substances in a very specific and hence good diagnostic way. Using carbon nanotubes (also discussed below) as wires to conduct current, and coating some with these antibodies, can alter electrical current flow detectably and so detect binding. In fact, as shown by Charles Lieber and coworkers at Harvard, such a system can detect even a single virus particle.

HEALTH RECORD BIOCHIPS

Batelle Technology, Applied Digital Solutions, a Palm Beach technology vendor, has developed subdermal RFID tags, called VeriChips, that are about the size of a grain of rice and can be inserted under a person's skin. Their vision is that within the next 10 years, we all will be carrying our health and medical records with us, either as jewelry or as implanted chips that can be easily read and understood in a medical emergency. These biochips, or bio IDs, will carry our vital statistics and our DNA to help identify our medical needs.

Ultimately advanced computation will be implemented on the biochip to monitor (1) patient status, (2) security, and (3) release of signaling molecules from the chip, such as natural hormone releasing factors that work at very low concentrations. Substantial developments are already taking place in nanotechnology in regard to electronic systems, storage, and sensors. In fact subcomponents of computer chips are built on the nanoscale. One terabyte can be stored per square inch and future developments in storage will include use of molecules to store information just as does DNA, or specific atom placement of substrata. As the preliminary proofs-of-concept, storage has been achieved at a bit spacing of 1.5 nanometers along the tracks and 1.7 nanometers between tracks (as demonstrated as feasible by Professor F. J. Himpel, University of Wisconsin Madison). When scalable, this amounts to a data storage density of 250 trillion bits per square inch, and it is roughly comparable in density and read-speed to DNA. Such developments would be equivalent to storing the contents of 6,650 DVDs in one square inch of material.

BIONICS AND BIOROBOTICS—EASIER TO UNDERSTAND, HARDER TO ACCEPT?

As we move to still more drastic replacements, the road becomes for a while much easier to travel. At least the basic ideas of an area variously called *bionics* and *biorobotics* are familiar to us all through science fiction. Remember *The Six Million Dollar Man*, the popular American TV series of the 1970s based on the book *Cyborg* by Martin Caidin? We can rebuild him. We have the technology. We have the capability to make the world's first Bionic man." Building humans better, stronger, and faster is an achievable technology, already proved with more basic artificial limbs that need not be explored in detail.

The notion of human enhancement by mingling with machine on the larger scale is a strange ethical area. No one would fail to be happy to see a disabled person now being able to leap 6-foot high walls and run at 60 miles an hour. But if friends who are not thus disabled were to jealously desire the same superior abilities, it is a much thornier area of ethics. That is perhaps because this area seems entangled with ancient, even archetypal, notions in our brain that address it in terms of larger-than-life superheroes, supervillains, and aliens.

Greek legends are full of body-enhancing gifts. Perseus went to three blind witches that shared one "prosthetic" eye among them. By stealing the eye, Perseus made them tell him where to find the nymphs of the north. Along with a magic sword and shield, they gave him winged sandals, an infinite-capacity magic bag, and a cap that made him invisible. These latter are perhaps "add-ons" rather than intimately bonded with the body (but then so are prosthetic limbs today). On the whole, the most ancient legends tended to take a positive view of prosthetics, and it may be said that the drive for a human to live an enhanced more effective life with such gifts of the gods is as old as the human condition.

These persistent notions survive today in comic books, movies, and TV, and with many more recent foundations than just the ancient Greeks. As medical science has evolved over the last few decades, many writers have grasped the potential and provided further fuel for thought. The thought has not always been positive, however. Frankenstein's monster is an early eighteenth-century fictional creation but so enduring a theme that it has been recreated many times in moves and modern literature, as in Brian Aldiss' *Frankenstein Unbound*. He (it?) was a construct from parts so cursed and mixed that it lost its soul—usually such stories carry a message about the dangers of meddling with nature or the human soul. In fact, somewhere between the ancient classical world and Frankenstein, stories and legends have not commonly seen half human, half robot-like entities in a rosy light. There are many legends of golems or robot-like entities driven by an unholy intimate human mind or spirit. However, the distaste seems far less to arise when the guiding force within is a hero with a healthy, public spirited human consciousness, whence, like Persus, they become superheroes.

The works of fiction reflect the ethics, or ethical controversies, in a human culture, and again can provide important clues about public future reactions to new technologies. Robots and hybrid entities in Japanese *manga* (comics culture) are built in the style of the Samurai, and for the most part are good guys. In extension of the Samurai tradition, heroes of the manga and Robert A. Heinlein's *StarShoop Troopers*, can wear sophisticated performance-enhancing body armor. While admittedly Heinlein's ironclad troopers are warrior citizens of a somewhat fascist state, they are comparatively very much the good guys against a very definitely evil, insect-like, enemy that in comparison evolved biological solutions for all its technology needs, including armor, weapons capable of hitting targets in outer space, and communications. Mechanical science and engineering is often the relatively "good guy," yet a mingling of life and machine is sometimes made to seem more appropriate to the villain or alien warrior. H. G. Wells' tripods were definitely a kind of "smart body armor" extending the power of the Martians to invade Earth. Not the stuff of the well-meaning, self-respecting biped primate!

These examples suggest that all is forgiven if the enhancement is more like an add-one exoskeleton. But that itself does not bear up to deeper analysis as a key issue. For the true superhero rather than routine brave warrior, *unsolicited enhancement* seems the crux of the matter. In the modern tradition of heroes and legends as continued in the comic books, Spiderman's villainous archrival "Doc Ock" is enhanced by mechanical octopus-like arms, but not at the expense of his own limbs. In comparison, Spiderman is himself more fundamentally enhanced, but even this state is for him more excusable. That is because like the Six Million Dollar man, and also the Incredible Hulk, the Flash, and many other comic book heroes, enhancement is the result of an accident. Only the current top hero Batman remains fully human, untransformed by any physical accident but enhanced by gadgets and body armor. Still there were psychological accidents: a child falling and being stranded in a cave of bats, and witnessing the murder of his parents. It is notable that he remains an ambiguous figure, almost an anti-hero, dark and tortured by the past.

As noted above, the public perception seems much more tolerant of a person with super-abilities acquired through augmentation after an accident. Consider a very recent news item, reported on Fox News and http://www.foxnews.com/story/0,2933,289450,00.html: "The prosthetic legs double-amputee sprinter Oscar Pistorius uses provide less air resistance than normal legs, the IAAF said Monday. Pistorius, who wears curved, carbon-fiber prosthetic legs, finished second in Rome on Friday and last against elite able-bodied athlete at the British Grand Prix on Sunday. He hopes to compete at the 2008 Beijing Olympics. The International Association of Athletic Federations has been *reviewing footage from two high-definition cameras that filmed Pistorius in Rome to determine if his prosthetic racing legs give him an unfair advantage.*"

At time of writing, with much Internet "blogging" on the topic, it is clear that Oscar Pistorious wins a lot of respect even if eligibility to compete is

controversial. But what if there was no accident, and amputation and augmentation was done by choice? These issues have possibly been best expressed in
fiction by Bernard Wolfe. In 1952 he published *Limbo 90*. The book was well
received at the time: "More satisfying than Orwell's *1984* or Mr. Huxley's
Brave New World" (*The Saturday Review*). The comparisons with relatively
dark or cynical works might suggest that like many historical predecessors,
Wolfe also took a cynical view of playing with technology, and that he was
endorsing appreciation of the dangers of transgressing the natural and the
artificial. Indeed there are some different interpretations of the novel, and
some are more pessimistic. For example, Wolfe's notion of humans having
voluntary amputation in order to obtain superior prosthetic limbs makes it
seem pretty much that Wolfe was trying to raise an unfavorable gut reaction
from the reader. Critics have pointed out, however, that for the most part, the
machines and devices are not the bad guys of the book. Human greed and
naivety are the villains. At very least, Wolfe was seeing a future world in which
fusion of human and machine was the inevitable canvas, for better or for worse
(but frequently better), against which the usual human dramas would be
played out, albeit at an excitingly augmented level. He also considered,
however, that human bodies are weak and capable of useful extension by
machines and prosthetic limbs, yet that the human mind will remain more
powerful than any such artificial aid. Human brains would adapt and grow to
be able to handle very complex devices. These could lie yet close to or within
the brain's physical boundaries. The above-mentioned recent experiences with
artificial devices such as hearing devices support this, where the human brain
adapts to be able to decode alien new messages from computer chips and treat
those messages as if they were their natural counterparts. The positive part of
Wolfe's message seems therefore to be that the human mind can rise above
the perils and complexities of intimate marriage with machines.

Is enhancement when not needed fundamentally distasteful, do mechanical
solutions seem better or worse than biological ones, and when are they appropriate? So given the good intentions, heart and soul of Perseus and the Six
Million Dollar Man, could any of us become mechanically and/or biologically
augmented superheroes today? Six million dollars went a long way in those
days of the TV series. It would not get us very far now. But there is a continuing argument that if there were sufficient interest and funds, then formidable
technologies could be mobilized and many people could not only be cured or
live greatly prolonged life spans but become super-beings. This argument will
be addressed later, below. What mythology and modern comic books teach us
is that it is better to have superpowers (relative to the rest of society) thrust
upon you than self-elected, but either way, the superhero needs character. It
distinguishes him or her from the supervillain. The dictionary definitions of
"character" are something like (1) the inherent complex of attributes that
determine a persons moral and ethical actions and reactions, (2) a characteristic property that defines the apparent individual nature of something. Bill
Hybels (the founding and senior pastor of Willow Creek Community Church

in Illinois, and an author of a number of Christian books, especially on the subject of Christian leadership) defined "character" as "a will power to do a right thing at any cost" in his book titled *Who You Are When No One's Looking*. We would somewhat similarly define "character" as a will power to do a right thing as a good-faith return to the society without anticipating any rewards or recognition in any circumstances and at any cost. And, as Spiderman was taught, "With great power comes great responsibility."

The next likely advance seems oddly more acceptable to many, perhaps because in its fullest vision it is indistinguishable from magic. We are reminded of the adage due to science fiction guru Arthur C. Clarke that a sufficiently advanced technology is indistinguishable from magic.

NANOTECHNOLOGY

When the great American comic book heroes were created, their super-attributes were acquired by a variety of scientific accidents reflecting the state of science at the time, and all the better if the science involved mechanisms that are not well understood, like mutation caused by radiation. Strangely, it is not so long ago that patients were exposed to radiation to improve well-being, and the notion that exposure to UV does so persists to this day (if only to make one look like he or she has a healthy outdoor life!). Spiderman was in the original comics the result of a radioactive spider bite, for example. But we know a lot more now about the risks and benefits of radiation, and in the modern movie versions, the technology that many perceive as in a comparable "weird mechanism" is *nanotechnology*. The latest movie Spiderman was bitten by a spider, but it wasn't radioactive. It was carrying small nanotechnological devices called *nanobots* (from *nano-robots*) developed by human research.

We will return to nanobots later, as a more futuristic theme. They are a long-term feature of nanotechnology that we do not require in our armory in order that nanotechnology may be useful right now. In fact nanotechnology gained more public visibility outside of fiction on December 3, 2003 when President Bush signed a law authorizing federal research and development subsidies of $3.7 billion over the four years as of October 2004. Nanogen, one of a handful of publicly traded start-up companies, received a patent for a nanoscale manufacturing method that is claimed to make advanced micro-chips and flat-panel displays. The US National Science Foundation (NSF) predicts that nanotechnology will contribute $1 trillion a year to the United States economy by 2015.

So outside of science fiction, what is this nanotechnology that seems to have such diverse facets from the bizarre to the practical? The prefix "nano" in terms like "nanotechnology" or "nano-scale" simply means very small. The original Greek word "nano" means "very small" or "dwarf." However, its modern more specific use is to indicate a scale of a billionth of a meter (i.e., 10^{-9} or 0.000000001 meters). That is, nanotechnology draws its name from the nanometer, 100,000th of a human hair in diameter and the length of 10 hydrogen atoms joined up in a row. Another "scientists' style" definition that comes to the same thing but avoids actual numbers is to say it concerns technologies that operate on the range of scale between atomic distances and the wavelength of visible light. In 1974 Norio Taniguchi of Tokyo Science University first coined the term nanotechnology. Taniguchi was interested in the problem of manufacturing materials with nanometer tolerances. The term was used in his papers "Nanotechnology: integrated processing systems for ultra-precision and ultra-fine products" and "On the Basic Concept of Nanotechnology"[1] His basic definition of nanotechnology stands up pretty well today too: "'Nanotechnology' mainly consists of the processing of separation, consolidation, and deformation of materials by one atom or one molecule."

The basic idea then is not to study atoms but to manipulate atoms. It is important to understand the thinking that went before in order to see the important distinction. In a way chemists and physicists have been thinking about and even manipulating atoms for centuries, but in vast collections and not at an atom at a time, to assemble heterogeneous systems with vast information density in their seeming infinite detail. The basic understanding of atoms is, in contrast, far from new and takes us back again to the ancient Greeks. As long ago as the fifth century BC, Democritus and Leucippus conceived that matter was made up of tiny, indivisible particles in constant motion. Aristotle disagreed, and his influence at that time was such that the idea was developed in detail until the 1600s, when Sir Isaac Newton proposed an atomic model in "The Mathematical Principles of Natural Philosophy," more commonly known as *The Principia*. John Dalton (1766–1844) developed the first useful atomic theory of matter around 1803. Some of the finer details of Dalton's atomic theory have since been dethroned. However, the central concepts (that chemical reactions can be explained by the linkage and separation of atoms with different characteristic properties) are used today. British physicist, J. J. Thomson (1856–1940) at the Cavendish Laboratory at Cambridge University, discovered that electrons made up almost all of the volume of atoms. Previously scientists thought that the atom was indivisible, being the most fundamental unit of matter; remember the Greek word "atom" means indivisible. Thomson also discovered the isotope (i.e., atoms of the same chemical element whose nuclei have the same atomic number but different atomic weights). The atomic number corresponds to the number of protons in an atom, and isotopes of each element contain the same number of protons. Different atomic weights among elements are the result of the differences in the number of neutrons in the nuclei. In 1911 Thomson's student, Ernest Rutherford, suggested a more refined model for the atom in which there was a center of the atom, now known as the nucleus around which electrons revolved. Rutherford also discovered the proton and neutron. Three years later Swedish physicist Niels Bohr advanced atomic theory further in discovering that electrons

---

[1] Proc. Intl. Conf. Prod. Eng. Tokyo, Part II, Japan Society of Precision Engineering, 1974.

traveled around the nucleus in fixed energy levels, laying the basis of, among other things, theoretical chemistry for drug design, and the understanding of the forces and linkages from which things could be built with atoms.

Basically all these essential founding efforts were restricted by a seeming law of nature that, as far as individual atoms were concerned, "You can look but you better not touch!" Following the work by Bohr and others, quantum mechanics and statistical mechanics became computational means of calculating the observed properties of populations of billions of molecules. But consideration of such massive collections seemed to place an even greater barrier between the commonsense world and the world of individual particles. Individual atoms became not only (almost) officially untouchable, but downright weird in their behavior, neither here nor there but smears of probability in space–time, forever beyond human ken.

Against the background of that troublesome philosophy, the great late twentieth-century physicist Richard P. Feynman (Nobel Prize winner for physics in 1965) is celebrated as being the thought-father of *the manipulation of individual atoms*. Unlike his intellectual successor Norio Taniguchi, he never used the word nanotechnology, but it is clear that he had the same concept in mind and in even more general and powerful way. It started with an interest in what exactly were the physical challenges in working with the very small. He could not see an obvious insurmountable barrier. He stated in the 1960s: "It would be interesting in surgery if you could swallow the surgeon. You put the mechanical surgeon inside the blood vessel and it goes into the heart and 'looks' around. ... Other small machines might be permanently incorporated in the body to assist some inadequately-functioning organ." Likely this inspired *Fantastic Voyage*, a (1966) book by Isaac Asimov, then a biochemistry professor in Texas, who shifted the focus of the time from outer space to inner space— the world within our bodies. In this book a miniaturization technology has been developed. Five scientists in a futuristic submarine who were miniaturized and injected into a patient's body destroyed a blood clot. As with so many of Asimov's visions, this was prophetic. Although we do not even remotely see how to miniaturize whole people, we probably will be able to make miniaturized whole components even down to the molecular scale. Researchers hope to develop blood cell size nanobots to be sent into the human body on vital health missions.

There is no doubt that in thinking about the very small, Feynman was thinking about manipulating atoms. Feynman's famous lecture "There's Plenty of Room at the Bottom," was pre-suspected by a few to be a complaint about his place in the hierarchy of academe. In fact it turned out that he was asking further relevant questions about engineering the world of the incredibly small, such as: "Why cannot we write the entire 24 volumes of the *Encyclopaedia Britannica* on the head of a pin?" The talk Feynman gave was later published in the February 1960 issue of Caltech's Engineering and Science, which many say represents the first statement on nanotechnology. Feynman also asked questions such as "What are the limitations as to how small a thing has to be before you can no longer mold it?" Essentially he saw the prevailing manufacturing processes of cutting, soldering, stamping, and drilling as crude. Final products took up too much space and needed huge amounts of energy to function. He also asked whether human engineers couldn't manufacture things at the same level as living cells. Indeed why we couldn't manufacture not only at the cellular level, but better still, at the atomic level? Could one make machines out of atoms? Feynman was more than well aware of the problems surrounding the notion of building with atoms. As we noted above, he was raised in the era of quantum mechanics and statistical mechanics, and the near-doctrine of "untouchable atoms." Things do not simply scale down in proportion, and the laws of quantum mechanics, chemistry, and physics would come into question.

But what does it all really mean for us? Quite a lot! Feynman-like thinking became an accepted biomedical research topic by the mid-1990s. The National Institutes of Health were quick to see the medical applications, defining nanotechnology as "the creation of functional devices, materials and systems through the control of matter of 1 to 100 nanometers, and the exploitation of novel properties and phenomena at the same scale." Here are some "nano disciplines" and "nano products" that are already becoming of interest to industry:

1. Nanomaterials science for interfacing with living tissues, for delivery of pharmaceuticals, tissue-engineering scaffolds, wound repair, adhesion prevention, and other biological agents and medical devices.
2. Nanoimaging for real-time imaging of structure, function, properties, and metabolism inside cells.
3. Nanoscale research on cellular processes, including macromolecules, multimolecular assembly, membranes, organelles, and macromolecules.
4. Biosensing and biosignaling.
5. Nanomotors for understanding structure/function and self-assembly and primary and secondary power supply.
6. Mechanical, chemical, and cellular implant nanotechnologies to repair or replace tissues.
7. Nanobioprocessors for implantable nanoscale processors to modify biological pathways and processes.
8. Nanosystem design and application as fundamental principles and tools to measure and image the biological processes of health and disease, and methods to assemble nanosystems.
9. "Nanoplumbing" components such as valves, microfluidic channels, and pumps.
10. New methods for probing biological properties and phenomena not well understood at the nanometer scale and for characterizing nanoscale materials.

11. Smarter fluorescent probe devices at the nanometer scale for monitoring biochemical processes in and on cells.
12. "Smart" biocompatible nano materials for self-assembling techniques and self-patterning materials.
13. Biosensor nanotechnologies for detection and analysis of biologically relevant molecular and physical targets in samples from body fluids in vitro, or even for use in vivo, within in the living body.

With further exploitation of advanced biotechnology, IT, and nanotechnology we may one far-off day not only enjoy prolonged disease-free healthy lives but also be able to perfect ourselves by enhancing our brains for higher analytical thinking and reasoning abilities, and for higher controlling skills for solving mathematical problems, learning multiple languages, and playing musical instruments. In addition the facial features can be genetically enhanced to perfect them for beautiful faces through cell rejuvenation. Implanted nanodevices will compensate the functions of heart to pump superstrong bloodstreams, of eyes for not only 20–20 vision without eyeglasses but also for telescopic and microscopic vision … the Six Million Dollar man and woman, a trillion fold! Will these blessings fall only upon a controlling elite or wealthy few? It is hard to eliminate entirely the sin of greed and "divine right for me, not for you" instinct of humans, but hopefully healthcare IT will level the playing field and help set the proper tone for equal rights for all in matters of health and well-being. But note anyway that the price falls for technology that gets used. The original human genome projects are said to cost about $3 billion, all told, yet we are close to the $1,000 genome! The Honeywell Datamatic 1000 computer, first introduced in 1957 cost several million dollars, filled a 6,000 square-foot room, required a cooling system that used 1,000 gallons of water per minute, and did less than your laptop. What makes the difference is when something can be made automatically in bulk, and as discussed below, that may well be the *forte* of nanotechnology.

FIRST REAL STEPS IN NANOTECHNOLOGY

There are already things in nature on the nanoscale known to our forebearers, and some have even been tools. Obsidian blades carved by our prehistoric ancestors had blade edges so fine that they were on the nanoscale, and such blades are made and used for surgery even today. In more recent history Kodak found out in the 1930s a way to insert a layer of nanoscale silver particles in its film to filter light. Similarly vesicles of partially oily partially water-liking molecules called liposomes are produced by agitation in water but are often found naturally: the trick is to make them homogeneous in size. They become important vehicles for delivering certain drugs.

Another major contribution well-found in nature comes from soot. Richard Smalley discovered C60, the soccer-ball-like sphere made of 60 carbon atoms

C60 (Buckminsterfullerene, also known as the "buckyball"). Along with other fullerenes such as C70, they constitute a cage-like class of molecules now constituting third allotropic form of carbon (after graphite and diamond). Smalley was the founding director of the Center for Nanoscale Science and Technology (at Rice University) from 1996 to 2002. He is now director of the new Carbon Nanotechnology Laboratory at Rice university, Houston, Texas. The *buckytubes* he now studies are elongated fullerenes that are essentially a new high tech polymer, following on from nylon, polypropylene, and Kevlar. When very long, they are usually called *nanotubes*. They conduct electricity and are likely to find applications in several areas of electronics. In February 2000 this research led to the start-up of a company called Carbon Nanotechnologies, Inc. Carbon nanotubes were discovered in 1991 by S. Iijima. They are unique for their size, shape, and remarkable physical properties, which are still being researched and discovered. Carbon nanotubes are extremely thin, hollow cylinders made of carbon atoms. Their diameter is about 10,000 times smaller than a human hair. Nanotubes, depending on their structure, can be metals or semiconductors. They are also extremely strong materials and have good thermal conductivity. The characteristics above have generated strong interest in their possible use in nanoelectronic and nanome-chanical devices. For example, they can be used as nanowires or as active components in electronic devices such as the field-effect transistor.

As it happens, the electronics and IT industries have made major contribu-tions to the birth of nanotechnology, a future they may help see through to the "end of days." Magnetic recording for computers and other digital equip-ment had been increasing its data density at a rate of 60% a year, doubling every 18 months, just like a celebrated Moore's law of transistor or microchip density and performance. The main way of storing computer data seemed likely to reach physical limits in the next decade or so, to a level that made it difficult to keep the tiny data bits stable. So researchers began exploring poten-tial successor technologies, including atom sensing and manipulation tech-niques, that seemed as if data densities might be enabled well beyond the current storage density of magnetic recording. Strangely the devices resulting were relatively simple instruments operating on laboratory benchtops: the scanning tunneling microscope (STM), and later the atomic force microscope (AFM) discussed below. The STM was developed by G. Binnig and H. Rohrer at an IBM Research Lab in Zurich, Switzerland, during the late 1970s and early 1980s. The central component is an extremely sharp needle or tip made from a metal, such as tungsten, nickel, or gold, mounted within an array of ceramic piezoelectric elements. These can control the needle's position in three dimensions because they contract or expand by small amounts when a voltage is applied to them. The movements induced by the voltage may be smaller than a tenth of a nanometer. This allows the extremely fine control necessary for successful imaging and manipulation at the atomic and molecular level. In addition there are means of "feeling" the atoms that the tip is in contact with. At such minute distances the electron clouds of the atoms in the tip begin to overlap with those of the atoms on the surface of the sample. When a voltage is applied, these quantum effects permit electrons to "tunnel" across the gap. The voltage creates a minute but detectable "tunneling current" that is extremely sensitive to the distance between the tip and the surface. Because the current increases rapidly as the distances decreases, changes of less than a tenth of a nanometer in the position of the tip can be detected. Although it is often said the STM can see individual atoms, what the instrument is actually imaging is the structure of the electron clouds of the surface atoms in the sample. To generate an image, such a tip scans the surface by adjusting its height continually so as to keep the tunneling current constant, while rising to glide over nano-hills and dropping down into nano-valleys. These movements generate a topographic map of a small part of the surface. The STM was therefore initially used as an imaging device.

However, the STM has also been used in an increasingly sophisticated manner to manipulate atoms and clusters of atoms. When it happened, it got international press coverage: IBM researchers used AFM to arrange 35 xenon atoms to spell "IBM," creating the world's smallest logo. Donald Eigler and Erhard Schweizer accomplished this feat with a carefully prepared nickel surface as a substrate and xenon atoms as a working material. The surface corrugations between rows of nickel atoms are large enough to keep xenon atoms in place during STM imaging, yet small enough to permit the xenon atoms to be pulled along the surface during fabrication. To move a xenon atom, the researchers positioned the STM tip over the atom using the imaging mode, and then switched to atom-moving mode by lowering the tip toward the xenon atom until the tunneling current increased significantly. The xenon atom, attracted to the tip, could be dragged by moving the STM tip horizontally. Reducing the tunneling current retracted the tip and left the xenon atom in a new location on the nickel.

Progress continues. Since the STM is only seeing an "electronic" surface, in a sense it only has a kind of "night vision"; it cannot really distinguish very well subtle hues, meaning here the differences between atoms of different elements (except for hints based on size and density). To overcome this and other limitations, Gerd Binnig, along with Calvin Quate of Stanford University and Christopher Gerber from IBM Zurich, developed a modified version of the STM. This was an atomic force microscope (AFM) that did not rely on electron flow. Instead, the tip of the scanning needle is brought into contact with the sample surface, albeit with a very light touch. The downward force is exerted by a finely calibrated, spring-like micromachined cantilever mechanism. Images are again generated by scanning the tip across the surface. However, instead of adjusting the height to maintain a constant current, the AFM adjusts the height to maintain a constant force of impact. As with the STM, these movements are used to build up a sort of atomic-scale map of the surface. The maps are getting better, and the rush is now on to construct more elaborate methods capable of making more elaborate nano-structures than an IBM logo!

Nanotechnology promises very long-term benefits for everyday life. At the turn of the new millennium, nanotechnology of a perhaps simpler kind already became a significant force in industry. The new generation of advanced materials is already changing our traditional approaches for many products, even by borrowing from nature or at least nature's ideas. For example, coatings made with aluminum-titanium nanoparticles add to the durability of boiler components and submarine periscopes for the United States Navy; carbon nanotubes add stiffness to tennis rackets; nanoscale clay particles strengthen car bodies; and pants are being made with techniques that alter the structure of cotton to create nanoscale whiskers and make the fabric more stain resistant. However, some promising concepts, like computers that replace silicon transistors with single molecules and new materials (e.g., the carbon nanotubes) that are many times stronger than steel, still have a long way to go to be materialized for commercial use. So what is in this development for medicine? In parallel has grown an industry in *biomaterials*, new smarter materials that will mix well with our bodies to strengthen and repair them.

The nanoscale is rapidly becoming no longer the exclusive domain of nature. Increasingly we need less and less to borrow from nature's helpful gifts and clues like obsidian shards, metallic particles, oily droplets, and soot. That all said, however, there is an even larger area of nature's gifts that remain yet to be exploited.

NANOTECHNOLOGY AS BIOTECHNOLOGY

A glaring omission in the above is that biology already provides beautiful examples of nanotechnology, and moreover also provides us also with ready-made nano-scale tools such as enzymes and antibodies for research and therapy. In a very real sense it *is* nanotechnology. It is a nanotechnology evolved through trial and error over nearly five billion years.

Some natural large biomolecules or well-defined molecular assemblies on the nano-scale are already poised to enter the arena of drug delivery, and incidentally have roles in the pharmaceutical industry and the *cosmoceutical* industry, a new hybrid of the pharmaceutical and cosmetic products. Liposomes, microsomes, and micelles are bodies derived from fats. More generally, such lipid vehicles are balloon-like entities with a lipid skin and water-filled interior, but they can have many skins as an onion, where a water-compatible drug may still be accommodated between the skins. Such vehicles are already being used in drug delivery. Some are all skin—the lipid fills the entire phase, an obvious attraction in the use of fat-soluble drugs that cannot dissolve well in water. Both types of vehicle are, in principle, able to merge with a target cell membrane (the targeting could be done by specially prepared antibody components) and enter the cell, typically in an in-tucking of the cell membrane, which becomes the cell's endosome. A dendromer is an alternative that is throughout more or less exposed to water but consists of highly branched polymers looking more like a fur ball. By "more or less" is meant that some parts may contain small amounts of high structuralized water—structuralized—by having very few water molecules bound to the arms of the polymer. One consequence is that the drug molecule or molecules can be conveniently trapped in the structuralized water. Another is that under certain physical conditions or by simple chemical reaction, the polymer can be made to swell like a gel and release the drug.

All such seem to fall short, however, of the dazzling capabilities of proteins. Proteins are long chains of amino acids. They are shining examples to the nanotechnology industry. In a way that is instructed by the specific order of 20 types of amino acid in those long chains, they can fold up themselves in a second or less into little machines. These machines catalyze chemical reactions (as enzymes in metabolism), carry molecules and chromosomes to required destinations, detect and emit light, detect electrical fields, move electrons like microcircuitry (in the chloroplasts and mitochondria of cells) to sniff out the mate to an insect by detecting tiny traces of pheromones, move molecular levers and hence ultimately cilia and muscle fibers, and (in their role as antibodies) to recognize and attack invading molecules and organisms.

Human inventions of nanotechnology and biotechnology promise to mix very well with each other and with nature's own efforts. New industry terms even reflect this. Bio-nanotechnology and nano-biotechnology are important and only vaguely distinct terms that combine the science of nanotechnology with biotechnology. Rather like bionic prosthetics, they may involve joining of natural proteins and nucleic acids with synthetic components, but now all on the nano-scale.

An incentive to the nanotechnology industry is that the flow is not all from molecular-scale engineering to biology. It can flow the other way too. Andrew McMillan and his team at the NASA Ames Research Center in California started with natural molecular structures. These were "heat shock" proteins from microbes that live in hot springs. These proteins naturally assemble into cage-like structures called chaperonins. They allow the microbes to survive the high temperatures of hot springs. In the lab the team steered the proteins to form lattices, with a lattice spacing of 20 nanometers. They then engineered the proteins so that they could trap tiny magnetic particles in a regular array. That is a potential basis for a computer memory 100 times as compact as today's hard disks, said McMillan. He noted that if you could make each 10-nanometer particle represent a bit of data, you'd have an incredible high-density computer "disk," close to Feynman's idea of *Encyclopaedia Britannica* on the head of a pin.

The importance of all this research is that it leads to (or gives ideas about) smaller and ever more intelligent biochips in our bodies, including our brains. Susan Lindquist, director of the MIT Whitehead Institute for Biomedical Research, is working on very small computer chips. She is doing the requisite nanotechnology for this with the help of aberrant shapes of proteins, the *prions* that are responsible for mad cow disease and Creuzfeldt-Jacob disease in humans but are safe when they are the form found in yeast. She genetically engineered these fiber-forming prions so that they could bind to gold and silver particles of nano size, forming ultrafine conductive wires for nano-scale computer circuits. Her neighbor Angela Belcher at MIT manufactured semiconductor materials into circuits less than a hundredth the size of devices on a standard microchip. She, however, used viruses called bacteriophages (viruses that normally infect bacteria), engineered in her Biomolecular Materials Group laboratory to have "plug-in points" that can bind and handle 30 different molecular-scale devices. Viruses are little more than DNA with a protein coat, but they have one aspect reminiscent of the nanobot dream of nanotechnology: they reproduce or replicate. Belcher makes viruses to reproduce in millions. Typical of the character of much current work, the natural molecules involved (here in Belcher's viruses) are modified to bind to certain materials, metals being the recurrent material in much contemporary work. After much breeding and selection of viruses, not unlike that in breeding new varieties of animal and plant, she made new viruses that bind to a semiconductor and trigger the semiconductor materials to adhere all over their protein coats, forming tubular wires.

TOWARD QUANTUM COMPUTING

Nature so far is much better at the ability to have components that recognize and dock with each other, the essential basis for the built-in instructions for the nanoengineer's construction kit. So fortunately nanotubes can be combined with biological components, say proteins and DNA, to aid assembly. Like proteins, DNA has recognition too. The double strands of DNA zip together in a precise way, with each strand seeking and linking to another strand containing a matching sequence of genetic code. Erez Braun and his team at the Technion, Israel Institute of Technology, recently exploited this to make circuits out of carbon nanotubes. We may recall that nanotubes have extraordinary electrical properties that could make them the basis of future nanoelectronics. Braun and his team described how they used DNA, along with certain proteins, as "smart Velcro" to connect nanotubes to minuscule electrodes. The result was a set of the basic components of a minute computer chip, but fabricated in a "test tube."

Space does not permit detailed discussion of all the interesting variants in DNA nanotechnology and DNA/RNA computing, which seemed to have multiplied explosively in very recent years. They include quite complex logic processing with loops of nucleic acids using G to C and A to T pairing, and innate catalytic activity. There are also the peptide nucleic acids, or PNAs, that is, nucleic acid with a protein-like, instead of nucleic acid-like, backbone. Though it is reasonable to say that they are totally artificial in architecture, the DNA/RNA pattern matching code is retained, that is, G with C, A with T, and it has been conjectured that their great stability makes them a possible candidate for the "molecule of life" on very early, and hence hot, Earth. If this rate of process keeps up, we might see soon the electrical, pattern-matching, and catalytic properties of nucleic acids and PNAs combined in some quite complex artificial structures with remarkable functions.

A very potent means of computation on computer chips of this scale would be to use them for quantum computing. Already in the microscopic world, and for a short time, multiple universes can occur for an event, and this promises an extraordinarily high degree of parallelism for extremely efficient computing. It unlikely to develop soon until a bottleneck problem called "decoherence" is overcome, in which these multiple universes collapse to one and give us the common sense world we see. With advances in quantum computing there will come smaller, more powerful computers and electronics that will allow appliances and other products to make intelligent decisions for us. But it is very difficult to establish a timeline: 2010? 2030? 2050?

PRACTICAL BIONANOTECHNOLOGY NOW, USING ANTIBODIES AND MIRRORS!

Nanotechnological work flowing into medicine has perhaps been slower, not least because of strict requirements of the food and drug authorities. An exception is the use of those proteins that we call antibodies. They are also of interest to nanotechnology with the aim of exploiting nature's solution to a very difficult problem. In nanotechnology the parts must find right partners, assemble, and then recognize the appropriate place in the body with which to interact. So how does one build a surface complex enough to recognize uniquely another surface, and also to bind to precise molecular targets in the body? The quick biotechnology answer is to make specific antibodies to order by presenting a sheep or cow, for example, with the molecular target required (or an analogue thereof) and, stimulated by known methods, the animal's immune system will make the antibody required to fit. While antibodies are a great shortcut, the newly arising problem is that they are biological and look like invading biological material, raising a defensive or adverse reaction from the patient. W. Wait Gibbs published an article in the *Scientific American* (August 2005) on "nanobodies," which are much smaller versions of normal antibodies that are produced by camels and llamas (for the readers who is a molecular biologist, this means that these antibodies lack the "light chain"). Nanobodies can be produced much the same as normal antibodies from mice, rabbits, sheep, and other animals, to hit specific targets and, potentially, human tumors. The natural camel and llama products already have shown great penetration and survival skills when injected into human patients as the basis of a therapeutic, but a form cloned by genetic engineering in an animal of choice is being explored to allow for more refinement and tweaking.

The reaction of the body's defenses to bio-like materials is nonetheless a persistent general problem for many contemporary things on the nanoscale.

Proteins recognized by the T-system (thymus-based immune system) of the body as not our own are subject to attack from protein-degrading enzymes, and visible and vulnerable to our immune systems. That is the problem with transplants. Primarily the teeth of this self/nonself recognition system lies in the protein products of genes known as HLA genes. To our natural defenses, most nanoscale devices right now simply look too much like invading organisms.

To slip past the body's defenses, one of the authors (BR) led a team that was concerned with borrowing the nano-design plan from nature, but not the material. The ability of Steve Kent from the Scripp's Institute to chemically synthesize whole proteins allowed us to do adopt that chemistry under his guidance without help from any living material. Once one has that power, proteins can be made with many useful chemical modifications. Notably they can be made using D-amino acids, mirror images of the normal forms. Indeed they can be made entirely of mirror images. The protein then folds and functions, in its otherwise normal biological way but all in reverse image. The body does not recognize such molecules: they are more like plastics. However, ancient mechanisms for dealing with D-amino acids in peptides do eventually cut in so that the plastic is biodegradable, not like a silicone. The remaining problem is to get the molecule to act in the biological way when what it targets, sees, and acts on is biological, but to its own "eyes" now looks like a mirror image of what nature intended it to be. A patent application was filed for that nano design. If the target is made in mirror image, then normal antibodies are raised to recognize it, and the antibody heads are synthesized chemically in mirror image. Here again, the antibodies are used as the "good guys," not part of the defense system that one is trying to elude. The essential message is that there are tricks that allow us to borrow from nature's ideas without actually using the same material. It is the information content that nature has evolved over billions of years that really matters. Most of the biological molecules we see are only minutes to months old, anyway.

ANY ADEQUATELY EQUIPPED BIONANOTECHNOLOGICAL DEVICE STARTS LOOKING LIKE A TINY ROBOT

In molecular devices for medical application, typically speaking the principle actor is only one component, the payload, namely the repair equipment or the drug. The rest of the structure is to get the payload material where it needs to be, from gut to blood, from blood to tissue, and from cell surface to cellular compartment, and maybe into the chromosome. There is effectively a series of distinct keys to be used, a bit like those you must win to get you to your goal in a computer-based adventure game. Most such structures functioning as elaborate "antibiotics" are injected into the bloodstream, and they recognize, bind to, and possibly enter an infecting bacterium, parasite, or cancer cell. Those that enter the cell also may need to have features that allow them to escape from that intracellular organelle known as the endosome, which encapsulates many kinds of natural and unnatural cell visitors. When the payload is a gene or gene section, as in gene therapy, the construct must also target another intracellular organelle, in that case the nucleus, enter it, and insert the payload DNA into that of the patient. To do that, gene therapy requires the construct to contain or otherwise utilize an enzyme and associated proteins or nucleic acids that help position and insert the new genetic component in the precise manner required into the patient's chromosome.

All the steps above require some distinct molecular component, each analogous to a key or other tool. Thus, if many imminent agents are not actually yet like a machine, they can at least look like a complex multi-tool, like a Swiss Army Knife®. In most cases the carrying function part can be distinguished as a component called the *vehicle*. Such a "trucking role" sounds fairly simple. It could be simple molecules with attachment points like chemical hooks. But it could be a more complex protein construct like a virus, the exterior of which provides also the support for the other tools. Under the electron microscope, it would start looking more like a nanobot from science fiction.

THE COMING AGE OF NANOBOTS?

The IT industry can provide powerful computers to help design nanotechnological materials, but can it return to a more central role, such as nano-scale robotics? We introduced nanotechnology by reference to nanobots because these are a familiar theme in contemporary science fiction. Can such science fiction ever be fact? Let us not lose the significance of the challenge and take things for granted just by overuse of the word "nano." Nanobots, sometimes called *nanites*, are after all robots whose key features will be measured in billionths of a meter!

There are many researchers who not only expect that day, but pray fervently for it. To some the fact that nanotechnology has been so far a kind of biotechnology plus a science of obsidian, metallic particles, oily droplets, soot, metal-coated prion, and so on, is a disappointment and a severe limitation. A bigger picture, they feel, is needed to unleash nanotechnology's full power. To this end, nanotechnology has its own philosophy and to some, it even has a hint of religion. To its most orthodox high priests, starting as above from biology's gifts is a kind of cheating, even when medicine is the aim. The reason seems to be that in borrowing from nature, and especially from biology, we are much like peasants in the Dark Ages, living among ruins and borrowing stones from sophisticated structures left by the Romans. We ought to know how to do things ourselves, to design and build our own structures atom by atom. The argument is that science and technology have so far been working mainly "top down." But now we will be building from the bottom up, building with atoms as building blocks. And as Feynman said, "There is plenty of room at the bottom."

If Feynman was the prophet and workers we noted above were among the converted, Eric Drexler was the ultimate evangelist. Eric Drexler took the word "nano" and explored the subject in much greater detail. In 1986 he published the celebrated and important *Engines of Creation: The Coming Era of Nanotechnology*. However he was not actually the first to use the term. Interestingly Drexler did not yet have his PhD when he wrote his book, but it was the basis of a postdoctoral thesis in 1991 called *Nanosystems: Molecular Machinery, Manufacturing, and Computation*. So MIT awarded Drexler the first ever PhD in molecular nanotechnology. Although Drexler was not the first to consider the notion of molecular-scale machines, and indeed there were several independent efforts. But thanks to him, nanotechnology became a buzzword for a then hypothetical discipline that spawned much fervor in the late 1990s.

The novel idea introduced by Drexler was the seeming need for nano-machines to replicate; otherwise, we would have to painfully manufacture countless millions of them to have a significant affect on large-scale matter, such as human patients. Actually, his contribution was to develop an idea in greater detail that he would have learned from a 1980 NASA study on advanced automation for space missions, by request of then President Jimmy Carter, at a cost of nearly $12 million, even though the program caught no great attention. The study called for a self-replicating automated lunar factory system: "… designing the factory as an automated, multiproduct, remotely controlled, reprogrammable Lunar Manufacturing Facility (LMF) capable of constructing duplicates which would themselves be capable of further replication. Successive new systems need not be exact copies of the original, but could, by remote design and control, be improved, reorganized, or enlarged so as to reflect changing human requirements." In the study NASA gave Hungarian-American mathematician John von Neumann most of the credit for the conception of self-reproducing machines in 1966. He had noted that the basic principles are (1) follow instructions to make machinery, (2) copy the instructions, (3) divide the machinery, providing a sufficient set in each half, (4) assign a set of instructions to each half, and (5) complete the physical separation. This conceptually follows the process in living cells.

We are now in what is sometimes called the third generation of robotics, perhaps the fourth or fifth will involve robots on the nano-scale. However, some primitive nanotechnology devices have been tested. An example is a sensor having a switch approximately 1.5 nanometers across, capable of counting specific molecules in a chemical sample. Advanced sensors, nanotechnology, fuel cell development, and studies in neural network processing are all leading toward a future where robots not only do heavy lifting and carry freight in unattended autonomous vehicles, they also will be used in space exploration, national defense, and even injected into your bloodstream to conduct medical procedures for diagnosis, treatment, or monitoring. They will be the size of bacteria, covered with a protein-like skin that makes them look like human blood cells to the human body. Injected into the body, these tiny sensors circulate harmlessly in the bloodstream, recording body chemistry, blood flow and pressure, and whatever else they had been programmed to monitor. They will report the information to outside monitors by constructing characteristic information signatures easily detected by the inexpensive monitors in the shape of scanners, perhaps built into the next generation of "smart clothing."

The ultimate medical nanobots are nano-electromechanical surgeons and nurses that some day our physicians will be able to inject into our bloodstream or implant in our body. Most likely, such nanobots will be powered (not by a normal battery) but by chemical energy such as that provided by the hydrolysis of adenosine triphosphate (ATP, the energy coin molecules of the living cell) molecules into adenosine diphosphate (ADP, the burned-out form) molecules. Robots, as defined by the Robotics Institute of America, are "reprogrammable multifunctional manipulator(s) designed to move material, parts, tools, or specialized devices through various programmed motions for performance of a variety of tasks."

Although we won't literally be shrinking ourselves to ride inside these nanobots as in Asimov's imaginary tale, we will be able to control their movements and actions remotely as soldiers today control smart weapons systems. Control of the nanobots could be by on-board nanoscale computers, by external control, or a combination of the two. So alternatively, or as well, these devices could be controlled by artificial intelligence in tiny on-board computers, but they will almost certainly communicate somehow with external supercomputers that "beam" the itinerant software into the nanobots instructing them to smooth things around inside our body and keep us healthy. At the very least, a degree of external control is desirable; it must to compensate for errors, and stop the nanobots "running amuck." The growing "urban legend" among scientists is that these things could run amuck and reduce all around us to a "gray goo."

JUST A FEW NANO-PROBLEMS TO SOLVE FIRST

Seemingly obvious in the connection between nanobots and computers is that their communication will be by radio with external computers, rather like NASA space missions guided by the computers in Houston. Great idea! But any direct contact by radio seemed out of the picture. The difficulty is not just because nanobots are weak signal strength emitters, it is that they are very small and likely to be sparsely populating the body; thus overall the signal is very weak and also the signal strength varies. The fact is that electromagnetic radiation, including cosmic rays, X rays, ultraviolet, visible light, infra red, microwaves, and radio waves—here on order of increasing wavelength, and decreasing frequency and hence decreasing energy—can only interact with objects of size comparable with their wavelength. So, to send and receive a signal, the aerial you use must be of the same size of the wavelength of electromagnetic radiation with which you wish to communicate. You have probably noticed how big your radio and TV aerials are. However, see the article by Ed Regis (Scientific American, March 2009 (Vol. 300, no.3). Nonotubes are tiny radios!

Criticisms have been raised from time to time by the editors of *Scientific American*, not a big fan of the wilder fringe thinkers of nanotechnology (although the issues raised in this book are less insurmountable). As the *Scientific American* put it, how would these nanobots see to carry out their tasks? How would they report back to us?

If we push up through infrared and microwave, then we also have some chance of interacting directly with the motions of molecular arms, and the like, attached to the nanomachines. Likely the noise from the vibrations and rotations of all the other molecules in the body will drown out the signal, and increasing the strength to that approaching the strength of a microwave oven may get a signal to your nanobots but does not seem like a cool idea. Water at 70% of the human body provides the worst absorbance, in the infrared. Attention must be paid to the "water window" at 800 to 1300 nanometers. Nanospectra Biosciences, Inc. use minute glass beads with attached gold particles that can absorb light at 810 nm and cook cancer cells to which they are targeted by attached antibodies. Infrared does transmit well short distances at 650 to 1050 nm. Near the skin surface bright visible light has some chance at 700 to 900 nm—fireflies emit it from their luciferase enzymes interacting on luciferin (actually that is the ATP molecule well known to biochemists as the "energy coin" or energy rich molecule of the cell)—but again release can only be fairly near the body surface. Magnetic interactions with small metallic attachments might work—passenger pigeons were supposed to have such objects in their brain cells to help navigate in the Earth's magnetic field. Indeed using modified MRI (magnetic resonance imaging) machines and special chemical organometallic groups might have some hope of getting the signal in, but the effect of the drowning noise of the body in getting a signal out would still be a problem. Somehow electromagnetic radiation can be used, even though generally it seems easier to get a strong signal in than a weak one out. Very small RFID-style chips might act as signal relay stations and local command posts. They might even be conceived as tiny "aircraft carriers" that launch and collect the nanobots.

Somehow or other it will be done. We know at least one working communication method, the one used between nature's own nanodevices: signaling molecules, like those found in every living organism, released from one source and detected by another. Embedded microchip sensors might detect molecules released from a nanobot, or the nanobot itself, and the same chip, or a simple injection or a skin-contact diffusion pad might do the releasing.

The second major connection is that nanobots could rely minimally on external control and carry their own programs. They would be the computers. How could that be done? The best way we know on the nano-scale is to use DNA or its natural relative RNA as a kind of "magnetic tape" carrying the instructions that, by its interactions with other molecules, could have a variety of chemical, mechanical, electrical, and even electromagnetic-radiation-releasing effects. Early nanobots might work on this basis, even be modified viruses or intracellular structures like ribosomes. For such systems we already know proteins that naturally interact with DNA or RNA to deliver the information encoded in it, and more to act on it. But these will also look like viruses, and the human body has enzymes and antibodies that might recognize and destroy them. One alternative is a totally new design not borrowed from nature but using new classes of polymer. Another is to use mirror image proteins referred to earlier above, and mirror image DNA or RNA. These would not be readily recognized by the body's defenses. They could be manufactured by artificial chemical synthesis, but one could imagine a time in the not so far future where synthesizing the basic construction machinery of the cell just once in mirror image (for the initiated: the RNA, the tRNA, the ribosome, and all the associated proteins) would result in a system churning out the mirror image material on demand. And in the farther future, why not make whole bacteria in mirror image, as mirror image device construction plants?

AND A POTENTIAL BIG PROBLEM ... A NANOPATH TO DESTRUCTION?

What about the risks posed by nanobots going out of control? That possibility reminds us of the Greek legend of Icarus who died for the folly of rising above the mortal, or even the German classic story written by Goethe, in which the main character Faust sold his soul to the devil in exchange for a paradise (of power and knowledge, in Goethe's version). In other words, will things ultimately be highly likely to go "pear shaped" like a bad business deal? There must be many opportunities for things to go wrong. The above-mentioned 1980 NASA study did not ignore the risks and dangers of self-replicating machines. The combination of artificial intelligence and self-replicating machines, NASA warned, could become adversarial. Without further research, there was no telling what kinds of behavior such a machine might evolve. The mandate should be "improve, protect, and increase the productivity of human society," the study reported. In the most extreme case, nanobots could, it has been perceived, run amuck much like cells do when they become cancerous, and begin manipulating atoms on a disorganized basis. That might not only harm us, but reduce all matter on Earth to a disorganized "gray goo" mentioned above. If you consider that unlikely, recall two things: (1) on the cellular scale, that is what cancer is, and (2) it is easier to imagine that something can go wrong if involves a nanotechnological weapon specifically designed to reduce an enemy to a gray goo.

The current view is that the process of self-replication can be made inherently safe, but free-roaming replicators are notably absent from current plans for developing and using molecular manufacturing. The problem is, however, that it is not that hard to imagine an unstoppable nano-scale system, even without replication cability. At first glance, the problem would be this: how could something have a specificity so broad or adaptable that it could take out many of the proteins in our body. Now consider the "mirror imaging" technology of natural proteins chemosynthesized in the same sequence but only with D-amino acids. There are some enzymes in our bodies that do destroy proteins with D-amino acids naturally, not least because flipping of the handedness of amino acids happens spontaneously all the time. It is part of aging. The amino acid called aspartic acid is particularly prone. These enzymes are very nonspecific in order to carry out their task generally. Still it is unlikely that this mechanism would work efficiently on a protein made entirely of D-amino acids. So now imagine that it is precisely this D-amino protein destroying enzyme that is made in mirror image, of D-amino acids. The rules of the mirror game is that it will now attack the mirror image of its normal D-amino acid target, namely the healthy L-amino acids that make up all our proteins. It is nonspecific, but now nonspecific to normal proteins. Our internal defenses might be useless against it. Protease enzymes cannot attack it, nor can the T-immune system that depends on protease action. The kidneys may filter it out, but the kidneys also recycle proteins from our urine (proteins are recovered—proteins in the urine are a sign of disease). Although many are degraded to free amino acids by proteases in the kidney and recycled only as such, those L-amino acid proteases again cannot work on the D-target. Many barriers like the blood–brain barrier also rely at least partly on a rejection system, including protease action, and in any event, peptides (small proteins) containing a few amino acids are known to cross such barriers; they might not be able to bar the D-invader. Although the body does have defenses (e.g., the peroxisomes), studies on the beneficial pharmaceutical properties of other D-systems suggest that they could persist in the blood and tissue for some three to six days, adequate time for a good D-protein therapeutic to do good, and adequate time for a bad one to wreak much destruction.

So some kind of molecular juggernaut on the rampage might be hard to stop. And so is our message that "nanotechnology must be stopped?" No! Bionanotechnology is inevitable, and its close relative biotechnology is already well established. Even the simplest nanotechnology, like the D-protein described above, could run amuck. In general, like any clumsy first effort, simple injudicious first attempts at bionanotechnology are intrinsically *more likely* to go wrong, with our body's natural defenses less able to stop them. All that might be able to stop them is a more *sophisticated* nanotechnology. Who knows: perhaps again military and security issues could be the driver to keep ahead of the game, and give us tools with powerful and peaceful applications. This is a gloomy view of human motivations, as for the first payload V-rockets, and the research into the atom bomb. Fortunately a gloomy view is not the prevalent one.

A REALISTIC NANOPATH TO IMMORTALITY?

Assuming the difficulties mentioned above can be overcome, most people interested in the further visions of nanotechnology have a kind of missionary zeal. Many people interested in nanotechnology take an essentially humanist perspective, but also as a route to personal immortality in a way that is somewhat at right angles to that. Several nanotech fans have arranged to have their heads frozen (after death) on the ground that future civilizations will rebuild and resuscitate them using nanotechnology. Why such a future civilization would want to do that is unclear, but certainly the chance that they will do so is higher than if you have yourself cremated or buried.

That chance, of revival after your death, would nonetheless still be very small. Would you want to revive your great grandfather? And at the end of the day, would he thank you for it? Moreover longevity seems less controversial that artificial enhancement, but not to all. Author Francis Fukuyama, for example, considers research that might extend human longevity by artificial means beyond its current fourscore years to be immoral. Prolonging life by say five hundred years does seem to carry some moral issues, but a hundred and fifty does not seem destined to be quite as controversial (discussions on Medicare apart!).

But there is a loophole to success and immortality that seems less distasteful, and more enticing, to most of us. Just stay healthy! Well, that has not led to immortality in the past, but things have changed. From our store of knowledge about nutrition we could simply use the acceptable best health principles at the time to keep going. So technology need not be perfect right now; we just need to keep going long enough until the technology *is* good enough. That might include a naturally prolonged life when nanotechnology will come of age and be acceptable while we are still living. How could we hope to benefit from advanced forms of such technology within that life span? Ray Kurzweil spent several decades studying and modeling technology trends and their impacts on society. He notes that the rate of change is itself accelerating. This means that the past is not a reliable guide to the future if done on a linear basis. The twentieth century was not 100 years of progress at today's rate but, rather, was equivalent to about 20 years because we've been speeding up to current rates of change. And we'll make another 20 years of progress at today's rate, equivalent to that of the entire twentieth century, in the next 14 years. And then we'll do it again in just 7 years. Because of this exponential growth, the twenty-first century will equal 20,000 years of progress at today's rate of progress—1,000 times greater than what we witnessed in the twentieth century, which itself was no slouch for change. The result will be profound changes in every facet of our lives, from our health and longevity to our economy and society, even our concepts of who we are and what it means to be human.

So how long would it take for technology to be available for all? In 2010, 2015, 2020, 2030, or even 2070? If the latter, surely we could never hope to live so long (being the age that we are). But recall again the Six Million Dollar

Man. Six million dollars went a long way in the 1970s, but there is today an argument that if there were sufficient interest and funds, then formidable technologies could be mobilized and many rich people could be cured or live greatly prolonged life spans.

So is hope now only for the rich? Some don't think so. A mere 150 years ago, life expectancy was 37 years; we now live longer. In *Fantastic Voyage: Live Long Enough to Live Forever* published in 2004, Ray Kurzweil got together with physician Terry Grossman to argue that if you can just keep yourself healthy long enough by current techniques, even those available on a routine basis and a simple as improve nutrition, then techniques really are getting better all the time, and at an accelerating rate. In consequence, as long as you can keep going long enough to catch the next wave in technology that is publicly available and financially acceptable, then you could end up living forever. Ultimately that next wave will be the technology of nanobots.

The road to extending longevity, say Kurzweil and Grossman, can be considered as involving three big bridges. It is not accidental that their book has the same main title as Asimov's, because nanotechnology relates to one of the last bridges to cross if you want to live forever, as well as referring to the fantastic voyage of current humans through to immortality. Their book is intended to serve as a guide to using lifestyle and nutrition to live long enough in good health and spirits, allowing you to cross bridge 1. Bridge 2 will allow you to take advantage of the full development of the biopharmaceutical technology revolution: personalized medicine, pharmacogenomics, and the like. This, in turn, will lead to what is referred to as nanotechnology (supported by IT, including artificial intelligence). This "nanotechnological" bridge 3, say the authors, has the potential to allow us to live forever.

Ray Kurzweil and Terry Grossman's ideas, if not entirely novel (it is a popular science fiction theme), are coherently and elegantly expressed, and worth thinking more about. Much attention is given to the idea of living healthily enough to make it to the point when we can be salvaged forever— should we wish it. Many other experts also believe that within a decade we will be adding more than a year to human life expectancy every year. At that point, with each passing year, your remaining life expectancy will move further into the future. Expert Aubrey de Grey believes that we will successfully stop aging in mice—who share 99% of our genetic code—within 10 years, and that similar therapies for humans (to halt and reverse aging) will follow 5 to 10 years after that. A small minority of older baby boomers will make it past this impending critical threshold. The reader could be among them.

And if you live forever, what will it mean?

THE UNIVERSE AS OUR HEALTHCARE SYSTEM?

What will this mean for healthcare in billions of years? If our engineers, or a superior race of our computational gods, do the best they can for us, then our far future will look very different. Computers will be so ubiquitous and pervasive that they will be all around us, part of the universe, and perhaps part of us, and we part of them. What we even think of as a computer, and how we distinguish it from normal "stuff," will change dramatically. The universe itself may become the ultimate engine of Hippocrates.

How would that be achieved? The means to this end we can only think of the means as being nanobots, effectively "smart matter" that can spread out and convert all other matter to its ever-evolving self. Somehow, given eons of time, shorter time with the discovery of means to beat the speed-of-light barrier (more correctly, the maximum-speed-of-information-transmission barrier), or the ability to tunnel through wormholes in space, nanobots will spread. They could have cosmological impact, rather like Tipler's vision at the end of Chapter 1. At the very least, however far we actually get, we will take our nanotechnology with us. In the *2001* series of films based on the writings of Arthur C Clarke, an alien black obelisk or "slab" has the power to transform humans, act as a gateway through time and space, to replicate and also convert planets. Like augmented superheroes, such themes may strike an "archetypal chord" in human memory, since the story is not unlike one from ancient Egypt in which a singing obelisk also taught early humans to use tools. In Clarkes's near future, however, these black obelisks created life on Europa, and replicated on Jupiter, to transform it to a sun to warm that life. Of course, these black obelisks are a lot larger than nanobots. But they are clearly intricate machines and very smart. So who knows what they are made of, if not nanobots?

Will we lose our identity? Not for a long time. And in the far future we will think differently. We will be as different in billions of years as we are now from the primordial soup. For a long time to come, we will not be "sucked into" the every machinery that cares for us but will stand for the most part distinct from the pieces outside and within us. However, there is a price to pay in keeping ourselves exactly as we are. To really look after us in a really smart way, and to control and receive information from these robotic and nanotechnology components, there is likely to be much computing power required outside ourselves. The laws of physics say that there is only so much smartness that can be compressed into the volume typical of the mass of a human being. A computer, for example, cannot monitor and correct everything about itself. To oversee a human being will probably require a larger mass, and certainly more energy and information. Still there may be a point beyond that in which, for the common good of all patients and the system protecting them, the distinction does vanish and we are really at one with the machine.

And is such thinking distasteful, irreligious, even sacrilege? It is impossible to avoid the religious implications, and there have been those who have been both scientists and priests or monks who have expressed similar ideas very positively, although not necessarily so specifically as in nanobot-like terms. Certainly many have been cosmologists. George Lemaitre, who promoted with mathematical and physical argument the "Big Bang" and the "primordial atom" as origins of creation, was a priest from Belgium. Addressing the opposite end of time, Pierre Teilhard de Chardin was a French Jesuit and paleontologist who conceived of the evolution of the universe toward an *omega point*. This is an ultimate final state at the end of time in which life and consciousness converge on a single mind and consciousness in God, reminiscent of the very much older Hindu tradition. They are not alone. In the first chapter we first mentioned the thoughts of Frank Tippler and Pierre Teilhard de Chardin, and even a name for the science of thinking about it: *eschatology*.

Although the word "healthcare" is not used by such authors who include IT in that vision, the all-embracing computers (or one giant supercomputer) are, of course, supposed to look after us. So it comes to the same thing. The problem is that it is not everyone's idea of heaven. Some visions do not look so nice to all of us now, but whatever happens, evolution teaches us that we will change too if we are lucky enough to survive as a line of biological descent at all. As noted above, possible future scenarios may seem very alien and unwholesome to many of us, but, again, as living organisms we are very different from those simple cells in a primordial soup billions of years ago, and in billions of years we will similarly be so much more than we are today. Over hundreds and thousands and millions of years to come, our thinking and sense of what is natural will inevitably change, for better or worse. Our mindset and worldview today is far from that of a metabolic mélange or primordial one-celled organism, to say the least! Incidentally, before the reader raises an objection to that, there are indeed people who argue that thought and spirit may not be confined only to neurons but may reside in anything that can compute: digital devices, flows of water, springs, cogs and levers, and yes, metabolic soup, and cells and organisms talking chemically or otherwise to each other. Perhaps there is even a flow of information embracing all life on Earth. Such a *Gaia hypothesis* was first scientifically formulated in the 1960s by the independent research scientist James Lovelock, as a consequence of his work for NASA regarding methods of detecting life on Mars. He initially published the Gaia hypothesis in small articles in the early 1970s, followed by his 1979 book *Gaia: A New Look at Life on Earth*. But Lovelock and many others appear to feel that humans have become detached from that communion, putting the biosphere, including ourselves, at risk. If so, then the former seemingly unpalatable aspects of our superhuman future are merely restoring us to our rightful, global, and potentially universal way of thinking. Perhaps what seems an unnatural future is much more like what nature intended!

Another perspective is that not only becoming at one with the computer for our health is inevitable, but that it was already the case eons ago (in a sense different to the above, but at least showing that a computational universe is far from impossible). Many theoretical physicists who call themselves cosmologists or information theorists have argued that the universe already is a computer, and we are immersed in its program. That may come as no shock to a generation so immersed in cyberspace, virtual reality, and business and leisure environments like Second Life (a virtual world developed by Linden

Lab that launched in 2003 and is accessible at http://secondlife.com) that they almost forget that there is a first life. But the issue remains, is the first life that we perceive really the first life anyway? After all, quantum mechanics teaches that as we look deep down to the world of the very small, there are essentially digital computations going on with its digits working in the realm of the physical constant h discovered by Max Planck. Moreover it teaches that rather like a computer simulation today as a snapshot of a tiny interesting part of reality, say a simulation modeling protein and drug interactions to help design new drugs, there are processes that appear to be in one place to the simulation but are really distributed all over the computer. Everything is not where and when it seems but only simulated to so seem. Some of the effects in the universal computer leak through to the experimental studies of scientists who, for example, refer to *entanglement* of things and *spooky action at a distance*. Some might argue that illogical superstitions are real, just bugs in the master program. It sounds very much that we are in a holistic system and very much at one with the universe, and indeed in the latest cosmology thinking the whole universe is a hologram.

The implication seems to be that we are already in the mind of a computer that we did not create, and this computer-cum-universe does not look like anyone's idea of a healthcare system. But perhaps we have been planted in that universal program as the seeds of greater beings to come who will refine, improve, and maintain the universal master computer and so necessarily themselves and each other. We are all in the same computational "boat." On the universal scale the medical ethical principle of solidarity versus patient autonomy has unavoidable dominance. We are, to be sure, our brother's keepers.

How powerful is the universal machine and how long can it run? Seth Lloyd, the physicist who argued that a black hole can be considered a kind of computer, claimed in 2001 that the whole universe was too. He estimated that it has so far performed 10^{120} binary operations (the basic unit of computer processing). Three years later Lawrence Krauss and colleagues did the same calculation for the amount of computing processing that the universe can still do in the future. It came to about the same (very roughly). If such estimates and the timescales set by cosmologists give something like the correct picture, then the program is about half run, and we all know, give or take a few billion years, the most optimistic estimate possible of the day of our death.

To take that long road will clearly demand that the difficulties described earlier for the design of nanobots can be overcome, but there are other practical issues too for nanobots working on the cosmic scale. We will assume that spaces can be spanned fast enough; else we will be confined to a much smaller, colder, local universe with the rest of the universe expanding away and fading from contact forever. But perhaps that "lonely island" will be the sanctuary of the human race, and perhaps one of more manageable proportions.

One challenge is that constructing and running computers on both a submicroscopic and superplanetary scale will, by the inviolable laws of thermodynamics, generate a great deal of heat. In asking the question as to what kind of things need to be done in the latter part of the 10^{120} or so binary operations that are left to us, a big part of the answer could be "keep cool." The brain runs at a temperature 37 °C (98 °F). Theoretically a 1 by 1 cm object consuming 1 watt will reach about 610 °C, a 1 by 1 mm about 2000 °C, and 1 by 1 mm will reach about 64,800 °C, somewhat more than 10 times hotter than the surface of the sun. So ideally, from the point of view of temperature, we would "want" matter converted to computer elements of the same density of computation per volume as the brain and running about the temperature of the Earth, and yet each of those could be still dissipating of the order of 1 watt of energy into space.

The simple take home messages are that although there will be heat, it will be too long in the future to worry about it yet, and we may by then become smart enough to find our ways around, and even exploit, the problem. Moreover, by the time we have to worry about the heat on a cosmological scale, the universe may be well expanded, and very cold. The stars are thinly spread and dim, and the microwave heat from the Big Bang is all but gone, so space is almost as cold as true nothingness. Indeed any evidence of the Big Bang is lost, stars are billions of light years apart, losing all evidence of the universe's past because the radiation of that can never reach us. It could be that advanced civilizations are presently hugging the fires of their suns, enclosed in gigantic artificial spheres, as envisaged by the physicist Freeman Dyson. Creating heat may be a good thing, and a natural consequence of making the absolute best of the little matter that is locally accessible to us. At that distant point in time we will have plenty of time to think of something even better than nanotechnology.

SOMETHING BETTER TO COME AFTER?—FEMTOTECHNOLOGY

Nanotechnology seems to be as small as one can go for engineering, at least in any way that we can think about in roughly classical (even classic quantum mechanical) terms. However, a comparable kind of femtotechnology, meaning a much smaller hypothetical technology at subatomic scale, may ultimately be possible as the successor to nanotechnology. Right now, it does *not* seem to us possible in any comparable way. That is not least because subatomic particles lack dispersion forces for sophisticated interaction and recognition. This is essentially the "stickiness" between atoms. Nanotechnology tends to have focused on strong chemical bonds. The weaker atomic stickiness is often regarded as a hindrance to nanotechnology in that it causes atoms to stick around in places where you don't want them to. However, life uses them ubiquitously to huge advantage in its own natural nanotechnology, in protein folding, structure assembly, binding of hormones, neurotransmitters, and other signaling molecules to target receptors on the cell surface. These same forces that cause atoms to stick together are directly or indirectly responsible for, among many other things, biological structures at the cellular level, including the folding of proteins to achieve specific functional forms. So it is a bad omen that they are missing on the femto scale.

Yet, it may simply be that femtotechnology would make use of nuclear weak and strong forces in ways that we cannot yet conceive but that our enhanced descendents can. Folding and channels believed to exist in the extra small dimensions of high-energy physics seem to be part of a precise topological form. The deepest level of structure is made already by nature in the folding and origami of the very fabric of existence. Our descendents may be able to bend the tinier hidden dimensions, and time and space itself, in service to the master computation as our ultimate healthcare system.

A DAY IN THE EVENING OF TJI LI CHAN

On his balcony, in little trays and pots, and like his ancestors so long ago, Tji Li Chan keeps a modest herb garden. He steps through the curtains, sniffs the night air, and walks to the little silver herb pot. He cups in his hands the little herb, admiring its small but intricate blue flowers. The night breeze is warm on the balcony. There is a gentle tinkle of leaves from the gardens below, and a soft scent of jasmine. Bright fireflies in the corner dance in an undulating spiral to a faint melody on distant pipes. Tji Li Chan feels at peace. Not least, he loves the little herb. It bears his name.

He looks up. The stars are growing dim now, dimmer than he remembers them as a much younger man. Although he feels so much at peace, for just a moment, Tji Li Chan feels his age, and a little sad.

Although the stars are growing dim, Tji Li Chan's eyes, and mind, are not. It is the stars themselves that dim because this is all in our far distant future. He has watched them grow dim for seven billion years now, and his memory is perfect. Though it has long since vanished, he could point out without hesitation the point in the heavens where Earth's sun used to be.

He looks down again at the little herb. The herb knows him. The herb knows every essence of him. The herb is very smart, a product of engineering when the human race was learning the ultimate truths about the nature of life, space, and time. It continued to gain wisdom as humankind changed the very nature of what physical reality and well-being means. It knows that Tji Li Chan is no longer really here, and in a sense neither is the herb, but it knows every tiny twist of space that codes for both of them. It monitors those twists of space, and if the foam of the fabric of space–time undulates just a little too much, and those twists are torn, it repairs them.

This is not just nanoengineering. The little herb is an excellent femtoengineer, a level of subatomic resolution far beyond nanoengineering. It can drill deep into the substructure of the universe to fulfill its tasks. It has immense wisdom. It can work magic. It is the perfect guru, physician, and nurse, personally assigned to Tji Li Chan, and at the same time it is part of him.

One day, the herb knows, Tji Li Chan may die. Tji Li Chan may die because the universe may die. But perhaps not all is as inevitable, or at least not quite as final, as would seem. A few hours later, once again, just before dawn, just before the twin suns rise, the herbs will break from their normal duties and confer, as they have done for millennia before. They are indeed worried that the universe, and so Tji Li Chan and all others under their keep, may die. But they are working on it.

GLOSSARY

Abstract syntax   A description of a data structure that is independent of system hardware structures and encoding rules in computer science.

ACID   Properties of transaction processing: atomicity, consistency, isolation, and durability.

Active problem list   List of current medical problems that are identified by patients or doctors to be linked to a specific medical diagnosis. The certainty of that diagnosis may vary.

Adverse drug reaction (ADR)   A response to a drug that occurs at doses normally used or tested in humans but is noxious and unintended. The medical complications range from mild (e.g., nausea/vomiting) to severe (e.g., kidney damage).

Allergy   Immune reaction to a drug/antigen/allergen (e.g., rash, hives); hypersensitivity reaction.

Amino acid   Small molecule chemical building blocks of peptides and proteins.

ANDF (architecture neutral distribution format)   A set of standard formats for software developers to create a single version of application that can run on heterogeneous platforms.

Antibody   A protein produced by the immune system in response to the introduction of an antigen.

The Engines of Hippocrates: From the Dawn of Medicine to Medical and Pharmaceutical Informatics, by Barry Robson and O.K. Baek
Copyright © 2009 by John Wiley & Sons, Inc.

Antigen   A substance that causes the formation of an antibody.

API   Application programming interface.

Applet   A unit of a program written in Java programming language. An applet can be downloaded onto a client platform along with a web page over a computer network and executed within its virtual environment called the Java Virtual Machine.

Assay   A biochemical analysis technique used to measure the activity of drugs and to identify candidate drugs.

Authentication   Verification of the identity of a user or a computer program for information technology security.

BI (business intelligence)   The use by an organization of its data assets to improve decision making and organizational performance.

Bioinformatics   The science of storing and analyzing information in biological research and development.

Biological markers   A physiologic or pharmacologic measure used to predict function or dysfunction in cells, tissues, or organs of animals or humans.

Biomarker   An increasingly popular term the implication of which is somewhat different from "biological marker." Used generally, this means any experimental parameter describing the status of the patient and that, for example, might be used in data mining. It includes clinical laboratory results ("blood work"), medical images, and genomic and proteomic data. Used more specifically, it implies a genomic biomarker, and an SNP (q.v.) of particular value in diagnosis, risk assessment, or selection of therapy.

BLAST   Basic local alignment search tool for discovery of matching patterns of DNA or protein sequences.

Cache   A buffer storage to store frequently accessed instructions and data. A cache is used to reduce access time.

CDISC   Clinical Data Interchange Standards Consortium for defining data standards related to clinical trials.

cDNA (complementary DNA)   DNA synthesized from mRNA or DNA by reverse transcriptase often synthesized from a cellular extract.

Clinical Practice Guidelines (CPG)   Systematically developed statements to help physicians and patients make decisions about appropriate healthcare for specific clinical circumstances; The guidelines involve a synthesis of best available medical evidence and recommended methods to identify and treat a specific medical problem.

Clinical Prescription Guidelines   Same as Clinical Practice Guidelines above but with a focus on prescriptions.

Compendium of Pharmaceuticals and Specificities (CPS) Manual   Drug reference for health professionals that provides lists of drugs by generic names and trade names with the manufacturer's product insert reproduced. The manuel includes a therapeutic guide, manufacturer's index, drug listing by generic name, and a clinical information section (providing ADR, drug interactions, regulation, poison control, and dietary guidance). It also includes information for the patient demographics and monographs.

CPAF (cell pathway analysis factory) An automated, industrial biochemical processing system that analyzes protein complexes in cell-signaling pathways using mass spectrometry.

CRF Case report form in clinical trials.

Chromosomes Part of a cell that contains genetic information. Most multicellular organisms have several chromosomes that together comprise the genome. Sexually reproducing organisms have two copies of each chromosome, one from the each parent.

Cube A structure in which data are arranged along various dimensions and are used to support OLAP functions.

Daemon A long-lived computer process that runs unattended to perform continuous or periodic systemwide functions. Some daemons are triggered automatically to perform their tasks, while others operate periodically.

Datamart A database, often sourced from an enterprise data warehouse, that serves the advanced data analysis needs of a particular group of business intelligent users within an organization.

DCF Data clarification format in clinical trials.

Diagnostics Tests used to identify diseases including, but not limited to, the use of biological markers.

DICOM Digital imaging and communication in medicine.

Dispatcher The program in an operating system that places jobs or tasks into execution.

DNA (deoxyribonucleic acid) A complex molecule found in the chromosomes of almost all organisms that comprises the genetic code. DNA is a double-stranded polymer of nucleotides. The two strands are held together by hydrogen bonds between base pairs of nucleotides. The four nucleotides in DNA contain the bases: adenine (A), guanine (G), cytosine (C), and thymine (T).

Dosage range checking Ensure that the correct dose is administered based on patient-specific data such as age, weight, diet, smoking habits, concurrent drugs, metabolic/excretory ability (renal and liver function), and changing disease state. At the minimum, dosage range checks should be based on age, weight, or elimination ability.

Double doctoring Patient using more than one prescriber in order to obtain multiple prescriptions for the same or similar drug without informing each prescriber about the other.

DPR Digital patient record, essentially the same as EHR (electronic health record) and EMR (electronic medical record).

Drug identification number (DIN) Unique number used to identify a specific drug.

Drug interaction checking   Verifying that the prescribed drug does not compete or interact in an unintended fashion with another drug on the patient's current drug profile.

Drug profiles   List of drugs taken by a patient with the drug (brand), fill date, prescriber, directions, refills (dates taken and remainder), initials of pharmacist filling Rx, quantity dispensed, and drug plan information.

Drug targets   Proteins that are used to find new drug candidates or the actual cell proteins affected by drugs.

Drug utilization evaluation (DUE)   An evaluation of prescribing patterns to specifically determine appropriateness of drug therapy. The evaluation may be performed at the time when the prescription is written or dispensed (prospective DUE), during the course of therapy (concurrent DUE), or after the therapy has been completed (retrospective DUE). The evaluation includes dosage range and drug interaction checking and can be expanded to best choice or therapeutic guideline.

Drug utilization review (DUR)   An authorized structured and continuing program that reviews, analyzes, and interprets patterns (rates and costs) of drug usage in a given health delivery system against predetermined standards. Utilization and costs are reviewed retrospectively and used at the various levels: individual prescriber, pharmacy, plan, or region.

EBM (evidence-based medicine)   A relatively recent movement in medicine, starting with Archie Cochrane in 1972, and promoted by David Sackett and colleagues. It emphasizes the importance of objective use of best possible evidence in making medical decisions, as opposed to personal experience, anecdotal evidence, and so-called expert opinion. The motivation is to reduce the medical accident rate due to bad diagnoses and therapy decisions, and hence it is of considerable current interest. Information-based medicine may be considered EBM as assisted by IT (and it is now hard to imagine EBM without it).

ECG   Electrocardiogram.

e-Commerce   General term for business transactions performed over the Internet. It includes ordering as well as contacting between individual companies.

EDC   Electronic data capture in clinical trials.

EDI (electronic data interchange)   An ISO standard for exchange of documents among computer systems.

EDW (enterprise data warehouse)   A database used as the foundation for comprehensive business intelligence infrastructure, typically characterized by a data-centric (as opposed to application-centric) database design.

EHR (electronic health record)   Essentially same as DPR (digital patient record) and EMR (electronic medical record).

EMR (electronic medical record)   Essentially same as DPR (digital patient record) and EHR (electronic medical record).

Enzyme   A protein that catalyses a biological reaction.

EST (expressed sequence tag)   Unique identifier for cDNA clones.

ETL   Extract, transform, and load of data usually from an operational data store into a data warehouse for analyses.

Eukaryote   Cell or organism with membrane-bound, structurally discrete nucleus, and other well-developed subcellular compartments. Eukaryote includes all organisms except viruses, bacteria, and blue-green algae.

Event record   A record specific to a patient but focused only on specific visits and events at hospitals.

FDA (Food and Drug Administration)   US regulatory governing body that approves medical therapeutics for human use.

FISH (fluorescence in situ hybridization)   Diagnostic approach through molecular probes by using DNA sequences of differing sizes, complexity, and specificity, coupled with technological enhancements (direct labeling, multicolor probes, computerized signal amplification, and image analysis).

Founder mutation   Basically an SNP (q.v.) or biomarker (q.v.) in a gene arising from a mutation in an ancestor and that has been inherited with surrounding DNA, which may be identified by further SNPs as being the DNA of the ancestor. The surrounding DNA gets progressively shorter over many generations. The change in the gene itself may be the cause of a certain genetic disease, but founder genes survive because historically or prehistorically, the disease may be outweighed by some advantage.

Gene   A segment of DNA that codes for the manufacture of a specific protein.

Gene expression   The process by which a gene's DNA sequence is converted to a protein.

Gene sequence   The order of deoxyribonucleotides (DNA) present in a gene.

Genetics   The study of the patterns of inheritance of specific traits.

Genome   The entire genetic information present in the chromosomes of a particular organism.

Genomics   The study of genomes, including genome mapping, gene sequencing, and structure and functional expression of the genome.

GPS   Global positioning system used to track the location of mobile object using the satellite.

Health record   The data and information regarding a patient's health events and history, and also all information and data needed to run the health system in support of the patient's well-being (i.e., we have chosen to not separate the supporting information and roles from the direct service delivery). The personal health record is a specific portion of the patient's entire health record that is designed to be shared.

High-throughput screening (HTS)   Analysis of drug target interactions in a high-capacity manner.

Human Genome Project   A public, government-sponsored project to determine the nucleotide sequence of all the human genes.

HPC   High-performance computing for complex mathematical calculations.

HTS   High-throughput screening process used in the pharmaceutical industry to identify drug-like chemical compounds.

IEEE   Institute of Electrical and Electronics Engineers.

IETF   Internet Engineering Task Force, which is responsible for solving short-term engineering needs of the Internet.

IMAGE   Integrated molecular analysis of genomes and their expression.

Internet   A worldwide association of interconnected networks based on the TCP/IP protocol.

Intranet   A private network based on the TCP/IP protocol.

Internet protocol   The network protocol for routing data packets in a concatenated network, such as the World Wide Web.

Internet TV   While connecting a television to a PC has been relatively easy for years, many providers are now trying to find a way of using televisions to display Internet contents, for example, web pages transmitted via a TV signal or access to the network via a second channel.

Internet telephony   Data previously transmitted over telephone lines such as faxes and voice data are now being directed through the Internet.

ISO   International Organization for Standardization.

Java   A programming language based on C++ to achieve the IT industry objective of developing software once to run on any platform. Java also provides an architecture-independent platform (Java Virtual Machine) to provide automatic code distribution with a network security.

JVM (Java Virtual Machine)   An operating system developed by Sun Microsystems as the runtime environment for Java programs.

Kerberos   An authentication technique (for information technology security) developed at the Massachusetts Institute of Technology. It is named after the three-headed dog of Greek mythology that guarded the gates of Hades.

Levinthal's paradox   As there are an astronomical number of conformations possible, an unbiased search would take too long for a protein to fold, and yet most proteins fold in seconds!

Lexical analyzer   A program that analyzes input data and breaks it into categories, such as numbers, letters, and operators.

Ligand   A molecule that interacts or binds to a specific site on a protein or another molecule, usually involving an interaction between a small molecule and a protein.

LIMS   Laboratory information management system for keeping track of experimental data in a biological or chemical laboratory.

Longitudinal health record A health record that spans across many features of the patient's health and across the patient's entire life, in being essentially lifelong.

Mass spectrometry A rapid and sensitive technique for separating and determining the structure of molecules by very accurate measurement of their mass/charge ratio.

MDP (message driven processing) Application processing that utilizes messaging for intersystem communication mechanism in a distributed environment, where application status information can be carried within the messages, and application flow and context can be managed outside the application.

Medical data standards (ICD-9CM, ICD-10CM) Topography of standardized medical diagnosis and procedures sanctioned by the World Health Organization (WHO) as the international standard.

Metabolism The total sum of chemical processes in a living cell.

Microarray A microarray (or slide) refers to the physical substrate to which biosequence reporters (cDNA or oligonucleotide) are attached. Microarrays are hybridized with labeled samples and then scanned and analyzed to generate data.

Microarray experiment An experiment to study a microarray system under controlled conditions while some conditions are changed. In gene expression, one parameter is varied, such as time, drug, developmental stage, or dosage on a sample. The sample is processed and labeled with a detectable tag so that it can be used in hybridization with microarray.

MIME (multipurpose Internet mail extensions) Extension of electronic mail encoding for exchange of multimedia mail, including support of audio and video data.

Minimum data set The minimum set of data elements or data attributes necessary to be shared to support a particular purpose. All data elements must have a stated reason for collection, so the collection of data already available or derivable from existing data must be avoided. Each data element needs to be defined with sufficient clarity that different individuals can consistently record measures or observations with acceptable reliability and specificity. A description of the context in which data are captured must also be recorded.

MOLAP (multidimensional OLAP) The analysis of data in prebuilt Cubes that are stored in a proprietary, nonrelational data structure.

Molecular biology A branch of biology that studies genes and gene products in relation to cell structure and function.

MRI (magnetic resonance imaging) Medical imaging technology to scan tissues without using radiation and without enclosing patient.

mRNA (messenger RNA) A specialized form of RNA that serves as a template to direct protein biosynthesis. The amount of any particular type of mRNA in a cell reflects the extent to which gene has been expressed.

Nonclinical   Does not involve the direct provision of medical care to a client.

Nonprescription   Drugs (over the counter drugs and herbal remedies) that do not require a prescription for purchase.

Nucleotide   The basic building blocks of DNA: adenine, thymine, cytosine, and guanine.

Object orientation   Software engineering approach for organizing software component as a collection of discrete objects that incorporate both data structure and behavior.

ODA (open document architecture)   An ISO standard describing a complex document and the format for exchanging a document with another system.

ODBC (open database connectivity)   A database-independent application interface to enable applications to access data stored in heterogeneous relational and nonrelational databases.

ODP (open distributed processing)   An ISO standard defining the framework and architecture for distributed processing in an OSI environment.

Oligonucleotide   A short sequence of nucleotides (less than 80 base pairs), always single stranded and often chemically synthesized to be used as probes or spots.

OLAP (online analytical processing)   The sophisticated manipulation of data for analytic purposes, often using data organized into the cube structure.

OLTP   Online transaction processing.

OMO (observational medical outcome)   A parameter obtained from a patient record of which an adverse drug reaction (q.v.) is of particular, but not sole, interest. Usually OMOs are collected from many patient records and used in outcome analysis (q.v.).

OMOP (observational medical outcomes partnership)   Used generically, any partnership, usually of pharmaceutical companies, applying pharmacosurveillance (q.v.) or pharmacovigilance (q.v.) to patients. Sometimes elsewhere in the literature the "P" stands for pilot, process, or procedure.

Ontology   Domain of knowledge structured through formal rules so that it can be interpreted and used by computers, such as GOBO (global open biological ontology) and GO (gene ontology).

OQL (object query language)   A SQL-like query language with special features dealing with complex objects, values, and methods. OQL is an object-based version of SQL, and the key differences between OQL and traditional SQL are (1) OQL has the ability to support object referencing within tables and allows objects to be nested within objects, (2) not all SQL keywords are supported within OQL such as irrelevant keywords removed from the syntax, and (3) OQL has the ability to perform mathematical computations from within OQL statements.

Outcomes analysis Analysis of the relationship between therapies given to many patients and the responses to, i.e. consequences, of them. An important aspect of EBM (q.v.).

Over the counter (OTC) drugs Drugs obtained from a pharmacy without a written prescription (e.g., cough syrup, aspirin).

PACS (picture archival and communication system) Medical image management system for diagnostics.

PET (positron emission tomography) Doppler ultrasound systems in color for searches of cancers, obstetrical studies, or direction of blood flows.

Pharmacogenomics The study of the genetic basis of individual patient responsiveness to a drug substance.

Pharmacoproteomics The study of individual patient phenotype information to analyze drug efficacy and toxicological profiles.

Pharmacotherapy The use of drugs in the prevention and treatment of disease.

Pharmacosurveillance Monitoring the effects of drugs in patients prescribed by physicians and hence post-market, as opposed to a patient in a clinical trial. The reason is both to protect the public and learn new facts about the drug, and to help in pricing and other uses of the drug.

Pharmcovigilance In current WHO use, this is the same as pharmacosurveillance, but in the pharmaceutical industry, it is the part of pharmacosurveillance that focuses on the adverse drug reactions.

Pharmacy practice guidelines Same as clinical practice guidelines specific to the storage and dispensing of drugs.

Phenotype The physiological and biochemical characteristics of a biological organism.

Phish [pronounced same as fish] The verb representing the act of sending an email to a user, falsely claiming to be an established legitimate enterprise in an attempt to scam the user into surrendering private information that will be used for identity theft.

Phishing [pronounced same as fishing] The act of sending an email to a user, falsely claiming to be an established legitimate enterprise in an attempt to scam the user into surrendering private information that will be used for identity theft.

Plug and play A computer's ability to automatically detect programs or devices, without requiring manual installation of computer programs or computer devices.

Prescriber Any person permitted by legislation to write a prescription.

Prescription renewal Extension for an identical prescription due to a time limit placed on the initial prescription.

Protein A biological molecule that consists of many amino acids chained together by peptide bonds. Proteins perform most of the enzymatic and structural roles within living cells.

Protein expression   The process and result of transcribing the DNA sequence of a gene into messenger RNA, and subsequently the translation of the RNA into a protein.

Proteome   The complete library of proteins and protein sequences encoded by the genome of the organism.

Proteomics   The study of the proteins encoded by the genome, with focus on the high-throughput systematic separation, identification, and structural and functional characterization of proteins.

p-**Value**   A measure of evidence against the null hypothesis in a statistical test.

Rationale for therapy   An attempt to describe the thought processes that led to a particular therapeutic choice.

RNA (ribonucleic acid)   A class of nucleic acids that consist of nucleotides containing the bases adenine (A), guanine (G), cytosine (C), and uracil (U). An RNA molecule is typically single stranded and can pair with DNA or with another RNA molecule.

ROLAP   Relational OLAP characterized by the dynamic building of cubes using data sourced from relational database.

Schema   A formal representation with a defined set of symbols and rules governing the formation of a representation using the symbols.

Snowflake schema   Similar to a star schema but with larger dimensional tables that have been de-normalized into sets of smaller tables.

SNP (single nucleotide polymorphism or simple nucleotide polymorphism)   A difference in DNA that occurs between individuals, which could be as simple as one base change, say an A to a C. Those of specific interest in medicine by being directly involved in a gene of interest, or lying elsewhere but statistically associated with it, are usually called *genomic biomarkers* or just *biomarkers* (q.v.). SNPs are also of interest in that the number of differences in DNA between two individuals is a measure of how long ago they had a common parent. They also define founder genes (q.v.), which have one or more base changes and are inherited along with a stretch of surrounding DNA.

SQL (structured query language)   A language designed by IBM for using relational databases.

SQL-X   An extension of SQL that provides a set of operators to compose queries against a relational database, producing complex XML documents with a style reminiscent of report generation languages.

Star schema   A database design, often used to improve OLAP performance, that features a central fact table linked to associated dimensional tables by way of surrogate keys.

Substitute therapies (drugs)   Use of another drug similar to that prescribed in order to achieve the same clinical benefit. Drug substitutes can be therapeutic substitutions (drugs are not identical but produce an identical effect) or generic substitutions (active ingredients are identical but supplied by different companies). The substitute may have some advantage such as fewer side effects or lower cost.

Taxonomy Names and phrases in higher level categories used as formal knowledge representations for autonomic inferences and certain types of reasoning. Exemplified by the taxonomic tree classifying animals and plants (pp. 29, 30).

Therapeutic duplication Use of two or more drugs of the same class or type in the same person for the same medical indication. Prescriber may or may not be aware of duplication.

Trial prescriptions Program to prescribe/dispense a short initial drug course (7–14 days) in order to assess the patients response to the new therapy (e.g., the patient may be unable to tolerate side effects). This program lessens the waste of nonconsumed prescribed drugs. The program is aimed at encouraging the dispensing of prescriptions in two parts and is expected to reduce the incidence of drug-related problems and reduce drug costs by minimizing wastage.

Triplicate prescription Mandatory program of providing duplicate prescriptions for controlled substances. Duplicates are sent to the College of Physicians and Surgeons.

Unintended duplication Same as therapeutic duplication, but in this case prescriber is unaware of the duplication.

Working diagnosis A chosen diagnosis that has the highest probability of describing a patient's current problem, based on a variable level of evidence to permit an immediate intervention recognizing that forthcoming information may alter the final diagnosis.

XQuery (XML Query) Flexible query facilities used to extract data from real and virtual documents by way of XML notation in a file system or on the World Wide Web. XQuery consequently provides interaction and data exchange between the web world and the database world and ultimately enables collections of XML files to be accessed like databases. The XML Query project of the W3C Consortium includes not only the standard for querying XML documents but also the next-generation standards for doing XML selection (XPath2), for XML serialization, for full-text search, for a possible functional XML data model, and for a standard set of functions and operators for manipulating web data.

CLINICAL TRIAL TERMS

Phase 0. Recently introduced to speed up the development of promising treatments, or applications that requires small doses (esp. molecular imaging), this new phase of trial tests extremely small doses on a subject group.

Phase I. Researchers test a new treatment in a small group of subjects (20–90) to test its safety, identify the maximum tolerated dose, find a safe dosage range and identify adverse effects.

Phase II. The treatment is given to a larger group of subjects (100–300) to see if it is effective, to further evaluate safety and to gather additional information regarding the best dose range.

Phase III. The treatment is given to large groups of subjects (1,000–3,000) to confirm its effectiveness, monitor side effects, compare it to commonly used treatments and collect information that will allow the treatment to be used safely.

Phase IV. Researchers look for additional data regarding the treatment's risks, benefits, and best use. This may occur after the drug or treatment has been approved for use by the FDA.

Phase V. Broader trials, usually after marketing of a treatment, may be conducted to refine dosage guidelines and formulations, for indications for different strata of the populations, for repurposing (new indications), or for pricing (drug cost) studies.

The Engines of Hippocrates: From the Dawn of Medicine to Medical and Pharmaceutical Informatics, by Barry Robson and O.K. Baek
Copyright © 2009 by John Wiley & Sons, Inc.

Cross Over. To be fair to all subjects and to give an equal chance of cure, best ethical practice is that one group takes the real treatment and one the placebo, and later they switch.

Double Blind. Neither researcher nor subject is aware of which is the placebo and which the real treatment.

NOTES, BIBLIOGRAPHY, AND FURTHER READING GUIDE

CHAPTER 1

History of Humans and the Universe

Some intentionally popular sources are as follows. All are good, with McNeill's as the most formal and scholarly, but still easy reading. Bryson is a popular humorist and witty observer of British and US cultural differences. From 1990 to 1997 Gonick penned a bimonthly "Science Classics" cartoon for *Discover* Magazine. Science fiction writers and science popularizers have often undertaken similar tasks to give themselves "the big picture" and share it with the public. It is also worthwhile to hunt out Isaac Asimov's *Chronology of the World*, and H. G. Well's much earlier classic *A Short History of the World*.

- B. Bryson. 2003. *A Short History of Nearly Everything*. New York: Doubleday.
- L. Gonick. 1994, 1997. *The Cartoon History of the Universe*, 2 vols. New York: Main Street Books.
- W. H. McNeill. 1967. *In the Beginning: A World History*, 4th ed. New York: Oxford University Press. Reprint 1999.

Readers who like a challenging mathematical and physical perspective on the evolution of the universe, with some connection to the entropy and information theme, should try:

- R. A. Treumann. 1993. Evolution of the information in the universe. *Astrophysics and Space Science* 201(1):135–147.

Early Civilizations and First Cities

Early civilizations are covered in Chapter 2 in the human migration and genomics context, and recommended reading is on page 535. Besides the cities mentioned in Chapter 1, some of the very earliest known at time of writing include Tell Brak and Tell Hamoukar, Uruk, Jericho, Catal Huyuk, Suberde, and Tepe Yaha. Catal Huyuk is interesting as a Stone Age culture city built with all the houses piled together with streets on top like human-made caves. Not all the names of the cities are as they are known to their inhabitants today. "Tell" or "Tel" simply means hill: The modern city of "Tel Aviv" translates as "Spring Hill" in Hebrew. In archeology, "Tell" typically means the hill as it is seen before excavating it reveals that under that mound is really a city, so the term is almost synonymous with "excavation site." The tendency was, of course, to build cities on hills for defense purposes.

Concerning the History of Ideas and Discovery

Some classics and popular works are as follows. Friedman means by "flat" that the world is connected by IT, so globalized in culture, science, and markets.

- T. L. Friedman. 2007. *The World Is Flat*. New York: Picador.
- A. O. Lovejoy. 1936. *The Great Chain of Being: A Study of the History of an Idea*. Cambridge: Harvard University Press. Reprint 2005. New York: Harper.
- S. F. Mason. 1956. *A History of the Sciences*. New York: Collier Books.
- F. Crick. 1988. *What Mad Pursuit? A Personal View of Scientific Discovery*. New York: Basic Books.

Our brief discussion of famous scientists and engineers who ultimately had an impact on medicine and medical computing can be expanded upon by reading:

- J. G. Simmons. 2000. *The Scientific 100: A Ranking of the Most Influential Scientists, Past and Present*. New York: Citadel Press.

However, Simmons's widely quoted listed does not include Hippocrates, whom the author apparently chose not to consider a scientist. The list is often reproduced with added religious faith affiliations due to http://www.adherents.com/people/100_scientists.html. Adherents.com provides a growing collection of over 43,000 adherent statistics and religious geography citations, with references to published membership/adherent statistics and congregation statistics for over 4,000 religions, churches, denominations, and religious bodies. Most great scientists seem to have been religious, though nonconformists. The top twenty from his list are well worth a read. Among these is Paul A. M. Dirac, a quiet man who has not received the same general public awareness as Einstein, Schrödinger, Planck, or Heisenberg, yet he essentially "polished and finalized" quantum mechanics as we know it today. Fortunately for him, his widow Margit Dirac was keen to emphasize the importance of his contributions to medical and veterinary science, along with their applications to drug design. The top twenty scientists are:

1. Isaac Newton, the founder of classical physics
2. Albert Einstein, founder of quantum mechanics and relativity
3. Neils Bohr, the quantum mechanical explanation of the atom
4. Charles Darwin, evolution
5. Louis Pasteur, the germ theory of disease
6. Sigmund Freud, psychology of the conscious
7. Galileo Galilei, astronomy and cosmology
8. Antoine Laurent Lavoisier, revolutionized chemistry
9. Johannes Kepler, motion of the planets
10. Nicolaus Copernicus, the heliocentric universe
11. Michael Faraday, the classical field theory
12. James Clerk Maxwell, the electromagnetic field
13. Claude Bernard, founder of modern physiology
14. Franz Boas, founder of modern anthropology
15. Werner Heisenberg, uncertainty principle and quantum theory
16. Linus Pauling, theoretical chemistry
17. Rudolf Virchow, the cell doctrine as founder of cytology
18. Erwin Schrödinger, wave mechanics as quantum mechanics
19. Ernest Rutherford, the structure of the atom
20. Paul Dirac, refinement of quantum mechanics through relativistic quantum electrodynamics

An Introduction to Medical Informatics

- E. H. Shortliffe, L. E. Perrault, G. Wiederhold, and L. M. Fagan, eds. 2000. *Medical Informatics: Computer Applications in Health Care and Biomedicine.* New York: Springer.

Concerning IT and the Growth of Medical Information— The Petabyte Explosion

Genomic and proteomic data will add large amounts of data to our knowledge base, but medical imaging will reign supreme. See Table B.1. Fortunately IT seems to be keeping up helped by compression (Table B.1).

- Siemens Innovation Report. 2008. *IBM and Siemens Work Together to Deliver Medical Imaging Management Systems for Healthcare Industry ... Over 150 Petabytes of Medical Images Are Created Annually Worldwide.* http://www.innovationsreport.de/html/berichte/informationstechnologie/bericht-31907.html.
- M. Martin. 2002. *Supersize IT: From Megabytes to Petabytes: Scientific Research, Particularly in Astronomy and Biology, Is Very Data-Intensive.* http://www.sci-tech-today.com/perl/story/19162.html.
- R. Godomski. 2004. The incredible shrinking petabyte: how compression technologies are helping store more data in less space, *Computer Technology Review,* June 1 (also at http://findartides.com/p/articles/mi_m0BRZ/is_/).

World Information-Based Medical Storage Estimates per Major Center[2], 2010–2012

Table B.1

Object	Uncompressed	Average Compression
Text, lab data, cross-refs manual, and automated annotation	$1 \times E8^1$	$1 \times E7$
Time series data	$1 \times E6$	$6 \times E4$
Proteomics	$1 \times E9$	$3–4 \times E8$
Whole DNA	$3 \times E10$	$1 \times E10$
High-resolution radiology grayscale	$1.1 \times E7$	$5 \times E6$
Color histology, etc.	$1 \times E6$	$6 \times E4$
3D-MRI,CT, PET,US	$1 \times E8$	$4 \times E7$
4D imaging	$1 \times E11$	$1 \times E10$
Detailed 4D recording of patient-physician and operating rooms procedures	$6 \times E10$	$1 \times E9$
Total		

[1]$E8 = 10^8$. [2]Globally it will be hundreds of petabytes.

Research Papers Exemplifying Advanced Analysis of Brain Image Data

Although there is inadequate space to discuss further the important topic of medical imaging, save for the outstandingly heavy petabyte (in Chapter 1), bandwidth and processing demands (in Chapter 3), medical imaging is a dominant issue in the sharing of anonymous medical data. Brain imaging is one of the most intensive and of importance to future research, as the brain is the last frontiers of human biology. In July 2005, École Polytechnique Federale de Laussanne and IBM announced an exciting new research initiative, Blue Brain, a project to create a biologically accurate, functional model of the brain using IBM's BlueGene supercomputer. *Blue Brain* should provide significant advance in understanding of brain function and disease. By 2007, the Blue Brain project had created a model of the basic functional unit of the brain, the neocortical column. The model could reconstruct biologically accurate neurons based on detailed experimental data, and automatically connect them in a biological manner, a task that involves positioning around 30 million synapses in precise 3D locations. In late 2007, the Blue Brain project reached an important milestone and the conclusion of its first phase, with the announcement of an entirely new data-driven process for creating, validating, and researching the neocortical column. For more details of output per major center, see:

Number per Patient	Projected 5-Year Estimate	Notes
100	$1 \times E9$	Compression ratio depends on usage (e.g., lossy, lossless), not on data representation notation
100	$6 \times E6$	EKG, ECG, etc.
30–50	$1 \times E10$	Assuming million probe locations per array
1	$1 \times E10$	3 Giga base pairs, plus mtDNA, somatic mutations/immune system somatic, plus annotation, error correction, and privacy features
100	$5 \times E8$	$2,048 \times 2,577$ pixels
100	$6 \times E6$	Usage expected to increase
10	$4 \times E8$	Brain and body, 1.5 mm slice distance; repeated 10 times in life
5	$5 \times E10$	Beating heart, joint and spine movements, etc. $1.5\,mm \times 0.1\,s$ slice
10	$1 \times E10$	6–24 Megabytes per minute 1,200 frame/min, circa one hour per operation
	$82 \times E9$	Assume accessible $5 \times E7$ adult population, gives 4,100 petabytes

- EPFL. 2008. *The Blue Brain Project Is the First Comprehensive Attempt to Reverse-engineer the Mammalian Brain, in order to Understand Brain Function and Dysfunction through Detailed Simulations.* http://bluebrain.epfl.ch.

On the day of our writing this bibliographic section, there was noted substantial progress at the Stanford Research Institute in direct reading of the mind by computer:

- Time/CNN. 2008. *Mind-Reading Computer.* http://www.time.com/time/magazine/article/0,9171,942916,00.html.

Some solid pioneering efforts in the field of brain imaging and analytics include functional analytics (ultimately allowing "mind reading"). The sources provided below are examples of research on this and other brain-related topics:

- G. J. Carman, H. A. Drury, and D. C. Van Essen. 1995. Computational methods for reconstructing and unfolding the cortex. *Cerebral Cortex* 5(6):506–517.
- D. L. Collins, P. Neelin, T. M. Peters, and A. C. Evans. 1994. Automatic 3-D inter-subject registration of MR volumetric data in standardized talairach space. *Journal of Computer Assisted Tomography* 18(2):192–205.

- D. P. Corina, S. L. McBurney, C. Dodrill, K. Hinshaw, J. Brinkley, and G. Ojemann. 1999. Functional roles of broca's area and smg: Evidence from cortical stimulation mapping in a deaf signer. *Neuroimage* 10:570–581.
- A. M. Dale, B. Fischl, and M. I. Sereno. 1999. Cortical surface-based analysis: I. Segmentation and surface reconstruction. *Neuroimage* 9(2):179–194.
- C. Davatzikos and R. N. Bryan. 1996. Using a deformable surface model to obtain a shape representation of the cortex. *IEEE Transactions on Medical Imaging* 15(6):785–795.
- B. Fischl, M. I. Sereno, and A. M. Dale. 1999. Cortical surface-based analysis: II. Inflation, flattening, and a surface-based coordinate system. *Neuroimage* 9(2): 195–207.
- K. P. Hinshaw, R. B. Altman, and J. F. Brinkley. 1995. Shape-based models for interactive segmentation of medical images. In *SPIE Medical Imaging 1995: Image Processing*. San Diego: Academic Press, pp. 771–780.
- K. P. Hinshaw and J. F. Brinkley. 1997. Shape-based interactive three-dimensional medical image segmentation. In K. M. Hanson, ed., *SPIE Medical Imaging: Image Processing,* Vol. 3034. Newport Beach, CA: Academic Press, pp. 236–242.
- J. L. Lancaster, P. T. Fox, H. Downs, D. S. Nickerson, T. A. Hander, M. El Mallah, P. V. Kochunov, and F. Zamarripa. 1999. Global spatial normalization of human brain using convex hulls. *Journal of Nuclear Medicine* 40(6):942–955.
- D. MacDonald, N. Kabani, D. Avis, and A. C. Evans. 2000. Automated 3-D extraction of inner and outer surfaces of cerebral cortex from MRI. *Neuroimage* 12(3):340–356.
- B. Modayur, J. Prothero, G. Ojemann, K. Maravilla, and J. F. Brinkley. 1997. Visualization-based mapping of language function in the brain. *Neuroimage* 6:245–258.
- G. Ojemann, J. Ojemann, E. Lettich, and M. Berger. 1989. Cortical language localization in left, dominant hemisphere. *Journal of Neurosurgery* 71:316–326.
- A. V. Poliakov, K. P. Hinshaw, C. Rosse, and J. F. Brinkley. 1999. Integration and visualization of multimodality brain data for language mapping. In *Proceedings, American Medical Informatics Association Fall Symposium*. Washington, DC: SIG Publications, pp. 349–353.
- S. M. Smith. 2000. BET: Brain extraction tool. Technical report TR00SMS2a. Oxford Centre for Functional Magnetic Resonance Imaging of the Brain. Oxford University.
- D. C. Van Essen, H. A. Drury, J. Dickson, J. Harwell, D. Hanlon, and C. H. Anderson. 2001. An integrated software suite for surface-based analysis of cerebral cortex. *Journal of the American Medical Association* 8(5):443–459.
- A. V. Poliakov, E. Albright, D. Corina, G. Ojemann, R. F. Martin, and J. F. Brinkley. 2001. Server-based approach to web visualization of integrated 3-D medical image data. In *Proceedings, American Medical Informatics Association Fall Symposium*. Washington, DC: AMIA. pp. 533–537.

Concerning Our Ultimate Fate

Stephen Hawking's classic is an overview of the origin of the universe with reflections on its fate. Frank Tipler's classic view discussed in this chapter is but one example of many scientists' religious convictions and attempts to interpret religion in scientific terms. However, in reading such eschatological interpretations of the cosmos, concerning the end of things for our future descendants and their transformative states of being, we cannot escape whatever are the author's religious convictions.

- S. Hawking. 1998. *A Brief History of Time*. New York: Bantam.
- F. J. Tipler. 1994. *The Physics of Immortality: Modern Cosmology, God and the Resurrection of the Dead*. New York: Doubleday.

CHAPTER 2

SNPs and Genomic Biomarkers

Simple nucleotide polymorphisms (SNPs) are usually small local changes in our DNA that help predict our risks to diseases and responses to drugs, as well as many other things as well as behavior. We say "predict" because the effect is not necessarily direct on the gene with the modified action but is merely carried with it statistically, as part of a so-called haplogroup or haplotype, including in humans' ancient migrations. Basically, in the evolution jargon, SNPs as *single* nucleotide polymorphisms became *simple* nucleotide polymorphisms, and then biomarkers. The ultimate medical reason for considering any biomarker data for medical purposes is reviewed from the clinical biomarker, pharmacogenomic, and pharmaceutical *industry* perspective in:

- M. Svinte, B. Robson, and M. Hehenberger. 2007. Biomarkers in drug development and patient care. *Burrill 2007 Personalized Medicine Report* 6(8):3114–3126.

Many people disagree about details of how genetics, meaning primarily SNPs/biomarkers, determines the response to diseases and to therapies. The case of the single biomarker that has a major effect on eye color is the exception, not the rule. So most of this debate is in regard to how many genes in complex diseases such as cardiovascular disease and cancer interact with each other and the environment and lifestyle of the individual so as to involve tens or hundreds of biomarkers. This puts the problem still within reach of science and medicine, albeit it is a challenging problem for data analysis (e.g., see Chapter 9). However, such analysis tends to overlook the fact that over 8,500 genetic disorders known to medicine are characterized, more or less, by individual differences in single genes, although not necessarily involving a single nucleotide/base pair change. For more on this new, see:

- A. Milunsky. 2002. *Your Genetic Destiny: Know your Genes, Secure your Health, Save your Life*. New York: Perseus Books.

Two good sources of information on SNPs/biomarkers are Harvard University and Harvard–Partners Center for Genetics and Genomics (www.hpcgg.org) and the Broad Institute for the Study of Postgenomic Human Genetics and Medicine (www.wi.mit.edu/nap/features/nap_feature_broadinstitute.html). Additional reference data sources for SNP/biomarker Mapping include:

1. Snp.cshl.org
2. Press2.nci.nih.gov/sciencebehind/snps_cancer/snps_cancer().htm

3. www.niehs.nih.gov/envgenom/home.htm
4. www.genome.utah.edu/genesnps
5. www.ncbi.nlm.nih.gov/SNP
6. Egp.gs.Washington.edu
7. Gai.nci.nih.gov
8. Snp.ims.u-tokyo.ac.jp
9. Dbsearch.sanger.ac.uk/HGP/help/overview.shtml
10. www.imm.ki.se/CYPalleles

Concerning Recent Human Evolution and Genomic Biomarkers

Recent work such as the genographic project by the National Geographic Society and IBM has been deliberately nonclinical, concentrating on the biology. There are two must-read classics:

- L. L. Cavalli-Sforza. 2001. *Genes, Peoples, and Languages*. Berkeley: University of California Press.
- L. L. Cavalli-Sforza and F. Cavalli-Sforza. 1995. *The Great Human Diasporas: The History of Diversity and Evolution*. New York: Perseus Books.

Cavalli-Sforza focused on mitochondrial DNA, which we all have and which is passed down through the maternal line. His student Spencer Wells (subsequently a founder and major force in the above-mentioned genographic project) moved on to focus on the male Y chromosome:

- S. Wells. 2002. *The Journey of Man: A Genetic Odyssey*. Princeton: Princeton University Press.

See also:

- S. Olson. 2003. *Mapping Human History*. Boston: Mariner Books.
- E. Mayr. 1982. *The Growth of Biological Thought: Diversity, Evolution, and Inheritance*. Cambridge: Belknap Press/Harvard University Press.
- R. Lewin. 1993. *The Origin of Modern Humans*. Sun Francisco: Freeman.

Otherwise, we skip straight to recommending treatment of very latest developments:

- R. DeSalle and I. Tattershall. 2008. *Human Origins: What Bones and Genomes Tell Us about Ourselves*. Austin: University of Texas Press.
- N. Wade. 2006. *Before the Dawn*. London: Penguin Books.
- S. Wells. 2006. *Deep Ancestry: Inside the Genographic Project*. Washington, DC: National Geographic.
- G. Stix. 2008. Traces of a distant past: DNA furnishes an ever clearer picture of the multimillennial trek from Africa all the way to the tip of South America. *Scientific American* 299(1):56–63.

Research Papers on Recent Developments in Human Genomics

More formal reading on current developments in understanding our genomic basis includes:

- T. D Weaver and C. C. Roseman. 2008. New developments in the genetic evidence for modern humans. *Evolutionary Anthropology* 17:69–80.
- J. H. Relethford. 2008. Genetic evidence and the modern human origin debate. *Nature Heredity* 100:555–563.

Concerning Early Agriculture, and More on Cities

- C. Tudge. 1998. *Neanderthals, Bandits and Farmers: How Agriculture Really Began.* London: Weidenfeld and Nicolson.
- J. R. Harlan. 1998. *The Living Fields: Our Agricultural Heritage.* Cambridge: Cambridge University Press.

Arnold Toynbee's historical classic followed by two valuable more recent works:

- A. Toynbee, ed. 1967. *Cities of Destiny.* New York: McGraw-Hill.
- J. M. Kenoyer. 1998. *Ancient Cities of the Indus Valley Civilization.* New York: Oxford University Press/Karachi.
- P. Bairoch. 1988. *Cities and Economic Development: From the Dawn of History to the Present.* Chicago: University of Chicago Press.

Concerning Epidemics and the Origin of Disease

A classic is:

- A. Nikiforuk. 1993. *The Fourth Horseman: A Short History of Epidemics, Plagues, Famine and Other Scourges.* Canada: Penguin Group and New York: M. Evans.

Influence keeps changing and defeating vaccines largely by a characteristic of an RNA processor mixing called reassortment. Researchers at MIT have explained why two *mutations* in the H1N1 avian flu virus enabled viral transmission in humans during the 1918 pandemic outbreak that killed at least 50 million people. They showed that the 1918 influenza strain developed two mutations in the virus surface protein hemagglutinin (HA, the H in H1N1 and other strain numbers) that allowed it to bind tightly to receptors in the human upper respiratory tract:

- Scientist Live Web Page. 2008. *Explaining the 1918 flu.* http://www.scientistlive. com/lab/?/Genetics/2008/02/19/19813/Explaining_the_1918_flu.

There are continuing efforts to understand where other plagues come from, for example:

- T. H. Maugh. 2002. An empire's epidemic: Scientists use DNA in search for answers to 6th century plague. *Los Angeles Times*, May 6, p. A14.

Recent Research Studies on Origins of Infectious Disease

The research concerns the process of *escape from restriction* in animals to humans. But note also:

- P. Daszak, A. A. Cunningham, and A. D. Hyatt. 2001. Anthropogenic environmental change and the emergence of infectious diseases in wildlife. *Acta Tropica* 78(2):103–116.

Lest the reader doubt that pathogens jumping to humans is a fairly common occurrence, read the following (see also our Chapter 9):

- H. Krauss, A. Weber, M. Appel, B. Enders, A. v. Graevenitz, H. D. Isenberg, H. G. Schiefer, W. Slenczka, and H. Zahner. 2003. *Zoonoses: Infectious Diseases Transmissible from Animals to Humans*, 3rd ed. Washington, DC: ASM Press.

Concerning Ancient Greece

Good general background sources are:

- C. Freeman. 1996. *Egypt, Greece and Rome*. Oxford: Oxford University Press.
- C. R. Beye. 1975. *Ancient Greek Literature and Society*. Garden City, NY: Anchor Press.
- A. Konstam. 2003. *Historical Atlas of Ancient Greece*. Hove East Sussex, UK: Thalamus Publishing.

On Greek medicine, the first following is a classic, the other two excellent orientations:

- L. Cohn-Haft. 1956. *The Public Physicians of Ancient Greece*. Northampton: Mass., Department of History of Smith College.
- J. Longrigg. 1993. *Greek Rational Medicine: Philosophy and Medicine from Alcmæon to the Alexandrians*. London: Routledge.
- H. F. J. Horstmanshoff, M. Stol, and C. Tilburg. 2004. *Magic and Rationality in Ancient Near Eastern and Graeco-Roman Medicine*. Leiden: Brill Publishers.

Hippocrates

The end of this chapter brings us to Hippocrates, key to our book, so we must mention:

- J. Jouanna. 1999. *Hippocrates*, transl. by M. B. DeBevoise. Baltimore: Johns Hopkins University Press. Original edition: *Hippocrates*. Paris: Fayard, 1992.

Otherwise, there is a relative scarcity of books (other than his teachings) on Hippocrates, since not too much is known about his personal life. Nonetheless, there is a large collection of his works in eight volumes in the Loeb Classical Library (1923–1988) series: *Hippocrates. Hippocratic Collection*. Cambridge: Harvard University Press.

Of most interest here is probably volume 1:

- Loeb Classical Library. 1923. *Hippocrates: Ancient Medicine. Airs, Waters, Places. Epidemics 1 and 3. The Oath. Precepts. Nutriment.* Volume I in the eight-volume *Hippocratic Collection.* Cambridge: Harvard University Press.

Ancient Greek Understanding of Genetics

We perhaps played down the grasp that the ancient Greeks had of genetics. The level of Hippocratic understanding of genetics, both with its minuses and substantial plusses, is well indicated in "Airs, Waters, and Places" attributed to Hippocrates. It is in part one of the earliest studies of population genetics. For example, there is an entry concerning a tribe called the Macrocephali who performed the curious practice of head-binding on new born children to elongate the head. It was argued that at first this constitution was the result of force, but that in the course of time, it was formed naturally. "Children with bald heads are born to parents with bald heads, children with blue eyes to parents who have blue eyes, and the children of parents having distorted eyes usually squint also. If the same may be said of other forms of the body, what is to prevent it from happening that a child with a long head should be produced by a parent having a long head?" This sounds exactly like Lamarckism, Jean-Baptiste Lamarck being the nineteenth century biologist-philosopher who proposed that giraffes have long necks because for generations they stretched to reach the leaves on trees. But to be fair, these Hippocratic observations could be taken as consistent with Darwinism, which might postulate that children with already long heads were either less susceptible to the trauma or (more likely) that people with longer heads were considered more beautiful and more marriage-worthy. It is also interesting, however, that "Airs, Waters, and Places" subsequently states that long heads now do *not* seem to be passed on genetically, and that this might be due to the Macrocephali interbreeding with other tribes. Half right!

CHAPTER 3

Concerning the History of Medicine in Society

There are many sources on medical history, ever a popular topic. We like:

- R. Porter. 2002. *Blood and Guts: A Short History of Medicine.* New York: Norton.
- R. Porter. 1997. *The Greatest Benefit to Mankind: A Medical History of Humanity from Antiquity to the Present.* New York: Norton.
- G. S. Rousseau. 2003. *Framing and Imagining Disease in Cultural History.* Basingstoke: Palgrave Macmillan.

For general background:

- J. Diamond. 1997. *Guns, Germs, and Steel: The Fates of Human Societies.* New York: Norton.
- W. H. McNeill. 1963. *The Rise of the West: A History of the Human Community.* Chicago: University of Chicago Press.

See also on the Internet the *Encyclopaedia Britannica*, "History of Europe." http://www.britannica.com/EBchecked/topic/195896/history-of-Europe.

Christianity and Science

As hinted in this chapter, there have been some odd tensions between religion and medicine, and science generally, in Europe. Comment was often, and apparently continues to be, "official." According to the recent National Post "blogging" article, http://network.nationalpost.com/np/blogs/posted/archive/2008/01/28/pope-vs-science.aspx, "Pope Benedict has once again come out swinging against science, re-igniting a science-versus-religion debate by telling an academic gathering that science is not capable of fully understanding the mystery of human beings." It states that the Pope said: "In an age when scientific developments attract and seduce with the possibilities they offer, it's more important than ever to educate our contemporaries' consciences so that science does not become the criteria for goodness. ... Man is not the fruit of chance or a bundle of convergences, determinisms or physical and chemical reactions." Pope Benedict is said to have urged the meeting of scientists at the Paris Academy of Sciences and Pontifical Academy of Sciences to accompany current science by with "research into anthropology, philosophy, and theology" to give insight into "man's own mystery, because no science can say who man is, where he comes from or where he is going." There is much wisdom in these purported words by the Pope, and the apparent support of anthropology is pleasing in view of the important discoveries of molecular anthropology described in Chapter 2. However, the last statement on "man's own mystery" does seem strangely at odds with it. The following is an enduring essay on the Catholic church and science of the past hundreds of years, stopping short just before the dawn of quantum mechanics and what we see as modern medicine.

- J. J. Walsh. 1908. *The Popes and Science: The History of the Papal Relations to Science during the Middle Ages and Down to Our Own Time*. Whitefish, MT: Kessinger Publishing. Reprinted 2003.

Concerning Medieval Arabic and Chinese Medicine

The authors' mindsets are necessarily Western (BR) and Eastern (OB), but it is good to also emphasize and drill into the important Arab contribution:

- D. W. Tschanz. 1997. Arab roots of European medicine. *Saudi Aramco World* 48(3):20–31, at http://www.saudiaramcoworld.com/issue/199703/the.arab.roots.of.european.medicine.htm.
- B. Saad, H. Azaizeh, and O. Said. 2005. Tradition and perspectives of Arab Herbal medicine: A review. *Evidence-Based Complementary and Alternative Medicine* 2(4):475–479.

There are many sources on Chinese medicine. The words *ancient*, *Chinese*, and *medicine* get over a third of a million Google hits. Ancient Chinese medicine is not without its recent critics, and amazingly this popular cat-lover's website was fifth on the Google list today, stating that "this ridiculous black art of Chinese medicine is practiced at the expense of many wild animals" (http://cat-chitchat.pictures-of-cats.org/2008/06/ancient-chinese-medicine.html). The *Britannica Concise Encyclopaedia* (2007) also declares that "Use of certain animal remedies has seriously contributed to the endangered-species status of some animals (including tiger and rhinoceros)." It is unfortunate that some of the more controversial exotic animal ingredients of traditional Chinese medicine (apart perhaps from the naturally shed skin of reindeer antlers) may be of questionable value, while the thousands of mineral sources such as these described in Chapters 2 and 3, and iron (for anemia, as apparently discovered by the Chinese) and chaulmoogra oil (for leprosy), do seem to be beneficial. It is probable that sources such as tiger and rhinoceros were exotic medicines for emperors and high ranking officials and warriors, and so became attractive by lack of their common availability to the general ancient Chinese population. The following have good content describing Chinese medicine it developed over the time period of this Chapter 3:

- V. Lo. 2005. *Medieval Chinese Medicine: The Dunhuang Medical Manuscripts*. London: Routledge Curzon.
- N. Wiseman and A. Ellis. 1995. *The Fundamentals of Chinese Medicine*. Taos, NM: Paradigm Publications.
- D. Bensky and R. Barolet. 1990. *Chinese Herbal Medicine: Formulas and Strategies*. Seattle, WA: Eastland Press.

Concerning the History of Modern Biochemistry and Molecular Biology

The following two sources fill in some gaps in our discussion of the development of aspects of the basic biomolecular sciences. The first is also a good guide to the history of biochemistry, with an emphasis on the understanding of the role of proteins that is so important to pharmacology and now pharmacogenomics. The second focuses on the modern knowledge on the same theme.

- P. R. Srinivasan, J. S. Fruton, and J. T. Edsall, eds. 1979. The origins of modern biochemistry: A retrospect on proteins. *Annals of the New York Academy of Sciences USA* 325.
- J. S. Fruton. 1999. *Proteins, Enzymes, Genes: The Interplay of Chemistry and Biology*. New Haven: Yale University Press.

The following are mainly for historical researchers. It would not be complete without reading about Sir Hans Krebs and his founding contributions to modern biochemistry. Volume 1 is about his early life, so volume 2 is a better choice for reading about his methods and the conclusions that stand today regarding the core of metabolism of most living things.

- F. L. Holmes. 1993. *Hans Krebs*. Volume 2: *Architect of Intermediary Metabolism, 1933–1937*. Oxford: Oxford University Press.
- M. Morange. 1998. *A History of Molecular Biology*. Cambridge: Harvard University Press.
- F. H. Portugal and J. S. Cohen. 1972. *A Century of DNA: A History of the Discovery of the Structure and Function of the Genetic Substance*. Cambridge: MIT Press.
- G. Wolf. 2003. Friedrich Miescher: The man who discovered DNA. *Chemical Heritage* 21(2):10–11, 37–41.

- F. W. Stahl, ed. 2000. *We Can Sleep Later: Alfred D. Hershey and the Origins of Molecular Biology*. Cold Spring Harbor: Cold Spring Harbor Laboratory Press.
- F. L. Holmes. 2001. *Meselson, Stahl, and the Replication of DNA: A History of the Most Beautiful Experiment in Biology*. New Haven: Yale University Press.
- J. Cairns, G. S. Stent, and J. D. Watson. 1992. *Phage and the Origins of Molecular Biology*. Cold Spring Harbor: Cold Spring Harbor Laboratory Press.
- E. Chargaff. 1978. *Heraclitean Fire: Sketches from a Life before Nature*. New York: Rockefeller University Press.
- T. Hager. 1995. *Force of Nature: The Life of Linus Pauling*. New York: Simon and Schuster.
- L. Pauling. 1970. "Fifty Years of Progress in Structural Chemistry and Molecular Biology." *Dædalus* 99(4):988.
- T. Krude, ed. 2004. *DNA: Changing Science and Society*. Cambridge: Cambridge University Press.
- S. de Chadarevian. 2002. *Designs for Life: Molecular Biology after World War II*. Cambridge: Cambridge University Press.
- G. S. Stent. 1970. DNA. *Dædalus* 99(4):909.
- R. J. Dubos. 1976. *The Professor, the Institute, and DNA*. New York: Rockefeller University Press.
- M. Eigen. 1987. *Stufen Zum Leben: Die Frühe Evolution im Visier der Molekularbiologie*. Munich: R. Piper.
- L. E. Kay. 2000. *Who Wrote the Book of Life? A History of the Genetic Code*. Stanford: Stanford University Press.
- S. Brenner. 2001. *My Life in Science*. London: Science Archive.
- H. F. Judson. 1979. *The Eighth Day of Creation*. New York: Simon and Schuster.

A Quick Primer on the Central Dogma (DNA Makes RNA Makes Protein)

DNA has a form of double helix and contains nearly 3 billion base pairs, each of which consists of one of four types of nucleotides such as adenine, thymine, cytosine, and guanine. The human genome, the complete human DNA, would be equivalent to about 250 volumes of Manhattan phone directories when it is printed. Figure B.1 illustrates the processes associated with protein synthesis: transcription, translation, posttranslation modification (PTM), and folding.

Concerning the Double Helix

This paradigm—among many exciting discoveries in basic biomedical research—deserves special attention. We compiled these sources because of their interesting *evolving* views of the personal and establishment ecosystem dynamics around Crick and Watson and their discovery of the DNA double helix.

- J. Watson and F. Crick. 1953. Molecular structure of nucleic acids: A structure for deoxyribose nucleic acid. *Nature* 171:737–738.
- R. Olby. 1970. Francis Crick, DNA, and the central dogma. *Dædalus* 99(4):938.

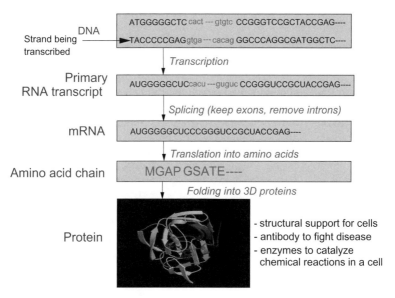

Figure B.1   From genes to proteins

- D. A. Chambers, ed. 1995. *DNA: The Double Helix. Perspective and Prospective at Forty Years. Annals of the New York Academy of Sciences USA* 758.
- S. Chomet, ed. 1995. *DNA: Genesis of a Discovery*. London: New-Hemisphere.
- W. Fuller. 2003. Who said "helix"? Right and wrong in the story of how the structure of DNA was discovered. *Nature* 424:876–878.
- G. B. Kauffman. 2003. DNA structure: Happy 50th birthday! *Chemical Educator* 8:219–230.

Concerning the History of Computers and the Internet

Computers are worth a whole history library, from counting-stones and notched sticks to abacus on to today's supercomputer. It is likely that very sophisticated devices in ancient Greece were lost from history by the fires in the great library in ancient Alexandria. However, a serious contender to the medieval computer mentioned in this chapter is the *antikythera mechanism*, the clockwork style device discovered more than 100 years ago in a Roman shipwreck and thought to have been used by ancient Greeks to read astronomical cycles.

See, for example, http://news.bbc.co.uk/1/hi/sci/tech/6191462.stm. The reader interested in the further historical development of the idea should look up Charles Babbage and Ada Lovelace, a daughter of Lord Byron who learned of Babbage's analytic engine and described how it could be programmed. More recent are the contubutions of Claude Shannon and Alan Turing, and of Gregory Chaitin today. For a discussion of the machines used, a friendly introduction is given in:

- J. Kopplin. 2002. *An Illustrated History of Computers*. http://www.computer-sciencelab.com/ComputerHistory/History.htm.

Extensive sources can be also found in:

- Yahoo. 2008. *Computers and Internet History in the Yahoo Directory*. http://dir. yahoo.com/Computers_and_Internet/history.

On the history of computer networks and the Internet, the following are useful. The first is in regard to an individual who may be less well known to the general reader but has made important contributions as an inventor at Stanford Research Institute (now SRI International). Douglas Engelbart and his team generated key ideas in the 1960s that led to the computer mouse, hypertext linking, real-time text editing, online journals, shared-screen teleconferencing, and remote shareware or collaboration technology. His work is regarded as the foundation of personal computing and the Internet. An example historical document is:

- D. C. Engelbart. 1962. Augmenting human intellect: A conceptual framework. Summary report AFOSR-3223 under Contract AF 49(638)-1024, SRI project 3578 for Air Force Office of Scientific Research. Stanford Research Institute, Menlo Park, CA.
- K. Hafner. 1998. *Where Wizards Stay up Late: The Origins of the Internet*. New York: Simon and Schuster.
- J. Markoff. 1999. *Internet Pioneer Ponders the Next Revolution*, NCBI. http:// partners.nytimes.com/library/tech/99/12/biztech/articles/122099outlook-bobb. html.

For a discussion of the technology of networking in general, as it was at least until recently and still mostly is, see:

- A. S. Tanenbaum. 1996. *Computer Networks*. Englewood Cliffs, NJ:Prentice-Hall.

CHAPTER 4

Concerning Revolutions and Transitions in World Industry

The following are some key books on transitions in industry and their effects on society, including the industry's globalization. No list would be complete without many works by Alvin Toffler (born 1928). He is known for his works on the digital, communications, corporate, social, military, and economic transitions arising from science and engineering advances. A former associate editor of *Fortune* magazine, his interests evolved from technology assessment in the shorter term to its broader social impact.

- A. Toffler. 1970. *Future Shock*. New York: Bantam Books.
- A. Toffler. 1975. *The Eco-Spasm Report*. New York: Bantam Books.
- A. Toffler. 1980. *The Third Wave*. New York: Bantam Books.
- A. Toffler. 1985. *The Adaptive Corporation*. New York: McGraw-Hill.
- A. Toffler. 1990. *Powershift: Knowledge, Wealth and Violence at the Edge of the 21st Century*. New York: Bantam Books.
- A. Toffler. 1995. *War and Anti-War*. New York: Warner Books.

- A. Toffler. 2006. *Revolutionary Wealth*. New York: Knopf.
- D. Landes. 1999. *The Wealth and Poverty of Nations: Why Some Are So Rich and Some So Poor*. New York: Norton.
- K. Pomeranz. 2000. *The Great Divergence: China, Europe and the Making of the Modern World Economy*. Princeton: Princeton University Press.
- S. L. Croucher. 2004. *Globalization and Belonging: The Politics of Identity a Changing World*. Lanham, MD: Rowman and Littlefield.
- J. Bhagwati. 2004. *In Defense of Globalization*. New York: Oxford University Press.
- A. Dreher, N. Gaston, and P. Martens. 2008. *Measuring Globalisation: Gauging Its Consequences*. Berlin: Springer.

Concerning the Limits and Frontiers of Scientific Discovery

In the spirit of the books listed above, the need for innovation is on the lips of every government. One of the authors (BR) participated in the following, effectively a Whitepaper to the White House.

- Panel on the National Innovation Initiative. 2004. *Innovate America*. Washington, DC: The Council on Competitiveness.

The 2004 Whitepaper covered medical as well as many other aspects, but note in particular:

- S. J. Heinig, J. Y. Krakower, H. B. Dickler, and D. Korn. 2007. Sustaining the engine of U.S. biomedical discovery. *New England Journal of Medicine* 357:1042–1047.

Whether we can keep discovering and inventing at the same rate, the following list will give food for thought. The last three should be read in the hindsight of reading the first, though for different reasons.

- J. Horgan. 1996. *The End of Science: Facing the Limits of Knowledge in the Twilight of the Scientific Age*. North Reading, MA: Helix Books/Addison Wesley.
- Scientific American Special Report. 2008. *The Future of Physics*. February.
- V. K. McElheny. 2003. *Watson and DNA: Making a Scientific Revolution*. New York: Perseus Books.
- R. Penrose. 1989. *The Emperor's New Mind: Concerning Minds and the Laws of Physics*. New York: Oxford University Press.

Concerning the History of Healthcare and Health Insurance

This is a selection of US managed healthcare and health insurance themes along with the themes of largely socialized UK healthcare for comparison. Compare finally the study on Canadian healthcare, typically seen as a kind of hybrid between the above.

- H. E. Sigerist. 1934. *The History of American Medicine*. New York: Norton.
- J. E. Murray. 2007. *Origins of American Health Insurance: A History of Industrial Sickness Funds*. New Haven: Yale University Press.

- G. Rivett. 1998. *From Cradle to Grave: Fifty Years of the NHS*. London: Kings Fund.
- Socialist Health Association. 2008. *NHS Reform*. http://www.sochealth.co.uk/news/NHSreform.htm.
- P. Hewitt. 2005. Even Nye Bevan's NHS saw a role for the private sector. *The Guardian*, February 7 (available at http://www.guardian.co.uk/politics/2005/jul/02/society.publicservices).
- M. Davidmann. 1985. *Reorganising the National Health Service: An Evaluation of the Griffiths Report*. http://www.solhaam.org/articles/nhs.html.
- Editors of Scientific American. 2008. Pay for what works: Presidential candidates must address unneeded medical technology and procedures as part of health care reform. *Scientific American* Vol. 298 (Special Report on the Future of Physics, February 2008):32.
- C. P. Shah. 2003. *Public Health and Preventative Medicine in Canada*, 5th ed. Toronto: Elsevier.

Concerning Medical Errors

Although the epidemiological scale of medical errors worldwide had been appreciated for some time, the first of these references on medical errors was seen as one among several a blockbuster announcements as to how bad things really are. The Amercian Rifle Association was quick to point out how many times it is safer to keep a gun at home, based on current statistics. The reader might indulge in some Internet research on the latter because a decimal point error in calculations seems to have cropped up and got propagated through the Internet, giving the impression of guns being thousands of times safer than medical care. Nonetheless, the statistics are startling.

- Institute of Medicine. 2000. *To Err Is Human: Building a Safer Health System*. Washington, DC: National Academy Press.
- T. P. Hofer, MD. 2000. *What Is an Error? Effective Clinical Practice Effective Clinical Practice*, 2000:3:261–269.
- S. Weingart, W. R. Wilson, R. Gibberd, and B. Harrison. 2000. *Epidemiology of Medical Error*. London: BMJ Publishing Group.
- R. A. Hayward. 2001. Estimating hospital deaths due to medical errors: Preventability is in the eye of the reviewer. *Journal of the American Medical Association* 286:415–420.
- S. Irwin, C. Fazan, and R. Allfrey. 1995. *Medical Negligence Litigation: A Practitioner's Guide*. London: Legal Action Group.

Research Studies in Drug Response

Two views on drug response, the first is on when things go wrong, and the second about the extent to which they can go right for the wrong reasons.

- J. Lazarou, B. H. Pomeranz, and P. N. Corey. 1998. Incidence of adverse drug reactions in hospitalized patients: a meta-analysis of prospective studies. *Journal of the American Medical Association* 279:1200–1205.

- F. Benedetti, G. Maggi, and L. Lopiano. 2003. Open versus hidden medical treatments: The patient's knowledge about a therapy affects the therapy outcome. *Prevention and Treatment* Vol 6(1), June 2003, ArtID 1a.

CHAPTER 5

Concerning Advanced Digital Medical Records

Electronic health records, and digital patient records generally, are important and inevitable:

- HealthCare IT News. 2006. We've got to adopt health information technology, and get on with it. http://www.healthcareitnews.com/printStory.cms.

But the electronic health records issue is still continually controversial. See:

- R. Pear. 2007. Warnings over privacy of U.S. health network. *New York Times*, February 18.
- R. Stein. 2004. Implantable medical ID approved by FDA. *Washington Post*, October 14, p. A01.

The medical ID idea is the basis for a potential implantable on-a-chip record. On digital patient records generally, it is good to read these in temporal sequence, to note the evolving positive mood.

- S. Kaihara. 1998. Realisation of the computerised patient record: Relevance and unsolved problems. *International Journal of Medical Informatics* 49:1–8.
- A. Shabo, P. Vortman, and B. Robson. 2001. *Who's Afraid of Lifetime Electronic Medical Records?* In *Proceedings of Towards Electronic Health Records Conference*, London: TEHRE.
- C. Parish. 2006. Edging towards a brave new IT world. *Nursing Standard* 27:15–16.
- American Health Information Management Association. 2007. *The Value of Personal Health Records: A Joint Position Statement for Consumers of Health Care.* Bethesda, MD: American Medical Informatics Association.
- D. Smaltz and E. Berner. 2007. *The Executive's Guide to Electronic Health Records.* Chicago: Health Administration Press, p. 3.

Research Papers Regarding Digital Medical Records

- J. A. Linder, D. W. Bates, B. Middleton, and R. S. Stafford. 2007. Electronic health record use and the quality of ambulatory care in the United States. *Arch Internal Medicine* 167:1400–1405.
- D. J. Ringold, J. P. Santell, and P. J. Schneider. 2000. American Association of Health Stem Pharmacists national survey of pharmacy practice in acute care settings: Dispensing and administration—1999. *American Journal of Health-System Pharmacy* 57(19):1759–1775.

- B. Raymond and C. Dold. 2001. Clinical information systems: Achieving the vision. In *The Benefits of Clinical Information Systems*. Oakland, CA: Kaiser Permanent Institute for Health Policy.
- D. Gans, J. Kralewski, T. Hammons, and B. Dowd. 2005. Medical groups' adoption of electronic health records and information systems. *Health Affairs (Project Hope)* 24(5):1323–1333.
- C. D. Carr and S. M. Moore. 2003. IHE: A model for driving adoption of standards. *Computerized Medical Imaging and Graphics* 27:1–10.
- B. Robson and R. Mushlin. 2005. The genomic messaging system language including command extensions for clinical data categories. *Journal of Proteome Research (Am. Chem. Soc.)* 4(2):275–299.
- F. Cao, H. K. Huang, and X. Q. Zhou. 2003. Medical image security in a HIPAA mandated PACS environment. *Computerized Medical Imaging and Graphics* 27:1–12.
- E. N. Barthell and K. R. Pemble. 2003. The National Emergency Extranet Project. *Journal of Emegency Medicine* 24(1):95–100.
- D. Lekkas, S. Gritzalis, and S. Katsikas. 2002. Quality assured trusted third parties for deploying secure internet-based healthcare applications. *International Journal of Medical Informatics* 65:79–96.
- Editorial. 2002. A healthy prognosis for biometric technologies. *Biometric Technology Today* 10(3):9–11.
- P. Degoulet, L. Marin, M. Lavril, C. Le Bozec, E. Delbecke, J.-J. Meaux, and L. Rose. 2002. The HEGP component-based clinical information system. *International Journal of Medical Informatics* 73(2):97–100.
- J. J. Cimino, V. L. Patel, and A. W. Kushniruk. 2002. The patient clinical information system (PatCIS): technical solutions for and experience with giving patients access to their electronic medical records. *International Journal of Medical Informatics* 68:113–127.
- C. Bolchni and F. A. Schreiber. 2002. Smart card embedded information systems: a methodology for privacy oriented architectural design. *Data and Knowledge Engineering* 41:159–182.
- M. Tsiknakis, D. G. Katehakis, and S. C. Orphanoudakis. 2002. An open, component-based infomation infrastructure for integrated health information networks. *International Journal of Medical Informatics* 68:3–26.
- D. C. Chou and A. Y. Chou. 2002. Healthcare information portal: A web technology for the healthcare community. *Technology in Society* 24:317–330.
- S. D. Goold and G. Klipp. 2002. Managed care members talk about trust. *Social Science and Medicine* 54:879–888.
- L. Janczewski and F. X. Shi. 2002. Development of information security baselines for healthcare information systems in New Zealand. *Computers and Society* 21(2):172–192.
- A. J. Rohm and G. R. Milne. 2002. Just what the doctor ordered: The role of information sensitivity and trust in reducing medical information privacy concern. *Journal of Business Research* 5757:1–12.
- A. Riva, K. D. Mandl, D. H. Oh, D. J. Nigrin, A. Butte, P. Szolovits, and I. S. Kohanne. 2001. The personal internetworked notary guardian. *International Journal of Medical Informatics* 62:27–40.

- G. Stalidis, A. Prentza, I. N. Vlachos, S. Maglavera, and D. Koutsouris. 2001. Medical support system for continuation of care based on XML web technology. *International Journal of Medical Informatics* 64:385–400.
- B. Blobel, P. Pharow, V. Spiegel, K. Engel, and R. Engelbrecht. 2001. Securing interoperability between chip card based medical information systems and health networks. *International Journal of Medical Informatics* 64:401–415.
- C. Dobbing. 2001. Paperless practice: Electronic medical records at island health. *Computer Methods and Programs in Biomedicine* 64:197–199.
- B. Sadan. 2001. Patient data confidentiality and patient rights. *International Journal of Medical Informatics* 62:41–49.
- L. G. Kun. 2001. Telehealth and the global health network in the 21st century: From homecare to public health informatics. *Computer Methods and Programs in Biomedicine* 64:155–167.
- A. M. Thornett. 2001. Computer decision support systems in general practice. *International Journal of Infomation Management* 21:39–47.
- B. Stanberry. 2001. Legal ethical and risk issues in telemedicine. *Computer Methods and Programs in Biomedicine* 64:225–233.
- B. M. Dickens and R. J. Cook. 2000. Law and ethics in conflict over confidentiality? *International Journal of Gynecology and Obstetrics* 70:385–391.
- C. Safran and H. Goldberg. 2000. Electronic patient records and the impact of the Internet. *International Journal of Medical Informatics* 60:77–83.
- J. Smith. 2000. Towards a secure EPR: Cultural and educational issues. *International Journal of Medical Informatics* 20(60):137–142.
- E.-H. W. Kluge. 2000. Professional codes for electronic HC record protection: Ethical, legal, economic and structural issues. *International Journal of Medical Informatics* 60:85–96.
- R. Cook and B. M. Dickens. 2000. Recognizing adolescents' "evolving capacities" to exercise choice in reproductive healthcare. *International Journal of Gynecology and Obstetrics* 70:13–21.
- R. Schoenberg and C. Safran. 2000. Internet based repository of medical records that retains patient confidentiality. *British Medical Journal* 321:1199–1203.
- J. G. Anderson. 2000. Security of the distributed electronic patient record: A case-based approach to identifying policy issues. *International Journal of Medical Informatics* 60:111–118.
- A. Donaldson. 2000. Policy for cryptography in healthcare—A view from the NHS. *International Journal of Medical Informatics* 60:105–110.
- K. Ishikawa. 2000. Health data use and protection policy; based on differences by cultural and social environment. *International Journal of Medical Informatics* 60:119–125.
- R. Neame. 2000. Communications and EHR: Authenticating who' s who is vital. *International Journal of Medical Informatics* 60:185–190.
- J. Brender, C. Nohr, and P. McNair. 2000. Research needs and priorities in health informatics. *International Journal of Medical Informatics* 58–59:257–289.
- B. Blobel. 2000. Advanced tool kits for EPR security. *International Journal of Medical Informatics* 60:169–175.
- A. Ohrn and L. Ohno-Machado. 1999. Using Boolean reasoning to anonomize databases. *International Journal of Medical Informatics* 15:235–254.

- J. D. Halamka, C. Osterland, and C. Safran. 1999. CareWeb, a web-based medical record for an integrated health care delivery system. *International Journal of Medical Informatics* 54:1–8.
- D. B. Baker and D. K. Masys. 1999. PCASSO: A design for secure communication of personal health information via the Internet. *International Journal of Medical Informatics* 54:97–104.
- E. Smith and J. H. P. Eloff. 1999. Security in health-care information systems current trends. *International Journal of Medical Informatics* 54:39–54.
- G. S. Meyer. 1999. Privacy versus progress: The international debate over medical records research. *Nutrition* 15(1):81–82.
- K. Louwerse. 1998. The electronic patient record; the management of access-case study: Leiden University Hospital. *International Journal of Medical Informatics* 49:39–44.
- A. L. Espinosa. 1998. Availability of health data: Requirements and solutions. *International Journal of Medical Informatics* 49:97–104.
- H. Takeda, Y. Matsumura, T. Okada, S. Kuwata, and M. Inoue. 1998. A Japanese approach to establish an electronic patient record system in an intelligent hospital. *International Journal of Medical Informatics* 49:45–51.
- F. de Meyer, P.-A. Lundgren, G. de Moor, and T. Fiers. 1998. Determination of user requirements for the secure communication of electronic medical record information. *International Journal of Medical Informatics* 49:125–130.
- E.-H. W. Kluge. 1998. Fostering a security culture: A model code of ethics for health information professionals. *International Journal of Medical Informatics* 49:105–110.
- C. I. McDonald, J. M. Overhage, P. Dexter, B. Takesue, and J. G. Suico. 1998. What is done, what is needed and what is realistic to expect from medical informatics standards. *International Journal of Medical Informatics* 48:5–12.
- C. Lovis, R. H. Baud, and J.-R. Scherrer. 1998. Internet integrated in the daily medical practice within an electronic patient record. *Computers in Biology and Medicine* 28:567–579.
- D. Gritzalis. 1997. A baseline security policy for distributed healthcare information systems. *Computers and Security* 16:709–719.
- T. C. Rindfleisch. 1997. Confidentiality, information technology, and health care. *Communications of the Association of Computing Machinery* 40(8):93–100.
- A. B. King. 1996. Safeguarding patient records. *Nutrition* 12(10):726–727.
- H. Lærum, T. H. Karlsen, and A. Faxvaag. 2003. Effects of scanning and eliminating paper-based medical records on hospital physicians' clinical work practice. *Journal of the American Medical Informatics Association* 10:588–595.
- K. D. Mandl, P. Szolovits, and I. S. Kohane. 2001. Public standards and patients' control: How to keep electronic medical records accessible but private. *British Medical Journal* 322:283–287.

CHAPTER 6

Concerning Medical Ethics

The first of the directives given below is a true historical classic. The next two remain, comprising the ACP Ethics manual, and are still valid.

- T. Percival. 1849. *Medical Ethics*. Oxford: Parker, Oxford University.
- American College of Physicians Ethics Manual. 1989. Part 1: History; the patient; other physicians. American College of Physicians. *Annals of Internal Medicine* 111:245–252.
- American College of Physicians Ethics Manual. 1989. Part 2: The physician and society; research; life-sustaining treatment; other issues. American College of Physicians. *Annals of Internal Medicine* 111:327–335.

Research Papers, Reports and Advanced Studies in Ethics in Research and Pharmaceutical Collaboration

Pure medical research ethical issues and the sometimes controversial issue of the physician dealing with pharmaceutical companies is an odd mix. Today the physician might also work with pharmaceutical companies in regard to the success, or otherwise, of drugs, and this is something at which a physician can make a fair amount of extra money. Some medical schools appear to be teaching evidence-based medicine research and other research, in part so that this can be executed and reported correctly, and presumably the pharmaceutical companies like physicians to be trained this way. While part of the feedback from physicians is to allow monitoring of drug safety and also to look for alternative uses for marketed drugs, another is to assign appropriate prices to drugs, based on use. Generally speaking, the public thinks the prices are too high. See:

- Malcolm Gladwell. 2004. High prices: How to think about prescription drugs. *New Yorker*. http://www.newyorker.com/archive/2004/10/25/041025crat_atlarge.

This arrangement may be in a state of flux, however, in view of the emerging initiatives to formalize and augment by IT the process by involving pharmaceutical consortia with the FDA. That matter has received some ongoing Internet research.

- Commission on Research Integrity. 1995. *Integrity and Misconduct in Research: Report to the Secretary of Health and Human Services*. House Committee on Commerce and the Senate Committee on Labor and Human Resources. Washington, DC: US Department of Health and Human Services, Public Health Service.
- S. E. Lind. 1988. Innovative medical therapies: Between practice and research. *Clinical Research* 36:546–551.
- R. J. Levine. 1986. *Ethics and Regulation of Clinical Research*, 2d ed. Baltimore: Urban and Schwarzenberg.
- American College of Physicians. 1989. Cognitively impaired subjects. *Annals of Internal Medicine* 111:843–848.
- S. E. Lind. 1990. Finder's fees for research subjects. *New England Journal of Medicine* 323:192–195.
- O. R. Goodenough. 2004. Responsibility and punishment. *Philosophical Transactions of the Royal Society: Biological Sciences* (Special Issue: Law and the Brain) 359:1805–1809.
- L. Snyder and A. L. Hillman. 1996. Financial incentives and physician decision making. In L. Snyder, ed., *Ethical Choices: Case Studies for Medical Practice*. Philadelphia: American College of Physicians, pp. 105–112.

- Council on Ethical and Judicial Affairs. 1992. Conflicts of interest. Physician ownership of medical facilities. American Medical Association. *Journal of the American Medical Association* 267:2366–2369.
- American College of Physicians. 1990. Physicians and the pharmaceutical industry. *Annals of Internal Medicine* 112:624–626.
- Royal College of Physicians. 1986. The relationship between physicians and the pharmaceutical industry. *Journal of the Royal College of Physicians* 20:235–242.

Research Papers, Reports, and Advanced Studies in Clinical Ethics

Here is a widespread selection of common and diverse ethical issues in medical practice.

- P. M. Dunn, T. H. Gallagher, M. O. Hodges, T. J. Prendergast, G. D. Rubenfeld, and S. W. Tolle. 1994. Medical ethics: An annotated bibliography. *Annals of Internal Medicine* 121:627–632.
- G. Povar and J. Moreno. 1988. Hippocrates and the health maintenance organization: A discussion of ethical issues. *Annals of Internal Medicine* 109:419–424.
- F. W. Peabody. 1927. The care of the patient. *Journal of the American Medical Association* 88:877–882.
- F. A. Rozovsky. 1990. *Consent to Treatment: A Practical Guide*, 2d ed. Boston: Little, Brown.
- G. Geller, J. R, Botkin, M. J. Green, N. Press, B. B. Biesecker, B. Wilfond, et al. 1997. Genetic testing for susceptibility to adult-onset cancer: The process and content of informed consent. *Journal of the American Medical Association* 277:1467–1474.
- A. R. Jonsen. 1990. *The New Medicine and the Old Ethics*. Cambridge: Harvard University Press.
- S. J. Reiser, A. J. Dyck, and W. J. Curran. 1977. *Ethics in Medicine: Historical Perspectives and Contemporary Concerns*. Cambridge: MIT Press.
- D. J. Rothman. 1991. *Strangers at the Bedside: A History of How Law and Bioethics Transformed Medical Decision Making*. New York: Basic Books.
- R. M. Veatch. 1981. *A Theory of Medical Ethics*. New York: Basic Books.
- T. L. Beauchamp and J. F. Childress. 1994. *Principles of Biomedical Ethics*, 4th ed. New York: Oxford University Press.
- J. Katz. 1997. *The Silent World of Doctor and Patient*. New York: Free Press.
- President's Commission for the Study of Ethical Problems in Medicine and Biomedical and Behavioral Research. 1982. *Making Health Care Decisions: A Report on the Ethical and Legal Implications of Informed Consent in the Patient-Practitioner Relationship*. Washington, DC: Government Printing Office.
- President's Commission for the Study of Ethical Problems in Medicine and Biomedical and Behavioral Research. 1983. *Securing Access to Health Care: A Report on the Ethical Implications of Differences in the Availability of Health Services*. Washington, DC: Government Printing Office.

- President's Commission for the Study of Ethical Problems in Medicine and Biomedical and Behavioral Research. 1983. *Screening and Counseling for Genetic Conditions: A Report on the Ethical, Social, and Legal Implications of Genetic Screening, Counselling, and Educational Programs.* Washington, DC: Government Printing Office.

- President's Commission for the Study of Ethical Problems in Medicine and Biomedical and Behavioral Research. 1982. *Splicing Life, A Report on the Social and Ethical Issues of Genetic Engineering with Human Beings.* Washington, DC: Government Printing Office.

- President's Commission for the Study of Ethical Problems in Medicine and Biomedical and Behavioral Research. 1983. *Deciding to Forgo Life-Sustaining Treatment: A Report on the Ethical, Medical, and Legal Issues in Treatment Decisions.* Washington, DC: Government Printing Office.

- L. Snyder and J. Weiner. 1996. Ethics and Medicaid Patients. In L. Snyder, ed., *Ethical Choices: Case Studies in Medical Practice.* Philadelphia: American College of Physicians, pp. 63–70.

- American College of Physicians. 1989. Health care needs of the adolescent. *Annals of Internal Medicine* 110:930–935.

- J. F. Burnum. 1991. Secrets about patients. *New England Journal of Medicine* 324:1130–1133.

- D. L. Roter, M. Stewart, S. M. Putnam, M. Lipkin Jr, W. Stiles, and T. S. Inui. 1997. Communication patterns of primary care physicians. *Journal of the American Medical Association* 277:350–356.

- T. E. Quill and P. Townsend. 1991. Bad news: delivery, dialogue, and dilemmas. *Archives Internal Medicine* 151:463–468.

- American Academy of Pediatrics Committee on Adolescence. 1989. Counseling the adolescent about pregnancy options. *Pediatrics* 83:135–137.

- J. Weiner. 1996. *The duty to treat HIV-positive patients.* In L. Snyder, ed., *Ethical Choices: Case Studies for Medical Practice.* Philadelphia: American College of Physicians, pp. 71–78.

- Health and Public Policy Committee, American College of Physicians; and the Infectious Diseases Society of America. 1988. The acquired immunodeficiency syndrome (AIDS) and infection with the human immunodeficiency virus (HIV). *Annals of Internal Medicine* 108:460–469.

- R. H. Murray and A. J. Rubel. 1992. Physicians and healers-unwitting partners in health care. *New England Journal of Medicine* 326:61–64.

- M. O. van Deventer. 2008. Meta-placebo: Do doctors have to lie about giving a fake treatment? *Medical Hypotheses* 71(3):335–339.

- W. Zinn and N. Furutani. 1996. Physician perspectives on the ethical aspects of disability determination. *Journal of General Internal Medicine* 11:525–532.

- Council, on Ethical and Judicial Affairs. 1991. Sexual misconduct in the practice of medicine. American Medical Association. *Journal of the American Medical Association* 266:2741–2745.

- J. Weiner and S. W. Tolle. 1996. Sex and the single physician. In L. Snyder, ed., *Ethical Choices: Case Studies for Medical Practice.* Philadelphia: American College of Physicians, pp. 53–60.

Research Studies on Ethical Handling of Seriously Ill Patients

In contrast to the mixed bag above, ethical handling of seriously ill patients deserves its own focus. It includes, for example, the ever-thorny issue of euthanasia.

- The SUPPORT Principal Investigators. 1995. A controlled trial to improve care for seriously ill hospitalized patients. The Study to Understand Prognoses and Preferences for Outcomes and Risks of Treatments (SUPPORT). *Journal of the American Medical Association* 274:1591–1598.
- Institute of Medicine. 1997. *Approaching Death: Improving Care at the End of Life*. Washington, DC: National Academy Press.
- C. K. Cassel and B. C. Vladek. 1996. ICD-9 code for palliative or terminal care. *New England Journal of Medicine* 335:1232–1234.
- M. L. Buchan and S. W. Tolle. 1995. Pain relief for dying persons: Dealing with physicians' fears and concerns. *Journal of Clinical Ethics* 6:53–61.
- L. Snyder. 1990. Life, death, and the American College of Physicians: The Cruzan case. *Annals of Internal Medicine* 112:802–804.
- G. J. Annas. 1991. The health care proxy and the living will. *New England Journal of Medicine* 324:1210–1213.
- S. W. Tolle, W. M. Bennett, D. H. Hickm, and J. A. Benson Jr. 1987. Responsibilities of primary physicians in organ donation. *Annals of Internal Medicine* 106:740–744.
- Council on Scientific Affairs and Council on Ethical and Judicial Affairs. 1990. Persistent vegetative state and the decision to withdraw or withhold life support. *Journal of the American Medical Association* 263:426–430.
- Executive Board, American Academy of Neurology. 1998. Position of the American Academy of Neurology on certain aspects of the care and management of the persistent vegetative state patient. April 21, 1998, Cincinnati, Ohio. *Neurology* 39:125–126.
- American Thoracic Society and ATS Board of Directors. 1991. Withholding and withdrawing life-sustaining therapy. *American Review of Respiratory Disease* 144(3 Pt 1):726–731.
- New York State Task Force on Life and the Law. 1994. *When Death Is Sought: Assisted Suicide and Euthanasia in the Medical Context*. Albany.
- Report of the Task Force on Physician-Assisted Suicide of the Society for Health and Human Values. 1995. Physician-assisted suicide: Toward a comprehensive understanding. *Academic Medicine* 70:583–590.
- S. W. Tolle and L. Snyder. 1996. Physician-assisted suicide revisited: comfort and care at the end of life. In L. Snyder, ed., *Ethical Choices: Case Studies for Medical Practice*. Philadelphia: American College of Physicians, pp. 17–23.

Other Issues in Healthcare Ethics

A broad range of issues for the most part affect healthcare somewhat more in the large but also address, for example, ethics consultation, the physician as an expert witness, patient referrals, and so on.

- J. LaPuma, D, Schiedermayer, and M. Seigler. 1995. Ethical issues in managed care. *Trends Health Care Law Ethics* 10:73–77.
- D. Mechanic and M. Schlesinger. 1996. The impact of managed care on patients' trust in medical care and their physicians. *Journal of the American Medical Association* 275:1693–1697.
- Ethics case study. 1997. Deciding how much care is too much. *ACP Observer* 17:1, 30–31.
- United Nations. 1955. First Congress on the Prevention of Crime and the Treatment of Offenders. *Standard Minimum Rules for the Treatment of Prisoners.* New York.
- J. C. Fletcher and M. Siegler. 1996. What are the goals of ethics consultation? A consensus statement. *Journal of Clinical Ethics* 7:122–126.
- Joint Commission on Accreditation of Hospitals. 1992. *Accreditation Manual for Hospitals*, Vol. 106. Chicago: Joint Commission on Accreditation of Healthcare Organizations.
- American College of Physicians. 1990. Guidelines for the physician expert witness. *Annals of Internal Medicine* 113:789.
- A. Varki. 1992. Of pride, prejudice, and discrimination: Why generalizations can be unfair to the individual. *Annals of Internal Medicine* 116:762–764.
- F. K. Conley. 1993. Toward a more perfect world-eliminating sexual discrimination in academic medicine. Editorial. *New England Journal of Medicine* 328:351–352.
- L. Snyder. 1996. Referrals and patients' wishes. In L. Snyder, ed., *Ethical Choices: Case Studies in Medical Practice.* Philadelphia: American College of Physicians, pp. 35–40.
- J. Weiner and L. Snyder. 1996. The impaired colleague. In L. Snyder, ed., *Ethical Choices: Case Studies in Medical Practice.* Philadelphia: American College of Physicians, pp. 79–84.

CHAPTER 7

Personalized and holistic medicine integrating physical medicine with psychological, lifestyle, cultural, and social aspects of the patient not so controversial, but introducing personalized and holistic medicine as a development of traditional alternative medicine is controversial. According to Richard L. Nahin, writing for the *American Medical Women's Association on* http://www.amwa-doc.org/index.cfm, Harold Varmus director of the NIH, suggested five strategies to improve the nation's health, in his speech to the 1997 graduating class of Stanford School of Medicine. First on his list was to "eliminate the divide between alternative and conventional [medicine] … Let's adopt another mindset: There are methods that work and methods that don't. Or methods that have been properly tested, so we know whether they work."

Concerning Alternative Medicine, Pros and Cons

A selection of sources and recommended further reading must include the pro-alternatitive medicine lobby as well as the ant-alternatitive medicine lobby so that the intersted reader can draw an independent conclusion. Note that the prestigious Mayo

Clinic below does support the alternatitive option by patients, and it is by no means a "lunatic fringe" issue in modern medical prcatice. For the most part, the more negative sources or potentially contra themes are placed at the end of this list.

- S. Bratman. 1997. *The Alternative Medicine Sourcebook*. Los Angeles, CA: Lowell House.
- Mayo Clinic. 2007. *Mayo Clinic Book of Alternative Medicine: The New Approach to Using the Best of Natural Therapies and Conventional Medicine*. Parsippany, NJ: Time Inc Home Entertainment.
- L. Galland. 1998. *Power Healing: Use the New Integrated Medicine to Cure Yourself*. New York: Random House.
- L. A. Wisneski and L. Anderson. 2005. *The Scientific Basis of Integrative Medicine*. Boca Raton, FL: CRC Press.
- S. Crompton. 2004. Back to the future: Complementary therapies get real. *Times Online*. Times Newspapers, Ltd., January 17.
- I. Illich. 1976. *Limits to Medicine. Medical Nemesis: The Expropriation of Health*. London: Penguin Books.
- B. Goldberg, J. Anderson, and L. Trivieri. 2002. *Alternative Medicine: The Definitive Guide*. Berkeley, CA: Ten Speed Press.
- K. Trudeau. 2006. *Natural Cures "They" Don't Want You to Know About*. Birmingham, AL: Alliance Publishing Group.
- W. D. Hand. 1980. Folk magical medicine and symbolism in the West. In W. D. Hand, *Magical Medicine*. Berkeley: University of California Press, pp. 305–319.
- M. Murray and J. Pizzorno. 1997. *Encyclopedia of Natural Medicine*. New York: Three Rivers Press.
- B. R. Cassileth. 1996. Alternative and complementary cancer treatments. *Oncologist* 1(3):173–179.
- P. Stevens Jr. 2001. Magical thinking in complementary and alternative medicine. *Skeptical Inquirer Magazine* (November–December):20–25.
- J. Alcock. 1999. Alternative medicine and the psychology of belief. *Scientific Review of Alternative Medicine* 3(2).
- F. E. Planer. 1988. *Superstition*. Buffalo, NY: Prometheus Books.
- R. Barker Bausell. 2007. *Snake Oil Science: The Truth About Complementary and Alternative Medicine*. New York: Oxford University Press.

Research Papers and Reports on Alternative Medicine

Some of the preceding references give rather annecdotal evidence. Appropiately the following are more rigorous studies that report on the two points of view.

- White House Commission. 2002. *Complementary and Alternative Medicine Policy*. ch. 2. Washington, DC: Government Printing Office.
- House of Lords Select Committee on Science and Technology. 2000. *Complementary and Alternative Medicine*. London: The Stationery Office.
- M. Angell and J. P. Kassirer. 1998. Alternative medicine: The risks of untested and unregulated remedies. *New England Journal of Medicine* 339:839.

- E. Ernst. 1995. Complementary medicine: Common misconceptions. *Journal of the Royal Society of Medicine* 88(5):244–247.
- D. Feinstein and D. Eden. 2008. Six pillars of energy medicine: Clinical strengths of a complementary paradigm. *Alternative Therapies in Health and Medicine* 14(1):44–54.
- D. M. Eisenberg. 1997. Advising patients who seek alternative medical therapies. *Annals of Internal Medicine* 127:61–69.
- F. Benedetti, G. Maggi, and L. Lopiano. 2003. Open versus hidden medical treatments: The patient's knowledge about a therapy affects the therapy outcome. *Prevention and Treatment* 6(1) (at http://psycnet.apa.org and also *Pain* 117(1):241.
- J. Diamond. 2001. Snake oil and other preoccupations. Foreword by Richard Dawkins. Reprint in R. Dawkins, *A Devil's Chaplain*. Boston: Houghton Mifflin, 2003.
- A. M. Downing and D. G. Hunter. 2003. Validating clinical reasoning: A question of perspective, but whose perspective? *Manual Therapy* 8(2):117–119.
- C. R. Joyce. 1994. Placebo and complementary medicine. *Lancet* 344(8932): 1279–1281.
- M. R. Tonelli and T. C. Callahan. 2001. Why alternative medicine cannot be evidence-based. *Academic Medicine: Journal of the Association of American Medical Colleges* 76(12):1213–1220.
- D. S. Sobel. 2000. The cost-effectiveness of mind-body medicine interventions. *Progress in Brain Research* 122:393–412.
- D. W. Saxon, G. Tunnicliff, J. J. Brokaw, and B. U. Raess. 2004. Status of complementary and alternative medicine in the osteopathic medical school curriculum. *Journal of the American Osteopathic Association* 104(3):121–126.
- K. J. Thomas, J. P. Nicholl, and P. Coleman. 2001. Use and expenditure on complementary medicine in England: A population based survey. *Complementary Therapies in Medicine* 9(1):2–11.
- M. V. Fenton and D. L. Morris. 2003. The integration of holistic nursing practices and complementary and alternative modalities into curricula of schools of nursing. *Alternative Therapies in Health and Medicine* 9(4):62–67.
- A. Kellehear. 2003. Complementary medicine: is it more acceptable in palliative care practice? *Medical Journal of Australia* 179(6 suppl):S46–S48.
- D. O. Weber. 1998. Complementary and alternative medicine: Considering the alternatives. *Physician Executive* 24(6):6–14.

Research Study Concerning Unconventional Medicine as an Industry

The following stands out as an essentially economic study:

- D. M. Eisenberg, R. C. Kessler, C. Foster, F. E. Norlock, D. R. Calkins, and T. L. Delbanco. 1993. Unconventional medicine in the United States: Prevalence, costs, and patterns of use. *New England Journal of Medicine* 328:246–252.

Acupuncture

Acupuncture has enduring popularity. So we provide some further discussion here.

Hua Tuo made many innovative contributions to the field of acupuncture. A patient sought medical treatment from Hua Tuo because he had problems with his feet and couldn't walk. After checking the pulse, Hua Tuo marked several acupuncture points on his back, and applied moxibustion seven times on each spot. The patient began to walk quickly after the treatment. Based on his own experience in acupuncture, Hua Tuo discovered the "Jia Ji acupuncture point," an acupuncture point that nips the spine. Today the acupuncture point in this area is still referred as "Hua Tuo point."

Guo Yu was from Guanghan County in the eastern Han dynasty, which is known today as Xindou County or Guanghan County in Sichuan province. He was the most famous medical doctor during the reign of Emperor He in the Han dynasty and served as the imperial physician. He wrote two books of medical theories, *The Classics of Acupuncture* and *Practical Approaches to Diagnosis through Feeling the Pulse*. Both were circulated widely all over China.

On Ying and Yang

Emperor He had a feeling that Guo Yu (the same man as above) was more than a regular physician, and he wanted to test his skill. One day Emperor He asked an imperial concubine, as well as his favorite man servant whose hands resembled those of a lady, to sit behind an opaque curtain. He asked the concubine to stretch out her hand, and the servant sitting beside her to stretch out the other hand, so that from the front of the curtain it looked as if the hands belonged to one person. Emperor He then asked Guo Yu to feel the pulse for "his concubine." After Guo Yu felt the pulse on both wrists, he said, "The left hand has the pulse of Yin; the right one has the pulse of Yang. Judging from the pulses, there should be a man and a woman. I do not understand why this is happening." After hearing Guo Yu's diagnosis, the Emperor He admired Guo Yu a great deal.

Modern View on Mysticism

- J. Horgan. 2003. *Rational Mysticism*. Dispatches from the border between Science and Spirituality. New York: Houghton Mifflin.

Concerning Zen

Zen texts are numerous; at time of writing the word *Zen* alone gets 114 million Google hits. Here are some useful first sources.

- T. Merton. 1967. *Mystics and Zen Masters*. New York: Farrar, Strauss and Giroux.
- H. Dumoulin. 2005. *Zen Buddhism: A History, Vol. 1: India and China*. World Wisdom.
- C. Prebish. 1975. *Buddhism: A Modern Perspective*. University Park: Penn State University Press.

Concerning Existentialism

The word *existentialism* in comparison gets just short of 3 million hits on Google. Here are but two example sources.

- W. Kaufmann. 1956. *Existentialism: From Dostoevsky to Sartre*. Cleveland: World Publishing.
- R. Aronson. 1980. *Jean-Paul Sartre: Philosophy in the World*. London: NLB.

Sources Used in Regard to "Automization" of the Human Mind

- J. Austin. 1978. *Chase, Chance and Creativity*. New York: Columbia University Press.
- J. Austin. 1998. *Zen and the Brain*. Cambridge: MIT Press.
- A. Deikman. 1999. Is there a voice in the night? *Times Literary Supplement*, August 6, p. 30.
- A. Deikman. 1999. Deautomization and the mystic experience. pp. 34–57 In C. Tart, ed., *Altered States of Consciousness*. New York: Harper Colins.
- A. Deikman. 2000. A functional approach to mysticism. *Journal of Consciousness Studies* 7:75–92.

More Bibliography Concerning Consciousness and Free Will

This is an mportant theme in behavioral and holistic healthcare. The first sets a rather different background, concerning the essentially material, chemical basis of our emotions. Although we have not investigated it in this book, it is plausible that various Zen and existential states we described are associated, at least in the subjective feel of it, with brain hormones such as neuropeptides. The works listed below relate to such a broad selection of themes.

- C. B. Pert. 1997. *Molecules of Emotion: Why You Feel the Way You Feel*, New York: Scribners.
- R. Penrose. 1994. *Shadows of the Mind: A Search for the Missing science of Consciousness*. New York: Oxford University Press.
- A. Sloman. 1993. The mind as a control system. In C. Hookway and D. Peterson, eds., *Philosophy and the Cognitive Sciences*. Cambridge: Cambridge University Press, pp. 69–110.
- P. Van Inwagen. 1986. *An Essay on Free Will*. New York: Oxford University Press.
- M. Velmans. 2003. *How Could Conscious Experiences Affect Brains?* Exeter, UK: Imprint Academic.
- D. Wegner. 2002. *The Illusion of Conscious Will*. Cambridge: MIT Press.
- C. Williams. 1980. *Free Will and Determinism: A Dialogue*. Indianapolis: Hackett Publishing.
- C. Koch and S. Greenfield. 2007. How does consciousness happen? *Scientific American* 297(4):76–83.
- B. Libet, A. Freeman, and K. Sutherland, eds. 1999. *The Volitional Brain: Towards a Neuroscience of Free Will*. Exeter, UK: Imprint Academic.

Research Papers in Models of Thought

These two examples are of interest in their own right, but the authors have also struck a chord in regard to neurological or systems models of Zen and existentialism.

- A. Nowak, R. R. Vallacher, A. Tesser, and W. Borkowski. 2000. Society of self: The emergence of collective properties in self-structure. *Psychological Review* 107: 39–61.
- H. A. Simon. 1979. Motivational and emotional controls of cognition. In *Models of Thought*. New Haven: Yale University Press, pp. 29–38.

Overview of Current Psychotherapies

- R. J. Corsini and D. J. Wedding, eds. *Current Psychotherapies*. Boston: Wadsworth Publishing.

Personalized Molecular Medicine

A personal scientific and molecular view of how *personalized* medicine will evolve is given in:

- B. Robson and J. Garnier. 2002. The future of highly personalized health care. *Studies Health Technology Information* 80:163–174.

CHAPTER 8

On architecting in general, the following is a good source, with much philosophy transferable to the world of IT:

- P.-A. Johnson. 1994. *The Theory of Architecture: Concepts Themes and Practices.* New York: Wiley.

On architecting *computer systems* for general application there are of course also many examples. Many concepts and terms about computer systems architecture can be found in the following:

- P. A. Laplante. 2001. *Dictionary of Computer Science, Engineering, and Technology.* Boca Raton, FL: CRC Press, pp. 94–95.

Distinguish architecting IT systems from *architecting a computer*; that said, however, the following is of interest because (although the title refers to the architecture of the individual computer not of the systems that embeds it) the author studies many quantifiable aspects relevant to the interacting role of the computer in the larger system:

- J. L. Hennessy and D. A. Patterson. 2003. *Computer Architecture: A Quantitative Approach*, 3rd ed. San Francisco: Morgan Kaufmann.

This chapter is specifically about *architecting* healthcare information systems, but not specifically architecting references are given elsewhere, especially for Chapter 5. There is no shortage of commercial organizations pursuing the opportunity and offering what they see as local or global healthcare IT systems solutions, from all the main computer companies, and through Phillips, GE, Cerner, SAS, and many others, and no shortage of descriptions of healthcare organizations planning for such systems. A good book is, however:

- M. K. Bourke. 1995. *Strategy and Architecture of Health Care Information Systems.* New York: Spinger.

Example research and other works with an architectural theme, explicit or implict, include the following:

- J. R. Scherrer Jr. and S. Spahni. 1999. Healthcare information system architecture (HISA) and its middleware models. *Proceedings American Medical Information Association Symposium*, Washington, DC: AMIA, pp. 935–939.
- F. F. Massimo. 1998. The standard "Healthcare Information Systems Architecture" and the DHE middleware. *International Journal of Medical Informatics* 52(1):39–51.
- W. J. Song, M. K. Cho, I. S. Ha, and M. K. Choi. 2006. *Healthcare System Architecture, Economic Value, and Policy Models in Large-Scale Wireless Sensor Networks in Computer Safety, Reliability, and Security.* New York: Springer.
- D. Peters. 2008. *Building a GIS: System Architecture Design Strategies for Managers.* Jacksonville, FL: ESRI Press, Ingram Publishers.
- J. Dudeck. 1997. *New technologies in hospital information systems.* Amsterdam: IOS Press.
- T. Bratan and M. Clarke. 2005. Towards the design of a generic systems architecture for remote patient monitoring in engineering in medicine and biology. *IEEE-EMBS 2005. 27th Annual International Conference of the Engineering in Medicine and Biology Society.* IEEE Publications, pp. 106–109.
- J. Bergmann, O. J. Bott, I. Hoffmann, and D. P. Pretschner. 2005. An eConsent-based system architecture supporting cooperation in integrated healthcare networks. *Studies in Health Information Technology Informatics* 116:961–966.
- J. Bergmann, O. J. Bott, D. Pretschner, and R. Haux. 2006. An eConsent-based shared system architecture for integrated healthcare networks. *International Journal of Medical Informatics* 76(2):130–136. See also *Studies in Health Technology Information* 2006, 116:961–966.
- A. Ailamaki, Y. E. Ioannidis, and M. Livny. 1998. Scientific workflow management by database management. In *Proceedings, 10th International Conference on Scientific and Statistical Database Management.* pp. 190–199.
- R. M. Jakobovits and J. F. Brinkley. 1997. Managing medical research data with a web-interfacing repository manager. In *Proceedings, American Medical Informatics Association Fall Symposium.* Nashville: American Medical Informatics Association, SIG Publications, pp. 454–458.
- B. Robson and R. Mushlin. 2004. Genomic messaging system for information-based personalized medicine with clinical and proteome research applications. *Journal of Proteome Research* 3(5):930–948.

Quick-Check Glossary Relating to Chapter 8 and the Readings Above

> **OLAP**   Online analytical processing; the sophisticated manipulation of data for analytic purposes, often using data organized into Cube (q.v.) structure.

Cube   A structure in which data are arranged along various dimensions and used to support OLAP functions.

ROLAP   Relational OLAP; characterized by the dynamic building of cubes using data sourced from a relational database.

MOLAP   Multidimensional OLAP; involving the analysis of data in prebuilt Cubes that are stored in a proprietary, nonrelational data structure.

Datamart   A database, often sourced from an EDW (q.v.), that serves the advanced data analysis needs of a particular group of business intelligent users within an organization.

BI   Business intelligence; an analysis needed by an organization of its data assets to improve decision making and organizational performance.

EDW   Enterprise data warehouse; a database that is the foundation for a comprehensive business intelligence infrastructure, typically characterized by a data-centric (as opposed to application-centric) database design.

Star schema   A database design, often used to improve OLAP performance, that features a central fact table linked to associated dimensional tables by way of surrogate keys.

Snowflake   Similar to a star schema, but with larger dimensional tables that have been de-normalized into sets of smaller tables.

"Languages" for Unified Access to Multidimensional Heterogeneous Data

The language SQL-X is an extension of SQL that provides a set of operators to compose queries against a relational database and produce complex XML documents, with a style reminiscent of report generation languages. A query is represented by a tree with the following kind of nodes:

<Root>   The tree root, and represents the whole document, containing a set of elements corresponding either to tuples or to group of tuples.

<Rel>   A database relation (obtained in general through an SQL query), whose tuples are converted into elements of its immediate container.

Moreover the user can specify if tuple fields are converted to attributes, instead of elements, the ordering of sequences, as well as other details of the conversion process.

<Att> (child of <Rel>)   A column whose value is used as element of its container.

<Nest>   The tuples of a relation that are associated, with a join operation, to a tuple of its container, and which will become roots of subtrees.

<Group>   The grouping of the tuples of a child node by some expression; each group is an element containing the tuples of the group as elements.

XQuery (XML Query) provides flexible query facilities to extract data from real and virtual documents using XML notation in a file system or on the World Wide Web, and consequently provides interaction and data exchange between the web world and the database world and ultimately enables collections of XML files to be accessed like databases. The XML Query project of the W3C Consortium includes not only the standard for querying XML documents, but also the next-generation standards for doing XML selection (XPath2), for XML serialization, for Full-Text Search, for a possible functional XML Data Model, and for a standard set of functions and operators for manipulating web data.

OQL is a SQL-like query language with special features dealing with complex objects, values and methods. OQL is an object-based version of SQL. The key differences between OQL and traditional SQL are (1) OQL has the ability to support object referencing within tables and allows objects to be nested within objects, (2) not all SQL keywords are supported within OQL (e.g., irrelevant keywords have been removed from the syntax), and (3) OQL has the ability to perform mathematical computations from within OQL statements.

A little More on Mobile Software Agent as a General Concept

The mobile software agent technology, also known as itinerant software technology, allows software components to travel to the system where the data to be processed reside, as opposed to sending the data to the program that processes the data. This concept is depicted in Fig. B.2. In general, this mobile software idea can be applied to a whole variety of types of medical software. For example, suppose that a physician in an ambulance is trying to retrieve a CT (computed tomography) image from a laboratory at another hospital for an unconscious patient being transported to a hospital emergency to check an abnormality. It is unlikely for the physician to be able to retrieve the large volume of CT image in time over the error-prone low-speed wireless network. In this case a program that is designed to check abnormalities in CT images could be sent to the laboratory. The program would visit the lab system and check the CT images for an abnormality and return only the result to the physician in the ambulance. Consequently the need to transfer the large amount of CT images across the network would be obviated.

Traditional Approach

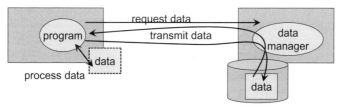

Mobile Agent Approach

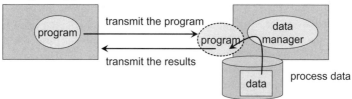

Figure B.2 Distributed computing based on mobile agents

The notion of mobile or itinerant software agents has evolved from the sheer demand for tools to help us manage the explosive growth of information we are experiencing currently, and that we will continue to experience henceforth. Information agents perform the role of managing, manipulating, and collating information from many distributed sources. Another motivation for developing mobile or itinerant software agents is the financial benefits to be gained through a proactive, dynamic, adaptive, and cooperative information manager, or information agents, for the World Wide Web. The information agents would have to be capable of knowing where to look, how to find the relevant information, how to negotiate the information management systems, and how to collate the results and send back to the original requester.

Mobile agents are computational software processes capable of roaming wide area networks (WANs) such as the Internet, interacting with foreign hosts, gathering information on behalf of its owner and coming back home with the final results after accomplishing the planned mission. Mobile software agents are autonomous and cooperative, albeit differently to collaborative agents. The anticipated benefits of mobile software agents are as follows:

1. Automatic assurance of data security as the data are not transmitted across a network but stay at the source.
2. Compliance to the statutory requirements for protection of privacy as the data can be captured once and stay at the source.
3. Management of intellectual property rights as the intellectual properties can stay at the source of origin.
4. Higher performance as the relatively small binary programs travel across and interact with the data across high-speed parallel channels, as opposed to low-speed serial network communication medium.
5. Reduced communication costs by obviating the need for costly network connections among remote computers and time-consuming data transmission across a network.
6. Asynchronous computing by setting off mobile agents and doing something else until the results are back at some later time and also by enabling disconnected operation.

Clinical and Clinical Genomic Messaging

However well the software can move to the data in the future, highly confidential clinical and genomic data also have to move sometimes. Special precautions are required once the software is potentially exposed in transit. The genomic messaging system is concerned with storage and transmission of clinical and/or genomic information across and between architectures as described in:

- B. Robson and R. Mushlin. 2004. Genomic messaging system for information-based personalized medicine with clinical and proteome research applications. *Journal of Proteome Research* 3(5):930–948.

A more detailed follow-up, including the basic binary codes used and extensions of it, is:

• B. Robson and R. Mushlin. 2005. The Genomic Messaging System Language Including Command Extensions for Clinical Data Categories. *Journal of Proteome Research* 4(2):275–299.

The first of these two was acclaimed in a press release from the American Chemical Society and as "One of Nine Top Healthcare Technologies to Watch" in the *Healthcare Technology* journal.

To carry the patient's wishes and consent with controlled levels of access to privacy, and physician's warnings and other annotations, GMS has a universal language called GMSL (GMS language) that converts XML records to GMSL on transmission, and back to XML on receipt if that is required. However, XML does not need to be involved at all, and the system is good at converting a variety of types of legacy data provided that someone writes a short program script to plug into GMS. Thus the GMS language is sufficiently rich that with appropriate software such as the GMS "system" or "engine" it can help convert legacy clinical patient record data and add DNA data, transmit, reconstitute and manage XML (including HL7) documents, handle layered security, combine manual and fully automated annotation of DNA consensus sequence features and the protein consensus sequence features of the implied protein sequence, and initiate statistical analysis, data mining, and computational biology techniques such as modeling of patient polymorphic proteins.

The GMS language (GMSL) could be thought of as a means of representing DNA sequences with embedded annotation, including not just comments of biomolecular and medical interest but also instructions to direct display and use of the DNA data. These functionalities have been retained, although DNA data do not have to be present. A simple sequence of bases ("base pairs," units) such as GATTACAGATTAC (i.e., lacking any such annotation) is also valid GMSL. An example with intrinsic GMSL annotation features that is also valid GMSL is GATTACA deletion GATA snp CGAT insertion (TACA) insertion GG, where the site of a deletion is noted, a section TACA highlighted as inserted, and C is highlighted as a SNP. An important feature is 64 types of bracket that can be overlapped (as opposed to solely nested) and associated with annotation, to describe overlapping sequence features: GATTAC "B epitope in protein:" (AGAT "T epitope in protein=" (20TACACATTAGA) ATT)20ACA. Incidentally, although the previous account (1) required a semicolon or line break (carriage return, new line) to terminate each command, and (2) the annotation required introduction by a command such as "data" and associated square brackets the equivalence of the above is a matter of relatively straightforward parsing, and the terminators and other features are not fundamental. Indeed the conversion from other forms, including legacy patient records and/or XML, is a function of cartridges plugged into the GMS system (see below).

The GMS system provides facilities to invoke a variety of clinical, bioinformatics, and computational biology tools that are routinely used to demonstrate the value of the approach and to test new developments. These include tools for the modeling of weakly homologous and patient-specific changes to proteins, for assessment of the model, and for clinical and genomic data mining. Genomic messaging can be seen as the glue that binds such diverse tools together, and importantly to the source data in archives of patient records. GMSL instructions and many other kinds of data can be outside (around, before, or after) as well as inside a DNA sequence (if present). A sequence of DNA data and/or instructions that is transmitted or stored is called the

"GMS stream," or just "stream" for short. Briefly, an incoming stream of GMSL, as received by, for example a researcher, can be considered as series of data and commands in machine code. A further feature is that except for data in specific data statements, the DNA sequence data and all GMS commands can considered as *instructions* at an equal rank level of implementation. For those familiar with computational theory, it is helpful to consider these data and instructions existing on the tape of a Turing machine represented by GMS as being a Turing machine, save that the tape cannot be rewound and the machine contains more internal states (variables) to memorize relevant data read as a basis for future action. For privacy or if the patient has consented only one-off use, incoming information could be destroyed as it is acted upon, byte by byte. GMSL uses a detailed code (e.g., in terms of bit patterns 01001000) that represents a byte, and each byte represents a unit of data or a basic command. Hence the reader familiar with "machine code" (the basic language of computers into which programs are complied or interpreted) might reasonably think of it as a kind of machine code, albeit medically specialized. Also the code does not contain mathematical operations, although any other kind of computer program feature including whole programs, can be carried along by GMSL, optionally activating and running on receipt of the GMS message.

For a program sent to be recognized and run, it must be inside a special GMS data statement. Data statements of many kinds are an important feature of GMSL. They show when certain data, such as a medical image, start and when they stop. GMS data can be a generic statement, or of a variety of statement types, indicating the kind of data they carry. Additional data in data statements may include applets and other executable code. This could be used to profoundly alter the behavior or mode of use of the GMS system, so here we refer to standard practice, as exemplified in the previous report. Apart from comprising part of the transmission, extra instructions in GMSL or other languages can be plugged into the GMS system as so-called cartridges. These are not transmitted in the stream but are used to assign specialized functions to the GMS system at any installation site or at any node in a bioinformatics network. GMS is usually set up to process one medical record at a time, although it is not a restriction on (or of) GMSL. While not common practice, there is nothing to stop a GMSL message for one patient record containing a larger archive of record summaries that could be used on receipt to perform, say, a diagnosis of the specific patient. Even in the single mode, the GMS system can, of course, be used multiple times to access or build, transmit, and manage many records, which are then used to assemble an archive of multiple records to be analyzed. Some patient records are becoming very rich and contain multiple data, such as time courses of calcium efflux in cardiac tissue, and these could of course be subjected to data analysis.

The GMS system or engine is in two parts. The user who "encodes" or sends a stream of data is the "sender" or "transmitting user," and this might typically be a clinical bioinformaticist working at the physician's office, hospital, or service site preferably within the physician's office or institutional firewall. The user who "decodes" or receives the data is the "receiver" or "receiving user," and this might be a paramedic at an accident site, a researcher, or clinical genomicist who must proofread and sign off on the content. The process of sending may, however, be one of storage and recovery, rather than actual transmission over a long distance. Both sending and receiving components are available to the sender. The system on sending will always automatically attempt a local receive, in the manner analogous to compilation, and so allow the users to verify that correct encoding and decoding will take place. The receiving component and possibly the sending mode will be accessible to the receiver, but (if present) the sending mode will be inactive when receiving occurs.

CHAPTER 9

Concerning Our Detailed Nature

Charles and Ray Eames made a 1968 ten-minute documentary film, *Powers of Ten*, showing the universe at different scales, from the cosmic scale down through the human DNA, its atoms, and beyond. The Philip and Phylis Morrison were scientific advisors on the movie, which Philip Morrison narrated. It was elected in 1998 for preservation in the National Film Registry, which selects "culturally, historically or aesthetically significant motion pictures" for preservation. The resulting book is:

- P. Morrison and P. Morrison 1994. *Powers of Ten*. New York: Freeman.

For an information-perspective scale of things, Treumann's paper mentioned in regard to Chapter 1 teaches that we cannot start by an enduring information content value for the universe and look down to human scale and below, since the information content of the universe changes, "initially from enormous rate of 10^{44} bits per second from an initial value of at least 2π (seven) bits at Planck time. Treumann notes that it can reach its contemporary value only if one or more inflationary phases have been passed by the universe in the course of its evolution." Various other information sources on the Internet put the current information value at about 10^{88}. In any event, with such vast numbers in mind, note that Warren D Smith (2006) collates some more local scale comparisons in terms of information content in *Information Content of Human Intelligence and Life* (http://www.math.temple.edu/~wds/homepage/dnainfo.pdf):

Human DNA 5.8×10^9

Human "non-junk" (regulatory and coding) DNA, 10^8

Proteomic state, 2×10^6

Number of synapses in human brain, 2×10^{14}

Number of cells in human body, 10^{13} to 10^{14}

Visual sensory information input and processed during human lifetime, 4×10^{15}

Amount of information output by human by writing 100 books, 10^9

Amount of information output by vocal human by talking during life, 10^{13}

Information storable in a human's memory, 10^{10} to 10^{13}

Information stored in books in world libraries, 10^{13}

The following sources include a number of statements, often pithy, about the nature of our biology in terms of information and molecules:

- M. Perakh. 2003. *Unintelligent Design*. Amherst, NY: Prometheus Books.
- L. Larson. 2000. Genomics: Medicine's future in our molecules. *Trustee* 53(1):8–12.
- F. Crick. 1968. *Of Molecules and Men*. Seattle: University of Washington Press.

Concerning Caring Robots and Artificial Intelligence

The first of these sources is a work of fiction, but the one that gave rise to the term robotics, and Asomov's famous Three Laws. The second is a classic by Minsky, regarded by many as the father of artificial intelligence. The third by AI and agents guru Sloman is an interesting issue in regard to personality in AI and may be important in healthcare applications.

- I. Asimov. 1950. *I, Robot*. New York: Gnome Press.
- M. L. Minsky. 1987. *The Society of Mind*. London: Heinemann.
- A. Sloman. 1995. What sort of control system is able to have a personality? In R. Trappl, ed., *Proceedings of Workshop on Designing Personalities for Synthetic Actors*. Vienna.

Research Papers in Artificial Intelligence and Caring Agents

The concept of a *caring agent* due to Marvin Minsky was expressed by him more verbally than in writing but propagated by one of his students Renata Busko, chair of the *Future of Health Technology Institute* (http://www.fhti.org). Although we did not overlabor the point, the notion of an IT entity in hardware or software that is an independent agent capable of taking responsibility over human patients is what underlies the theme. Here are a selection of references from a pioneering period is this field:

- P. N. Johnson-Laird. 1993. *The Computer and the Mind*, 2d ed. London: Fontana Press.
- J. M. Epstein. 1999. Agent based models and generative social science. *Complexity* 4(5):41–60.
- J. Bates, A. B. Loyall, and W. S. Reilly. 1991. Broad agents. *Sigart Bulletin* 2(4):38–40.
- L. M. Botelho and H. Coelho. 1996. Emotion-based attention shift in autonomous agents. In J. P. Meuller and M. J. Wooldridge, eds., *Intelligent Agents III. Proceedings of the Third International Workshop on Agent Theories, Architectures, and Languages (ATAL-96)*. Heidelberg: Springer, pp. 40–50.
- N. R. Jennings and R. A. Brooks. 1991. How to build complete creatures rather than isolated cognitive simulators. In K. VanLehn, ed., *Architectures for Intelligence*. London: LEA Pubs, pp. 225–239.
- R. A. Brooks. 1991. Intelligence without representation. *Artificial Intelligence* 47:139–159.
- D. N. Davis, A. Sloman, and R. Poli. 1995. Simulating agents and their environments. Cognitive Science Research Report CSPP-10-95, School of Computes Science, September 1995.
- I. A. Ferguson. 1995. Integrated control and coordinated behaviour: A case for agent models. In M. J. Wooldridge and N. R. Jennings, eds., *Intelligent Agents. Proceedings of the ECAI94 Workshop on Agent Theories, Architectures, and Languages (ATAL-94)*. Heidelberg: Springer, pp. 32–38.
- S. Franklin and A. Graesser. 1996. Is it an agent, or just a program? A taxonomy for autonomous agents. In M. J. Wooldridge and N. R. Jennings, eds., *Intelligent Agents III. Proceedings of the Third International Workshop on Agent Theories, Architectures, and Languages (ATAL-96)*. Heidelberg: Springer-Verlag.

- M. P. Georgeoff and A. L. Lansky. 1987. Reactive reasoning and planning. In *Proceedings of the Sixth National Conference on Artificial Intelligence*, Vol. 2. Seattle,WA, pp. 677–682.
- B. Hayes-Roth. 1993. Intelligent control. *Artificial Intelligence* 59:213–220.
- A. Newell. 1990. *Unified Theories of Cognition*. Cambridge: Harvard University Press.
- N. J. Nilsson. 1994. Teleo-reactive programs for agent control. *Journal of Artificial Intelligence Research* 1:139–158.
- T. J. Norman and D. Long. 1996. Alarms: An implementation of motivated agency. In M. J. Wooldridge, J. P. Müller, and M. Tambe, eds., *Intelligent Agents II. Proceedings of the Second International Workshop on Agent Theories, Architectures, and Languages (ATAL-95)*. Heidelberg: Springer, pp. 219–234.
- A. Sloman, L. Beaudoin, and I. Wright. 1994. Computational modeling of motive-management processes. In Frijda, ed., *Proceedings of the Conference of the International Society for Research in Emotions*. Washington, DC: ISRE Publications.
- A. Sloman and R. Poli. 1995. Sim agent: A toolkit for exploring agent designs. In M. J. Wooldridge, J. P. Müller, and M. Tambe, eds., *Intelligent Agents II. Proceedings of the Second International Workshop on Agent Theories, Architectures, and Languages (ATAL-1995)*. Heidelberg: Springer.
- A.K. Mackworth. 1977. Consistency in networks of relations. *Artificial Intelligence* 8:99–118.

Bioinformatics and Drug Design

The reason for combining bioinformatics with drug design is its potential importance in identifying exactly the target molecules in our body, normally proteins (especially receptors and enzymes). However, overall, the sparseness of evidence on the Internet about the success of bioinformatics with regard to the pharmaceutical industry is conspicuous to date. We have not given the attention to bioinformatics and drug design that we would have liked, despite the number of publications to which author BR has contributed on these themes. But that is really a matter for another kind of book.

- J. Li and B. Robson. 2000. Bioinformatics and computational chemistry in molecular design: Recent advances and their application. In R. R. Reid, ed., *Peptide and Protein Drug Analysis*. New York: Dekker, pp. 285–307.

As a starter the following on bioinformatics and drug design are useful texts:

- T. Attwood. 1999. *Introduction to Bioinformatics*. Englewood Cliffs, NJ: Prentice-Hall.
- H. John Smith, ed. 2005. *Smith & Williams Introduction to Drug Design and Action*. CRC Publications, Taylor & Francis Group.

There are a number of journals focusing on, reasonably enough, our molecules in relation to the artificial visitor molecules that we call drugs. *Chemical Biology and Drug Design*, edited by Tomi K. Sawyer, published by Wiley-Blackwell, is one example. In the spirit of the opening parts of this chapter regarding our detailed nature and the knowing of it, the following sources further highlight drug design in terms of molecules that will fit protein targets in our bodies:

- J. Greer, J. W. Erickson, J. J. Baldwin, and M. D. Varney. 1994. Application of the three-dimensional structures of protein target molecules in structure-based drug design. *Journal of Medicinal Chemistry* 37(8):1035–1054.
- K. Gubernator and H. J. Böhm. 1998. *Structure-Based Ligand Design, Methods and Principles in Medicinal Chemistry*. Weinheim: Wiley-VCH.

Protein modeling consequently is of interest when the 3D structure of the exact protein target has not been determined experimentally. *Introduction to Proteins and Protein Engineering* by Barry Robson and Jean Garnier is mentioned elsewhere, and seems a good start. For an update perspective on the underlying "protein-folding problem," namely the difficulty in understanding how proteins fold, see B. Robson and A. Vaithilingam, "Protein Folding Revisited," *Progress in Molecular Biology and Translational Science* 84:161–202. Not least, look at the many chapters by other authors in this book. Two further (somewhat arbitrary) examples illustrating different heuristic, bioinformatic, and simulation approaches to the problem, plus assessment of quality of results, are as follows:

- J. F. Brinkley, R. B. Altman, B. S. Duncan, B. G. Buchanan, and O. Jardetzky. 1988. Heuristic refinement method for the derivation of protein solution structures: validation on cytochrome b562. *Journal of Chemical Information and Computer Sciences* 28(4):194–210.
- B. Robson, A. Curioni, and T. Mordasini. 2002. Studies in the Assessment of Folding Quality for Protein Modeling and Structure Prediction. *Journal of Proteome Research* 1(2):115–133.

Research Papers on Biomedical Modeling

Going further up the scale from molecular modeling, here are some pioneering papers in relation to medical modeling. For the current status, look, for example, at the Visible Human Project on http://www.nlm.nih.gov/research/visible/data2knowledge.html, and the Digital Human Project on http://www.fas.org/dh/.

- R. B. Altman and J. F. Brinkley. 1993. Probabilistic constraint satisfaction with structural models: Application to organ modeling by radial contours. In *Proceedings, 17th Symposium on Computer Applications in Medical Care*. Washington, DC, pp. 492–497.
- J. Bloomenthal. 1985. Stanford Technical Report KSL-85-33. Knowledge-driven ultrasonic three-dimensional organ modeling. *Pattern Analysis and Machine Intelligence* 7(4):431–441.
- J. F. Brinkley. 1992. *Hierarchical geometric constraint networks as a representation for spatial structural knowledge*. In *Proceedings, 16th Annual Symposium on Computer Applications in Medical Care*. pp. 140–144.
- J. F. Brinkley. 1993. A flexible, generic model for anatomic shape: Application to interactive two-dimensional medical image segmentation and matching. *Computers and Biomedical Research* 26:121–142.

- K. P. Hinshaw. 2000. Seeing structure: Using knowledge to reconstruct and illustrate anatomy. PhD thesis. University of Washington.
- L. Markosian, J. M. Cohen, T. Crulli, and J. F. Hughes. 1999. Skin: A constructive approach to modelling free-form shapes. In *Proceedings, SIGGRAPH*, pp. 393–400.
- W. E. Lorensen and H. E. Cline. 1987. Marching cubes: A high resolution 3-D surface construction algorithm. *ACM Computer Graphics* 21(4):163–169.
- S. Sandor and R. Leahy. 1997. Surface-based labeling of cortical anatomy using a deformable atlas. *IEEE Transactions on Medical Imaging* 16(1):41–54.

Notes on Expert Systems

A key document for the Stanford work on MYCIN, and a review of all preceding efforts, is:

- B. G. Buchanan and E. H. Shortliffe. 1984. *Rule Based Expert Systems: The MYCIN Experiments of the Stanford Heuristic Programming Project*. North Reading, MA: Addison Wesley.

A decade later the European Commission initiatives of the early 1990s provide much detailed pioneering technical analysis, for example:

- P. Barahona and J. P. Christensen, eds. 1994. *Health Telematics for Clinical Guidelines and Protocols*. Amsterdam: OIS Press.
- C. Gordona and J. P. Christensen. 1995. *Knowledge and Decisions in Health Telematics*. Amsterdam: IOS Press.

Data and Data Mining

The modern way to get rules into an Expert System is not by human experts, but by data mining.

- P. Cabena, P. Hadjnian, R. Stadler, J. Verhees, and A. Zanasi. 1997. *Discovering Data Mining: From Concept to Implementation*. Englewood Cliffs, NJ: Prentice-Hall.
- C. J. Date. 2000. *Introduction to Database Systems*. Boston: Addison Wesley Longman.
- W. Frawley, G. Piatetsky-Shapiro, and C. Matheus. 1992. Knowledge discovery in databases: An overview. *AI Magazine*, pp. 213–228.
- I. M. Mullins, M. S. Siadaty, J. Lyman, K. Scully, C. T. Garrett, W. G. Miller, R. Muller, B. Robson, C. Apte, S. Weiss, I. Rigoustsos, D. Platt, S. Cohen, and W. A. Knaus. 2006. Data mining and clinical data repositories: Insights from a 667,000 patient data set. *Computers in Biology and Medicine* 36(12):1351–1377.

While the following are examples associated with one of the authors, they give fairly comprehensive references to relevant data analytics methods, and are somewhat unusual in highlighting some new applications of number theory. The specific argument is that number theory relating to prime numbers maps effectively to issues of data management and data mining, allowing development of new algorithms. A similar approach was used (along with two others mining methods) in the paper above by Irene Mullins et al., and there are still at time of writing very few proven examples of data mining of large numbers of patient records, and of programs specialized to do that.

- B. Robson. 2004. The dragon on the gold: Myths and realities for data mining in biotechnology using digital and molecular libraries. *Journal of Proteome Research* 3(6):1113–1119.
- B. Robson and R. Mushlin. 2003. Clinical and pharmacogenomic data mining: 1. The generalized theory of expected information and application to the development of tools. *Journal of Proteome Research* 2:283–301.
- B. Robson and R. Mushlin. 2004. Clinical and pharmacogenomic data mining: 2. A simple method for the combination of information from associations and multivariances to facilitate analysis, decision and design in clinical research and practice. *Journal of Proteome Research* 3(4):697–711.
- B. Robson. 2005. Clinical and pharmacogenomic data mining: 3. Zeta theory as a general tactic for clinical bioinformatics. *Journal of Proteome Research* 4(2): 445–455.
- B. Robson. 2008. Clinical and pharmacogenomic data mining: 4. The FANO program and command set as an example of tools for biomedical discovery and evidence based medicine. *Journal of Proteome Research* 7(9):3922–3947.

A more controversial paper, arguing that quantum mechanics might also be best practice in medical inference, provided that one mathematical change is made.

- B. Robson. 2007. The new physician as unwitting quantum mechanic: Is adapting Dirac's inference system best practice for personalized medicine, genomics and proteomics? *Journal of Proteome Research* 6(8):3114–3126.

Concerning Difficulty of Defense against Natural Biothreat

See also readings for Chapter 2. This reading predates the more recent concerns about SARS and avian flu, illustrating how prophetic such concerns can be.

- L. Garrett. 1995. *The Coming Plague: Newly Emerging Diseases in a World out of Balance*. London: Penguin Books.

CHAPTER 10

Concerning Updates

A few "news updates" on latest understanding and events were given in this chapter. To receive news alerts on medical advances, take a look at journal@healthorbit.ca. Similarly, for alerts specific to current developments in healthcare IT, see *Digital Healthcare and Productivity*, digitalhcp@chimediagroup.com.

Human Genomics Update Regarding Toba Catastrophe Theory

The news and TV documentaries that have covered the Toba theory represent an explosion of awareness and interest following the publication of Stanley Ambrose's paper:

- S. H. Ambrose. 1998. Late Pleistocene human population bottlenecks, volcanic winter, and differentiation of modern humans. *Journal of Human Evolution* 34(6):623–651.

A number of Internet sites provide information and report on the latest developments. See, for example, http://www.bradshawfoundation.com/stanley_ambrose.php.

Concerning Stem Cell Research and Regrowing Human Tissue

We wanted to be brief on the well worn topic of stem cells, but this paper gives a clear picture of a direction in which the research can take us:

- K. Muneoka, M. Han, and D. M. Gardiner. 2008. Regrowing human limbs. *Scientific American* 298:57–63.

Bionics

What you probably think of as bionics is this kind of thing:

- C. Gray, ed. 1995. *The Cyborg Handbook*. London: Routledge.

But in fact the original meaning is said to go back to the work of Jack E. Steele and the following early symposium on borrowing enegineering ideas from Nature:

- Bionics Symposium. 1960. Living Prototypes—The Key to New Technology, 13–15 September. *Wadd Technical Report*, pp. 60–600.

The original intended sense of "bionics" is explained in:

- K. M. Passino. 2005. *Biomimicry for Optimization, Control, and Automation*. Berlin: Springer.

Concerning Protein Engineering and Bionanotechnology

It may be a sweeping generality of annoyance to many authors, but protein engineering has been relatively quiet of late, especially in regard to novel protein design. The high profile PEGS series of conferences have kept up interest, and the proceedings for any current year as well as DVDs of the presentations can be obtained at http://www.pegsummit.com. On the design of proteins from near-to-scratch, see:

- C. Sander, G. Vriend, F. Bazan, A. Horovitz, H. Nakamura, L. Ribas, A. V. Finkelstein, A. Lockhart, R. Merkl, L. J. Perry, S. C. Emery, C. Gaboriaud, C. Marks, J. Moult, C. Verlinde, M. Eberhard, A. Elofsson, T. J. P. Hubbard, L. Regan, J. Banks,

R. Jappelli, A. M. Lesk, and A. Tramontano. 1992. Protein design on computers. Five new proteins: Shpilka, Grendel, Fingerclasp, Leather and Aida. *Proteins* 12:105–110.

EGAD is a computer program for designing, or more strictly evolving, proteins by a genetic algorithm. See http://egad.ucsd.edu/EGAD_manual/index.html.

On protein engineering generally, the following describes the history of the field and contains a significant bibliography on the topic:

- B. Robson and J. Garnier. 1984. *Introduction to Proteins and Protein Engineering.* Dordrecht: Elsevier.

Sources for other related issues are given in the main text. A justification for including the author's publications as the next two readings, however, is (1) that there just aren't many sources relating to proteins made synthetically *entirely* from D-amino (mirror image) amino acids, that fold and function in mirror image and do not suffer from quick degradation by proteases, or immune response, and (2) that, in that author's view at least, show significant if unappreciated promise in bionantechnology. A few more references can be found on nanotechnology sites such as http://www.nanodot.org/search. php?np=11&q=abstracts.

- B. Robson. 1999. Beyond proteins. *Trends Biotechnology* 17:311–315.
- B. Robson. 1996. Doppelganger proteins as drug leads. *Nature Biotechnology* 14:892–893.

Concerning Health, Longevity, and Nanotechnology

These themes are interwoven in trendy nanotechnology thinking. Eric Drexler's book gives the classic argument, while Ray Kurweil and Terry Grossman link nanotechnology by an interesting further argument. Isaac Asimov's book is the work of fiction from which these authors derive their title.

- K. E. Drexler. 1986. *Engines of Creation: The Coming Era of Nanotechnology.* New York: Anchor Books. Reprint 1990. Oxford: Oxford University Press.
- I. Asimov. 1966. *Fanstastic Voyage.* New York: Bantam Books.
- R. Kurzweil and T. Grossman. 2004. *Fantastic Voyage: Live Long Enough to Live Forever.* Emmaus, PA: Rodale Books.

Concerning the Universe as a Computer, Information, Entropy, and Space–Time

The first source below relates in scholarly detail the conception of the universe as a computer of sorts. The book is particularly useful for original source references; otherwise, it would take us too far afield to discuss this analogy, except to note that how "easy" it might be for our descendants to make the universe become a computer. At least that is the thinking of Frank Tipler whose book we referenced above in regard to Chapter 1.

- C. Seife. 2006. *Decoding the Universe: How the Science of Information Is Explaining Everything in the Cosmos, from Our Brains to Black Holes.* London: Penguin Books.

The second is an example covering some aspects of the fabric of space and time, and other aspects that may be relevant to our ultimate destiny:

- D. Deutsch. 1997. *The Fabric of Reality: The Science of Parallel Universes, and Its Implications*. London: Allen Lane/Penguin Press.

Two additional sources are:

- P. D. B. Collins, A. D. Martin, and E. J. Squires. 1989. *Particle Physics and Cosmology*. New York: Wiley-Interscience.
- W. H. Zurek, ed. 1990. *Complexity, Entropy, and the Physics of Information*. North Reading, MA: Addison Wesley.

Final Note

Finally, from data like that on page 565, a physician (arguably) holds about $10^{7\text{-}8}$ bits of medical information in his or her head. Some of this may be unique and worth sharing. But most of the patient records are worth sharing, because they take on new meaning when pooled and analyzed globally, a meaning that one physician is unlikely to spot.

INDEX

The Engines of Hippocrates: From the Dawn of Medicine to Medical and Pharmaceutical Informatics, by Barry Robson and O.K. Baek
Copyright © 2009 by John Wiley & Sons, Inc.